Foundations
of Epidemiology

THIRD EDITION

Revised by

David E. Lilienfeld
M.D., M.S. Eng., M.P.H., F.A.C.E.
Senior Epidemiologist, EMMES Corp.

Paul D. Stolley
M.D., M.P.H., F.A.C.E., F.A.C.P.
Professor and Chairman,
Department of Epidemiology
and Preventive Medicine
University of Maryland School of Medicine

Original edition by Abraham M. Lilienfeld,
M.D., M.P.H., D.Sc. (Hon.), F.A.C.E.

New York   Oxford   **Oxford University Press**   1994

Oxford University Press

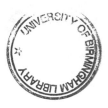

Oxford   New York   Toronto
Delhi   Bombay   Calcutta   Madras   Karachi
Kuala Lumpur   Singapore   Hong Kong   Tokyo
Nairobi   Dar es Salaam   Cape Town
Melbourne   Auckland   Madrid

and associated companies in
Berlin   Ibadan

Library of Congress Cataloging-in-Publication Data
Lilienfeld, David E.
Foundations of epidemiology.—3rd ed.
revised by David E. Lilienfeld, Paul D. Stolley.
p. cm.
Rev. ed. of: Foundations of epidemiology
Abraham M. Lilienfeld and David E. Lilienfeld. 2nd ed. 1980.
Includes bibliographical references and index.
ISBN 0-19-505035-5
ISBN 0-19-505036-3 (pbk.)
1. Epidemiology.
I. Stolley, Paul D.
II. Lilienfeld, David E. Foundations of epidemiology.
III. Title.   [DNLM:
1. Epidemiologic Methods.
2. Epidemiology.
WA 950 L728f   1994]
RA651.L54   1994   614.4—dc20
DNLM/DLC for Library of Congress   93-5963

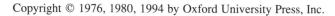

1939 8514

9 8 7 6 5 4 3 2 1

Printed in the United States of America
on acid-free paper

To Jo Ann and the luck of the Castel Felice (P.D.S.)

To Karen and Sam (D.E.L.)

PREFACE

The purpose of this book is to present the concepts and methods of epidemiology as they are applied to a variety of health problems. The broad scope of epidemiology is liberally illustrated with studies of specific diseases. Emphasis is placed on the integration of biological and statistical elements in the sequence of epidemiologic reasoning that derives inferences about the etiology of disease from population data. The epidemiologist's role in integrating knowledge obtained from a variety of scientific disciplines is described.

A knowledge of biostatistics is indispensable in the conduct of epidemiologic studies and the analysis of their results. This information is found in many textbooks of biostatistics. To provide the minimal background necessary for understanding the epidemiologic methods that are discussed, however, the statistical appendix has been expanded to cover correlation, regression, life tables and survivorship analysis, comparison of two sample means, and the kappa statistic.

This book has been designed as a text for introductory courses in epidemiology wherever they are offered. Thus, it can be used in schools of medicine, public health, allied health sciences, dentistry, nursing, and veterinary medicine, as well as in environmental health sciences and other programs offered by colleges of arts and sciences. To facilitate such use, a new chapter on the use of epidemiologic information in clinical settings has been added to this edition. This chapter includes a discussion of how health care providers should critically read reports in the medical literature.

The text has been divided into four parts. In Part I ("Introduction to Epidemiology"), Chapters 1 to 3 review the historical background and conceptual basis for epidemiology. Chapters 4 to 7 make up Part II ("Demographic Studies"); they discuss mortality and morbidity, and their application to epidemiologic problems. The next four chapters, 8 to 11, constitute Part III ("Epidemiologic Studies"); both experimental and observational epidemiologic studies are considered. The last section, Part IV ("Using Epidemiologic Information"), consists of Chapters 12 and 13. The ways in which the types of data obtained from the various demographic and epidemiologic studies are integrated into a conceptual whole and focused on the derivation of biologic inferences are described in Chapter 12, and the use of epidemiologic information in health care settings is discussed in the last chapter.

Several changes have been made in this edition. Many chapters have been extensively revised to include findings from recent epidemiologic studies. New examples illustrating a greater variety of epidemiologic problems, including such public health challenges as AIDS, have been included. In the discussion of morbidity and mortality, descriptions of surveillance and kappa as a measure of inter- and intra-observer variability have been added. The sequence of material on epidemiologic studies has also been changed: experimental studies are discussed before observational studies, cohort investigations before case-control studies. These revisions will assist students in their understanding of the epidemiologic study and should facilitate their assimilation of the material.

To enhance the teaching value of the book, answers to the study problems for the chapters have been added at the end of the text. The problem sets also have been revised to reflect current epidemiologic challenges. The problems give students an opportunity to apply the methods and reasoning process that constitute epidemiology. Some of them invite broad consideration of various epidemiologic issues and viewpoints.

Some Comments on Terminology. We have made some changes in the terms used in the previous edition to describe the different types of demographic and epidemiologic studies and their resultant measures. The changes are intended to reflect current terminology and to minimize confusion, and they are consistent with the second edition of the *Dictionary of Epidemiology* edited by John Last. It may be helpful to list some synonyms of commonly used terms here:

1. *Case-control studies,* in addition to being called ''retrospective'' studies, are also referred to as ''case-referrent'' studies.
2. *Cohort studies* are also termed ''prospective studies'' as well as ''longitudinal'' studies. What we call ''non-concurrent cohort'' studies are also referred to as ''historical cohort,'' ''retrospective cohort,'' ''retrospective longitudinal,'' and ''historical retrospective'' studies.
3. *Relative risk* is also termed ''risk ratio.''
4. *Attributable fraction,* as the term is used in this book, is synonymous with ''attributable risk'' and ''population attributable risk.''

This book was written for both students and practitioners of epidemiology. It seeks to present the reasoning used by epidemiologists in the context of both recent epidemiologic activity and classical epidemiologic investigations. It is through understanding these studies, and the concepts and methods on which they are based, that we can prepare to deal with the public health and medical challenges of the future.

February, 1994   D.E.L.
Baltimore, Md.   P.D.S.

ACKNOWLEDGMENTS

Dr. Tamar Lasky, co-author of Chapter 13, was of invaluable assistance in the preparation of this edition and her care and hard work are gratefully acknowledged. Her astute comments and suggestions have greatly improved the book. We thank Drs. Jack Mandel, Curt Meinert, Roger Sherwin, David Vlahov, J. Michael Sprafka, and Sankey Williams for their reviews of selected chapters and suggestions. Drs. Ellen Fisher, L. Ronald French, James Godbold, and Michael Osterholm also gave us some very helpful comments, and for that we thank them. Mr. Edward Parmalee assisted us with some of the questions for the book and Mrs. Hildred Griffeth typed the manuscript with her usual tact, efficiency, and good humor (sometimes sorely taxed). We greatly valued the advice and help we received from Jeffrey House of the Oxford University Press.

CONTENTS

I

INTRODUCTION TO EPIDEMIOLOGY

The first three chapters provide an introduction to the epidemiologic view of disease. The many facets of epidemiologic inquiry are explored in Chapter 1. The ways in which epidemiologic data may be used by clinicians, other health care providers, public health officers, or epidemiologists are also discussed. The essence of the epidemiologic approach to disease, which is focused on the occurrence of disease in *populations,* is described in the context of a food-borne outbreak.

Chapter 2 gives a brief account of the history of epidemiology, attempting to show how epidemiology evolved into its present form. The major figures in the development of epidemiology are mentioned. Many of the more notable historical examples of the uses of epidemiology, such as John Snow and the Broad Street Pump, are presented.

Chapter 3 deals with general epidemiologic principles in the study of diseases. One such principle, the triad of "time, place and persons," permits the epidemiologic description of a disease. Another triad, "agent, host, and environment," provides insight into the relationship between the agent or cause of a disease, the host in whom the disease develops, and the environment that facilitates the interaction of the agent and the host. The incubation period (also known as a latent period when studying chronic diseases) is used to determine the probable time of exposure to the agent for both infectious and noninfectious diseases. The epidemiologic importance of subclinical cases of disease is highlighted by the concept of a disease spectrum. Health care providers see only those cases that manifest clinical symptoms and require treatment, but epidemiologists are concerned with all cases of disease as they develop in the population. The chapter concludes with a discussion of herd immunity, the epidemiologic basis for the vaccination policies of several nations.

1

LAYING THE FOUNDATIONS: THE EPIDEMIOLOGIC APPROACH TO DISEASE

Epidemiology is concerned with the patterns of disease occurrence in human populations and the factors that influence these patterns. Epidemiologists are primarily interested in the occurrence of disease as categorized by **time, place, and persons.** They try to determine whether there has been an increase or decrease of the disease over the years, whether one geographical area has a higher frequency of the disease than another, and whether the characteristics of persons with a particular disease or condition distinguish them from those without it.

The personal characteristics that concern epidemiologists are:

1. Demographic characteristics such as age, gender, race, and ethnic group.
2. Biological characteristics such as blood levels of antibodies, chemicals, and enzymes; cellular constituents of the blood; and measurements of physiological function of different organ systems.
3. Social and economic factors such as socioeconomic status, educational background, occupation, and nativity.
4. Personal habits such as tobacco and drug use, diet, and physical exercise.
5. Genetic characteristics such as blood groups.

Much of this is encompassed by Hirsch's definition of historical and geographical pathology as a "science which ... will give, firstly, a picture of the occurrence, the distribution and the types of the diseases of mankind, in distinct epochs of time and at various points of the earth's surface; and secondly, will render an account of the relations of these diseases to the external conditions surrounding the individual and determining his manner of life" (Hirsch, 1883;

Frost, 1941). This statement has commonly served as a base for defining epidemiology as the "study of the distribution of a disease or a physiological condition
in human populations and of the factors that influence this distribution" (Lilienfeld, 1978). A more inclusive description was given by Wade Hampton Frost,
one of the architects of modern epidemiology, who noted that "epidemiology is
essentially an inductive science, concerned not merely with describing the distribution of disease, but equally or more with fitting it into a consistent philosophy"
(Frost, 1941). Thus epidemiology can be regarded as a sequence of reasoning
concerned with biological inferences derived from observations of disease occurrence and related phenomena in human population groups. To this we can add
that epidemiology is an integrative, eclectic discipline deriving concepts and
methods from other disciplines, such as statistics, sociology, and biology, for the
study of disease in a population.

GENERAL PURPOSES OF EPIDEMIOLOGIC INQUIRIES

The information obtained from an epidemiologic investigation can be utilized in
several ways:

1. To elucidate the etiology of a specific disease or group of diseases by
   combining epidemiologic data with information from other disciplines
   such as genetics, biochemistry, and microbiology.
2. To evaluate the consistency of epidemiologic data with etiological
   hypotheses developed either clinically (at the bedside) or experimentally
   (in the laboratory).
3. To provide the basis for developing and evaluating preventive procedures
   and public health practices.

Examples of each of these three general purposes will be presented.

Etiological Studies of Disease

A simple example of the use of epidemiologic data to determine etiological factors
would be the investigation of an outbreak of food poisoning to determine which
food was contaminated with the microorganism or chemical responsible for the
epidemic. Another example would be the study of a disease that occurs with
higher frequency among workers in occupations exposing them to particular
chemicals, as illustrated in the study of aniline, ortho-toluidine, and bladder cancer
by Ward et al. (1991). Although the carcinogenicity of aniline-based dyes to the
human bladder has been known for the past four decades, that for aniline and a

related chemical, ortho-toluidine, is not yet established. At a western New York State plant in which aniline and ortho-toluidine were used to produce an anti-oxidant for tire production, the union had reported a cluster of bladder cancer cases among its members. During the subsequent investigation, lists were obtained of all employees in the plant since 1946. These workers were divided into three groups: those with definite exposure to these two chemicals (persons who worked in the department in which the chemicals were used), those with possible exposure to the chemicals (janitorial, maintenance, and shipping personnel), and those with no exposure (all other workers). Cases of bladder cancer among these employees were identified by the company and the union, with confirmation by review of medical records. Additional cases were ascertained from the New York State Cancer Registry. The observed numbers of cases were then compared with those that would be expected based on the bladder cancer incidence rates for New York State. A significantly larger number of bladder cancer cases (seven) was found to have occurred among the 708 persons definitely exposed to ortho-toluidine and aniline than would be expected (approximately one); for the 288 possibly exposed workers, there was also an excess number of cases, though less than for the definitely exposed group. The 753 persons not exposed had no significant excess in the number of bladder cancer cases. Further, this relationship between bladder cancer and exposure to aniline and ortho-toluidine showed a dose-response effect, i.e., the longer an employee was exposed to these two compounds, the greater was his or her chance of developing bladder cancer. The investigators concluded that a causal relationship existed between exposure to aniline and ortho-toluidine compounds and bladder cancer.

Only occasionally do investigators find that the increased exposure of individuals to certain agents results in a decreased frequency of disease. A classical example of this kind of relationship is that between the presence of fluorides in the water supply and dental caries. The investigation of this relationship is worth recounting as it illustrates in concise form how a sequence of studies can be conducted to develop a preventive measure for a disease.

By the late 1930s, it had been recognized that mottled enamel of teeth was due to the use of a water supply with a high fluoride concentration (Dean, 1938; Dean and Elvove, 1936; Dean et al., 1939). Earlier, a practicing dentist had formed a clinical impression that persons with mottled teeth had less caries than usual (Black and McKay, 1916; McKay, 1925; McKay and Black, 1916). This led the Public Health Service to conduct surveys of children 12–14 years old in thirteen cities in four states where the fluoride concentration in the water supply varied considerably (Dean et al., 1942). The results indicated that dental caries decreased with increasing content of fluoride in the water, thus suggesting that the addition of fluorides to the water supply should decrease the frequency of dental caries (Figure 1–1). This could best be demonstrated by comparative exper-

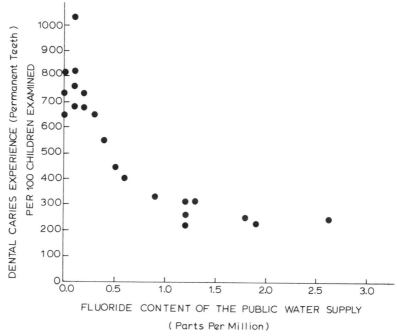

Figure 1–1. Relationship between the number of dental caries in permanent teeth and fluoride content in the public water supply. *Source:* Dean, Arnold, and Elvove (1942).

iment, where fluorides were added to the water supply of one community and the water supply remained untouched in a comparable community where the fluoride concentration was naturally low. The dental caries experience of school children in these communities could then be determined by periodic examinations over a number of years and compared. Several such studies were initiated, including one comparing Kingston and Newburgh, New York (Table 1–1) (Ast and Schlesinger, 1956). In the town with fluorides in the water supply, the index of dental caries (DMF) was found to be lower than in the one without fluorides. In this instance, a clinical impression led to both an epidemiologic survey and a comparative experiment, both of which demonstrated the relationship between a population characteristic, fluoride consumption, and a disease, dental caries.

Consistency with Etiological Hypotheses

The investigator attempts to determine whether an etiological hypothesis developed clinically, experimentally, or from other epidemiologic studies is consistent with the epidemiologic characteristics of the disease in a human population group(s). Many studies of the relationship between oral contraceptive use and various forms of cardiovascular disease illustrate this approach. Over a period of

Table 1–1. DMF* Teeth per 100 Children, Ages 6–16, Based on Clinical and Roentgenographic Examinations—Newburgh† and Kingston, New York, 1954–1955

	NUMBER OF CHILDREN WITH PERMANENT TEETH		NUMBER OF DMF TEETH		DMF TEETH PER 100 CHILDREN WITH PERMANENT TEETH§		
							PERCENT DIFFERENCE
AGE‡	NEWBURGH	KINGSTON	NEWBURGH	KINGSTON	NEWBURGH	KINGSTON	(N−K)/K
6–9‖	708	913	672	2,134	98.4	233.7	−57.9
10–12	521	640	1,711	4,471	328.1	698.6	−53.0
13–14	263	441	1,579	5,161	610.1	1,170.3	−47.9
15–16	109	119	1,063	1,962	975.2	1,648.7	−40.9

*DMF includes permanent teeth decayed, missing (lost subsequent to eruption), or filled.
†Sodium fluoride was added to Newburgh's water supply beginning May 2, 1945.
‡Age at last birthday at time of examination.
§Adjusted to age distribution of children examined in Kingston who had permanent teeth in the 1954–1955 examination.
‖Newburgh children of this age group were exposed to fluoridated water from the time of birth.
Source: Ast and Schlesinger (1956).

years, epidemiologic studies had shown a relationship between oral contraceptive use and both venous thromboembolism and thrombotic stroke (Collaborative Group for the Study of Stroke in Young Women, 1973; Vessey and Mann, 1978). Soon after these studies started to appear, the first of a series of case reports associated oral contraceptive use with myocardial infarction (Boyce et al., 1963). This stimulated several investigators to conduct epidemiologic studies of this issue (Mann et al., 1976a; Mann et al., 1976b). The statistically significant results of a study by Mann, Inman, and Thorogood (1976b) of women aged 40–44 who died from myocardial infarction are presented in Table 1–2.

Basis for Preventive and Public Health Services

Perhaps the simplest example of this objective is the epidemiologic evaluation of vaccines in controlled trials in human populations, such as the national study that was done to establish the effectiveness of the Salk vaccine in the prevention of poliomyelitis (Francis et al., 1955). In addition to controlled trials and the other types of epidemiologic studies already mentioned, information on the population distribution of a disease in itself provides the basis for developing certain aspects of community disease control programs. Knowledge of specific etiological factors is not essential for this purpose. For example, epidemiologic data on those persons with a higher frequency of a disease or a higher risk of developing one are useful

Table 1–2. Oral Contraceptive Practice Among Women Aged 40–44 Years Who Died from Myocardial Infarction (MI), and Controls

ORAL CONTRACEPTIVE PRACTICE	PATIENTS WITH MYOCARDIAL INFARCTION		CONTROLS	
	NO.	PERCENT	NO.	PERCENT
Never used	78	73.6	86	84.3
Current users (used during month before death or during same calendar period for controls)	18	17.0 ⎫	7	6.9 ⎫
		28 (26.4%)		16 (15.7%)
Ex-users (used only more than one month before death or during same calendar period for controls)	10	9.4 ⎭	9	8.8 ⎭
Total	106	100.0	102	100.0
Not known	2		8	
Comparison between users and women not currently using oral contraceptives	$\chi^2 = 4.35; P < 0.05$			

Source: Mann et al. (1976b).

to the physician or public health administrator in indicating those segments of the population where health care activities should be focused.

The familial aggregation of diabetes mellitus illustrates this point. In a study of diabetic patients admitted to the Mayo Clinic, Steinberg and Wilder (1952) obtained a history of the presence or absence of diabetes among their parents and siblings (Table 1–3). Whether one hypothesizes a genetic etiological mechanism or environmental factors common to family members as an explanation for the observed familial aggregation, the higher-than-usual frequency of the disease in certain families suggests to the physician that the examination of parents and siblings of known diabetic patients will provide for the early detection of diabetes in a high-risk group of the population.

CONTENT OF EPIDEMIOLOGIC ACTIVITIES

Epidemiologists engage in three broad areas of study, each involving different methods: experimental epidemiology, natural experiments, and observational epidemiology.

Table 1–3. Frequency of Diabetes Among Siblings and Parents of Diabetic Patients Admitted to the Mayo Clinic

DIABETES STATUS OF PARENTS	NUMBER FAMILIES	SIBLINGS TOTAL	DIABETES NUMBER	PERCENT
Both diabetic	22	100	16	16.0
One diabetic	370	1,620	185	11.4
Neither diabetic	1,589	6,664	311	4.7
Total families	1,981	8,384	512	6.1

Source: Steinberg and Wilder (1952). Reprinted by permission of The University of Chicago Press, Copyright © 1952. The American Society of Human Genetics, Waverly Press, Inc.

Experimental Epidemiology

In planned experiments, the investigator controls the population groups being studied by deciding which groups are exposed to a possible etiological factor or preventive measure. The Newburgh-Kingston dental caries study, for instance, was a planned, controlled experiment. An important feature of many experiments is that the investigator can randomly allocate subjects to experimental and control groups. This method is discussed in greater detail in Chapters 8 and 9.

Natural Experiments

Occasionally, the investigator is fortunate enough to observe the occurrence of a disease under natural conditions so closely approximating a planned, controlled experiment that it is categorized as a "natural experiment." Any inferences about etiological factors derived from such situations are considerably stronger than if they had been derived solely from an observational study. The studies in England by Doll, Hill, and Peto of the relationship between tobacco use and lung cancer illustrate this approach (Doll and Hill, 1950; Doll and Peto, 1976; Doll et al., 1980; Report of the Royal College of Physicians, 1971). In 1951, these investigators ascertained the smoking habits of British male physicians, aged thirty-five and over, and followed them to determine their mortality from different causes, in particular lung cancer. Initially, this study indicated that physicians who smoked cigarettes had a mortality rate from lung cancer that was about ten times that of nonsmoking physicians (Doll and Hill, 1950). Questionnaires were sent to these physicians again to determine their cigarette smoking habits in 1956,

1966, and 1971 (Doll and Peto, 1976; Report of the Royal College of Physicians, 1971). The findings of these surveys in terms of the ratio of number of cigarettes smoked by the male physicians to the numbers smoked by all British men in the same age group is shown in Figure 1–2. There was about a 50 percent decline in cigarette smoking among these male physicians. During this same period of time, the investigators continued to obtain information on the mortality experience of the physicians, comparing it with the mortality among all British men (Doll and Peto, 1976; Report of the Royal College of Physicians, 1971). Figure 1–3 presents the trend of the physicians' mortality experience from lung cancer and from all other cancer as a percentage of national mortality. There was an approximately 40 percent decline in mortality from lung cancer with essentially no decline in other cancer deaths.

Observational Epidemiology

This refers to the observation and analysis of the occurrence of disease in human population groups and to the inferences that can be derived about etiological factors that influence this occurrence. Appropriate methods for selecting specific groups in the population and for analyzing information obtained from them have been developed. Much of what the epidemiologist does falls into this category and, therefore, several of the later chapters as well as the Appendix deal with it. The studies of aniline- and ortho-toluidine-exposed employees, dental caries, and familial aggregation of diabetes already cited are examples of observational investigations.

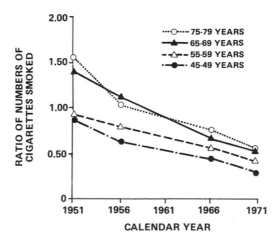

Figure 1–2. Trend in ratio of numbers of cigarettes smoked by male physicians of same ages, by age groups, 1951–1971. *Source:* Doll and Peto (1976).

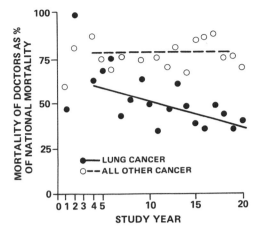

Figure 1-3. Trend in mortality of male doctors as percentage of national mortality of same ages for lung cancer and all other cancer, 1951–1971. *Source:* Doll and Peto (1976).

Development and Evaluation of Study Methods

As the scope of epidemiology has been broadened to include new and/or different types of diseases, epidemiologists have had to develop new methods of study. In some cases these methods have been adapted from other disciplines, such as sociology, statistics, biology, and demography. However, the appropriateness of such new methods for particular epidemiologic situations is not always apparent. Thus, they need to be evaluated for different epidemiologic circumstances to determine their utility.

One often hears the statement that there are "two epidemiologies," one for infectious diseases and the other for noninfectious diseases. This is a misconception. In general, the methods used and the inferences derived are the same for both disease groups; this will be illustrated throughout our discussions. The reader should note that epidemiology is essentially a *comparative* discipline. It is mainly concerned with studying diseases and related phenomena at different time periods, in different places, and among different types of people (i.e., "time, place, and persons") and then comparing them. This approach is used for all categories of disease, infectious and noninfectious alike (Lilienfeld, 1973).

THE SEQUENCE OF EPIDEMIOLOGIC REASONING

Epidemiology was defined at the beginning of this chapter in terms of a reasoning process. The observational study, one of the major tools of epidemiology, affords an excellent view of the reasoning process by which one achieves the objective of elucidating etiological factors of a disease. Basically, the epidemiologist uses a two-stage sequence of reasoning:

1. The determination of a statistical association between a characteristic and a disease.
2. The derivation of biological inferences from such a pattern of statistical associations.

The methods used to determine the statistical associations fall into one of two broadly defined categories: (a) associations based on group characteristics, and (b) associations based on individual characteristics. Although there is a certain degree of overlap between these two categories, their distinction has proved to be extremely useful.

In studying *group* characteristics, the epidemiologist concentrates on the comparison of the mortality and/or morbidity experience from a given disease in different population groups in the hope that any observed differences can be related to differences in the local environment, in personal living habits, or even in the genetic composition of these groups. In these **demographic studies,** information on the characteristics of the individual members of the population groups is not usually obtained. Generally, existing mortality and morbidity statistics are utilized. For example, let us assume that Community A has a higher mortality rate from cancer of the liver than Community B. Furthermore, Community A is engaged primarily in mining, while Community B is engaged in agriculture. Comparison would suggest that mining may be of etiological importance in liver cancer. Usually, the results of such studies provide *clues* to etiological hypotheses and serve as a basis for more detailed investigations. Such an observed relationship, generally termed an "ecological correlation," may suffer from an **"ecological fallacy"**; that is, the two communities differ in many other factors, and one or more of those may be the underlying reason for the differences in their observed mortality or morbidity experience (Goodman, 1953; Robinson, 1950; Selvin, 1958; Piantadosi et al., 1988). The various types of studies of group characteristics will be discussed in Chapters 4–7.

After an association has been established in a study of group characteristics, or when a lead has been developed from either clinical studies of patients, experimental work, or other sources, the investigator attempts to determine whether this association is also present among *individuals.* Answers will be sought to such questions as:

1. Do persons with the disease have the characteristic more frequently than those without the disease?

2. Do persons with the characteristic develop the disease more frequently than those who do not have the characteristic?

Such associations are established in epidemiologic studies, i.e., by cohort or case-control studies, which will be discussed in Chapters 10 and 11.

These two general methods of determining statistical associations—those between groups and those among individuals—must be distinguished since a relationship derived from a study of individuals is less likely to result from an ecological fallacy and is, therefore, more likely to be biologically significant than one derived from a study of group characteristics. Conversely, an association derived from studies of groups has a greater likelihood of being the result of a third common factor (Piantadosi et al., 1988).

AN EXAMPLE OF THE EPIDEMIOLOGIC APPROACH

The essentials of the epidemiologic approach in determining the specific etiological agent of a disease are perhaps best demonstrated by the investigation of the origin of a food poisoning outbreak. This usually includes ascertaining whether a statistical association is found between the consumption of a specific food at some event and the specific form of the disease. This is accomplished by computing food-specific attack rates, defined as follows:

$$\text{Food-specific attack rate} = \frac{\begin{array}{c}\text{Number of persons who ate} \\ \text{a specific food and became ill}\end{array}}{\begin{array}{c}\text{Number of persons who ate} \\ \text{the specific food}\end{array}},$$

and comparing them with attack rates for those who had not eaten the specific food. The report of a salmonellosis outbreak caused by *Salmonella typhimurium* DT4 illustrates this approach (Ortega-Benito and Landridge, 1992).

During late July, 1989, the guests and staff of a private club experienced a striking increase in gastrointestinal symptoms. Most of the people affected had eaten at the club between Saturday, July 22, and Monday, July 24. Those who had consumed hot foods did not appear to develop any illness. During that weekend, the club had also supplied sandwiches for tea break to members of a cricket team. Symptoms of gastrointestinal illness among team members began to increase on July 23, although regional public health officials were not notified until August 1, 1989. The limited nature of the exposure of the cricket team members suggested that the sandwiches (specifically, eggs or mayonnaise) may have contained the etiologic agent.

Two groups were selected for study: 129 club staff members who ate their meals at the club and 105 persons involved with the cricket team (team members, umpires, scorers, and guests). Each of these persons was given a self-administered questionnaire; 177 (110 club staff and 67 cricket group) completed questionnaires were returned. Since not all the members of the two groups completed questionnaires, one must assume that those who did so are a representative *sample* of all the members.

A case was defined as anyone who had diarrhea or vomiting or had *Salmonella typhimurium* isolated from his stools between July 20 and July 26, 1989. From the club staff group, 33 persons met the case definition, as did 35 cricket group members. A crude attack rate was computed:

$$\text{Crude attack rate} = \frac{\text{Number of persons ill with the disease}}{\text{Number of persons eating at the club}}.$$

The crude attack rate among club staff was 30 percent (33/110) and among the cricket team group, 5 percent (35/67). Meal-specific attack rates were computed for the club staff (Table 1–4). They showed a definite statistical association between salmonellosis and sandwiches. Additional analyses of the attack rates for consumption of specific sandwiches by the cricket group and on specific days for club staff were also calculated (Tables 1–5 and 1–6). Among the cricketers, statistical associations between illness and egg mayonnaise, tuna mayonnaise, and tuna and cucumber sandwiches were found. Among club staff, statistical associations between illness and egg mayonnaise sandwiches were found regardless of which day they were consumed; an association could also be discerned between illness and tuna and cucumber sandwiches consumed on July 24. The investigators concluded that only sandwiches containing mayonnaise were associated with the illness.

Laboratory investigations were undertaken to identify the specific form of salmonellosis. Salmonella was identified in 36 of 68 stool specimens examined. *Salmonella typhimurium* was the only type isolated. This information allowed the investigators to trace the source of the outbreak. Eggs, a component of mayonnaise, are often found to be contaminated in investigations of food-borne salmonellosis outbreaks. The eggs used in the mayonnaise had been provided by one supplier. Investigation of that supplier's environment did not reveal a source of the salmonella. However, that supplier had also used three supplementary sources for the eggs, which the investigators also examined. Two flocks in two farms were found to be infected with salmonella; one with *Salmonella enteritidis* and the other with *Salmonella typhimurium* DT4 in 2,580 infected birds. These

Table 1–4. Attack Rates by Meal and for Sandwiches among 110 Club Staff

	EATEN				NOT EATEN				DIFFERENCE IN ATTACK RATES
MEAL	ILL (1)	NOT ILL (2)	TOTAL (3)	ATTACK RATE (%) (4)	ILL (5)	NOT ILL (6)	TOTAL (7)	ATTACK RATE (%) (8)	(4)−(8)=(9).
Breakfast	9	20	29	31	24	45	69	35	−4
Lunch	18	42	60	30	15	23	38	39	−9
Dinner	11	19	30	37	22	46	68	32	5
Sandwiches	25	24	49	51	8	41	49	16	35*

*The only difference that was statistically significant (p=0.006) was for sandwiches.

Source: Adapted from Ortega-Benito and Landridge (1992).

Table 1-5. Attack Rates for Specific Sandwiches among 110 Club Staff on July 24, 1989[+]

| SANDWICH | EATEN | | | | NOT EATEN | | | | DIFFERENCE IN ATTACK RATES |
| | ILL | NOT ILL | TOTAL | ATTACK RATE (%) | ILL | NOT ILL | TOTAL | ATTACK RATE (%) | |
	(1)	(2)	(3)	(4)	(5)	(6)	(7)	(8)	(4)−(8)=(9).
Egg Mayonnaise	4	1	5	80	18	47	65	28	52*
Tuna Mayonnaise	2	1	3	67	21	47	68	31	36
Egg and Tomato	0	1	1	0	24	47	71	34	−34
Tuna and Cucumber	5	1	6	88	16	47	63	25	53*
Cheese and Tomato	1	0	1	100	23	48	71	32	68
Cheese and Pickle	0	1	1	0	24	47	71	34	−34
Lettuce and Tomato	0	1	1	0	23	47	70	33	−33
Turkey Salad	0	0	0	0	24	48	72	33	−33
Ham Salad	2	0	2	100	21	48	69	30	70
Roast Beef	2	0	2	100	23	48	71	32	68
Liver Sausage	0	1	1	0	24	47	71	34	−34

[+]For July 23 and July 25, similar results were found, except for the absence of an association between illness and tuna and cucumber.

*The only differences that were statistically significant were for egg mayonnaise (p=0.03), and tuna and cucumber (p=0.008).

Source: Adapted from Ortega-Benito and Landridge (1992).

Table 1–6. Attack Rates for Specific Sandwiches among 55 Cricketers

SANDWICH	EATEN				NOT EATEN				DIFFERENCE IN ATTACK RATES (4)−(8)=(9).
	ILL (1)	NOT ILL (2)	TOTAL (3)	ATTACK RATE (%) (4)	ILL (5)	NOT ILL (6)	TOTAL (7)	ATTACK RATE (%) (8)	
Egg Mayonnaise	14	3	17	82	7	18	25	28	54*
Tuna Mayonnaise	7	2	9	78	13	18	31	42	36
Egg and Tomato	3	0	3	100	18	21	41	44	56
Tuna and Cucumber	12	3	15	80	9	16	25	36	44*
Cheese and Tomato	6	6	12	50	16	15	31	52	−2
Cheese and Pickle	5	6	11	45	18	14	32	56	−11
Lettuce and Tomato	2	0	2	100	23	21	44	52	48
Turkey Salad	0	0	0	0	26	21	47	55	−55
Ham Salad	11	5	16	69	11	16	27	41	28
Roast Beef	2	0	2	100	22	20	42	52	48
Liver Sausage	1	0	1	100	25	21	46	54	46

*The only differences that were statistically significant were for egg mayonnaise (p=0.0017), and tuna and cucumber (p=0.017).

Source: Adapted from Ortega-Benito and Landridge (1992).

17

flocks were slaughtered. In summary, the findings were:

1. Chickens at two farms were infected with salmonella.
2. These eggs had not been pasteurized before use.
3. The eggs supplied by one of these farms were used by the club staff to make mayonnaise for sandwiches during the third weekend in July, 1989.
4. The contaminated mayonnaise was consumed by club staff and the cricket group.

The pattern of statistical associations and the laboratory findings showing that a flock which had provided some of the eggs was infected with the same type of *Salmonella typhimurium* that had been found among the ill club staff and cricketers clearly implicated the infected eggs as the cause of this epidemic.

SUMMARY

Epidemiology is a comparative science in which the occurrence of disease in population groups is related to the presence or absence of factors in those groups. Epidemiologists place these associations into a biological framework to provide insights into the causes of disease. Epidemiologic activities include experimental studies, in which the investigators control the exposure of the individuals to a factor; observational studies, in which the investigators follow the health experiences of individuals exposed and not exposed to a factor (the control of the individuals' exposures was beyond the investigators' control); and the development and evaluation of new study methods.

Factors studied by the epidemiologist include demographic characteristics, biological characteristics, social and economic characteristics, personal habits, and genetic traits. The factors may be associated with either an increased risk of disease (suggestive of a causal relationship) or a decreased risk (suggestive of a protective relationship). Such associations are best discerned in studies of individuals in a population. The finding of an association between a disease and group characteristics in a study of population (rather than individual) characteristics can lead to an "ecological fallacy." The determination of a statistical relationship between a characteristic and a disease is only the first step in epidemiologic reasoning. The second step is deriving a biological inference from the patterns of statistical associations.

Epidemiologists use two approaches to discern a statistical relationship between a characteristic and a disease. In one approach, the demographic study, the relationship between group characteristics and disease is examined. In the other approach, the epidemiologic study, the relationship between individual characteristics and disease is examined. An example of the latter can be found in the investigation of a food-borne outbreak. The source of an outbreak may be found by comparing the attack rates among persons who consumed a given food with those for persons who did not consume that food. The food item with the greatest disparity in attack rates among those who consumed it and those who did not consume it was the source of the outbreak.

STUDY PROBLEMS

1. What is the epidemiologic significance of the expression "time, place, persons"?
2. What is an "ecological fallacy"? Why is it important to the epidemiologist?
3. Why should epidemiologists be interested in population-based statistics such as mortality rates? Why should they be cautious in the use of such rates?
4. What are the major steps in an investigation of a food-borne outbreak?
5. An outbreak of food poisoning occurred at a Coast Guard training station a few hours after the communal breakfast meal. The symptoms were mainly nausea, vomiting and diarrhea. An investigation revealed the findings listed in the table below.

TYPE OF FOOD	CONSUMED FOOD			DID NOT CONSUME FOOD		
	NUMBER OF INDIVIDUALS	NUMBER ILL	ATTACK RATE (%)	NUMBER OF INDIVIDUALS	NUMBER ILL	ATTACK RATE (%)
Tomato juice	204	47		263	21	
Cantaloupe	290	53		177	15	
Chipped beef with sauce	147	60		320	8	
Potatoes	161	44		306	24	
Eggs	169	39		298	29	
Pastry	204	34		263	34	
Toast	238	46		229	22	
Milk	301	50		166	18	

(a) Calculate the attack rates for each food for those who consumed and those who did not consume each food item.
(b) Which food do you think is the likely cause of this "common source" epidemic? Explain your choice.

(c) What additional investigations could be done to determine the source of the likely microorganism?

(d) How can such food poisoning epidemics be prevented in the future?

REFERENCES

Ast, D. B., and Schlesinger, E. R. 1956. "The conclusion of a ten-year study of water fluoridation." *Am. J. Pub. Health* 46:265–271.

Black, G. V., and McKay, F. S. 1916. "Mottled teeth: an endemic developmental imperfection of the teeth, heretofore unknown in the literature of dentistry." *Dent. Cosmos.* 58:129–156.

Boyce, J., Fawcett, J. W., and Neal, E.W.P. 1963. "Coronary thrombosis and conovid." *Lancet* 1:111.

Collaborative Group for the Study of Stroke in Young Women. 1973. "Oral contraception and increased risk of cerebral ischemia or thrombosis." *New Eng. J. Med.* 288:871–878.

Dean, H. T. 1938. "Endemic fluorosis and its relation to dental caries." *Pub. Health. Rep.* 54:1443–1452.

Dean, H. T., and Elvove, E. 1936. "Some epidemiological aspects of chronic endemic dental fluorosis." *Am. J. Pub. Health* 26:567–575.

Dean, H. T., Jay, P., Arnold, F. A. Jr., McClure, F. J., and Elvove, E. 1939. "Domestic water and dental caries, including certain epidemiological aspects of oral *L. acidophilus.*" *Pub. Health Rep.* 54:862–888.

Dean, H. T., Arnold, F. A. Jr., and Elvove, E. 1942. "Domestic water and dental caries. V. Additional studies of the relation of fluoride domestic waters to dental caries experience in 4,425 white children, aged 12 to 14 years, of 13 cities in 4 states." *Pub. Health Rep.* 57:1155–1179.

Doll, R., and Hill, A. B. 1950. "Smoking and carcinoma of the lung: Preliminary report." *Br. Med. J.* 2:739–748.

Doll, R., and Peto, R. 1976. "Mortality in relation to smoking: 20 year's observations on male British doctors." *Br. Med. J.* 2:1525–1536.

Doll, R., Gray, R., Hafner, B., and Peto, R. 1980. "Mortality in relation to smoking: 22 years' observations on female British doctors." *Br. Med. J.* 1:967–971.

Francis, T. Jr., Korns, R. F., Voight, R. B., Boisen, M., Hemphill, F. M., Napier, J. A., and Tolchinsky, E. 1955. "An evaluation of the 1954 poliomyelitis vaccine trials: summary report." *Am. J. Pub. Health* 45:1–63.

Frost, W. H., 1941. "Epidemiology." In *Papers of Wade Hampton Frost, M.D.,* K.E. Maxcy, ed., New York: The Commonwealth Fund, pp. 493–542.

Goodman, L. A. 1953. "Ecological regressions and behavior of individuals." *Am. Soc. Rev.* 18:663–664.

Hirsch, A. 1883. *Handbook of Geographical and Historical Pathology, Vol. I.* London: New Sydenham Society.

Lilienfeld, A. M. 1973. "Epidemiology of infectious and non-infectious disease: some comparisons." *Am. J. Epidemiol.* 97:135–147.

Lilienfeld, D. E. 1978. "Definitions of epidemiology." *Am. J. Epidemiol.* 107:87–90.

Mann, J. I., Doll, R., Thorogood, M., Vessey, M. P., and Waters, W. E. 1976a. "Risk factors for myocardial infarction in young women." *Br. J. Prev. Soc. Med.* 30:97–100.

Mann, J. I., Inman, W. H., and Thorogood, M. 1976b. "Oral contraceptive use in older women and fatal myocardial infarction." *Br. Med. J.* 2:445–447.

McKay, F. S., and Black, G. V. 1916. "An investigation of mottled teeth." *Dent. Cosmos.* 58:477–484.

McKay, F. S. 1925. "Mottled enamel: A fundamental problem in dentistry." *Dent. Cosmos.* 67:847–860.

Ortega-Benito, J. M. and Landridge, P. 1992. "Outbreak of food poisoning due to Salmonella typhimurium DT4 in mayonnaise." *Public Health* 106:203–208.

Piantadosi, S., Byar, D. P., and Green, S. B. 1988. "The ecological fallacy." *Am. J. Epidemiol.* 127:893–904.

Report of the Royal College of Physicians. 1971. *Smoking and Health Now.* London: Pitman Medical and Scientific Publishing Co.

Robinson, W.S. 1950. "Ecological correlations and the behavior of individuals." *Am. Soc. Rev.* 15:351–357.

Selvin, H. C. 1958. "Durkeim's suicide and problems of empirical research." *Am. J. Soc.* 63:607–619.

Steinberg, A. G., and Wilder, R. M. 1952. "A study of the genetics of diabetes mellitus." *Am. J. Human Genet.* 4:113–135.

Vessey, M. P., and Mann, J. I., 1978. "Female sex hormones and thrombosis. Epidemiological aspects." *Br. Med. J.* 34:157–162.

Ward, E., Carpenter, A., Markowitz, S., Roberts, D., Halperin, W. 1991. "Excess number of bladder cancers in workers exposed to ortho-toluidine and aniline." *J. Nat. Cancer Inst.* 83:501–506.

2

AN OVERVIEW OF THE HISTORY OF EPIDEMIOLOGY

The development of epidemiology has spanned many centuries. As an eclectic discipline, epidemiology has borrowed from sociology, demography, and statistics, as well as other fields of study. Hence, the reader should not be surprised to learn that its history is interwoven with that of other scientific disciplines. It was not until the nineteenth century that the fabric of epidemiology was woven into a distinct discipline with its own philosophy, concepts, and methods.

This chapter first describes the social and medical environment within which epidemiology developed. The emergence of epidemiology in the 1800s as an area of medical inquiry is then discussed. Stimulated by the observation of patterns of disease in the population, nineteenth-century epidemiologists devised methods to investigate the causes of these diseases and the means by which they could be prevented. The overwhelming of this demographic focus by the rise of bacteriology in the 1880s and 1890s is then examined. Epidemiologists turned their attention from the occurrence of disease in a population to the spread of bacteria by individual contact. The reemergence of epidemiology in the early and mid-twentieth century, associated with the entry of demographers and sociologists into the field, is then described.

THE SOCIAL AND MEDICAL ENVIRONMENT

Humankind has experienced disease for as long as records of human culture have existed. Along with these plagues and pestilence there have been attempts, crude at first, to understand and prevent such occurrences. The fourteenth century witnessed perhaps the most severe plague in recorded history in Europe and Asia: a worldwide pandemic of bubonic plague called the Great Plague. It is estimated that as many as one-third of the inhabitants of Europe died during this plague. Agriculture, economic relationships, and family life itself were altered by this horrific epidemic. Explanations put forth at the time to explain the occurrence of the plague included person-to-person spread of some mysterious disease-causing agent, deliberate poisoning by the Jews of Europe, divine retribution, and so on. However, the state of medical science did not provide much understanding of the causes of the Great Plague. When the Great London Fire of 1666 killed the rodent population that had served as a reservoir of the etiologic agent, *Yersinia pestis,* epidemics of the plague declined in London.

The underlying logic for modern epidemiologic investigations evolved from the scientific revolution of the 1600s, which indicated that the orderly behavior of the physical universe could be expressed in terms of mathematical relationships (Mason, 1962). During this period, Francis Bacon developed the basis of inductive logic and, with it, the concept of "inductive laws" (Copleston, 1963). Many seventeenth-century scientists reasoned that if mathematical relationships could be found to *describe, analyze,* and *understand* the physical universe, then similar relationships, known as *"laws of mortality,"* must exist in the biological world (Lilienfeld, 1979b; Merz, 1976). Laws of mortality were considered to be generalized statements about the relationships between disease (as manifested by mortality) and man. These laws formed the basis of the life table, which attempted to both quantitate and express them mathematically. From this philosophical base, the epidemiologic study evolved.

For specific aspects of disease, such as epidemics, attempts were made to formulate "laws of epidemics." In fact, the contagium vivum theory was regarded in a like manner. It was a generalization of the observed facts that several diseases (smallpox, measles, cholera) were thought to be caused by contagia viva.

Inspired by Bacon's writings, the Royal Society of London was founded in 1662. Its initial members included Robert Boyle, for formulator of Boyle's Law, William Petty, one of the founders of economics, and John Graunt, a tradesman who was a close friend of Petty and one of the Society's financial patrons. That same year, Graunt published his *Natural and Political Observations Mentioned in a Following Index and Made Upon the Bills of Mortality,* a pioneering work in a comparative study of mortality and morbidity in human populations (Lorimer, 1959).

An intellectually curious man, Graunt collected the Bills of Mortality, which had been initiated in 1603 by the parish clerks, in London and in a parish town of Hampshire. After organizing the published Bills, he derived from them inferences about mortality and fertility in the human population, noting the usual excess of male births, the high infant mortality, and the seasonal variation in

Table 2–1. Life Table of Deaths in London
Adapted from Graunt's *Observations*

EXACT AGE	DEATHS	SURVIVORS
0	—	100
6	36	64
16	24	40
26	15	25
36	9	16
46	6	10
56	4	6
66	3	3
76	2	1
80	1	0

Source: Graunt (1662).

mortality. Graunt attempted to distinguish two broad causes of mortality, the acute and the "chronical diseases," and to discern urban-rural differences in mortality. From collected data, he constructed the first known life table, summarizing the mortality experience in terms of the number, percent, or probability of living or dying over a lifetime, a truly outstanding achievement (Table 2–1). Further, Graunt noted that one could attempt to formulate a law of mortality from such tables; he proposed that each country should prepare similar tables so that they could be compared to construct a general law of mortality (Lorrimer, 1959). Reviewing Graunt's work at the tercentenary of the publication of his *Observations,* D. V. Glass (1963) said:

> But, whatever the particular and varying emphases, demographers in general would agree that probably the most outstanding qualities of Graunt's work are first, the search for regularities and configurations in mortality and fertility; and secondly, the attention given—and usually shown explicitly—to the errors and ambiguities of the inadequate data used in that search. Graunt did not wait for better statistics; he did what he could with what was available to him. And by so doing, he also produced a much stronger case for supplying better data.

As mathematical principles developed during the late 1600s and early 1700s, Graunt's ideas were refined and extended. During this period, the idea of using comparative groups in studies also began to emerge. The control group was initially viewed as another group in which a law of mortality, formulated from a different ("experimental" or "study") group, could be tested. In light of this development, it is not surprising that the two noteworthy epidemiologic papers, each the first of its kind, appeared in the middle of the eighteenth century.

The first, a report of an experiment that was conducted in 1747 by James Lind (1753), who had developed certain hypotheses from epidemiologic observations regarding the etiology and treatment of scurvy. He decided to evaluate these hypotheses in the following way:

On the 20th of May, 1747, I took twelve patients in the scurvey, on board the SALISBURY at sea. Their cases were as similar as I could have them. They all in general had putrid gums, the spots and lassitude, with weakness of their knees. They lay together in one place, being a proper apartment for the sick in the fore-hold; and had one diet common to all, viz., water-gruel sweetened with sugar in the morning; fresh mutton broth often times for dinner; at other times puddings, boiled biscuit with sugar, etc.; and for supper, barley and raisins, rice and currents, sago and wine, or the like. Two of these were ordered each a quart of cyder a day. Two others took twenty-five gutts of elizir vitriol three times a day, upon an empty stomach; using a gargle strongly acidulated with it for their mouths. Two others took two spoonsful of vinegar three times a day, upon an empty stomach; having their gruels and their other food well acidulated with it, as also the gargle for their mouth. Two of the worst patients, with the tendons in the ham rigid (a symptom none of the rest had), were put under a course of sea water. Of this, they drank half a pint every day, and sometimes more or less as it operated by way of a gentle physic. Two others had each two oranges and one lemon given them every day. These they eat with greediness, at different times, upon an empty stomach. They continued but six days under this course, having consumed the quantity that could be spared. The two remaining patients took the bigness of a nutmeg three times a day, or an electuary recommended by a hospital-surgeon, made of garlic, mustard seed, rad raphan, balsam of Peru, and gum myrrh; using for common drink, barley-water well acidulated with tamarinds; by a decoction of which, with the addition of cremor tartar, they were gently purged three or four times during the course.

The consequence was, that the most sudden and visible good effects were perceived from the use of the oranges and lemons; one of those who had taken them being at the end of six days fit for duty. The spots were not indeed at that time quite off his body, nor his gums sound; but without any other medicine, then a gargarism of elixir vitriol, he became quite healthy before we came into Plymouth, which was on the 16th of June. The other was the best recovered of any in his condition; and being now deemed pretty well, was appointed nurse to the rest of the sick.

From these results, Lind inferred that citric acid fruits cured the scurvy and that this would also provide a means of prevention. The British Navy eventually accepted his analysis, requiring the inclusion of limes or lime juice in the diet on ships from 1795; hence, the nicknaming of British seamen as ''limeys.''

The other paper, an epidemiologic analysis, was published in 1760 by Daniel Bernoulli, a member of the noted European family of mathematicians. Having evaluated the available evidence, Bernoulli concluded that inoculation protected against smallpox and conferred life-long immunity. Using a life table, not unlike those of today, he determined that inoculation at birth would increase life expectancy.

EPIDEMIOLOGY EMERGES IN THE NINETEENTH CENTURY

The French Revolution at the end of the eighteenth century had a far-reaching influence on epidemiology. It stimulated an interest in public health and preventive medicine, thereby facilitating the development of the epidemiologic approach to disease. Furthermore, it permitted several individuals from the lower classes to assume positions of leadership in medicine. One such person was Pierre Charles-Alexandre Louis, one of the first modern epidemiologists. The characteristic that distinguished Louis's work was the comparison of groups of individuals.

Louis (1836) conducted several observational studies, the most famous of which demonstrated that bloodletting was not efficacious in the treatment of disease and, thus, helped reverse a trend toward its increasing use in medical practice. His approach to epidemiology is illustrated by a comment, in 1836, on the question of the inheritance of phthisis (tuberculosis) (Louis, 1837): "To determine the question satisfactorily, tables of mortality [life tables] would be necessary, comparing an equal number of persons born of phthisical parents with those in an opposite condition." Louis was not the first to use statistical methods in medicine, which he termed "la méthode numerique," but he pioneered in emphasizing their importance in medicine (Lilienfeld, 1979a; Lilienfeld, 1979b; Shyrock, 1947).

Louis was a well-known teacher with students from both England and the United States (Lilienfeld, 1979b). His influence was international and had an astounding impact on the growth of epidemiology that extends to the present (Lilienfeld, 1977a; Lilienfeld, 1977b; Lilienfeld, 1979b). Many of his students were from England and the United States. Lacking a vital statistics system to provide information on the health condition of the population, French epidemiology declined in the mid-1800s (Lilienfeld, 1980c), Louis's students, including William Farr and William Augustus Guy, assumed leadership in the field. They acted as "santiary physicians" involved in epidemiologic and other public health activities.

SANITARY PHYSICIANS—EPIDEMIOLOGY IN ACTION

Between 1835 and 1845, the center of epidemiologic activity moved from Paris to London (Lilienfeld, 1979b). For the following half century, Victorian epidemiology flourished. Physicians in London and elsewhere in England applied Louis's numerical method to the health problems of the day. Their activities were directed toward both disease prevention and treatment, including epidemiologic assessments of the efficacy of smallpox vaccination, specific medical practices, and the morbidity and mortality experiences of persons in various trades. Victorian epidemiology flourished, led by two institutions: the Registrar-General's Office and the London Epidemiological Society.

The Registrar-General's Office

In 1836, the Registrar-General's Office was legislated into existence by the English Parliament as a centralized registry for information on births, deaths, and marriages (Registrar-General, 1839; Szreter, 1991a). As Goldman (1991) noted, this action was a political one and it is not surprising that the first annual report of the Registrar-General (for 1837–1838) viewed the data collected and analyzed from the commercial perspective of life insurance companies. However, by the second such report, William Farr had assumed command of the office and had shifted the focus toward public health (Eyler, 1979). This orientation was to remain characteristic of the Registrar-General's Office and its successor agencies (e.g., the Office of Population Censuses and Surveys) up to the present.

Under Farr's direction, the Registrar-General's Office became a major force in the Victorian public health movement. It provided the statistical facts that were often necessary for initiatives to be developed in response to public health problems (Eyler, 1979; Wohl, 1983). An example of the Office's influence is illustrated by Farr's 1843 analysis of mortality in Liverpool (Szreter, 1991b). Farr found that barely half the native residents of this city lived to see their sixth birthday, while in England in general, the median age of death was 45 years. At the request of the municipal leaders of Liverpool, Parliament passed the landmark Liverpool Sanitary Act of 1846 (Frazer, 1947; Wohl, 1983). This act created a sanitary code for Liverpool, established a local public health authority to enforce it, and introduced the position of the "Medical Officer of Health," the physician who was charged with implementing the code and managing the authority. It served as a model for the organization of English local public health administration during the second half of the nineteenth century.

Farr also developed the concept of mortality surveillance, in which mortality data are regularly reviewed and analyzed to discern changes in the health of the public. These activities represent the first regular use of vital statistics and other demographic data for epidemiologic purposes, and they were a major reason for the vitality of Victorian epidemiology.

The London Epidemiological Society

Another institution of Victorian epidemiology was the London Epidemiological Society (LES) (Lilienfeld, 1979b). Among its founding members were Farr, William Augustus Guy (Dean of the King's College Medical School and a President of the Royal Statistical Society), Thomas Addison (describer of Addison's disease), and Richard Bright (who provided the first description of end-stage renal disease) (Lilienfeld and Lilienfeld, 1980a; 1980b; 1980c; Brockington, 1965). The influence of Louis was also apparent in this society when, at its inaugural, the President (Dr. Benjamin Babbington) remarked: "Statistics, too, have supplied us with a new and powerful means of testing medical truth, and we learn from the labours of the accurate Louis how appropriately they may be brought to bear upon the subject of epidemic disease" (Epidemiological Society, 1850).

The initial purpose of the London Epidemiological Society was to determine the etiology of cholera, but its activities quickly expanded. Its report on smallpox vaccination in 1853, for example, was the major reason for the passage of the Vaccination Act of 1853, mandating vaccination on a nationwide basis. One of the Society's founding members, John Snow (1936), conducted a series of classical studies of cholera. Snow, who was known for his administration of chloroform to Queen Victoria during childbirth, investigated the occurrence of cholera in London during 1848–1854 in addition to reviewing reports of epidemics occurring aboard ships and in Europe.

In London, several water companies were responsible for supplying water to different parts of the city. In 1849, Snow noted that the cholera rates were particularly high in those areas of London that were supplied by the Lambeth Company and the Southwark and Vauxhall Company, both of whom obtained their water from the Thames River at a point heavily polluted with sewage. Between 1849 and 1854 the Lambeth Company had its source of water relocated to a less contaminated part of the Thames. In 1854, when another epidemic of cholera occurred, an area consisting of two-thirds of London's resident population south of the Thames was being served by both companies. In this area, the two companies had their water mains laid out in an interpenetrating manner, so that houses on the same street were receiving their water from different sources. Snow ascertained the total number of houses supplied by each water company, calculated cholera death rates per 10,000 houses for the first seven weeks of the epidemic and compared them with those for the rest of London; the data were supplied to Snow by Farr (Table 2–2). His findings were indisputably clear; the mortality rates in the houses supplied by the Southwark and Vauxhall Company were between eight and nine times greater than those in homes supplied by the Lambeth Company. From these findings, integrated with his investigation of the Broad Street Pump cholera outbreak and his asssssment of other characteristics of

Table 2–2.   Deaths from Cholera per 10,000 Houses by Source of Water Supply,
London, 1854

WATER SUPPLY	NUMBER OF HOUSES	DEATHS FROM CHOLERA	DEATHS IN EACH 10,000 HOUSES
Southwark and Vauxhall Company	40,046	1,263	315
Lambeth Company	26,107	98	37
Rest of London	256,423	1,422	59

Source: Snow (1936).

cholera epidemics, Snow inferred the existence of a ''cholera poison'' transmitted by polluted water.

John Snow's achievement was based on his logical organization of observations, his recognition of a natural experiment, and his quantitative approach in analyzing the occurrence of a disease in a human population. The influence of his report was more widespread than has been realized. It led to legislation mandating that *all* of the water companies in London filter their water by 1857, only two years after the report's publication. (It was not until 1883 that Robert Koch identified the cholera vibrio).

A somewhat different approach to the epidemiologic study of disease is embodied in William Budd's studies of typhoid fever, which were published during the years 1857–1873 (Budd, 1931). Budd, an active member of the LES and a student of Louis, practiced medicine in his native village of North Tawton, a remote rural community in England. From his observations of the environmental conditions of the village, he argued against the miasmatic origin of typhoid fever.

> Much there was, as I can myself testify, offensive to the nose, but [typhoid] fever there was none. It could not be said that the atmospheric conditions necessary to [typhoid] fever was wanting, because while this village remained exempt, many neighbouring villages suffered severely from the pest. . . . Meanwhile privies, pig-styes, and dungheaps continued, year after year, to exhale ill odours, without any specific effect on the public health. . . . I ascertained by an inquiry conducted with the most scrupulous care that for fifteen years there had been no severe outbreak of this disorder, and that for nearly ten years there had been but a single case. For the development of this fever a more specific element was needed than either the swine, the dungheaps, or the privies were, in the common course of things, able to furnish.

From his epidemiologic observations of an outbreak of typhoid fever that occurred in North Tawton between July and November 1839, Budd inferred that it was a contagious disease. During this period, he saw more than eighty patients with typhoid fever. Noting instances of three or four successive cases occurring in the same household, he ascribed these to contagion. Considerably more important was his observation that three individuals who left the village during the epidemic for other villages spread the disease to some of their new contacts. He traced specific instances of person-to-person contact that resulted in the appearance of typhoid fever in villages previously free of the disease despite environmental conditions similar to North Tawton. Budd concluded that typhoid fever is a "contagious, or self-propagating fever," that the intestinal disturbance is its distinctive manifestation, and that "the contagious matter by which the fever is propagated is cast off, chiefly, in the discharges from the diseased intestine." It was not until 1880 that the typhoid fever bacillus was described.Other members of the LES were active in research on such issues as whether smallpox vaccination should be mandatory and whether occupation influenced health and if so, how. They also testified before Parliament and provided data for Parliamentary debates. The vitality in the field of epidemiology, however, diminished as the bacteriological revolution swept through medicine in the late nineteenth and early twentieth centuries.

THE BACTERIOLOGICAL REVOLUTION

The Bacteriological Revolution, in which the cause of various diseases was attributed to bacteria, marked a major change in the development of modern medicine (Shyrock, 1947). For the first time, there was a scientific understanding of the etiology of disease and thus a basis for public health efforts. However, the bacteriological revolution posed a major challenge for epidemiology. Once the cause of a disease was known, the major epidemiologic question was how the disease propagated itself in a population. In the late nineteenth and early twentieth centuries epidemiologists responded to this question by tracing the "point-contact spread" of infection; i.e., from which individuals did the cases of the disease become infected with the etiologic agents? In this manner, it might be possible to find out which individual brought the disease into the community so that contacts between this individual, those already infected, and uninfected persons in the community could be minimized (Eyler, 1986, 1989; Leavitt, 1992). Epidemiologic expertise could thus be brought to bear on disease control through knowledge of the etiologic agent. The focus on populations, an essential aspect of epidemiologic investigation into disease etiology that was characteristic of Victorian epidemiology, waned.

THE DEMOGRAPHIC FOCUS REESTABLISHED

The poulation focus in epidemiology regained strength during the first half of the twentieth century through the activities of demographer-sociologists and statisticians. Some of this impetus came from professionals in the life insurance industry, which had an economic interest in determining which individuals were at greatest risk of morbidity and mortality. Outside the life insurance industry, three individuals, Edgar Sydenstricker, A. Bradford Hill, and Harold Dorn, were of special importance. The epidemiologic activities of these individuals will be discussed briefly since they illustrate the role that population studies had in the reemergence of epidemiology in the early 1900s and in the expansion of epidemiologic activities to include noninfectious diseases during 1930–1970.

Sydenstricker, an economist and sociologist by training, joined the United States Public Health Service in 1915 (Wiehl, 1974). After some initial studies of sickness insurance in Europe, Sydenstricker was assigned to work with Dr. Joseph Goldberger in his studies of pellagra in South Carolina. Sydenstricker organized a series of surveys to discern the diets, illnesses, housing, sanitary conditions, and economic status of families living in cotton mill villages in South Carolina during 1916–1918. These extensive epidemiologic studies identified the etiology of pellagra and made it possible to develop interventions.

Toward the end of his pellagra studies, Sydenstricker was assigned to work with a young Public Health Service physician, Wade Hampton Frost, on the 1918 influenza pandemic. Sydenstricker quickly determined that existing data on the epidemiology of the disease were inadequate. He organized field studies to provide the necessary information. (During this collaboration, Frost was summoned to the Johns Hopkins University School of Hygiene and Public Health to direct the first epidemiology training program but Sydenstricker and Frost continued to collaborate despite this move.) Based on the successful conduct of the influenza studies, Sydenstricker was appointed to direct the Public Health Service's Office of Statistical Investigations. In this role, he undertook a series of morbidity surveys in Hagerstown, Maryland, which established a model for other workers to follow in determining public health priorities in a population.

A. Bradford Hill was an English statistician who, as a result of illness, was unable to pursue his desire to become a physician (Doll, 1993). His early work in the 1920s dealt with the analysis of vital statistics, particularly demographic characteristics such as the difference in mortality among urban and rural residents (e.g., Hill, 1925). Later he was instrumental in the development of the randomized clinical trial and its widespread adoption as a means of assessing the efficacy of a new treatment for a disease (Doll, 1993; Hill, 1990). He was also among the leaders in discerning the role of cigarette smoking in the epidemic of lung cancer. This work was completed with his colleague and student, Professor Richard Doll.

Harold Dorn was trained as a demographer and developed an interest in urban-rural differences in mortality (Dorn, 1934). As a result, he became familiar with the work of both Sydenstricker and Hill. Soon after he completed his doctoral work in 1936, Dorn joined the United States Public Health Service. As part of the Social Security Act of 1936, which created the Social Security system, the

Public Health Service had been given research funds with which it would undertake a national morbidity survey; one major concern was the morbidity related to cancer (Fox, 1987; Mountin et al., 1939). Dorn was appointed director of a national cancer survey to provide data on this issue. The result was the First National Cancer Survey in 1937, the predecessor of the current Surveillance, Epidemiology, and End Results (SEER) cancer surveillance system in the United States.

The National Cancer Institute was established in 1937 and Dorn was assigned to it. The First National Cancer Survey provided much information on the burden of cancer in the population, and Dorn sought to use it as the basis for an epidemiologic profile of cancer. To do so, he would need a biostatistics and epidemiology unit. World War II interrupted these efforts, and Dorn was not able to organize this group at the National Cancer Institute until the late 1940s (Ellenberg, 1993). The group that he recruited to the National Cancer Institute included Jerome Cornfield, Samuel Greenhouse, and Nathan Mantel. Many of the statistical and epidemiologic techniques now routinely used in epidemiologic work (e.g., the odds ratio estimate of the relative risk) were developed in Dorn's unit.

SUMMARY

The basis of epidemiologic inquiry evolved from the Scientific Revolution of the 1600s, which suggested an ordering of nature explicable in mathematical relationships. This concept was extended to biological phenomena and led to the development of the life table. However, until 1830, most epidemiologic activities were the result of isolated efforts by individuals such as John Graunt and James Lind. In the 1830s, the emergence of the Parisian school of medicine fostered the development of a quantitative comparative approach to investigations into the etiology of disease and the efficacy of medical practices. The major figure in this development was Pierre Charles-Alexandre Louis, who created the "numerical method" to undertake epidemiologic investigations. Louis's research and teaching attracted many foreign students, including several from England and the United States. It was Louis's English students who would assume leadership of epidemiology during the middle and late nineteenth century.

William Farr, the first director of the Registrar-General's Office, was one of Louis's English students. Under Farr's supervision, the Registrar-General's Office served as the national center for health statistics. It provided the statistical data that underlay many of the public health initiatives taken in Victorian England. In one instance, the data culled by Farr led to the development of the position of the Medical Officer of Health. Farr's activities were not restricted to the direction of the Registrar-General's Office; he was also a member of the London Epidemiological Society.

The London Epidemiological Society provided a forum for the discussion of epidemiologic activities by its members. The Society also investigated issues, such as vaccination, and issued reports of such work. One member of the Society, John Snow, investigated the relationship between consumption of water from one of the water companies in London and the development of cholera. His epidemiologic study suggested that such a relationship existed, and Snow inferred that a "cholera poison" was transmitted by the water. Another of the Society's members, William Budd, undertook an epidemiologic study of typhoid fever. Forty years before the discovery of the typhoid fever bacillus, he concluded that typhoid fever was propagated through "discharges from the diseased intestine."

The development of bacteriology in the late nineteenth century led epidemiologists to focus on the "point-contact spread" of the agents of disease, i.e., bacteria. With the agents of disease identified, however, the need for epidemiology lessened. It was not until demographers and sociologists, such as Edgar Sydenstricker, A. Bradford Hill, and Harold Dorn, began to undertake epidemiologic investigations in the early and middle twentieth century that epidemiology was reinvigorated. These individuals brought a population focus back into epidemiology. They also trained the next generation of leaders in epidemiology, many of whom are active in the field today.

REFERENCES

Bernoulli, D. 1760. "Mathematical and physical memoirs, taken from the registers of the Royal Academy of Sciences for the year 1760: An attempt at a new analysis of the mortality caused by smallpox and of the advantages of inoculation to prevent it." In *Smallpox Inoculation: An Eighteenth Century Mathematical Controversy. Translation and Critical Commentary* by L. Bradley, 1971. Nottingham, England: Univesity of Nottingham.

Brockington, C. F. 1965. *Public Health in the Nineteenth Century.* Edinburgh: E. & S. Livingstone.

Budd, W. 1931. *Typhoid Fever: Its Nature, Mode of Spreading and Prevention.* Original publication 1873. New York: American Public Health Association.

Copleston, F. 1963. *A History of Philosophy, Vol. 3, Pt. II.* Garden City, N.Y.: Image Books.

Doll, R. 1993. "Sir Austin Bradford Hill, 1897–1991." *Stat. Med.* 12:795–806.

Dorn, H. F. 1934. "The effect of rural-urban migration upon death-rates." *Population* 1: 95–114.

Ellenberg, J. 1993. "Remarks." Presented at: Conference on Current Topics in Biostatistics, National Institutes of Health, Bethesda, Md., January 25, 1993.

"Epidemiological Society." 1850. *Lancet* 2:641.

Eyler, J. M. 1979. *Victorian Social Medicine. The Ideas and Methods of William Farr.* Baltimore: Johns Hopkins University Press.

———. 1986. "The epidemiology of milk-borne scarlet fever: the case of Edwardian Brighton." *Am. J. Pub. Health* 76:573–584.

———. 1989. "Poverty, disease, and responsibility: Arthur Newsholme and the public health dilemmas of British liberalism." *Milbank Q.* 67(Suppl 1):109–126.

Fox, D. M. 1987. "Politics of the NIH extramural program, 1937–1950." *J. Hist. Med. Allied Sci.* 42:447–466.

Frazer, W. M. 1947. *Duncan of Liverpool.* London; Hamish Hamilton Medical Books.

Glass, D. V. 1963. "John Graunt and his natural and political observations." *Proc. Roy. Soc. (Biology)* 159:2–37.

Goldman, L. 1991. "Statistics and the science of society in early Victorian Britain: an intellectual context for the General Register Office." *Soc. Hist. Med.* 4:415–434.

Graunt, J. 1662. *Natural and Political Observations Mentioned in a Following Index, and Made Upon the Bills of Mortality.* London. Reprinted. Baltimore: The Johns Hopkins Press, 1939.

Hill, A. B. 1925. *Internal Migration and its Effects upon the Death-Rates: with Special Reference to the County of Essex.* Medical Research Council Special Report Series No. 95, London: HMSO.

———. 1990. "Memories of the British Streptomycin Trial in tuberculosis: the first randomized clinical trial." *Controlled Clinical Trials* 11:77–79.

Leavitt, J. W. 1992. " 'Typhoid Mary' strikes back: bacteriological theory and practice in early twentieth-century public health." *Isis* 83:608–629.

Lilienfeld, A. M., and Lilienfeld, D. E. 1979a. "A century of case-control studies: Progress?" *J. Chron. Dis.* 32:5–13.

———. 1980a. "The 1979 Heath Clark Lectures. 'The Epidemiologic Fabric.' I. Weaving the Threads." *Int. J. Epid.* 9:199–206.

———. 1980b. "The 1979 Heath Clark Lectures. 'The Epidemiologic Fabric.' II. The London Bridge—It Never Fell." *Int. J. Epid.* 9:299–304.

Lilienfeld, D. E. 1979b. "The greening of epidemiology: Sanitary physicians and the London Epidemiological Society (1830–1870)." *Bull. Hist. Med.* 52:503–528.

Lilienfeld, D. E., and Lilienfeld, A. M. 1977a. "Teaching preventive medicine in medical schools: An historical vignette." *Prev. Med.* 6:469–471.

———. 1977b. "Epidemiology: A retrospective study." *Amer. J. Epid.* 106:445–459.

———. 1980c. "The French influence on the development of epidemiology." In *Times, Places, Persons.* A. M. Lilienfeld, ed. Baltimore: The Johns Hopkins University Press.

Lind, J. 1753. *A Treatise on the Scurvy.* Edinburgh: Sands, Murray, and Cochran.

Lorrimer, F. 1959. "The development of demography." In *The Study of Population.* P. M. Hauser and O. D. Duncan, eds. Chicago: University of Chicago Press, pp. 124–179.

Louis, P.C.-A. 1836. *Researches on the Effects of Bloodletting in Some Inflammatory Diseases, and on the Influence of Tartarized Antimony and Vesication in Pneumonitis.* Translated by C. G. Putman with Preface and Appendix by James Jackson. Boston: Milliard, Gray and Co.

———. 1837. "Pathological researches on phthisis." *Amer. J. Med. Sci.* 19:445–449.

Mason, S. F. 1962. *A History of the Sciences.* New York: Collier Books.

Merz, J. T. 1976. *A History of European Scientific Thought in the Nineteenth Century, Vol. 2.* Glouceseter, Mass.: Peter Smith.

Mountin, J. W., Dorn, H. F., and Boone, B. R. 1939. "The incidence of cancer in Atlanta, Ga., and surrounding counties." *Pub. Health Rep.* 54:1255–1273.

Registrar-General. 1839. "First annual report of the Registrar-General on births, deaths, and marriages in England in 1837–8." *J. Stat. Soc. London* 2:269.

Shyrock, R. H. 1947. *The Development of Modern Medicine.* New York: Knopf.

Snow, J. 1936. "On the mode of communication of cholera." In *Snow on Cholera.* New York: The Commonwealth Fund, pp. 1–175.

Szreter, S. 1991a. "Introduction: the GRO and the historians." *Soc. Hist. Med.* 4:401–414.

———. 1991b. "The GRO and the public health movement in Britain, 1837–1914." *Soc. Hist. Med.* 4:435–463.

Wiehl, D. G. 1974. "Edgar Sydenstricker: a memoir." In *The Challenge of Facts.* R. V. Kasius, ed. New York: PRODIST.

Wohl, A. S. 1983. *Endangered Lives.* Cambridge, Mass.: Harvard University Press.

3

SELECTED EPIDEMIOLOGIC CONCEPTS
OF DISEASE

Many of the fundamental epidemiologic concepts have evolved from studies of infectious diseases, but they are equally applicable to noninfectious diseases and conditions. Only those that have proved to be of practical value will be considered in this chapter.

AGENT, HOST, AND ENVIRONMENT

Essentially, the epidemiologic patterns of infectious diseases depend upon factors that influence the probability of contact between an infectious agent and a susceptible person known as a host. The presence of the infectious material by which the disease may be transmitted varies with the duration and extent of its excretion from an infected person, the **environmental** conditions affecting survival of the **agent,** the route of entry into the **host,** and the existence of alternative reservoirs or hosts of the agent. The availability of susceptible hosts depends upon the extent of mobility and interpersonal contact within the population group and the degree and duration of immunity from previous infections with the same or related agents.

Relationships similar to those among infectious agents of disease, human hosts, and their environment also exist among noninfectious etiological agents, hosts, and environment. For example, whether or not a person develops a specific form of cancer may depend upon the extent of his exposure to the carcinogenic agent, the dose of the agent, and his susceptibility, which may be influenced by genetic and/or immunological factors. A classification of agent, host, and environmental factors is presented in Table 3–1 as a frame of reference in the search for determinants of disease occurrence in a population.

A specific scientific discipline is usually concerned with a particular category of the factors listed in Table 3–1. For instance, the geneticist concentrates on genetic factors; the microbiologist on infectious agents; the sociologist on human behavior, ethnic groups, and socioeconomic environments. The epidemiologist, however, attempts to integrate from diverse disciplines the data necessary to analyze a particular disease. The need for evaluating the *interaction* of these factors relative to **time, place,** and **persons** is the main reason for viewing this frame of reference as primarily an epidemiologic concept.

Table 3–1. A Classification of Agent, Host, and Environmental Factors That Determine the Occurrence of Diseases in Human Populations

I. *Agents of Disease– Etiological Factors*

Examples

A. Nutritive elements
    excesses — Cholesterol
    deficiencies — Vitamins, proteins
B. Chemical agents
    poisons — Carbon monoxide, carbon tetrachloride, drugs
    allergens — Ragweed, poison ivy, medications
C. Physical agents — Ionizing radiation, mechanical
D. Infectious agents
    metazoa — Hookworm, schistosomiasis, onchocerciasis
    protozoa — Amoebae, malaria
    bacteria — Rheumatic fever, lobar pneumonia, typhoid, tuberculosis, syphilis
    fungi — Histoplasmosis, athlete's foot
    rickettsia — Rocky mountain spotted fever, typhus, Lyme disease
    viruses — Measles, mumps, chickenpox, smallpox, poliomyelitis, rabies, yellow fever, HIV

II. *Host Factors* (Intrinsic Factors)—Influences Exposure, Susceptibility, or Response to Agents

Examples

A. Genetic — Sickle cell disease
B. Age — Alzheimer's disease
C. Sex — Rheumatoid arthritis
D. Ethnic group — —
E. Physiologic state — Fatigue, pregnancy, puberty, stress, nutritional state

(continued)

Table 3–1. A Classification of Agent, Host, and Environmental Factors That Determine the Occurrence of Diseases in Human Populations (continued)

F.	Prior immunologic experience	Hypersensitivity, protection
	active	Prior infection, immunization
	passive	Maternal antibodies, gamma globulin prophylaxis
G.	Intercurrent or preexisting disease	
H.	Human behavior	Personal hygiene, food handling, diet, interpersonal contact, occupation, recreation, utilization of health resources, tobacco use

III. *Environmental Factors* (Extrinsic Factors)—Influences Existence of the Agent, Exposure, or Susceptibility to Agent

		Examples
A.	Physical environment	Geology, climate
B.	Biologic environment	
	human populations	Density
	flora	Sources of food, influence on vertebrates and arthropods, as a source of agents
	fauna	Food sources, vertebrate hosts, arthropod vectors
C.	Socioeconomic environment	
	occupation	Exposure to chemical agents
	urbanization and economic development	Urban crowding, tensions and pressures, cooperative efforts in health and education
	disruption	Wars, floods

MODE OF TRANSMISSION

As is evident from Table 3–1, infectious diseases are usually classified by the etiological agent, such as a virus or a bacterium. This classification, based on the biological features of the agent, is satisfactory from many points of view, including that of potential preventive measures. However, it is also possible to classify diseases by their epidemiologic features. In many instances, this may be more advantageous for applying preventive measures than an etiological classification. Infectious diseases, for example, can be divided according to the way they are spread through human populations:

1. *Common-vehicle epidemics.* The etiological agent is transmitted by water, food, air, or inoculation (Table 3–2). Common-vehicle epidemics can result from a single exposure of a population group to the agent, from repeated multiple exposures, or from continued exposure over a period

of time. They are usually characterized by explosiveness of onset and limitation or localization in time, place, and persons. This type of epidemic can be illustrated by a food poisoning outbreak, which is the result of a single source of exposure.

2. *Epidemics propagated by serial transfer from host to host.* The agent is spread through contact between infected and susceptible individuals by means of the respiratory, anal, oral, genital, or other route; by serial transfer of infected blood or sera; by dust; or by insects and arthropods (vectors) (Table 3–2). The course of such an epidemic is illustrated in Figure 3–1.

This simple classification of infectious diseases by mode of transmission provides a basis for considering possible measures to prevent epidemics in the community. But several types of infections, particularly from viral and parasitic agents, may have more complicated modes of transmission. An example is given in Figure 3–2.

Table 3–2. Classification of Human Infections by Selected Epidemiologic Features*

	Examples
I. *Dynamics of Spread through Human Populations:*	
A. Spread by a ''common vehicle''	
ingestion with water, food or beverage	Salmonellosis
inhalation in air breathed	Legionnaire's disease
inoculation (intravenous, subcutaneous)	Hepatitis B
B. Propagation by serial transfer from host to host	
respiratory route of transfer	Measles
anal-oral route	Shigellosis Hepatitis B
genital route	Syphilis, AIDS
II. *Portal of Entry (and Portal of Exit) in Human Host:*	
Upper respiratory tract	Diphtheria
Lower respiratory tract	Tuberculosis
Gastrointestinal tract	Typhoid fever
Genitourinary tract	Gonorrhea
Conjunctiva	Trachoma
Percutaneous	Leptospirosis
Percutaneous (bite of arthropod)	Yellow fever

(continued)

Table 3–2.   Classification of Human Infections by Selected Epidemiologic Features*
(continued)

III. *Principal Reservoir of Infection:*

      Man   Hepatitis A

      Other vertebrates (zoonoses)   Tularemia

      Agent free-living (?)   Histoplasmosis

IV. *Cycles of Infectious Agent in Nature:*

      (arrows designate transfer to

        occasional host)

      Man-man   Influenza

      Man-arthropod-man   Malaria

      Vertebrate-vertebrate↘   Psittacosis

                    man

      Vertebrate-arthropod-   Viral encephalitis

        vertebrate↘

                    man

V. *Complex Cycles*—seen especially in certain helminth infections. For example, in paragonimiasis the cycle is as follows:

            Ovum——miracidium——cercaria——adult——ovum

                   (in snail)   (in crab,   (in man)

                           crayfish)

      The agent is free-living in fresh water during a part of its existence as ovum, miracidium, and cercaria.

---

*Some diseases may be classified in more than one category in this classification; the most usual situation is given in the examples cited.

THE INCUBATION PERIOD

One important epidemiologic feature of a disease is the incubation period, first described by Fracastoro in 1546 (Fracastoro, 1930). This is the interval between the time of contact and/or entry of the agent and onset of illness. In infectious diseases, it is generally thought of as the time required for the multiplication of the microorganism within the host up to a threshold point where the pathogen population is large enough to produce symptoms in the host.

    Each infectious disease has a characteristic incubation period, largely dependent upon the rate of growth of the organism in the host (Benenson, 1990). Other factors that play a role include the dosage of the infectious agent, its portal of entry, and the rate and degree of immune response by the host. An incubation period will vary among individuals; and, in a group of cases, its distribution will be asymmetrical, so that the part of the curve with longer incubation periods has a long "tail," that is, the curve is "skewed to the right" (Figure 3–3). Sartwell pointed out that this asymmetrical curve resembles a log-normal distribution. Indeed, when one graphs the frequency of incubation periods against the loga-

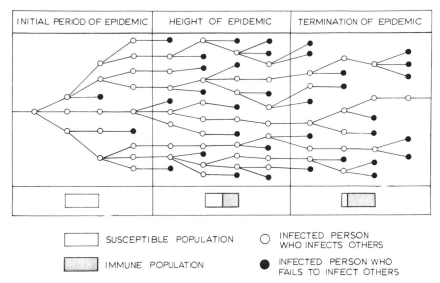

Figure 3–1. Course of a typical propogated epidemic in which the agent is transmitted by contact between individuals. *Source:* Burnet and White (1972).

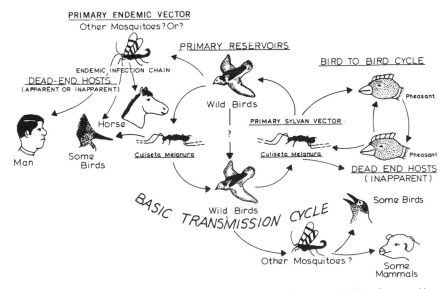

Figure 3–2. Summer infection chains for eastern equine encephalitis. *Source:* Hess and Holden (1958).

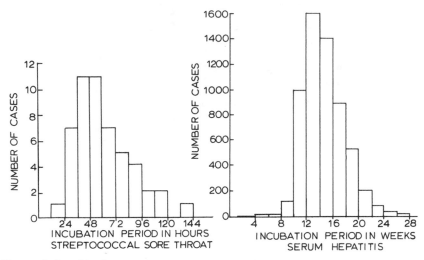

Figure 3–3. Distribution of incubation periods in an epidemic of food-borne strepto-coccal sore throat and a series of serum hepatitis following administration of icterogenic lots of yellow fever vaccine. *Source:* Sartwell (1950).

rithm of time, the skewness essentially disappears and the curve resembles a normal distribution; hence, the name "log-normal distribution" (Armenian and Khoury, 1981; Polednak, 1974; Sartwell, 1950, 1966).

In a graph of a common-vehicle epidemic from a single source, the curve resulting from plotting the times of onset of the disease also represents the distribution of incubation periods. Knowing the incubation period for a disease in a single-source common-vehicle epidemic enables one to estimate the time of exposure to the disease agent.

Only three factors are necessary to describe this type of epidemic:

1. Distribution of times and onset of illness, known as the **epidemic curve**.
2. The specific disease, which is characterized by its incubation period.
3. The time of exposure.

In practice, if only two of these factors are known, it is possible to deduce the third factor.

If one recognizes an infectious disease from its clinical characteristics, the incubation period is then also known. In a single-source common-vehicle epidemic, the epidemic curve represents the distribution of incubation periods and the median point on the curve represents the median incubation period (Figure 3–4). The median is preferred as a measure of central tendency because of the usual skewness of the distribution of the incubation periods. Using the median incubation period, one can estimate the time of exposure to the etiological agent

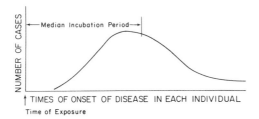

Figure 3–4. Distribution of times of onset of disease (the epidemic curve) and median incubation period in a single-source common-vehicle epidemic.

and investigate the events that occurred about that time to determine the cause of the epidemic. Likewise, if sufficient information is available to construct the epidemic curve and the time of exposure is known, one can determine the type of infectious disease if the incubation period of that disease is already known.

Although the prototype for this kind of reasoning is the previously described single-source food poisoning outbreak, it is also applicable to diseases caused by several possible etiological agents, one of which may be known (Armenian and Khoury, 1981). Cobb, Miller, and Wald (1959) attempted to apply this approach to leukemia, where exposure to radiation is recognized as one etiological factor for some forms of the disease. They analyzed the cases of leukemia that occurred after the 1945 atomic bomb explosion in Hiroshima, which can be regarded as a single exposure. Figure 3–5A compares the annual incidence of leukemia following explosion of the bomb among those who were located less than 1,000 meters (m) from the hypocenter (the location of the bomb in the air at the time of the explosion) with the incidence among those who were 2,000 m or more from the center, generally considered an unexposed group. The annual leukemia incidence rate proved to be higher in the first group, but interestingly, the peak incidence of leukemia occurred in 1951 or 1952, about six years after the radiation exposure. Admittedly, the data for the earlier years are probably incomplete, but, nonetheless, the shape of the curve resembles that of an epidemic curve observed in single-exposure common-vehicle epidemics. The incidence pattern for those who were between 1,000 to 1,999 m from the bomb site is similar although their rates are lower (Fig. 3–5B). Continued follow-up of these survivors still shows an excessive rate of leukemia in the exposed group.

Cobb, Miller and Wald also collated several reports of ankylosing spondylitis patients who developed leukemia following radiation treatment by either a single exposure or multiple exposures over a number of years. In the latter case, they determined the central point of the exposure period and adjusted for the size of the administered dose. Assuming the interval between the time of exposure and onset of leukemia to be the incubation period, they obtained the results presented in Figure 3–6. These results show that the curve peaks at about four years after

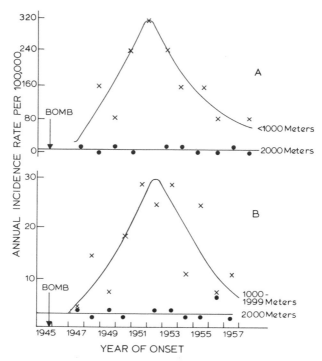

Figure 3–5.   Annual incidence rate of leukemia following the atomic bomb explosion among survivors who were residents of Hiroshima City at the time of diagnosis. (A) Persons less than 1000 meters from hypocenter compared with persons 2000 or more meters from the hypocenter at time of explosion. (B) Persons 1000 to 1999 meters from hypocenter compared with persons 2000 or more meters from hypocenter at time of explosion. *Source:* Cobb, Miller, and Wald (1959).

exposure to radiation and that 90 percent of the cases have occurred within nine years of such exposure.

If one is willing to assume from these data that the incubation period of leukemia induced by unknown factors is similar to that of leukemia caused by radiation, it would suggest that the search for etiological factors of leukemia should focus on the ten-year period before the onset of the disease in adults. However, data obtained from future studies may change these estimates. It is also of interest that the distribution of leukemia cases is skewed to the right, as in single-source common-vehicle epidemics of infectious diseases. The skewness in the ankylosing spondylitis data may partially reflect the number of patients who had multiple exposures over a period of several years.

An example of similar reasoning is the analysis of the changing pattern of mortality from leukemia among children under five years old in England and Wales between 1931 and 1953 (Hewitt, 1955). Hewitt noted the similarity between the shape of the mortality curve and the curves usually observed in

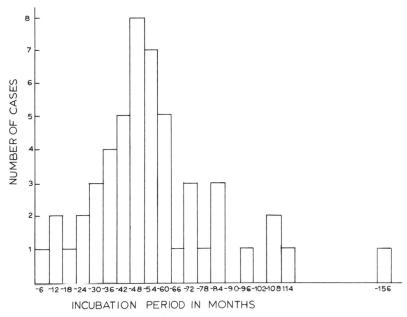

Figure 3–6. Distribution of incubation periods of leukemia cases following irradiation for ankylosing spondylitis. *Source:* Cobb, Miller, and Wald (1959).

incubation periods of infectious diseases. He also noted an increasing peak of mortality during this period at about three to four years of age (Figure 3–7). He postulated that the increased use of X-rays during this period, which were known to be leukemogenic, was one possible explanation. This analysis provided the basis for a field investigation of the possible influence of prenatal and postnatal X-rays and other procedures on the occurrence of childhood leukemia (Stewart, Webb, and Hewitt, 1958). Their finding of a connection between intrauterine radiation (mainly X-ray pelvimetry) and childhood leukemia stimulated many others to investigate this relationship (Diamond, Schmerler, and Lilienfeld, 1973; Graham et al., 1966; Kato, 1971; MacMahon, 1962). Several of these studies suggested that although the entire increase in death rates could not be explained by intrauterine radiation, a part of the increase could be so explained (Diamond, Schmerler, and Lilienfeld, 1973; Graham et al., 1966; MacMahon, 1962). It must be admitted, however, that there are still differences of opinion among those who have investigated the problem (Kato, 1971).

Armenian and Lilienfeld (1974, 1983) analyzed the incubation periods of certain neoplastic diseases, including several with known etiological factors and specific exposure times such as thyroid adenomas, cancers following childhood exposure to radiation, bronchogenic carcinoma in asbestos workers, and bladder tumors among dyestuff workers. Figure 3–8 shows the distribution of incubation

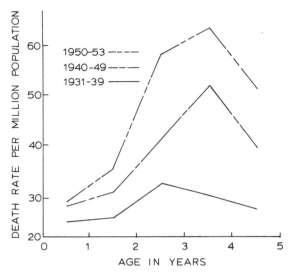

Figure 3–7. Age-specific death rates from leukemia among children under five years old, England and Wales, 1931–1953. *Source:* Hewitt (1955).

periods for 281 cases of bladder tumors that occurred among dyestuff workers. The shape of the distribution is skewed to the right and was demonstrated to be log-normal with a median incubation period of about seventeen years. Similarly, Armenian and Khoury (1981) analyzed the distribution of the ages at onset for various inherited conditions, such as familial hypercholesterolemia, and found that these distributions were log-normal; for diseases of known multifactorial etiology, the distribution of the age at onset was not log-normal (Armenian and Lilienfeld, 1983).

    If, in infectious diseases, the incubation period reflects the multiplication of an organism and its interaction with host defenses, it is interesting to speculate on the biological model that underlies the incubation period (or "latency" period, as investigators have called it) when exposure to a chemical carcinogenic agent is the etiologic factor. Doll and Pike have each postulated that the neoplastic transformation of a number of individual cells is necessary in order to produce a "nest" of transformed cells that constitute the beginning of a tumor (Doll, 1971; Pike, 1966). It is also possible that a carcinogenic agent initiates a malignant transformation that requires an additional promoting agent for further specific growth of the malignancy. Thus, an individual is exposed at a specific point in time to an initiating agent that transforms the cell, and only after an interval of years does exposure to a promoting agent occur, which stimulates growth leading to a malignant tumor (Armenian, 1987; Berenblum, 1941). To these concepts must be added the potentially important roles of oncogenes and immunogenetics

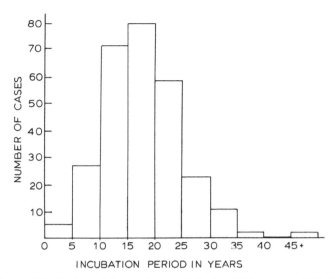

Figure 3–8. Distribution of incubation periods for 281 cases of bladder tumors among dyestuff workers. *Source:* Case et al. (1954).

in the genesis of cancer (Nowell, 1991). In cancer, the incubation period may result from the interaction between the growth of neoplastic cells and the development of immune responses by the host.

THE SPECTRUM OF DISEASE

The spectrum of disease may be defined as the sequence of events that occurs in the human organism from the time of exposure to the etiological agent until death, as shown in Figure 3–9 (Reimann, 1960). It has two broad components, subclinical and clinical. Whether an individual with the disease progresses through the entire spectrum depends upon the availability and efficacy of preventive and/or therapeutic measures that, if introduced at a particular point of the spectrum, will completely prevent or retard any further development of the disease. In the case of cancer of the cervix, the spectrum might consist of three main stages: dysplasia, carcinoma in situ, and invasive carcinoma. Similarly, cerebrovascular disease may have the following stages: atherosclerotic changes in carotid arteries, transient ischemic attacks, and stroke. The atherosclerotic changes in the carotid arteries are subclinical and can be ascertained only by special diagnostic tests such as carotid Doppler studies.

In infectious diseases, this spectrum is usually known as the ''gradient of infection,'' which refers to the sequence of manifestations of illness that reflect

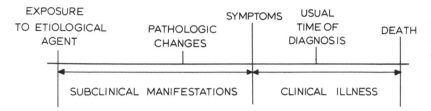

Figure 3–9.   Spectrum of disease.

the host's response to the infectious agent. This extends from "inapparent infections" at one extreme to death at the other (Figure 3–10). The frequency with which these different manifestations occur varies with the specific infectious disease. For example, in measles, the vast majority (over 90 percent) of infected persons exhibit clinical illness; in mumps, the proportion is somewhat less, approximately 66 percent; and in poliomyelitis, over 90 percent of the infections are not clinically apparent.

Clinicians and epidemiologists are usually only aware of a small part of the spectrum of a given disease or gradient of infection, the "tip of the iceberg" (Last, 1963). However, epidemiologists try to determine the entire range of the spectrum since it may provide a very different picture of a disease than that seen by clinicians in fully developed cases. Histoplasmosis is a case in point. From its first description in 1906 until the 1940s, histoplasmosis was regarded as a rare and usually fatal disease. Epidemiologic surveys by the Public Health Service in the 1940s, using the histoplasmosis skin test, completely changed this view. They revealed that most nonepidemic histoplasmosis infections produce no symptoms, or a mild influenzalike disorder, and rarely lead to a progressive systemic disease. In certain areas of the country (parts of Kentucky, Tennessee, Missouri, Indiana, Ohio, and Arkansas), the frequency of infection in the general population was found to be higher than 80 percent (Comstock, 1986). It should be emphasized that one of the major deterrents in elucidating the epidemiology of diseases of unknown etiology is the absence of methods to detect the subclinical state—the bottom of the "iceberg."

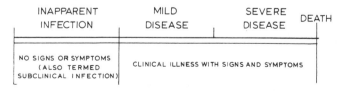

Figure 3–10.   Gradient of infection.

Inapparent infections are important because they play a role in the transmission of infectious agents. The spread of poliomyelitis, meningococcal meningitis, and other diseases can only be explained on this basis. To estimate the number of individuals in the population who have become immune to the infectious agent, the frequency of these clinically inapparent infected persons must be assessed by means of tests for antibodies or skin tests for a specific disease, if available.

Epidemiologists have to consider the role of latent, as well as inapparent, infections in the study of certain diseases, particularly viral diseases. Latent infection is distinguished from inapparent infection in that the host does not shed the infectious agent, which lies dormant in the host cells. A viral disease may occur early in life in one clinical form, and in later life, the dormant virus may produce a different clinical disease due to some (as yet unknown) mechanism; these are referred to as "slow virus diseases" (Fucillo, Kurent, and Sever, 1973; Gajdusek, 1977; Gajdusek and Gibbs, 1975). For example, investigations into the relationship of measles virus to subacute sclerosing panencephalitis suggest that the latter may represent a late manifestation of measles infections and may be a slow virus disease.

HERD IMMUNITY

Herd immunity is the resistance of a community to a disease (Last, 1990). Just as individual immunity decreases the probability that an individual will develop a particular disease when exposed to an infectious agent, "herd immunity" refers to the decreased probability that a group or community will experience an epidemic after the introduction of an infectious agent, although some persons in the group may be individually susceptible to the agent (Fox et al., 1971; Cliff et al., 1981; Cliff and Haggett, 1984; Anderson and May, 1990). This concept is helpful in understanding why an epidemic does not occur in a community and in explaining the periodic variation of some infectious diseases, particularly those that are transmitted from one person to another. It also is useful in the formulation of national vaccination policies. Herd immunity is measured in terms of the proportion of immune, or conversely, of susceptible, persons in a social group. Clearly, the presence of a large proportion of immune individuals in a community decreases the chances of contact between infected and susceptible persons. By acting as a barrier between the two, the immune population decreases the rate of spread of the infectious agent. The degree of herd immunity necessary to prevent the development of an epidemic varies with the specific disease. It depends upon such factors as the degree to which an infected individual is capable of transmit-

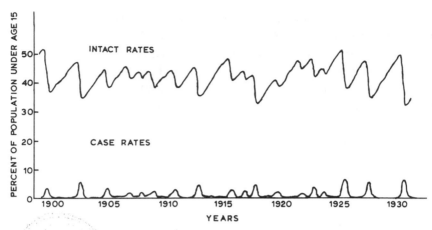

Figure 3–11. Estimated complete monthly attack rates from measles and intact rates (proportions not previously attacked for the population under fifteen, Old Baltimore, Md., July 1899–December 1931. *Source:* Hedrich (1933).

ting the infection, the length of time during which he is infectious, and the size and social behavior of the community.

The relationship between the proportion of susceptible individuals in a community and the periodicity of disease is illustrated by the analysis of case rates of measles in Baltimore for the period 1899–1931 (Figure 3–11) (Hedrich, 1933). The incidence of measles increases when the number of susceptible persons is highest and herd immunity is lowest. Mathematical models have shown that the smaller the community, the longer the interval between epidemics (Bartlett, 1957). (The smaller the community, the lower the probability of contact by a susceptible person with an infectious one.)

A very practical aspect of this concept of herd immunity is that an entire population (100 percent) does not have to be immunized to prevent the occurrence of an epidemic (Fox et al., 1971). For measles, for instance, Schlenker et al. (1992) suggested that transmission of the virus would stop if only 70 percent of the population were immunized. However, in the large metropolises of modern urban society, one must recognize that the interpersonal contacts necessary for the spread of an infectious agent occur in smaller neighborhood groups, not in the entire metropolis. Consequently, from the viewpoint of immunization and other public health practices, it is the herd immunity of these smaller groups that must be taken into consideration.

National differences in rubella vaccination policy illustrate the application of herd immunity. In the United States, girls and boys are vaccinated at around two years of age. This policy aims to block all transmission of the rubella virus and thereby prevent congenital rubella syndrome (CRS). However, there is no boosting of immunity by reexposure to the virus in the community. This policy is effective only if high levels of immunization are achieved (80–85 percent); in the United States, such high levels are met by requiring vaccination for school entry (Anderson and Nokes, 1991). Since 1964, when nationwide vaccination began, measles incidence has declined by more than 90 percent. CRS incidence has simlarly declined. In the United Kingdom, many other European countries, and Australia, a different approach has been taken: Girls are vaccinated at age 12 years. The result is natural immunity among children less than 12 years old and continued circulation of the virus in the community, allowing immunity to be boosted. Since the girls are vaccinated before menarche, CRS will presumably be prevented. This policy should be more effective at preventing CRS if the proportion of persons in the population who have been vaccinated is low (less than 60 percent), as was the case in the United Kingdom.

SUMMARY

The occurrence of disease reflects the interaction of the **agent,** the **host,** and the **environment.** The interaction may reflect a single exposure of a population to the agent, resulting in a **common-vehicle** outbreak. Another possibility is a disease spread by serial transfer of the agent from an affected individual to a susceptible host. Once the agent has been introduced to a susceptible host, a series of biological events takes place leading to either subclinical or clinically apparent disease. The gradient between a subclinical event and a severe clinical event (perhaps resulting in death) is the spectrum of disease. The time period from exposure to the agent until the appearance of clinical disease is the incubation period. Each disease has a characteristic incubation period. In the case of single-vehicle outbreaks, the incubation period is defined as the median time period from exposure to the agent until occurrence of the disease among all cases. The distribution of such time periods is known as the epidemic curve. It is log-normally distributed, regardless of whether the agent is infectious or noninfectious.

The concept of **herd immunity** provides a basis for population-based vaccination activities. As the proportion of the population immunized (either by previous exposure to the agent or by vaccination) increases, the opportunity for transmission of the agent within that population declines. For many infectious agents, the level of immunization within the population at which transmission ceases is less than 100 percent; it is as low as 70 percent in the case of measles. Herd immunity is one of the bases for current rubella vaccination policies in both the United Kingdom and the United States. The policy differences between these two countries reflect different levels of attained immunization in their respective populations.

STUDY PROBLEMS

1. Define the latency period for a non-infectious disease, such as ischemic heart disease or chronic obstructive lung disease. Give an example of a latency period.
2. Contrast the epidemic curves encountered in:
   (a) a common-vehicle single-exposure outbreak,
   (b) a common-vehicle continuous-exposure outbreak,
   (c) a serial-transfer propagated epidemic,
   (d) an outbreak resulting from a slow-virus disease.
3. Of what importance is the concept of herd immunity to the public health administrator?
4. Subclinical cases have always posed a problem in investigating the etiology of both infectious and noninfectious diseases. Discuss the reasons for this.
5. Hall and Barker (1984) noted that the distribution of the age of onset of Legg-Perthes disease (avascular necrosis of the head of the femur in children) in several case series was a log-normal one. What does this observation imply about the causal agent?
6. One often hears that there is a sexually transmitted disease epidemic in the United States today. Into what category (e.g., common vehicle, serial transfer) would you classify this epidemic?
7. A local health officer in a small community received reports from three physicians that they were taking care of persons who had diarrhea, abdominal cramps, vomiting, chills, and fever. From stools collected from several patients, a strain of salmonella *(S. typhimurium)* was isolated. A total of 119 patients were identified and the times of onset of the disease in this group were tabulated as follows:

JANUARY 7		JANUARY 8		JANUARY 9	
TIME	NO. OF ILL PERSONS	TIME	NO. OF ILL PERSONS	TIME	NO. OF ILL PERSONS
6–7 A.M.	2	12–1 A.M.	5	12–1 A.M.	3
8–9 A.M.	5	2–3 A.M.	3	2–3 A.M.	2
10–11 A.M.	11	4–5 A.M.	3	4–5 A.M.	0
12–1 P.M.	18	6–7 A.M.	3	6–7 A.M.	1
2–3 P.M.	10	8–9 A.M.	4	8–9 A.M.	0
4–5 P.M.	7	10–11 A.M.	6	10–11 A.M.	1
6–7 P.M.	5	12–1 P.M.	8	12–1 P.M.	0
8–9 P.M.	4	2–3 P.M.	4	2–3 P.M.	0
10–11 P.M.	4	4–5 P.M.	3		

JANUARY 7		JANUARY 8		JANUARY 9	
TIME	NO. OF ILL PERSONS	TIME	NO. OF ILL PERSONS	TIME	NO. OF ILL PERSONS
		6–7 P.M.	3		
		8–9 P.M.	2		
		10–11 P.M.	2		

(a) Make a graph of the epidemic curve.

(b) What type of outbreak does this curve resemble? Why?

(c) What are the possible reasons for the bimodality of this epidemic curve?

(d) Describe the investigation that the health officer should conduct.

8. Rose (1982) has noted that strong correlations could be found between serum cholesterol concentrations and systolic blood pressure measurements in 1958–1964 in men, ages 40–59, in population samples from Finland, Greece, Italy, Japan, the Netherlands, the United States, and Yugoslavia, and subsequent national mortality from coronary heart disease 10 years later. Both serum cholesterol concentration and systolic blood pressure are known risk factors for coronary heart disease. What does this finding imply about the latency period of coronary heart disease? What would be the next step in such an investigation?

REFERENCES

Anderson, R. M., and May, R. M. 1990. "Immunisation and herd immunity." *Lancet* 335: 641–645.

Anderson, R. M., and Nokes, D. J. 1991. "Mathematical models of transmission and control." In *Oxford Textbook of Public Health*. Second Edition. W. W. Holland, R. Detels, and G. Knox, eds. Oxford: Oxford University Press.

Armenian, H. K., 1987. "Incubation periods of cancer: old and new." *J. Chron. Dis.* 40(Suppl 2):9S–15S.

Armenian, H. K., and Khoury, M. J. 1981. "Age at onset of genetic diseases." *Am. J. Epidemiol.* 113:596–605.

Armenian, H. K., and Lilienfeld, A. M. 1974. "The distribution of incubation periods of neoplastic diseases." *Amer. J. Epid.* 99:92–100.

———. 1983. "Incubation period of disease." *Epi. Rev.* 5:1–15.

Bartlett, M. S. 1957. "Measles periodicity and community size." *J. Roy. Stat. Soc.* 120: 48–70.

Benenson, A. S. 1990. *Control of Communicable Diseases in Man*. 15th Edition. New York: American Public Health Association.

Berenblum, I. 1941. "The mechanism of carcinogenesis. A study of the significance of cocarcinogenic action and related phenomena." *Cancer Res.* 1:807–814.

Burnet, M., and White, D. O. 1972. *Natural History of Infectious Disease*. 4th Edition. Cambridge, England: Cambridge University Press.

Case, R.A.M., Hosker, M. E., McDonald, D. B., and Pearson, J. T. 1954. "Tumours of the urinary bladder in workmen engaged in the manufacture and use of certain dye-stuff intermediates in the British industry. Part I. The role of aniline, benzidine, alpha-napthylamine and beta-naphthalamine." *Brit. J. Ind. Med.* 11:75–104.

Cliff, A., and Haggett, P. 1984. "Island epidemics." *Sci. Am.* 250(5):138–147.

Cliff, A. D., Haggett, P., Ord, J. K., and Versey, G. R. 1981. *Spatial Diffusion. An Historical Geography of Epidemics in an Island Community*. Cambridge: Cambridge University Press.

Cobb, S., Miller, N., and Wald, N. 1959. "On the estimation of the incubation period in malignant disease." *J. Chron. Dis.* 9:385–393.

Comstock, G. W. 1986. "Histoplasmosis." In *Maxcy-Rosenau Preventive Medicine and Public Health*. 10th Edition. J. Last, ed. New York: Appleton-Century-Crofts.

Diamond, E. L., Schmerler, H., and Lilienfeld, A. M. 1973. "The relationship of intra-uterine radiation to subsequent mortality and development of leukemia in children: a cohort study." *Amer. J. Epidemiol.* 97:283–313.

Doll, R. 1971. "The age distribution of cancer: implications for models of carcinogenesis." *J. Roy. Stat. Soc.* 134:133–166.

Fox, J. P., Elveback, L., Scott, W., Gatewood, L., and Ackerman, E. 1971. "Herd immunity: basic concept and relevance to public health immunization practices." *Amer. J. Epidemiol.* 94:179–189.

Fracasatoro, H. 1930. *De contagione et contagiosis morbis et eorum curatione, Libri III*. Translation and notes by W. C. Wright. New York: G. P. Putnam and Sons.

Fucillo, D. A., Kurent, J. E., and Sever, J. L. 1974. "Slow virus diseases." *Ann. Rev. Microbiol.* 28:231–264.

Gajdusek, D. C. 1977. "Unconventional viruses and the origin and disappearance of kuru." *Science* 197:943–960.

Gajdusek, D. C., and Gibbs, C. J. 1975. "Slow virus infections of the nervous system and the laboratories of slow, latent, and temperate virus infections." In *The Nervous System, Vol. 2,* D. B. Tower, ed. New York: Raven Press, pp. 113–135.

Graham, S., Levin, M. L., Lilienfeld, A. M., Schuman, L. M., Gibson, R., Dowd, J. E., and Hempelman, L. 1966. "Preconception, intrauterine, and postnatal irradiation as related to leukemia." In *Epidemiological Approaches to the Study of Cancer and Other Chronic Diseases*. W. Haenszel, ed. National Cancer Institute Monograph No. 19. Washington, D.C.: United States Government Printing Office.

Hall, A. J., Barker, D.J.P. 1984. "The age distribution of Legg-Perthes disease: an analysis using Sartwell's incubation period model." *Am. J. Epidemiol.* 120:531–536.

Hedrich, A. W. 1933. "Monthly estimates of the child population 'susceptible' to measles, 1900–1931, Baltimore, Md." *Amer. J. Hyg.* 17:613–636.

Hess, A. D., and Holden, P. 1958. "The natural history of the arthropod-borne encephalitides in the United States." *Ann. N.Y. Acad. Sci.* 70:294–311.

Hewitt, D. 1955. "Some features of leukemia mortality." *Brit. J. Prev. Soc. Med.* 9:81–88.

Kato, H. 1971. "Mortality in children exposed to A-bombs while *in utero,* 1945–1969." *Amer. J. Epidemiol.* 93:435–442.

Last, J. M. 1963. "The iceberg: completing the clinical picture in general practice." *Lancet* 2:28–31.

————. 1990. *Dictionary of Epidemiology,* 2nd ed. New York: Oxford University Press.

MacMahon, B. 1962. "Prenatal X-ray exposure and childhood cancer." *J. Nat. Cancer Inst.* 28:1173–1191.

Nowell, P. C. 1991. "How many cancer genes?" *J. Nat. Cancer Inst.* 83:1061–1064.

Pike, M. C. 1966. "A method of analysis of a certain class of experiments in carcinogenesis." *Biometrics* 22:142–161.

Polednak, A. P. 1974. "Latency periods in neoplastic diseases." *Amer. J. Epidemiol.* 100: 354–356.

Reimann, H. A. 1960. "Spectrums of infectious disease." *Arch. Int. Med.* 105:779–815.

Rose, G. 1982. "Incubation period of coronary heart disease." *Br. Med. J.* 284:1600–1601.

Sartwell, P. E. 1950. "The distribution of incubation periods of infectious disease." *Amer. J. Hyg.* 51:310–318.

————. 1966. "The incubation period and the dynamics of infectious disease." *Amer. J. Epid.* 83:204–216.

Schlenker, T. L., Bain, C., Baughman, A. L., Hadler, S. C. 1992. "The association of attack rates with immunization rates in preschool children." *JAMA* 267:823–826.

Stewart, A., Webb, J., and Hewitt, D. 1958. "A survey of childhood malignancies." *Brit. Med. J.* 1:1495–1508.

II

DEMOGRAPHIC STUDIES

Chapters 4, 5, 6, and 7 deal with the conduct and interpretation of **demographic studies.** Demographic studies, focused on the occurrence of disease in *populations,* search for associations between disease frequency and the presence or absence of possible etiologic agents in those populations. These studies address such issues as whether a disease is increasing or decreasing in the population and whether the disease occurs more often in populations that have greater exposure to a potential cause. Also, the means by which the epidemiologist can assess the health status of a population from the perspective of morbidity and mortality are encompassed in the demographic study. Since demographic studies often can be conducted by using readily available vital and health statistics, they are often inexpensive and may be used as the first test of an etiologic hypothesis. **Epidemiologic studies,** in contrast, concentrate on the occurrence of disease among *individuals* in relation to possible risk factors and therefore are generally more expensive than demographic studies.

Chapter 4 shows how mortality statistics are assembled and describes the advantages and problems of working with such data. The means by which epidemiologists contend with the difficulties are also discussed. Chapter 5 addresses the use of mortality data. Such issues as the validity of mortality data, the assessment of temporal information about mortality in the population, and the demographic characteristics (e.g., age, sex, and race) of those who die from the disease are discussed. Although mortality data are often of direct interest to the epidemiologist, they can also serve as proxies for morbidity information about a population.

Chapter 6 applies many of the ideas presented in Chapters 4 and 5 to morbidity statistics. The possible sources of morbidity data (e.g., surveillance) are reviewed, with an emphasis on the cross-sectional survey. Ongoing national surveys, which provide information on the health status of a population, are also described. The accuracy and validity of survey data are important considerations in their use. The concepts of sensitivity and specificity of diagnostic tests are considered, as are their positive and negative predictive value. These four measures of screening and diagnostic test performance are important to both the clinician and the epidemiologist. Another measure of test performance, kappa (K), provides information on inter- and intra-observer variability, two sources of error in the interpretation of clinical data.

The means of analyzing morbidity data are discussed in Chapter 7. Examples of how such data provide important clues to the etiology of various diseases are presented. Usually the epidemiologist focuses on time, place, and persons. Sometimes a disease may occur in a cluster, defined either by time or by place. Even when examining the occurrence of clusters, however, the epidemiologist must remember that demographic studies may only suggest a hypothesis regarding the cause of a disease or provide an initial test of a hypothesis. For a more definitive assessment of a hypothesis, an epidemiologic study (discussed in Part III), in which the association between disease occurrence and exposure to a possible agent is assessed in individuals, is necessary.

4

MORTALITY STATISTICS

> Anyone can stop a man's life, but no one his death; a
> thousand doors open on to it.
> SENECA, Phoenissae, 152

The study of mortality provides information that may prevent early and perhaps needless deaths. What are the leading causes of death? How do they differ around the world and what are the important determinants of early death? These are the kinds of questions epidemiologists ask in an effort to diagnose the health problems of the community and generate hypotheses about the causes of those diseases that are important contributors to premature mortality. As biologists we recognize the inevitability of death, but as medical scientists we strive to delay it and to improve the quality of the longer life we seek. The study of mortality patterns is a fruitful way to pursue these goals.

SOURCES OF MORTALITY DATA

Death certificates were introduced not for epidemiologic studies, but rather as legal documents. Graunt's use of the Bills of Mortality and Farr's adaptation of the Registration System to portray the health and social conditions of the population (Chapter 2) initiated the broad epidemiologic use of data that were regularly collected. Although this chapter deals with mortality statistics, it should be noted that these are only part of a system of vital records existing today in most developed countries. In addition to deaths, such vital events as births, marriages, and divorces are also recorded. Such reporting systems, however, are most highly developed for births and deaths.

National death registration has been legally mandated in England and Wales since 1837. Mortality data are now compiled by the Office of Population Censuses and Surveys (OPCS), which regularly reports the annual tabulations of deaths, their causes, and the demographic characteristics (e.g., age, gender, residence) of those who died.

In 1902 the collection of copies of death certificates by a permanent U.S. Bureau of Census began as an annual procedure in ten states and in several additional cities that had an adequate registration system, thereby creating a Death Registration Area (Cassedy, 1965). This Area was predominantly urban and included about 40 percent of the U.S. population (Dorn, 1966). By 1933, the Death Registration Area covered the entire United States, and when Alaska and Hawaii became states they also entered this data system. These changes in the denominator may have affected mortality statistics in the United States over this century.

CLASSIFICATION OF CAUSE OF DEATH

A standard death certificate developed by the National Center for Health Statistics has been adopted, with only minor modifications, by most states (Figure 4–1); there is a separate certificate for fetal deaths. Information is requested on demographic factors such as place of residence, occupation, national origin, age, and sex, as well as cause of death. The cause of death as stated on the certificate must be accepted with caution. Figure 4–1 shows that the immediate cause is entered first, then any intermediate conditions, and finally the underlying cause. A separate space allows for the inclusion of other significant conditions. (In other countries, a similar death certificate, modeled on one developed by the World Health Organization, is used.) In official tabulations, the cause of death is, in fact, the underlying cause, classified according to the International Statistical Classification of Diseases, Injuries and Causes of Death (ICD), which is revised about every eight or ten years by the World Health Organization. Changes in ICD classification or patterns of diagnosis can cause artifactual changes in mortality trends.

A problem develops when the physician enters two or more causes on the death certificate. Before 1949, a *Manual of Joint Causes of Death,* specifying rules for assigning priorities to various causes, was used to assure standardization for selecting the cause of death based on both the sequence of pathophysiologic events accepted at the time and the information required for public health programs. This manual was updated periodically but ended when the sixth ICD revision was adopted in 1949 and the physician became responsible for determining the underlying cause of death. These changing methods of tabulating causes of death have affected the mortality trends of certain diseases, such as diabetes; but, for most diseases, the effects have been small (Dunn and Shackley,

1945; Faust and Dolman, 1963; Faust, 1964, 1965). Still, these facts must be kept in mind when interpreting mortality statistics.

The use of a single cause of death for routine statistical tabulations has been criticized as not providing a complete representation of events (Krueger, 1966). It has been suggested that epidemiologists should really be interested in ''those diseases that one dies with as well as from,'' i.e., a listing of multiple causes of death. Since 1978, multiple cause-of-death data have been available for all recorded deaths in the United States after 1968. Table 4–1 shows the number of deaths in the United States in 1979 in which selected causes of death were stated. For some diseases, such as hypertension, angina pectoris, and nutritional deficiencies, the condition is more often reported as a nonunderlying cause than as an underlying one. Other diseases, however, are mentioned on the death certificate more frequently as an underlying cause. In other countries, multiple cause-of-death data have recently been made available, i.e., for the years 1985 and 1986 in England and Wales.

Because the physician completing the death certificate may not have been the attending physician and therefore would be unfamiliar with the deceased's medical history, the reliability of statements of causes of death can be less than optimal. Even if an autopsy is performed, the results may not be available in time to be entered on the death certificate (which is required for burial).

Many studies have been conducted to evaluate the accuracy of the cause-of-death statements on the certificate (James et al., 1955; Moriyama et al., 1958; Moriyama et al., 1966; Pohlen and Emerson, 1942; Pohlen, 1943). With AIDS, for example, underreporting of the underlying cause of death on the death certificate has been noted (Hardy et al., 1987). On the other hand, overreporting occurs for stroke. In about 40 percent of deaths attributed to stroke in one study in Framingham, Massachusetts, no evidence of a stroke could be found (Corwin et al., 1982). Other studies have shown that differences among physicians in evaluating the same case histories lead to variation in the underlying cause of death stated on the death certificate (Moriyama, 1989; Moussa et al., 1990; Benavides et al., 1989).

Mortality data may be collected from sources other than death certificates such as autopsy, hospital, occupational, and financial records (e.g., insurance, pension funds). Death certificates can be linked to other data bases to form records that contain information about occupational history, outpatient pharmaceutical use, parental background, or hospital treatment before death. The National Death Index (NDI) is a computer file of all deaths in the United States and it can be linked to other databases through combinations of the Social Security number, name, and date of birth. This system began in 1979, but mortality databases have existed in other countries for decades; the Canadian mortality database was founded in 1950 (Last, 1987). All infant death certificate records (deaths occurring

STATE OF MARYLAND / DEPARTMENT OF HEALTH AND MENTAL HYGIENE
CERTIFICATE OF DEATH

FOR
STATE
REGISTRAR

1 -

REG. NO.

1. DECEDENT'S NAME (First, Middle, Last)

2. DATE OF DEATH			3. TIME OF DEATH
MONTH	DAY	YEAR	M

4. SOCIAL SECURITY NUMBER

5. SEX
1 ☐ M 2 ☐ F

6. AGE (In yrs. last birthday)
YRS.

IF UNDER 1 YEAR
MONTHS   DAYS

IF UNDER 24 HRS.
HOURS   MIN.

7. DATE OF BIRTH (Month, Day, Year)

8. BIRTHPLACE (State or Foreign Country)

9a. FACILITY NAME (If not institution, give street and number)

9b. CITY, TOWN OR LOCATION OF DEATH

9c. COUNTY OF DEATH

RESIDENCE OF DECEDENT

10a. STATE

10b. COUNTY

10c. CITY, TOWN OR LOCATION

10d. INSIDE CITY LIMITS?
1 ☐ YES 2 ☐ NO

10e. STREET AND NUMBER

10f. ZIP CODE

10g. CITIZEN OF WHAT COUNTRY?

11. MARITAL STATUS
1 ☐ Never Married   2 ☐ Married
3 ☐ Widowed   4 ☐ Divorced

12. WAS DECEDENT EVER IN U.S. ARMED FORCES?   1 ☐ YES   2 ☐ NO
IF YES, GIVE WAR OR DATES

13. WAS DECEDENT OF HISPANIC ORIGIN? (Specify Yes or No— If yes, specify Cuban, Mexican, Puerto Rican, etc.)
1 ☐ YES 2 ☐ NO   Specify:

14. RACE — American Indian, Black, White, etc.
Specify:

15. DECEDENT'S EDUCATION
(Specify only highest grade completed)
Elementary/Secondary (0-12)   College (1-4 or 5 +)

16a. DECEDENT'S USUAL OCCUPATION
(Give kind of work done during most of working life. Do NOT use retired.)

16b. KIND OF BUSINESS/INDUSTRY

17. FATHER'S NAME (First, Middle, Last)

18. MOTHER'S NAME (First, Middle, Maiden Surname)

19a. INFORMANT'S NAME (Type/Print)

19b. MAILING ADDRESS (Street and Number or Rural Route Number, City or Town, State, Zip Code)

20a. METHOD OF DISPOSITION
1 ☐ Burial   2 ☐ Cremation   3 ☐ Removal from State
4 ☐ Donation   5 ☐ Other (Specify)

20b. PLACE OF DISPOSITION (Name of cemetery, crematory or other place)

20c. LOCATION — City or Town, State

21. SIGNATURE OF FUNERAL SERVICE LICENSEE

22. NAME AND ADDRESS OF FACILITY

▲

TO BE COMPLETED BY FUNERAL DIRECTOR

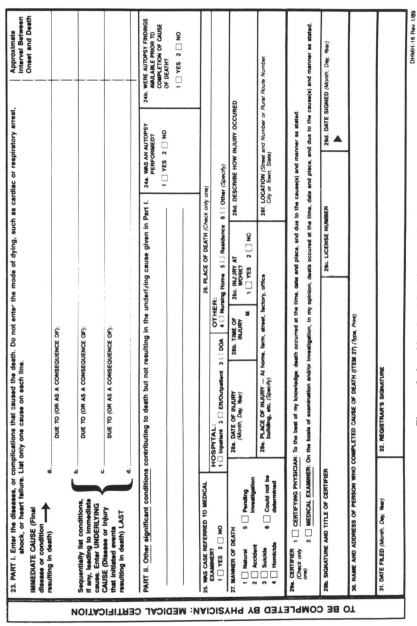

Figure 4–1. Maryland Certificate of Death.

63

Table 4-1. Number of Deaths with Any Mention of Specified Causes, with Specified Causes as Underlying Cause of Death, and Ratio of Reported to Underlying Cause in the United States, 1979 (examples from the National Center for Health Statistics "List of 72 Selected Causes of Death")

CAUSE OF DEATH (ICD-9 CODES)*	DEATHS WITH ANY MENTION OF SPECIFIED CAUSE	SELECTED AS UNDERLYING CAUSE	RATIO OF ANY MENTION TO UNDERLYING CAUSE
Septicemia (038)	52,154	8,024	6.50
Syphilis (090–097)	565	180	3.14
Malignant neoplasms of all other and unspecified sites (170–173, 190–199)	199,546	48,591	4.11
Diabetes mellitus (250)	128,373	33,192	3.87
Nutritional deficiencies (260–269)	22,111	2,210	10.00
Anemias (280–285)	27,465	3,171	8.66
Hypertension with and without heart disease ((401,403)	77,819	7,275	10.70
Angina pectoris (413)	4,113	500	8.23
All other forms of heart disease (415–423, 425–429)	675,733	142,942	4.73
Cerebral embolism (434.1)	3,314	850	3.90
Atherosclerosis (440)	160,086	28,801	5.56
Acute bronchitis and bronchiolitis (466)	1,846	554	3.33
Pneumonia (486)	147,089	44,426	3.31
Hernia of abdominal cavity and intestinal obstruction without mention of hernia (550–553, 560)	19,397	5,349	3.63
Hyperplasia of prostate (600)	4,096	810	5.06

*International Classification of Diseases, Ninth Revision.

Source: Israel et al., 1986.

in the first year of life) are linked to birth records in the United States and in many other countries to produce a set of data on maternal characteristics (i.e., age and pregnancy history), infant characteristics at birth (birth weight and other data), and cause of death.

Autopsy data, hospital records, and other sources of mortality data may provide accurate information about details omitted from death certificates, but they may not represent the general population. For example, autopsy series are selected from a hospital population but are not representative of that population or of the general population (Mainland, 1953; McMahan, 1962; Waife et al., 1952).

In view of such bias in selection, it may be impossible to correlate an autopsy series with any well-defined population at risk and therefore impossible to use such data to estimate the frequency of a disease. Despite the limitations of autopsy series for determining the frequency of a disease in a population, inferences made from an analysis of autopsy series may provide useful leads for more refined epidemiologic studies. For example, the observation that the relative proportion of lung cancer in different series of autopsies was increasing with time, and that the ratio of squamous cell carcinoma to adenocarcinoma was also increasing (while the proportion of adenocarcinoma remained fairly constant), led to the hypothesis that the total increase of lung cancer might be limited to squamous cell carcinoma (Cornfield et al., 1959; Kreyberg, 1954, 1962). Subsequent mortality and morbidity studies confirmed this.

MEASURES OF MORTALITY

Mortality Rates

The most frequently used measure of mortality is the mortality rate or death rate, which has three essential elements:

1. A specifically defined population group—the denominator.
2. A time period.
3. The number of deaths occurring in that population group during that time period—the numerator.

The numerator of the rate is the number of deaths that occurred in the specified population and the denominator is obtained either from a census or from estimates of that population:

$$\begin{matrix} \text{Annual death rate} \\ \text{from all causes} \\ \text{(per 1,000} \\ \text{population)} \end{matrix} = \frac{\begin{matrix} \text{Total number of deaths during} \\ \text{a specified twelve-month period} \end{matrix}}{\begin{matrix} \text{Number of persons in the} \\ \text{population at the middle of the} \\ \text{period} \end{matrix}} \times 1,000$$

The numerator and denominator are related to each other in that the numerator represents those individuals who died, and the denominator those who were at risk of death. For example, in 1988, in the United States there were 2,167,999 deaths in a population of 245,807,000. Thus:

$$\begin{matrix} \text{Annual death rate} \\ \text{in 1988 (per} \\ \text{1,000 population)} \end{matrix} = \frac{\text{2,167,999 deaths during 1988}}{\begin{matrix} \text{245,807,000 persons estimated} \\ \text{alive on July 1, 1988} \end{matrix}} \times 1,000 = \begin{matrix} \text{8.8 deaths per} \\ \text{1,000 population} \end{matrix}$$

The "crude" or unadjusted death rate is expressed in terms of a single year and a population of 1,000. The unit of time or the population can be selected by the investigator, but they should be specified. These rates can be made explicit for a variety of characteristics, such as age, gender, marital status, ethnicity, and specific causes. Two examples are shown below.

$$\begin{matrix} \text{Annual age-specific death} \\ \text{rate from all causes for} \\ \text{those less than 1 yr of age in} \\ \text{1988 (per 1,000 population)} \end{matrix} = \frac{\begin{matrix} \text{Number of deaths of individuals less than} \\ \text{1 yr of age in 1988} \end{matrix}}{\begin{matrix} \text{Number of individuals in the} \\ \text{population less than 1 on July 1, 1988} \end{matrix}}$$

$$= \frac{\text{38,910 deaths}}{\text{3,859,000 persons}} \times 1,000$$

$$= \begin{matrix} \text{10.1 deaths per 1,000 population less than 1} \\ \text{year of age} \end{matrix}$$

$$\begin{matrix} \text{Annual death rate from lung} \\ \text{cancer in 1989 (per 100,000} \\ \text{population)} \end{matrix} = \frac{\text{Number of deaths from lung cancer in 1989}}{\begin{matrix} \text{Number of persons in the population on} \\ \text{July 1, 1989} \end{matrix}}$$

$$= \frac{\text{133,284 deaths}}{\text{245,807,000 persons}} \times 100,000$$

$$= \text{54.2 deaths per 100,000 population}$$

Another type of rate, frequently and incorrectly termed a "mortality rate" in the clinical literature, is the "case-fatality rate":

$$\text{Case fatality rate (percent)} = \frac{\begin{array}{c}\text{Number of individuals dying during a} \\ \text{specified period of time after} \\ \text{disease onset or diagnosis}\end{array}}{\begin{array}{c}\text{Number of individuals with the} \\ \text{specified disease during that} \\ \text{period of time}\end{array}} \times 100$$

This rate represents the risk of dying during a defined period of time for those individuals who have a particular disease. Again, the period of time during which the deaths occurred should be specified. Case-fatality rates can also be made specific for age, gender, severity of disease, and any other factors of clinical and epidemiologic importance.

The proportionate mortality rate or ratio (PMR), which represents the proportion of total deaths that are due to a specific cause, is also frequently used:

$$\begin{array}{c}\text{Proportionate U.S. mortality} \\ \text{rate from cardiovascular} \\ \text{diseases in 1993}\end{array} = \frac{\begin{array}{c}\text{Number of U.S. deaths from} \\ \text{cardiovascular diseases in 1993}\end{array}}{\text{Total U.S. deaths in 1993}} \times 100$$

This rate is often multiplied by one hundred and expressed as a percentage, but it may also be expressed as a decimal fraction.

The proportionate mortality rate does not directly measure the risk or probability that a person in a population will die from a specific disease, as does a cause-specific mortality rate. To illustrate its limitation, let us assume that there are two countries, A and B, each with a population of one million. Furthermore, Country A had a death rate from all causes of death of 30 per 100,000 population in 1993, representing 300 deaths, and Country B had an all-cause death rate of 10 per 100,000 in 1993, representing 100 deaths. Each country had the same death rate from cardiovascular diseases of 5 per 100,000, representing 50 deaths, and a person's risk of dying from cardiovascular disease in each country was therefore the same. The proportionate mortality rates expressed as the percentage of all deaths from cardiovascular diseases in each country would then be as follows:

$$\text{Country A:} \quad \frac{50}{300} = 17 \text{ percent}$$

$$\text{Country B:} \quad \frac{50}{100} = 50 \text{ percent}$$

Clearly, this difference in proportionate mortality rates does not reflect the risk of dying from cardiovascular diseases in these countries—which is the same— but the difference in mortality from *other* causes of death. However, the proportionate mortality rate shows *within* any population group the relative importance of specific causes of death in the total mortality picture. This rate is useful to the epidemiologist in selecting areas for further study and to the health administrator in determining priorities for planning purposes.

Age Adjustment of Mortality Rates

Age is one of the main determinants of mortality (Figure 4–2). The age composition of a population will influence the total mortality rate; thus it is preferable to compare age-specific mortality rates in different geographical areas, population groups, or time periods. However, it is often useful to have a summary statistic of such comparisons that takes into account the differences in the age distribution of the population. This is accomplished by "age adjustment" or "age standardization." Of the several summary statistics that are available, two will be described here: the *direct* method of age adjustment, and the *indirect* method, the Standardized Mortality Ratio (SMR). Although age adjustment and standardization were originally developed to analyze and present mortality statistics and still are frequently used for this purpose, they can be applied to other types of rates such as morbidity or fertility rates. The same methods of adjustment can be used for taking into account other factors such as age, gender, social class, number of cigarettes smoked, or size of family.

An Example of Age Adjustment: Mortality Rates in Alaska and Florida

The overall or "crude" (not adjusted for age) mortality rates for Florida and Alaska in 1988 were 1,062.4 and 393.9 per 100,000, respectively (Table 4–2), and one's first conclusion is that the forces of mortality are stronger in Florida than in Alaska. The two states have very different age distributions, however (Figure 4–3); Florida is a retirement state for many elderly people, and Alaska draws many young people.

In the direct method of standardization, one applies the age-specific death rates from two populations with different age structures (Florida and Alaska) to a third "standard" population (e.g., the 1988 U.S. population). One multiplies the age-specific death rates from Florida and Alaska by the numbers in that age group for the U.S. population to produce an expected number of deaths in the standard population. The expected numbers of deaths are totaled and divided by the total standard population, in this case the total U.S. population, to produce a

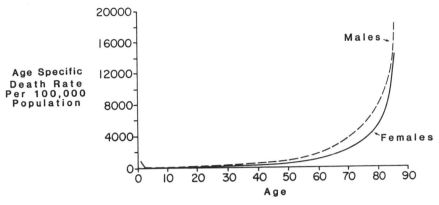

Figure 4–2. Age-specific death rates by sex, United States, 1987. *Source:* Vital Statistics of the United States (1990).

summary rate (the age-adjusted mortality rate) that would represent Florida and Alaska if each had the same age structure as the standard population. In this example, Florida would have an overall death rate of 812.0 per 100,000 population, not much different from Alaska's 764.4 or the U.S. overall rate of 882.0 (Table 4–3). Thus, the effect of the different age distributions is "adjusted" between the two states.

To use the indirect method of standardization, one applies the age-specific death rates from a standard population (here we used the death rates for the 1988 U.S. population) to the age-specific populations for Florida and Alaska. Multiplying death rates by population totals, one calculates the number of deaths in Florida and Alaska that might be expected if their populations were subjected to the same mortality experience as that of the standard population. Then one totals the age-specific expected deaths and compares them to the observed deaths; the expected number divided by the observed number multiplied by 100 produces the standardized mortality ratio (SMR). If the observed mortality is the same as expected, the SMR will be 100. An SMR greater than 100 indicates that mortality is higher than expected, and an SMR less than 100 indicates the opposite. In this

Table 4–2. Crude Mortality Rates in Florida and Alaska in 1988

	FLORIDA	ALASKA
Number of deaths	131,044	2,064
Total population	12,335,000	524,000
Crude (or overall) mortality rates	1,062.4 deaths per 100,000	393.9 deaths per 100,000

Source: Vital Statistics of the United States (1991).

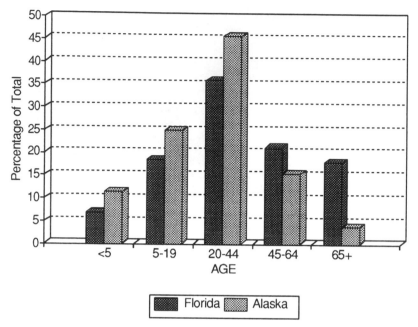

Figure 4–3. Percentage distribution of age groups in the Florida and Alaska populations, 1988. *Source:* Vital Statistics of the United States (1991)

Table 4–3. Age-Adjusted Mortality Rates for Florida and Alaska, 1988, Calculated by Direct Method

AGE GROUPS	AGE-SPECIFIC DEATH RATES/100,000		U.S. POP. (MILLIONS)	EXPECTED NUMBER OF DEATHS	
	FLORIDA	ALASKA		FLORIDA	ALASKA
<5	284	274	18.3	52,000	50,000
5–19	57	65	52.9	30,000	34,000
20–44	198	188	98.1	194,000	184,000
45–64	815	629	46.0	375,000	289,000
>65	4425	4350	30.4	1,345,000	1,322,000
			Total 245.7	1,996,000	1,879,000

$$\text{Expected death rate} = \frac{\text{Total expected deaths}}{\text{Total in standard population}} \times 100,000$$

$$\text{Expected death rate, Florida} = \frac{1,996,000}{245,800,000} \times 100,000 = 812.0$$

$$\text{Expected death rate, Alaska} = \frac{1,879,000}{245,800,000} \times 100,000 = 764.4$$

Source: Vital Statistics of the United States (1991).

example, Florida has an SMR of 110 and Alaska has an SMR of 111 (Table 4–4). They are virtually identical, and the mortality rate is not much higher than the overall U.S. mortality rate.

The crude rates, the direct adjusted rates, and the SMRs (indirect) for Florida and Alaska are shown in Table 4–5. Each method has advantages and disadvantages; the choice depends on the research question. An obvious disadvantage of the SMR is that it produces a ratio instead of a rate. It gives relative information but does not *describe* the mortality in the population. Both methods of adjustment depend on the choice of the standard population, and this is sometimes problematic. Texts are available that describe in more detail the technical methods used in age adjustment (Mausner and Bahn, 1974; Fleiss, 1981; Selvin, 1991). In our example, both methods show that the crude differences in mortality between Florida and Alaska are explained by differences in the age structure of the two populations. The direct age-adjusted mortality rates for both states are similar, and the SMRs are similar, demonstrating that mortality rates in Florida and Alaska are similar after adjusting for the differences in the age structures of the two states.

Both methods of adjustment can be used for other types of rates or variables. Studies of infant mortality often adjust for birth weight because birth weight distributions vary and birth weight is a strong predictor of infant deaths. Studies of pregnancy outcomes often adjust for the age of the mother because maternal age is a predictor of many birth outcomes.

Table 4–4. Calculations of Standardized Mortality Ratios (SMRs) for Florida and Alaska, 1988

AGE GROUPS	U.S. DEATH RATES*	POPULATION (MILLIONS)		EXPECTED DEATHS	
		FLORIDA	ALASKA	FLORIDA	ALASKA
<5	251.1	.85	.06	2,134	151
5–19	47.2	2.28	.13	1,076	61
20–44	161.8	4.41	.24	7,135	388
45–64	841.9	2.60	.08	21,889	674
>65	5,104.8	2.20	.02	112,305	1,021
		Total expected		144,539	2,295
		Total observed (from Table 4–2)		131,044	2,064
		SMR (ratio of expected to observed multiplied by 100)		110	111

*Per 100,000 population.

Source: Vital Statistics of the United States (1991).

Table 4–5.   Crude Death Rates and Age-Adjusted Rates for
Florida and Alaska, 1988

	FLORIDA	ALASKA
Crude death rates per 100,000	1062.4	393.9
Age-adjusted death rate per 100,000	812.0	764.4
Standardized mortality ratio	110	111

Source: Vital Statistics of the United States (1991).

Survival Analysis

Survival analysis (or life table analysis), as its name suggests, originated with studies of survivorship in actuarial populations for use by insurance companies to predict survivorship and set premium charges. It is used to make demographic predictions and to analyze data in clinical trials. Data describing the time from entry into the study until death or withdrawal from the study are collected for each patient or subject. The method allows one to compare groups and calculate a relative risk even when people are observed for different lengths of time. Survival analysis is commonly used in clinical trials to compare treatments, but it can be used in any study that measures time to a particular event. There are many texts describing the technique (Elandt-Johnson & Johnson, 1980; Lee, 1980) and computer programs to carry out the analysis. As with the other measures discussed above, it can be applied to data with endpoints other than death.

SUMMARY

Death certificate data are readily available, comprehensive, relatively uniform, and generally reliable. They constitute a major source of information for epidemiologists. Even so, trends in mortality data may be artifactual, reflecting changes in coding practices (e.g., ICD revisions, training of physicians), diagnostic capabilities (e.g., new tests, procedures for assigning diagnoses), and the denominator population (changing geographic coverage or census inaccuracies).

Mortality data are most often expressed as a rate, the number of deaths occurring in a given population over a specified period of time, and these rates can be specific for cause of death, for demographic characteristics such as age, gender, social class, residence, race, and ethnicity, or for any other variable of interest. Statistical techniques such as standardization (adjustment) can be used to adjust for differences in age or other variable distributions among populations. Epidemiologists can use mortality rates to develop and support hypotheses in mortality studies, the subject of Chapter 5.

STUDY PROBLEMS

Problems 1–5 refer to this table.

AGE GROUP	U.S. 1987 POPU-LATION	U.S. 1987 DEATHS FROM MALIG-NANT NEO-PLASMS	U.S. 1987 DEATHS FROM ACCI-DENTS	ALASKA 1987 POPU-LATION	ALASKA 1987 DEATHS FROM MALIG-NANT NEO-PLASMS	ALASKA 1987 DEATHS FROM ACCI-DENTS	FLORIDA 1987 POPU-LATION	FLORIDA 1987 DEATHS FROM MALIG-NANT NEO-PLASMS	FLORIDA 1987 DEATHS FROM ACCI-DENTS
<5	18,250,000	469	3,871	60,000	0	13	812,000	24	260
5–44	150,020,000	17,082	50,377	368,000	52	242	6,543,000	1,077	2,584
45–64	42,300,000	103,488	14,807	78,000	180	50	2,528,000	7,464	794
65+	29,840,000	242,617	25,838	19,000	210	15	2,140,000	21,599	1,482
Total	243,400,000	363,656	94,893	525,000	442	320	12,023,000	30,164	5,120

1. Calculate the death rate from all accidents in the age group 5–44 for the United States, Alaska, and Florida.
2. Calculate the death rate from all malignant neoplasms in the age group 65 and older for the United States, Alaska, and Florida.
3. Calculate the unadjusted death rates for the United States, Alaska, and Florida for (a) deaths from malignant neoplasms and (b) deaths from accidents.
4. Use the direct method of age adjustment to calculate mortality rates in Alaska and Florida for malignant neoplasms. The table below provides age-specific death rates from malignant neoplasms.

AGE GROUPS	AGE-SPECIFIC DEATH RATE FROM MALIGNANT NEOPLASMS PER 100,000 ALASKA	AGE-SPECIFIC DEATH RATE FROM MALIGNANT NEOPLASMS PER 100,000 FLORIDA	U.S. POPULATION	EXPECTED NUMBER OF DEATHS ALASKA	EXPECTED NUMBER OF DEATHS FLORIDA
<5	0	3.0	18,250,000		
5–44	16.5	14.1	150,020,000		
45–64	295.3	230.8	42,300,000		
65+	1009.3	1105.3	29,840,000		
Total			243,400,000		

5. Use the indirect method of age adjustment to calculate SMRs for Alaska and Florida deaths from accidents. The table below provides U.S. death rates.

	U.S. DEATH RATE PER 100,000	POPULATION		EXPECTED DEATHS	
		ALASKA	FLORIDA	ALASKA	FLORIDA
<5	21.2	60,000	812,000		
5–44	33.6	368,000	6,543,000		
45–64	35.0	78,000	2,528,000		
65+	86.6	19,000	2,140,000		
Total	39.0	525,000	12,023,000		

6. The crude (unadjusted) rates of death (per 100,000) from malignancies in Alaska and Florida are presented below. Compare them to the age-adjusted rates calculated in problem 4.

Alaska 84.2

Florida 250.8

7. The crude (unadjusted) rates of death (per 100,000) from accidents in Alaska and Florida are presented below. Compare them to the SMRs calculated in problem 5.

Alaska 61.0

Florida 42.6

8. Why is age adjustment especially useful in comparing patterns of mortality from malignancies and accidents in Alaska and Florida?

REFERENCES

Benavides, F. G., Bolumar, F., Peris, R. 1989. "Quality of death certificates in Valencia, Spain." *Am. J. Pub. Health* 79:1352–1354.

Cassedy, J. H. 1965. "Registration area and American vital statistics: Development of a health research resource, 1885–1915." *Bull. Hist. Med.* 39:221–231.

Cornfield, J., Haenszel, W., Hammond, E. C., Lilienfeld, A. M., Shimkin, M. B., and Wynder, E. L. 1959. "Smoking and lung cancer: Recent evidence and a discussion of some questions." *J. Natl. Cancer. Inst.* 22:173–203.

Corwin, L. I., Wolf, P. A., Kannel, W. B., McNamara, P. M. 1982. "Accuracy of death certification of stroke: the Framingham Study." *Stroke* 13:818–821.

Dorn, H. F. 1966. "Mortality." In *Chronic Diseases and Public Health*. A. M. Lilienfeld and A. J. Gifford, eds. Baltimore: The Johns Hopkins Press, pp. 23–54.

Dunn, H. L., and Shackley, W. 1945. "Comparison of cause of death assignments by the 1929 and 1938 revisions of the International List: Deaths in the United States, 1940." Vital Statistics—Special Reports 19:153–277, 1944. Washington, D.C.: United States Department of Commerce, Bureau of the Census.

Elandt-Johnson, R. C., and Johnson, N.L. 1980. *Survival Models and Data Analysis*. New York: John Wiley and Sons.

Faust, M. M., and Dolman, A.B. 1963. "Comparability of mortality statistics for the fifth and sixth revisions: United States, 1950." Vital Statistics—Special Reports, Selected

Studies 51: No. 2:133–178. Washington, D.C.: U.S. Government Printing Office, United States Department of Health, Education and Welfare, Public Health Services.

Faust, M. M. 1964. "Comparability ratios based on mortality statistics for the fifth and sixth revisions: United States, 1950." Vital Statistics—Special Reports, Selected Studies 51: No. 3:181–245. Washington, D.C.: United States Department of Health, Education and Welfare, Public Health Service.

————. 1965. "Comparability of mortality statistics for the sixth and seventh revisions: United States, 1958." Vital Statistics—Special Reports, Selected Studies 51: No. 4: 248–297. Washington, D.C.: United States Department of Health, Education and Welfare, Public Health Service.

Fleiss, J. L., 1981. *Statistical Methods for Rates and Proportions.* John Wiley & Sons, New York.

Hardy, A. M., Starcher II, E. T., Morgan, W. M., Druker, J., Kristal, A., Day, J. M., Kelley, C., Ewing, E., Curran, J. W. 1987. "Review of death certificates to assess completeness of AIDS case reporting." *Pub. Health Rep.* 102:386–391.

Israel, R. A., Rosenberg, H. M., and Curton, L. R. 1986. "Analytical potential for multiple cause of death data." *Am. J. Epid.* 124:161–179.

James, G., Patton, R. E., and Heslin, A. S. 1955. "Accuracy of cause-of-death statements on death certificates." *Pub. Health Rep.* 70:39 51.

Kreyberg, L. 1954. "The significance of histological typing in the study of the epidemiology of primary epithelial lung tumours: A study of 466 cases." *Brit. J. Cancer* 8: 199–208.

————. 1962. *Histological Lung Cancer Types: A Morphological and Biological Correlation.* Oslo, Norway: Norwegian Universities Press.

Krueger, D. E. 1966. "New enumerators for old denominators—multiple causes of death." In *Epidemiological Approaches to the Study of Cancer and Other Chronic Diseases.* W. Haenszel, ed. Natl. Cancer Inst. Monogr. No. 19. Washington, D.C.: United States Government Printing Office, pp. 431–443.

Last, J. M. (1987). *Public Health and Human Ecology.* Connecticut: Appleton and Lange.

Lee, E. T. 1980. *Statistical Methods for Survival Data Analysis.* Belmont, California: Lifetime Learning Publications.

Mainland, D. 1953. "Risk of fallacious conclusions from autopsy data on incidence of diseases with applications to heart disease." *Amer. Heart J.* 45:644–651.

Mausner, J .S. and Bahn, A. K. 1974. *Epidemiology: An Introductory Text.* Philadelphia, Pa.: W. B. Saunders.

McMahan, C. A. 1962. "Age-sex distribution of selected groups of autopsied cases." *Arch. Path.* 73:40–47.

Moriyama, I. M. 1989. "Problems in measurement of accuracy of cause-of-death statistics." *Am. J. Pub. Health,* 79:1349–1350.

Moriyama, I. M., Baum, W. S., Haenszel, W. M., and Mattison, B. F. 1958. "Inquiry into diagnostic evidence supporting medical certification of death." *Amer. J. Pub. Health* 48:1376–1387.

Moriyama, I. M., Dawber, T. R., and Kannel, W. B. 1966. "Evaluation of diagnostic information supporting medical certification of deaths from cardiovascular diseases." In *Epidemiological Approaches to the Study of Cancer and Other Chronic Diseases.* W. Haenszel, ed. Natl. Cancer Inst. Monogr. No. 19, Washington, D.C., United States Government Printing Office, pp. 405–419.

Moussa, M. A. A., Shafie, M. Z., Khogali, M. M., El-Sayed, A. M., Sugathan, T. N.,

Cherian, G., Abdel-Khalik, A. Z. H., Garada, M. T., Verma, D. 1990. "Reliability of death certificate diagnoses." *J. Clin. Epid.* 43:1285–1295.

Pohlen, K., and Emerson, H. 1942. "Errors in clinical statements of causes of death." *Amer. J. Pub. Health,* 32:251–260.

Pohlen, K. 1943. "Errors in clinical statements of causes of death: second report." *Amer. J. Pub. Health.* 33:505–516.

Selvin, S. 1991. "Statistical analysis of epidemiologic data." New York: Oxford University Press.

Szreter, S. 1991. "Introduction: the GRO and the Historian." *Soc. His. Med.* 4:401–414.

Vital Statistics of the United States. 1987. Volume II—Mortality, Part A. U.S. Department of Health and Human Services, Public Health Service, Centers for Disease Control, National Center for Health Statistics, Hyattsville, Maryland, 1990.

Vital Statistics of the United States. 1988. Volume II—Mortality, Part A. U.S. Department of Health and Human Services, Public Health Service, Centers for Disease Control, National Center for Health Statistics, Hyattsville, Maryland, 1991.

Waife, S. O., Lucchesi, P. F., and Sigmond, B. 1952. "Significance of mortality statistics in medical research: analysis of 1,000 deaths at Philadelphia General Hospital." *Ann. Intern. Med.* 37:332–337.

5

MORTALITY STUDIES

DISTRIBUTION OF MORTALITY IN POPULATIONS

Mortality statistics are routinely collected in many countries. They provide a readily available indicator of the frequency of disease as it occurs in *time, place,* and *persons* and therefore are important to the epidemiologist's view of disease.

Time: Trends in Mortality Rates

Figure 5–1 shows the age-adjusted mortality rates for selected sites of cancer in the United States from 1930 to 1987. These trends reveal considerable differences: lung cancer shows a marked increase; stomach and uterine cancer, a marked decrease; and primary liver cancer, a moderate but continuous decline. Slight but consistent increases are noted for pancreatic cancer and leukemia. Colon, rectum, and prostate cancer rates increased slightly until about 1950, after which the rates have remained essentially stable. Breast cancer mortality rates appear unchanged.

Trends over time are sometimes called *secular trends.* Epidemiologists constantly search for explanations of such trends. Table 5–1 provides a broad framework for considering possible reasons underlying changes in mortality trends.

One explanation to be considered immediately is that the trends may not be real, but rather artifactual—the result of errors in the numerator or denominator of the mortality rates. Improvements in medical services over any given period of time are reflected in improved diagnoses of disease and, in turn, in the accuracy of statements of the cause of death on death certificates. For example, the decline in mortality from primary liver cancer may have reflected diagnostic improve-

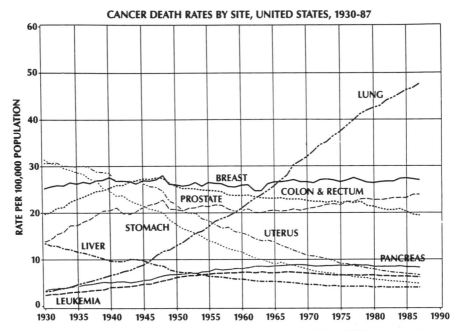

Figure 5–1. Cancer death rates by site, United States, 1930–1987. *Source:* American Cancer Society (1991).

Table 5–1. Outline of Possible Reasons for Changes in Mortality Trends of Disease

---

A. Artifactual
    1. Errors in the numerator due to
        (a) changes in the recognition of disease
        (b) changes in rules and procedures for classification of causes of death
        (c) changes in the classification code of causes of death
        (d) changes in accuracy of reporting age at death
    2. Errors in the denominator due to errors in the enumeration of the population

B. Real
    1. Changes in age distribution of the population
    2. Changes in survivorship
    3. Changes in incidence of disease resulting from
        (a) genetic factors
        (b) environmental factors

---

ments, since clinical experience indicates that many cancers spread to the liver from their primary sites. With improved diagnostic techniques, the original site will be diagnosed more frequently and the certifying physician will designate it as the underlying cause on the death certificate, even if metastases to other organs such as the liver have occurred. In order to determine the accuracy of site-specific cancer mortality statistics, Percy et al. (1974) investigated the extent to which the site of a malignancy was correctly listed on the death certificate. They ascertained cancer cases from the Third National Cancer Survey, a cancer incidence survey of ten population centers in the United States during 1969–1971. These workers found that in 65 percent of cancer deaths the site was accurately described on the death certificate. Death certificate information about the site of a malignancy tended to be less specific than hospital diagnosis information. If there is a marked change in a mortality trend, knowledge of specific diagnostic improvements in the disease category usually permits a judgment as to whether they are responsible for the change.

The International Classification of Diseases (ICD) is revised periodically to improve its efficiency in classifying causes of death. The revisions entail changes in code numbers and the addition of different disease entities to categories within a specific code. Special studies have been conducted to determine the effect of these changes, if any, on comparability of death rates in different years. When the United States National Center for Health Statistics began to use the Ninth Revision of the International Classification of Diseases in 1979, it investigated the effect of the change on the number of deaths coded to each cause. The procedure was to code the underlying cause of death for a sample of death certificates from 1976 (which had already been coded according to the Eighth Revision) using the Ninth Revision. The total number of deaths for each cause using the Ninth Revision would then be estimated from the sample. This number would then be divided by the number of deaths for that cause using the Eighth Revision to estimate the "comparability ratio." A comparability ratio of less than one indicates that the introduction of the Ninth Revision reduced the number of deaths coded to that cause; a ratio of more than one indicates the opposite. Some of the comparability ratios for the deaths coded to cardiovascular disease are shown in Table 5–2. For some causes (rheumatic heart disease, old myocardial infarction and other forms of chronic ischemic heart disease, and other diseases of arteries, arterioles, and capillaries), the comparability ratios are less than one, while those for other diseases (hypertensive heart disease, hypertensive heart and renal disease, and all other forms of heart disease) are greater than one. Fortunately, for acute myocardial infarction, angina pectoris, and cerebrovascular diseases, which are also common causes of death, the ratio is close to one. Although these differences are not large, they indicate that ICD revisions must be taken into account when evaluating mortality trends.

Table 5–2. Estimated Number of Deaths and Comparability Ratios for Selected Cardiovascular Diseases Using the Eighth and Ninth Revisions of the International Classification of Diseases, in 1976 in the United States

	NUMBER OF DEATHS		
	EIGHTH REVISION	NINTH REVISION	COMPARABILITY RATIO
Rheumatic heart disease	8,715	13,110	0.6648
Hypertensive heart disease	22,026	6,670	3.3022
Hypertensive heart and renal disease	4,872	4,020	1.2119
Acute myocardial infarction	319,562	319,477	1.0003
Other acute and subacute forms of ischemic heart disease	4,924	4,028	1.2224
Angina pectoris	195	186	1.0484
Old myocardial infarction and other forms of chronic ischemic heart disease	242,839	322,382	0.7533
Other diseases of the endocardium	5,154	4,195	1.2286
All other forms of heart disease	124,701	49,810	2.5035
Hypertension with or without renal disease	7,787	6,130	1.2703
Cerebrovascular diseases	189,553	188,623	1.0049
Atherosclerosis	31,273	29,366	1.0649
Other diseases of arteries, arterioles, and capillaries	19,583	26,432	0.7409
Total cardiovascular disease	981,184	974,429	1.0069

Source: Adapted from NCHS (1980).

Another approach to assessing the accuracy of mortality trends is to estimate whether an increase in mortality from one cause of death can be explained by a decline in another. For example, Gilliam (1955) attempted to determine whether the increase in death rates from lung cancer could be explained by errors in certification of deaths from other pulmonary diseases, such as tuberculosis. This hypothesis arose from the observation that during the period in which lung cancer mortality was increasing, mortality from tuberculosis was decreasing. Perhaps some of the deaths that had been attributed to tuberculosis in the earlier half of the twentieth century were actually due to lung cancer. Gilliam computed the degree of error in the certification of deaths from lung cancer, tuberculosis, and all respiratory diseases that would be necessary to produce the amount of the observed increase in lung cancer mortality from 1914 to 1950. He concluded that only a small part of the increase in mortality attributed to cancer of the lung since 1941 in the United States among white males and females could be accounted for by erroneous death certification of other respiratory diseases, ''without unreasonable assumptions of age and sex differences in diagnostic error.'' Since 1950, lung cancer mortality has continued to increase at a rate that is substantially greater than the decline in tuberculosis mortality, which confirms that earlier misdiagnoses could not explain the trend of increasing lung cancer mortality.

Another possibility is that artifacts in mortality trends may result from errors in the denominator of the rate, the population census, taken every ten years in the United States (Spiegelman, 1968). The degree of error in the census may differ from one decade to another. More important, however, is the observation that the errors in the census vary by age, sex, and race, and undoubtedly, other characteristics. This is illustrated in Table 5–3, which shows that young black males are more likely to be undercounted than any other subgroup. Thus, mortality rates among nonwhite males in this age group, assuming nearly complete death registration in the group, can be overestimated. If the degree of undercount changes in the different census years with no change in the quality of death certification, artifactual trends in mortality will result.

Other methods are available to evaluate trends. For example, one can determine whether the increases or decreases in mortality agree with the analyses of trends based on autopsies (Cornfield et al., 1959), or whether there is consistency between the sexes. If a mortality trend is real, it may be a result of changes in the age distribution of the population. It is preferable to make this assessment by analyzing the trends of age-specific death rates and then summarizing them by age adjustment. A decline in mortality might indicate an increase in survivorship, reflecting improvements in the treatment of a disease, or it might reflect a change in the incidence of the disease.

Once these possibilities of artifactual error are eliminated, two broad explanatory hypotheses for the trends must be considered in the search for the etiology of disease, namely, genetic and environmental causes. Environmental causes may

Table 5–3. Estimated Undercounting of the U.S. Population by Age, Sex, and Race for the 1980 Census, as a Percentage

AGE	WHITE		BLACK	
	MALE	FEMALE	MALE	FEMALE
<5	100%	100%	90%	91%
5–14	100	100	96	96
15–24	99	100	95	99
25–34	97	100	87	97
35–44	97	100	82	95
45–54	97	100	83	96
55–64	98	101	91	99
65–74	100	101	102	105

Source: Adapted from U.S. Bureau of the Census (1988).

include changes in personal living habits (e.g., smoking, diet), occupation, air and water pollution, and use of drugs.

Ordinarily, genetic factors, per se, do not produce marked mortality changes over a short period of time unless a specific genetic factor present in the population interacts with a newly introduced agent in the environment. Thus, large increases or decreases in mortality trends usually indicate that a new environmental agent has been introduced into or removed from the population undergoing the changing mortality. The pattern of mortality from AIDS illustrates the introduction into a specific population of a new virus that causes a fatal disease (Figure 5–2).

The relationship of asthma mortality to the use of pressurized aerosols is another example. Between 1959 and 1966, mortality attributed to asthma steadily increased in England and Wales, after remaining stable for a century (Figure 5–3) (Speizer et al., 1968). A detailed analysis led to the conclusion that the increase was not artifactual and that the mortality trend most likely resulted from a new method of treating asthma. A study of about 180 deaths attributed to asthma in persons 5–34 years old during 1966–1967 indicated that in 84 percent of the cases, pressurized aerosol bronchodilators were known to have been used, and probably in excess, whereas only about 66 percent had received corticosteroids (Speizer and Strang, 1968). The period of introduction of these bronchodilators, particularly isoprenaline, coincided with the increase in asthma mortality. These analyses confirmed previous clinical reports of several patients who died suddenly

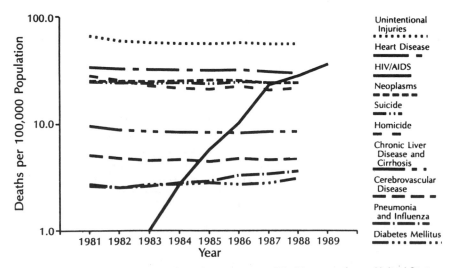

Figure 5–2. Leading causes of death among men 25–44 years of age, United States, 1981–1989. (The scale used for the *y*-axis, the death rate, is logarithmic. The slope of a line plotted on a logarithmic scale reflects percentage change. Hence, parallel lines in this graph reflect equivalent percentage changes.) *Source:* Centers for Disease Control (1991).

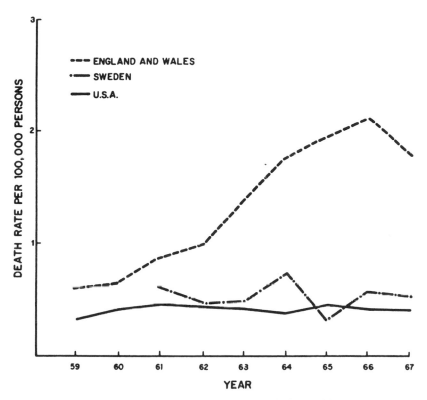

Figure 5-3. Annual mortality from asthma during 1959 to 1967 for persons 5–34 years old in England and Wales, the United States, and Sweden. *Source:* Stolley (1972).

following excessive use of aerosol inhalers (Greenberg, 1965; Greenberg and Pines, 1967; McManis, 1964). In June 1967, the Committee on Safety of Medicines issued a warning to all physicians in the United Kingdom, and in 1968 aerosols were made available by prescription only. Both deaths from asthma and aerosol sales declined and by 1969 asthma mortality had almost reached its earlier level (Inman and Adelstein, 1969). A further analysis of mortality rates from asthma in different countries, some showing a rise in asthma mortality and others not, strongly suggested a relationship between increased asthma mortality and high sales volume of a highly concentrated form of isoprenaline (isoproterenol) in pressurized aerosol nebulizers. The countries that did not show an increase in asthma mortality were those that had not licensed the concentrated nebulizers (Stolley, 1972). Subsequent pharmacologic studies provided information on the possible mechanism by which high concentrations of isoprenaline could result in asthma deaths (Conolly et al., 1971).

Mortality trends also provide a means of supporting hypotheses developed from other types of studies. A variety of epidemiologic studies, for example, showed a relationship between cigarette smoking and lung cancer (see Chapters

10 and 11). In light of the evidence of a marked increase in the consumption of cigarettes among males since 1920, one would expect to see a corresponding increase in lung cancer mortality, and this is shown in Figure 5–4.

Place

Mortality statistics from many countries are available for international comparisons in the compilations of national statistics that appear regularly in the World Health Organization Epidemiological and Vital Statistics Reports. With these data one may compare rates of diseases between countries. Figures 5–5 and 5–6 show the age-adjusted death rate for breast cancer in 15 different nations in 1987 and age-specific incidence of breast cancer in five different countries. In evaluating such reported international differences in mortality, one can follow the same sequence of reasoning that was used in evaluating mortality time trends (Table 5–1), substituting only the word "differences" for "changes." Again, one must determine whether the differences are artifactual, that is, due to distortions in the numerators and denominators of the mortality rates. International differences in the availability of medical services, diagnostic practices of physicians, and classification procedures may introduce distortions. Some countries do not conduct population censuses; also, it may be necessary to assess carefully the completeness of a census, particularly in a developing country.

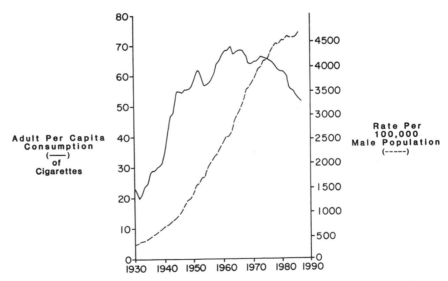

Figure 5–4. Adult per capita cigarette consumption and age-adjusted death rates from malignant neoplasms of the lung for males, United States, 1930–1980. *Source:* U.S. Department of Health and Human Services (1989).

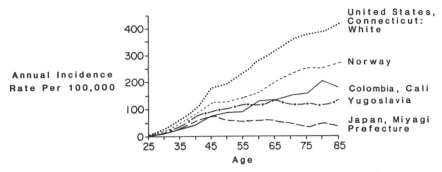

Figure 5-5. Age-adjusted death rates from malignant neoplasms of the breast among females in selected countries, latest available year, standardized to the 1989 world population. *Source:* World Health Organization (1989).

Comparability of coding practices is an example of the concerns an epidemiologist might have in comparing international death statistics. The degree of concern would depend on the disease being studied and the years and countries of interest. In work on ICD–9 and preparatory work on ICD–10 during the 1980s, the National Cancer Institute and the National Center for Health Statistics addressed the issue of cancer coding practices (Percy and Muir, 1989). They found a narrow range of variability in the coding of a sample of U.S. death certificates mentioning cancer when nine countries were given the opportunity to code them (see Table 5–4). The percentage of the sample coded for cancer as cause of death ranged from 87.2% in the United States to 95.8% in France.

If one can reasonably eliminate the possibility that mortality differences are artifactual and assume that they do reflect actual differences in disease frequency,

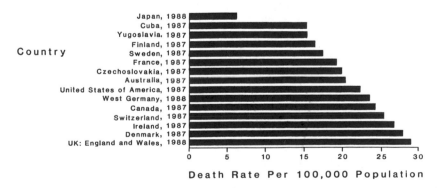

Figure 5-6. Average annual age-specific incidence rates of malignant neoplasms of the breast among females in selected countries, 1978–1982. *Source:* International Agency for Research on Cancer (1987).

Table 5–4.   Percentage of 1,243 Death Certificates Listing Cancer, Circulatory, or Other Diseases as Cause of Death That Mentioned Cancer

COUNTRY	CANCER %	CIRCULATORY DISEASES %	OTHER DISEASES %
United States	88.2	7.3	4.5
Canada	88.6	7.3	4.1
Federal Republic of Germany	91.6	5.7	2.8
New Zealand	90.5	6.6	2.9
England	91.6	5.5	2.9
France	95.8	3.0	1.2
Netherlands	90.9	6.1	3.0
USSR	90.1	7.5	2.1
Brazil	90.7	6.4	2.2

Source: Percy and Muir (1989).

it then becomes essential to resolve the issue of whether they are due to different environmental factors in the places studied or to different genetic compositions of the population. Migrant studies have been used for this purpose. These studies take advantage of the migration to one place by people from other places with different mortality experiences from many diseases. Comparisons are made between the mortality experience of the migrant groups and that of their place of origin and their current place of residence.

The rationale for these comparisons and the inferences derived from them can be stated in the following simplified form, where CO = country of origin, M = migrants, and CA = natives of the country of adoption.

1. If the change in environment is the explanation for an observed difference in death rates, one would expect that
   (a) CO rates would equal M rates and
   (b) M rates would approximate CA rates.
2. On the other hand, if genetic factors are of prime importance, one would expect that
   (a) CO rates would equal M rates and
   (b) CO and M rates will differ from CA rates.

Other factors that may influence these differences in mortality rates must also be taken into consideration:

1. *Premigration Environment.* If the premigration environment in the country of origin is of primary etiological importance, the mortality differences

would be erroneously interpreted as being genetically determined, according to the reasoning outlined above.

2. *Age at Time of Migration.* This may be significant since exposure to an etiological factor in the environment may occur, or be most likely, at a certain age or period of life. Such information would further determine whether genetic, premigration, or postmigration environmental factors are operating.

3. *Selective Factors.* Individuals who migrate may differ from those who remain in the country of origin in ways that influence the occurrence of disease. For example, the healthier and more physically fit would tend to migrate more often than those who are ill. Immigration laws of some countries may require potential migrants to pass a physical and mental examination.

Migration studies have been used within the United States to measure the effect of the environment on development of multiple sclerosis. This disease appears to vary with latitude; populations farther from the equator generally have higher incidences of multiple sclerosis than do populations closer to the equator (Kurland et al., 1965; Visscher et al. 1977). In a number of studies, researchers have shown that a migrating group can acquire the incidence rate in the geographic area to which they have migrated if they move at a young age, or can maintain the incidence rate of the place of origin if they move at an older age (about age 15 or over) (Alter et al., 1971; Dean, 1967). Detels et al. (1972) used death certificate data to compare age- and sex-adjusted death rates among four groups: migrants from high-risk areas of the United States (New England, Pacific, West–North Central, and East–North Central States) and migrants from low-risk areas of the United States (East–South Central and West–South Central) living in Washington (high risk) or California (low risk). These data, summarized in Table 5–5, show that migrants from high-risk areas have a higher death rate than

Table 5–5. Deaths from Multiple Sclerosis among Migrants to Washington and California

	CALIFORNIA		WASHINGTON	
	POPULATION AT RISK	AGE–SEX ADJUSTED RATE*	POPULATION AT RISK	AGE–SEX ADJUSTED RATE*
From northern areas:	3,597,993	0.81	784,897	1.35
From southern areas:	1,427,858	0.42	123,532	0.32

*Using the 1960 U.S. population, per 100,000.

Source: Detels et al., (1972).

migrants from low-risk areas when they move to either kind of area. Migrant studies help establish that there is an environmental contribution to a disease. Once an environmental effect is suggested, other studies are needed to measure and describe the effect.

There are geographical differences in mortality from many diseases, such as multiple sclerosis, coronary heart and cerebrovascular disease, anencephaly, and cancer of the esophagus (Gordon, 1966; Kmet and Mahboubi, 1972; Lilienfeld et al., 1972; Moriyama et al., 1971; Renwick, 1972; Tuyns, 1970). For some diseases, these regional differences within countries are as great as those between countries. Such a regional difference is illustrated by the reported mortality from cerebrovascular diseases in the United States (Figure 5–7).

This regional variation in cerebrovascular death rates may be artifactual. Inconsistency in coding cerebrovascular disease has been common historically (Table 5–6) but has been reduced by the development of more accurate diagnostic techniques. Between 1970 and 1980 computerized tomography improved the accuracy of the diagnosis of stroke. As part of the Minnesota Heart Survey, Iso et al. (1990) validated death certificate diagnosis of stroke in samples of deaths from 1970 and 1980. The proportion of death certificates that agreed with the independent review of medical records in assigning a diagnosis improved from 96 to 100 percent for the category of all types of stroke, from 59 to 82 percent for intracranial hemorrhage, and from 87 to 97 percent for nonhemorrhagic stroke (Table 5–7). Different areas of the country may have differed in the rate of access

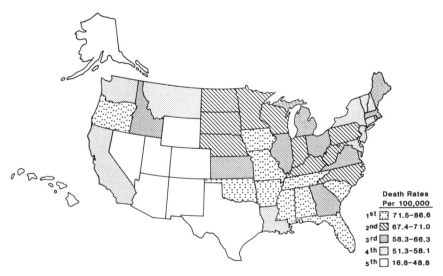

Figure 5–7. Annual state death rates from cerebrovascular disease by quintile rank, United States, 1987. *Source:* Vital Statistics of the United States (1990).

Table 5–6. Estimated Number of Cerebrovascular Disease Deaths Coded on Death
Certificates and Those Coded as Underlying Cause: United States, 1955

			CODED AS UNDERLYING CAUSE	
CAUSE OF DEATH	(ICD CODE)	TOTAL CODED CONDITIONS	NUMBER	PERCENT OF TOTAL
Cerebrovascular diseases (vascular lesions of the nervous system)	(330,334)	304,004	173,541	57.1
Subarachnoid hemorrhage	(330)	7,458	5,216	69.9
Cerebral hemorrhage	(331)	162,435	109,076	67.2
Cerebral embolism and thrombosis	(332)	67,308	41,326	61.4
Spasm of cerebral arteries	(333)	91	11	12.1
Other and ill-defined vascular lesions of the nervous system	(334)	66,712	17,912	26.8

Source: Vital Statistics of the United States (1965).

to diagnostic equipment and the rate with which physicians acquired new diagnostic skills. This would contribute to regional differences in the death rate from
cerebrovascular disease.

Persons

The third general category that may influence the distribution of mortality consists
of the characteristics of persons. In mortality data, the number of personal characteristics that can be analyzed is limited by the information available on death
certificates. They include age, gender, ethnicity, occupation, marital status, and
birth cohort (people born during specific years).

Age

Age is a major determinant of mortality. There is high mortality in the first
year of life, a decline in mortality in ages 1–5, lowest mortality in ages 5–24, and

Table 5–7. Percentage of Death Certificates Agreeing with
Independent Diagnoses, Minnesota Heart Survey, 1970 and 1980

YEAR	ALL TYPES OF STROKE	INTRACRANIAL HEMORRHAGE	NONHEMORRHAGIC STROKE
1970	96%	59%	87%
1980	100%	82%	97%

Source: Iso et al., (1990).

then a steady upward increase producing the well-known j-shaped curve (see Figure 4–2). Some diseases vary from the pattern of increasing mortality with age. AIDS, for example, affects young to middle-aged people more than elderly people because the behaviors leading to exposure occur more frequently in the young. Childbirth is another cause of death that is age-limited, occurring in women of child-bearing age but disappearing as women reach menopause.

Gender

Men have generally higher overall mortality than women at all ages and for many diseases. Figure 5–8 shows age-specific rates of mortality from ischemic heart disease on a semi-log scale for men and women aged 30–85 years. Even in the first year of life, male mortality is higher than female mortality, and this is found internationally, historically, for all ethnic groups, and throughout the first year of life (Table 5–8).

Of course, men and women experience different diseases and often die of different causes. Maternal mortality is a striking historical example of a gender-specific cause of death that has changed with time. United States maternal mortality declined from 1915–1919 rates of 727.9 per 100,000 live births to a 1949 rate of under 100, and to a 1988 rate of 8.4 per 100,000 live births (U.S. Vital Statistics, 1988). Antibiotics, sterile techniques and other technology have contributed to this decline, but so have changes in childbearing patterns. Changes in maternal mortality have affected overall female mortality rates and life expectancy.

In addition to biological factors, behavioral and occupational differences also affect mortality trends. The male mortality rate from accidents (motor vehicle

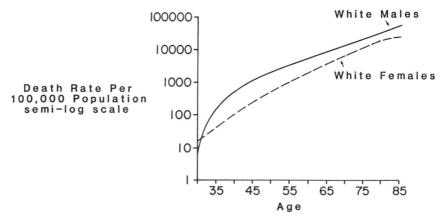

Figure 5–8. Annual age-specific death rates from ischemic heart disease by sex among whites, United States, 1987. *Source:* Vital Statistics of the United States (1990).

Table 5–8. Male and Female Infant Mortality by Ethnic Group and Age,
United States, 1988

ETHNIC OR RACIAL GROUP (PER 1000 LIVE BIRTHS)	MALE	FEMALE
White	9.5	7.4
Black	19.0	16.1
American Indian	9.5	8.6
Chinese	4.9	3.5
Japanese	4.2	3.5
Age at Death (per 100,000 live births)		
< 1 hour	112.1	95.6
1–23 hours	286.2	232.4
1–27 days	694.7	565.2
28–59 days	95.4	78.8

Source: Vital Statistics of the United States (1991).

and other) and homicides is twice as high as the rate for women (Table 5–9,
Figure 5–9). Tendencies to be present where violent behavior is occurring and
engaging in hazardous occupations may partially explain this difference. Behavioral variables such as seat belt use, driving speed, amount of time spent driving,
and likelihood of driving while intoxicated may be gender-related and may contribute to mortality differences related to motor vehicle accidents.

Race and ethnicity

In the United States race is recorded on the death certificate, but in other
nations indicators of ethnicity, national origin, or religion are sometimes recorded.
These indicators serve as markers of both "genetic background" and social class
characteristics, which are sometimes associated with particular diseases. Blacks
are more likely than whites to carry the gene for sickle-cell anemia; Jews have a
higher prevalence of the gene for Tay-Sachs disease than non-Jews.

In addition to genetic differences between ethnic or so-called racial groups,

Table 5–9. Death Rates per 100,000
Population for Accidents and Homicide by Sex,
1988, United States

CAUSE OF DEATH	MALE	FEMALE
Motor vehicle accidents	28.6	11.8
All other accidents	26.4	13.1
Homicide	14.0	4.2

Source: Vital Statistics of the United States (1991).

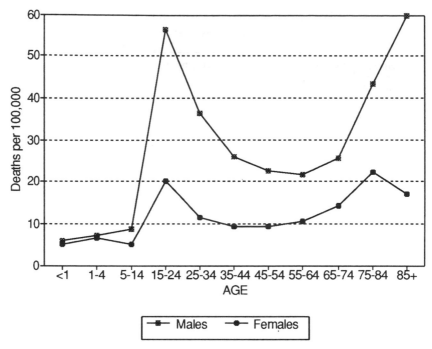

Figure 5–9. Male and female mortality from motor vehicle accidents by age groups, United States, 1988. *Source:* Vital Statistics of the United States (1991).

there are often differences in diet, life style, education, occupations, access to and use of health care, and many other characteristics. The interrelationship between these variables complicates the epidemiologist's effort to understand variations in mortality by race or ethnic group. Overall mortality in the United States is higher among blacks than among whites, as is infant mortality, maternal mortality, and mortality caused by malignant neoplasms, cardiovascular disease, diabetes, hypertension, and homicide (Table 5–10). These aggregate differences indicate the need for further investigation as it is quite unlikely that genetic explanations will account for much of the disparity.

Research on the relationship of race or ethnicity and social class to mortality has been insufficient. Social class may explain differences in mortality, but the definition of higher or lower social class may be different in specific racial or ethnic groups (Liberatos et al., 1988). There may also be an added stress related to membership in a minority that is subject to discrimination, and this stress may contribute to various illnesses, although solid evidence for this is lacking. Tyroler and James (1978) interpreted findings that darker skin color was associated with higher blood pressure among black males in Detroit (Harburg et al., 1978) to mean that "skin color in the U.S. black population may be an indicator of psy-

Table 5–10.   Some Mortality Differences between
Blacks and Whites in the United States per 100,000
Population, 1988

CAUSE OF DEATH (ICD-9 CODE)	BLACK	WHITE
All causes	788.8	509.8
Malignant neoplasms (140–208)	171.3	130.0
Cardiovascular disease (390–488)	293.0	199.2
Diabetes (250)	21.2	9.0
Hypertension (401, 403)	5.7	1.5
Homicide (E960–E978)	34.1	5.3
Maternal mortality*	19.5	5.9
Infant mortality**	17.6	8.5

*Per 100,000 live births.

**Per 1,000 live births.

Source: Vital Statistics of the United States (1991).

chological processes. . . related to blood pressure." The same data however, can be interpreted differently, without invoking the stress hypothesis.

Social class

Socioeconomic status or social class has become a more important variable to study as epidemiologists have turned their attention to diseases with multiple causes and to the contribution that "life style" makes to disease. Social class may be considered as an independent risk factor or as a variable associated with other risk factors for the disease in question. Table 5–11 presents some variables associated with socioeconomic status that may affect health outcomes.

Socioeconomic status is difficult to measure and is not generally recorded on death certificates (Liberatos et al., 1988). Max Weber (1946) developed a model of social class that had three components: class, status, and power. In the United States, sociologists have commonly used occupation, education, and income as indicators of social class. Britain has used and updated an index of social class that was first developed by the British Registrar General in 1911. Its five social classes are categorized on the basis of occupation. The British have changed this categorization of social class every 10 years so that historical data may not be comparable, and time trends within a social class category may be artifactual. International comparisons can also be difficult if different nations use different measures, or if an occupation varies in its relative social standing, remuneration, and associated risks. Occupations with higher income or prestige in one country may be lower in another country. An example is the physician, who is well paid in the United States and was poorly paid in what was once the U.S.S.R.

Table 5–11.   Some Health-Related Outcomes That Vary with Social Class

COMMON INDICATORS OF SOCIOECONOMIC STATUS	INTERMEDIATE VARIABLES	HEALTH OUTCOMES
Wealth	Access to health care	Detection and treatment of illnesses
	Access to dietary choices	Obesity, blood pressure, cholesterol levels
Education	Knowledge, attitude and and behavior about diet, smoking, alcohol, exercise, sexual practices, illegal drug use, family planning, prenatal care	Changes in risk factors for heart disease, lung cancer, AIDS, low birth weight
Occupation	Exposure to hazards, psychological stresses, physical activity	Cancer, heart disease, accidents, miscarriages, birth defects, other conditions

The United States does not collect social class information on its death certificates. Occupation is described with two entries (usual occupation, kind of business or industry), and more recently some states have begun requesting information on highest education level. Shai and Rosenwaike (1989) compared accuracy of education reporting in a group of Utah and New York middle-aged men who participated in studies and self-reported their educational level, then died and had their educational level described on their death certificates by a spouse. There was agreement in 68 percent of cases, varying with educational level. It is necessary to link death certificates to other databases in order to study social class and a particular mortality outcome because of the lack or inaccuracy of information on death certificates regarding social class, education, and occupation.

Social class may explain some of the "racial" differences observed in mortality. A study by Bassett and Krieger (1986) is one of the few that have controlled for social class in examining breast cancer survival among black and white women. When race is the "risk factor" and the analysis adjusts for social class, the risk of dying is similar for both races. When the "risk factor" is social class and the analysis is adjusted for race, breast cancer mortality is elevated by 52 percent in the lower social class.

Birth cohort

Analysis of data by birth cohort sometimes provides supporting evidence for other observations. An initial finding of seven cases of adenocarcinoma of the

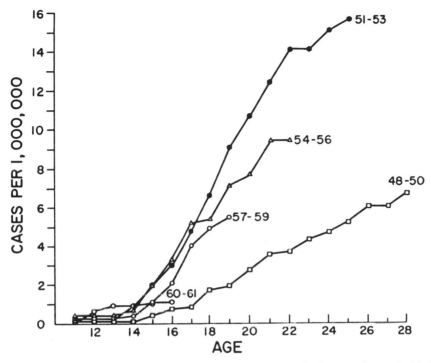

Figure 5–10. Cumulative risk for development of clear-cell adenocarcinoma by birth cohort (white females born in the United States). *Source:* Herbst et al. (1971).

vagina in women under 25 years of age was so unusual that it led to a case-control study that identified in-utero exposure to diethylstilbestrol (DES) as a highly probable cause (Herbst and Scully, 1970; Herbst et al., 1971). In a birth-cohort analysis the mortality rate for adenocarcinoma was compared with DES sales (Figure 5–10). The risk was lowest for females born in 1948–1950 and highest for those born in 1951–1953, declining with subsequent cohorts. This pattern follows the sales figures for DES, which were highest in the years 1950–1952 and declined in the following years. This helped confirm the causal role of in-utero DES exposure.

SUMMARY

After ruling out artifact as an explanation of mortality patterns, one can ascribe changes in mortality to genetic or environmental agents. Environmental agents include everything in a person's environment—culture, geography, accidents, smoking, chemical hazards, new drugs, viruses, diet, and all other exposures. Comparisons of mortality by time, place, and persons have been useful in suggesting hypotheses about the causes of disease and in providing evidence to support or reject them. In this chapter we have given examples of studies that have shown changes in death patterns over time. Such studies often highlight directions for public health concerns. An increase in mortality from a disease may indicate the need for a change in health policy or research. Geographic comparisons of death rates and correlations with other factors that vary with geography such as culture, diet, behavior, climate, or ethnicity often suggest hypotheses for future research. Death certificates generally contain information about the person who died, including age at death, gender, ethnicity, occupation, marital status, and birth cohort. Comparisons by such characteristics provide much information about subgroups at risk for different causes of death and help target public health efforts. Death rates vary widely with these personal characteristics, and almost all epidemiologic research can be informed by available mortality data.

STUDY PROBLEMS

1. Temporal patterns of mortality can be seen over years, by season, or by the day of the week. For example, deaths from homicide occur most frequently on Friday and Saturday nights, suggesting that alcohol consumption might contribute to the increase in homicides.

   The numbers of deaths in 1987 caused by motor vehicle accidents are listed below by the day of the week on which death occurred. Suggest three hypotheses to explain the increased number of deaths on Fridays, Saturdays, and Sundays.

   Sunday Monday Tuesday Wednesday Thursday Friday Saturday

   8,056   5,825   5,660   5,646   6,230   7,481   9,391

   Be sure to consider the full range of epidemiologic thinking including chance, artifact, confounding, and causality.

2. Geographic variation is another clue used by epidemiologists to understand the causes of a disease. The death rates from HIV infection are the result of transmission of a retrovirus through contact with the blood or body fluids of an infected person, most frequently because of intravenous drug use associated with needle sharing, unprotected sex, blood transfusions, or mother-to-infant transmission. The death rates from HIV infection in 1987 are given on the next page for the top five and lowest five states.

TOP 5 HIV DEATH RATES		LOWEST 5 HIV DEATH RATES	
STATE	RATE PER 100,000	STATE	RATE PER 100,000
Washington, D.C.	28.8	South Dakota	.3
New York	19.2	North Dakota	.4
New Jersey	13.8	Montana	.5
California	9.6	Wyoming	.6
Florida	9.2	Idaho/Iowa	.8

(a) Suggest three hypotheses to explain the geographic distribution of high or low HIV rates.

(b) What might explain Washington, D.C.'s rate of 28.8, which is 50% higher than that of New York State?

3. Most Western countries have shown sharp declines in infant mortality since 1900. In the United States, infant mortality has declined for both whites and blacks, but differences between the races have persisted over time. Variations over time and between racial groups can give information about several causes of infant mortality.

Infant mortality rates in the United States (deaths under 1 year of age per 1,000 live births) are listed below by year and race (problems 4–6 also refer to this table).

Infant Mortality (deaths under 1
year per 1,000 live births)

	WHITE	BLACK
1915–1919	92.8	150.4
1920–1924	73.3	117.3
1930–1934	55.2	90.5
1940	43.2	72.9
1950	26.8	43.9
1960	22.9	44.3
1970	17.8	32.6
1980	11.0	21.4
1987	8.6	17.9

(a) What are some arguments that the time trends are real, not artifactual?

(b) What effect would improved birth registration have on these data?

(c) What effect would improved death registration have on these data?

4. What might explain the decline in infant mortality between 1915 and 1960?

5. What might explain the decline in infant mortality between 1960 and 1987?

6. What are three hypotheses that might explain the differences in infant mortality between whites and blacks?

REFERENCES

Alter, M., Okihiro, M., Rowley, W., and Morris, T. 1971. "Multiple sclerosis among Orientals and Caucasians in Hawaii." *Neurology* 21:122–130.

American Cancer Society. 1991. *Cancer Facts and Figures.* Atlanta: American Cancer Society, Inc.

Bassett, M. T., and Krieger, N. 1986. "Social class and black-white differences in breast cancer survival." *Am. J. Pub. Health* 76:1400–1403.

Centers for Disease Control. 1991. *Morbidity and Mortality Weekly Report* 40(3):41–44, January 25.

Conolly, M. E., Davies, D. S., Dollery, C. T., and George, C. F. 1971. "Resistance to β adrenoceptor stimulants: a possible explanation for the rise in asthma deaths." *Brit. J. Pharmacol.* 43:389–402.

Cornfield, J., Haenszel, W., Hammond, E. C., Lilienfeld, A. M., Shimkin, M. B., and Wynder, E. L. 1959. "Smoking and lung cancer: Recent evidence and a discussion of some questions." *J. Natl. Cancer. Inst.* 22:173–203.

Dean, G. 1967. "Annual incidence, prevalence, and mortality of multiple sclerosis in white South-African-born and in white immigrants to South Africa." *Brit. Med. J.* 2:724–730.

Detels, R., Brody, J. A., and Edgar, A. H. 1972. "Multiple sclerosis among American, Japanese and Chinese migrants to California and Washington." *J. Chron. Dis.* 25:3–10.

Gilliam, A. G. 1955. "Trends of mortality attributed to carcinoma of the lung: Possible effects of faulty certification of death to other respiratory diseases." *Cancer* 8:1130–1136.

Gordon, P. C. 1966. "The epidemiology of cerebral vascular disease in Canada: An analysis of mortality data." *Can. Med. Assoc. J.* 95:1004–1011.

Greenberg, M. J. 1965. "Isoprenaline in myocardial failure." (Letter). *Lancet* 2:442–443.

Greenberg, M. J., and Pines, A. 1967. "Pressurized aerosols in asthma." (Letter). *Brit. Med. J.* 1:563.

Harburg, E., Gleibermann, L., Roeper, P., Schork, M. A., and Schull, W. J. 1978. "Skin color, ethnicity and blood pressure I: Detroit blacks." *Am. J. Pub. Health* 68(12):1177–1183.

Herbst, A. L., and Scully, R. E. 1970. "Adenocarcinoma of the vagina in adolescence." *Cancer* 25:745–757.

Herbst, A. L., Ulfelder, H., and Poskanzer, D. C. 1971. "Association of maternal stilbesterol therapy with tumor appearance in young women." *New Eng. J. Med.* 284(16): 878–881.

Inman, W.H.W., and Adelstein, A. M. 1969. "Rise and fall of asthma mortality in England and Wales in relation to use of pressurized aerosols." *Lancet* 2:279–285.

International Agency for Research on Cancer. 1987. *Cancer Incidence in Five Continents, Average Annual Age-Specific Incidence Rates of Malignant Neoplasms of the Breast among Females in Selected Countries.* 1978–82. 5(88). Lyon: World Health Organization.

Iso, H., Jacobs, D. R., and Goldman, L. 1990. "Accuracy of death certificate diagnosis of intracranial hemorrhage and non-hemorrhagic stroke." *Am. J. Epidemiol.* 132:993–998.

Kmet, J., and Mahboubi, F. 1972. "Esophageal cancer in Caspian Littoral of Iran: Initial studies." *Science* 175:846–853.

Kurland, L. T., Stazio, A., and Reed, D. 1965. "An appraisal of population studies of multiple sclerosis." *Ann. N.Y. Acad. Sci.* 122:520–541.

Liberatos, P., Link, B. G., and Kelsey, J. L. 1988. "The measurement of social class in epidemiology." *Epidemiol. Rev.* 10:87–121.

Lilienfeld, A. M., Levin, M. L., and Kessler, I. I. 1972. *Cancer in the United States.* Cambridge, Mass.: Harvard University Press.

McManis, A. G. 1964. "Adrenaline and isoprenaline: A warning." *Med. J. Aust.* 2:76.

Moriyama, I. M., Krueger, D. E. and Stamler, J. 1971. *Cardiovascular Diseases in the United States.* Cambridge, Mass.: Harvard University Press.

National Center for Health Statistics. 1980. Department of Health, Education and Welfare. Publication No. (PHS) 80-1120. Vol. 28, No. 11 Supplement, February 29.

Percy, C., and Muir, C. 1989. "The international comparability of cancer mortality data." *Am. J. Epidemiol.* 129:934–946.

Percy, C., Garfinkel, L., Krueger, D. E., and Dolman, A. B. 1974. "Apparent changes in cancer mortality. 1968." *Pub. Health Rep.* 89:418–428.

Renwick, J. H. 1972. "Hypothesis: Anencephaly and spina bifida are usually preventable by avoidance of a specific but unidentified substance present in certain potato tubers." *Brit. J. Prev. Soc. Med.* 26:67–88.

Shai, D. and Rosenwaike, I. 1989. "Errors in reporting education on the death certificate: Some findings for older male decedents from New York State and Utah." *Amer. J. Epidemiol.* 130:188–192.

Speizer, F. E., Doll, R., and Heaf, P. 1968. "Observations on recent increase in mortality from asthma." *Brit. Med. J.* 1:335–339.

Speizer, F. E., and Strang, L. B. 1968. "Investigation into use of drugs preceding death from asthma." *Brit. Med. J.* 1:339–343.

Spiegelman, M. 1968. *Introduction to Demography.* Rev. ed., Cambridge, Mass.: Harvard University Press.

Stolley, P. D. 1972. "Asthma mortality: Why the United States was spared an epidemic of deaths due to asthma." *Am. Rev. Resp. Dis.* 105:883–890.

Tuyns, A. J. 1970. "Cancer of the oesophagus: Further evidence of the relation to drinking habits in France." *Int. J. Cancer* 5:152–156.

Tyroler, H. A., and James, S. A. 1978. "Blood pressure and skin color." *Am. J. Pub. Health* 68(12):1170–1172.

U.S. Bureau of the Census. "Current Population Reports." Series P-25, No. 985, as cited in section 7, Technical Appendix of Vital Statistics of the United States, 1988.

U.S. Department of Health and Human Services. *Reducing the Health Consequences of Smoking: 25 Years of Progress: A Report of the Surgeon General.* Department of Health and Human Services, Public Health Service, Centers for Disease Control, Off. Smoking and Health, DHHS Publ. 89-8411, 1989.

Visscher, B. R., Detels, R., Coulson, A. H., Malmgren, R. M., and Dudley, J. P. 1977. "Latitude, migration, and the prevalence of multiple sclerosis." *Am. J. Epidemiol.* 106:470–475.

Vital Statistics of the United States. 1965. 1955 Supplement: Mortality Data, Multiple Causes of Death. United States Department of Health, Education and Welfare, Public Health Service, National Center for Health Statistics, Washington, D.C.: U.S. Government Printing Office.

Vital Statistics of the United States, 1987, Volume II—Mortality, Part A., U.S. Department of Health and Human Services, Public Health Service, Centers for Disease Control, National Center for Health Statistics, Hyattsville, Maryland, 1990.

Vital Statistics of the United States, 1988, Volume II—Mortality, Part A., U.S. Department of Health and Human Services, Public Health Service, Centers for Disease Control, National Center for Health Statistics, Hyattsville, Maryland, 1991.

Weber, M. 1946. "Class, status and party." In *From Max Weber: Essays in Sociology.* Geith, H., Mills, C. W. eds. New York: Oxford University Press.

World Health Organization. 1989. World Health Statistics Annual. Geneva: World Health Organization.

6

MORBIDITY STATISTICS

SOURCES

The limitations of mortality statistics and the need to obtain information on various aspects of illness in the population stimulated the collection of morbidity statistics. Morbidity statistics are essential to health agencies attempting to control disease, especially communicable diseases. Various tax-financed public assistance programs and medical care plans require knowledge of morbidity of the population groups they serve for purposes of planning and evaluation of health and social services. Industry is concerned with the effect of morbidity on its employees, particularly as it affects absenteeism and productivity. The planning and evaluation of public health activities and health facilities require knowledge of the extent of morbidity in the population. Morbidity statistics are sometimes the by-products of societal activities such as conscription for the armed services and enrollment in retirement plans. In recent years, increased reliance has been placed on a variety of morbidity statistics to maintain surveillance of the quality of medical care and to measure the utilization of health care facilities and services.

Table 6–1 presents an overview of some sources of morbidity statistics. Detailed consideration of them can be found in books on demography or vital statistics (Spiegelman, 1968; Alderson, 1988). In assessing the utility of any of these sources for epidemiologic studies, one must be aware of two factors: (1) the variety of definitions of illness used, and (2) the composition of the population that has served as the source of information. The definition of illness used in a particular instance is influenced by the nature of the program or activity for which the data were collected (Table 6–1). These data serve many different administra-

Table 6–1.   Various Sources of Morbidity Statistics

1. *Disease control programs*
   Disease reporting—communicable diseases; case registers of tuberculosis, cancer, cardiovascular disease, and other diseases; surveillance systems
   Case-finding programs in selected population groups
2. *Tax-financed public-assistance programs*
   Public assistance, aid to the blind, aid to the disabled
   State or federal medical care plans
   Armed forces, including preinduction records
   Department of Veterans Affairs
3. *Records of industrial and school absenteeism and preemployment and periodic physical examinations in industry and schools*
4. *Data accumulated as a by-product of insurance, prepaid medical care plans, and other health-related activities*
   Group health and accident insurance
   Prepaid medical care plans
   State disability insurance plans
   Life insurance companies
   Hospital insurance plans
   Railroad retirement board
   Selective Service records
   Clinics and hospitals
5. *Special research programs*
6. *Morbidity surveys on population samples for illness in general and for specific diseases*

tive purposes. Statistics derived from disability programs, for example, will vary according to the program's content and purpose (Lerner, 1974). Some programs are concerned with specific forms of disability such as blindness, whereas others consider a disabled person in terms of his physical or mental ability to support himself. Thus, disability may be defined with regard to specific types and/or according to a range from temporary and limited to permanent and total.

Determining whether a morbid condition or illness is present in an individual often depends upon the type and method of examination used. In a community case-finding program, for example, a single test such as an X-ray examination may be used to detect individuals with a high probability of having a specific disease, a process known as **screening.** Additional examinations would be necessary to determine whether they had the specific disease. Statistics derived from such programs provide information on presumptive diagnoses, whereas those obtained from hospitals and clinics usually represent the results of detailed examinations. Illness can also be determined by interview, i.e., by asking whether a person feels ill, or currently has or has had a specific disease. Thus, the various methods of determining the presence of illness will result in different definitions that must be considered in assessing the usefulness of such data for epidemiologic purposes.

Most sources of morbidity statistics, particularly items 2 to 5 in Table 6–1, only provide information on special population groups, i.e., the group covered by a particular health insurance plan or retirement program. In many instances, the population served by a facility, such as a hospital, is not even defined. Studies in the past have shown underreporting of communicable diseases (especially those transmitted sexually) by physicians. This, too, must be considered in evaluating the usefulness of such data (Schaffner et al., 1971; Sherman and Langmuir, 1952; Thacker and Berkelman, 1988). Underreporting of a variety of obstetrical conditions and congenital malformations on birth certificates has also been found (Milham, 1963; Lilienfeld et al., 1951). Case-finding programs have a similar limitation, and it has been particularly difficult to obtain even a 90 percent response to surveys for such chronic conditions as diabetes mellitus (McDonald et al., 1966; Colsher and Wallace, 1991; Nelson et al. 1990). Those who do respond to case-finding surveys may differ in important ways from those who do not. This may result in biased estimates of disease frequency in the population.

An approach that has proved extremely valuable in many areas of the United States and other countries is the population-based permanent or long-term registration system for a specific disease, such as cancer or one of the other chronic diseases (Bahn et al., 1965; Gordis et al., 1969; Gillum, 1978; Muir et al., 1987; Most and Peterson, 1969). A well-planned and well-operated registry can furnish a great deal of information on the frequency of a disease and can provide data for epidemiologic studies. An attempt is made through these registries to collect as much information as is practical on all newly recognized cases of the disease in a specific population. To achieve the desired degree of completeness, it is necessary to collect information from many sources, including hospitals, pathology laboratories, practicing physicians, and official death certificates.

Some registries require compulsory notification of cases by physicians; others depend on voluntary cooperation. In many instances, the reporting is limited to hospitalized cases (Most and Peterson, 1969; Gillum, 1978). If the registry is for a disease such as cancer where nearly all cases are hospitalized, registration is considered virtually complete.

The development of a case registry is costly. It is, therefore, essential to compare those costs and the benefits of having such data available with the costs and benefits for other methods of obtaining similar information, such as periodic population surveys. After its initiation, the survival of either a voluntary or compulsory case registry depends on maintaining the interest of cooperating physicians and hospitals. Interest in a registry generally can be sustained if the data collected are actually used as a basis for providing health and social services to patients or for research purposes.

SURVEILLANCE

The concept of surveillance derives from its French origins during the Napoleonic wars: to keep watch over a group of persons thought to be subversive (Eylenbosch and Noah, 1988). Until recently, epidemiologic surveillance focused on the identification of an infected individual, with the goal of isolation to minimize disease transmission (Langmuir, 1971; Thacker and Berkelman, 1988). In 1963, Langmuir shifted the focus to the status of a disease in a population, i.e., the "continued watchfulness over the distribution and trends of incidence through the systematic collection, consolidation and evaluation of morbidity and mortality reports and other relevant information" and the regular dissemination of such data to "all who need to know." An extension of epidemiologic surveillance is the use of data for disease prevention and control (Halperin and Baker, 1992). A surveillance system provides for the ongoing collection of data by a data center, the analysis of those data, the dissemination of the data and analyses, and the implementation of a response based upon the analyses.

There are three types of surveillance systems: *active, passive,* and *sentinel* (Table 6–2) (Eylenbosch and Noah, 1988; Thacker and Berkelman, 1988; Rut-

Table 6–2.   Advantages and Disadvantages of Different Types of Surveillance Systems

TYPE	CHARACTERISTIC	ADVANTAGES	DISADVANTAGES
Active	Regular periodic collection of case reports from health care providers or facilities	Data are more accurate than in other types of surveillance	Expensive
Passive	Reports of cases given by health care professionals at their discretion	Inexpensive	Data likely to underestimate the presence of disease in the population
Sentinel health event	Case report indicates a failure of the health care system or indicates that special problems are emerging	Very inexpensive	Applicable only for a select group of diseases

stein et al., 1976). **Active surveillance** depends on the periodic solicitation of case reports from health care providers or facilities. For example, the Connecticut Tumor Registry actively reviews hospital records throughout the state for new ("incident") cases of cancer and benign tumors (Heston et al., 1986). Hospitals outside the state are also under surveillance for such cases among Connecticut residents outside the state. Other cancer registries, in the United Kingdom for instance, exemplify active surveillance (Fraser et al., 1978; Muir et al., 1987).

In contrast, **passive surveillance** relies upon reporting of cases by health care professionals at their discretion. Reporting of cases of toxic shock syndrome in Wisconsin in the early 1980s exemplified this type of surveillance (Davis and Vergeront, 1982). Physicians and other community members (including patients) were asked to report cases to the state health department. One factor found to influence the level of reporting was media attention given to toxic shock syndrome.

In general, active surveillance requires more effort by the data collection center than does passive surveillance. It is therefore more expensive to maintain an active surveillance system than a passive one. On the other hand, active surveillance results in more complete and accurate data than does passive surveillance, because providers do not always report all cases to the data center. In an evaluation of active and passive surveillance systems for notifiable diseases in Vermont and in Pierce County, Washington, the physicians in the active system reported twice as many notifiable diseases per patient as did physicians in the passive one (Alter et al., 1987). Similar results have been reported by other researchers (Brachott and Mosley, 1972; Hinds et al., 1985; Thacker, et al., 1986; Marier, 1977; Vogt et al., 1983).

The third type of surveillance, **sentinel surveillance,** relies on reports of cases of disease whose occurrence suggests that the quality of preventive or therapeutic medical care needs to be improved (Rutstein et al., 1976; Rutstein et al., 1983). Such cases are termed "sentinel health events" since this occurrence serves as a warning to health officials. An example of a sentinel health event is a case of polio, which indicates the need for attention to immunization in the population. Similarly, the occurrence of malignant mesothelioma is a sentinel for past exposure to asbestos. Many European countries use sentinel surveillance systems to provide information on disease occurrence. Several developing countries have been encouraged by the Expanded Programme on Immunization of the World Health Organization to use sentinel surveillance systems for disease reporting (World Health Organization, 1985; World Health Organization, 1988). Although it is relatively inexpensive to maintain, sentinel surveillance lacks specificity regarding the cause of the disease and the risk factors to which the population has been exposed.

CROSS-SECTIONAL STUDIES

Cross-sectional studies, also known as "prevalence surveys," provide information on the frequency of disease in a population. Often the population is defined geographically, but it may also be defined by employment in a company or participation in a health care plan, for instance. In a cross-sectional study, the epidemiologist randomly selects a sample from the population of interest at one point in time (hence the name "cross-sectional"). Once the sample is selected, the epidemiologist determines the frequency of the disease(s) of interest in that population, as well as factors that may be associated with the presence or absence of the disease, such as age or gender (see Chapter 7).

When information on illness in a population is needed on a periodic or continuing basis, a morbidity survey, in which a cross-sectional study is repeatedly conducted in the same population, is established. Such surveys are also conducted because of the limitations of some of the sources of morbidity data mentioned above. This method was initiated on a large scale in continuous studies of all illnesses in a community by the United States Public Health Service in Hagerstown, Maryland, in 1921–1924 (Sydenstricker, 1974).

In general, community-wide morbidity surveys have collected information on population samples in two ways: by interview and by examination. Information obtained by interview can be elicited directly from the respondent or from a member of the household who reports the illnesses among all household members for a specified period of time. Information can be obtained by a complete physical examination or by examination of certain organ systems, e.g., cardiovascular, in a sample of the entire population or selected groups of the population, depending upon the purposes of the survey. Morbidity surveys can be carried out by a single visit to the household, a single examination of a person, or periodic visits or examinations.

Soon after the Hagerstown surveys, other national morbidity surveys were conducted in the United States for different purposes, but it was not until 1956 that a continuing program of surveying the health status of the United States population was begun. This was the United States National Health Survey, which is currently conducted by the National Center for Health Statistics (National Center for Health Statistics, 1963; Jekel, 1984). The National Health Survey includes three general programs of survey activities: the National Health Interview Survey (NHIS), the National Health and Nutrition Examination Survey (NHANES), and the National Health Record Survey (NHRS). National Center for Health Statistics findings from these surveys are reported in color-coded booklets, so that these reports have become popularly known as the "Rainbow Series" (Jekel, 1984).

The National Health Interview Survey is based on a sample of the noninstitutionalized population of the United States. It is conducted continuously by interviewing a sample of households each week and combining these findings to provide estimates of illness for longer periods of time. Among the specific items included in the NHIS are doctor visits and hospital stays, occurrence of reported acute and chronic conditions, health status indicators, and reported limitation of activities. Periodically, a supplemental set of questions is asked, such as knowledge and attitudes about AIDS, health promotion practices, and smoking habits (Chyba and Washington, 1990; Kovar, 1989; Jekel, 1984).

The National Health and Nutrition Examination Survey (NHANES) consists of examinations and a variety of physiological and psychological tests for specific diseases, carried out over a period of two or three years for a selected age group. Originally, the NHANES was organized as the National Health Examination Survey (NHES). The population groups examined in the three cycles of the NHES and the years that the examinations were conducted are shown in Table 6–3. In 1971, nutritional surveillance was added to the NHES and it became the National Health and Nutrition Examination Survey (Kovar, 1989). The sample is selected by methods similar to those of the Health Interview Survey, but it is much smaller. A special Hispanic Health and Nutrition Examination Survey (HHANES) was conducted in the 1980s to evaluate the health status of the Hispanic population in the United States (Kovar, 1989).

The Health Record Survey involves samples of institutions or facilities providing health or medical care services and is carried out on either a continuous or a periodic basis (Jekel, 1984; Kovar, 1989). Specifically, the National Hospital Discharge Survey, conducted annually since 1965, provides information about the diagnoses at discharge of a sample of patients admitted to short-stay hospitals. The complaints of patients and the diagnoses of physicians in their private offices are sampled by the National Ambulatory Medical Care Survey, conducted annually from 1974 to 1981 and then once every four years beginning in 1985.

Table 6–3. National Health Examination Surveys in the United States Since 1960

SURVEY	YEARS CONDUCTED	POPULATION SURVEYED
National Health Examination Survey		
NHES I	1960–1962	18–79 years of age
NHES II	1963–1965	6–11 years of age
NHES III	1966–1970	12–17 years of age
National Health and Nutrition Examination Survey		
NHANES I	1971–1974	1–74 years of age
NHANES II	1976–1980	6 months–74 years of age
NHANES III	1990–1993	6 months–74 years of age
HHANES	1982–1984	Hispanic Americans 6 months–74 years of age

Table 6–4.   Annual Report Incidence Rates (per 100 population) of Fractures and
Dislocations, and Sprains and Strains to the Musculoskeletal System,* United
States, 1989

AGE	PERCENTAGE INCIDENCE		
(YEARS)	FRACTURES AND DISLOCATIONS	SPRAINS AND STRAINS	TOTAL
<5	1.2	1.5	2.7
5–17	4.7	6.2	10.9
18–24	4.3	7.1	11.4
25–44	2.8	7.7	10.5
45–64	2.1	2.7	4.8
65+	2.6	2.9	5.5
All Ages	3.0	5.3	8.3

*Episodes associated with receipt of medical attention or with limitation of activity.
Source: Adams and Benson (1990).

In addition to these surveys, there is an ongoing program of data evaluation and
methodological research as well as a program of analytical studies of epidemiologic and statistical problems. Table 6–4 and Figure 6–1 show some examples of
the types of information provided by the National Health Survey Program (Adams
and Benson, 1990).

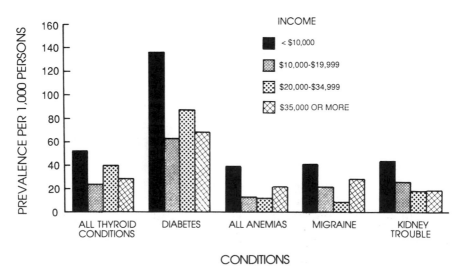

Figure 6–1.   Prevalence of selected chronic conditions per 1,000 persons 65 years
of age and older, by family income, National Health Survey, 1989. *Source:* Adams
(1990).

A continuing program of health status surveys, similar to the United States National Health Survey, was begun in Japan in 1953 (Soda, 1965; Soda and Kosaki, 1975). The Office of Population Censuses and Surveys has conducted an annual General Household Survey in the United Kingdom since 1971; it provides information on the health status of the population similar to that of the NHIS (Office of Population and Censuses and Surveys, 1973; Alderson, 1988). Various types of continuing national health survey systems have also been developed by other European countries, e.g., the Netherlands since 1981 (Alderson, 1988).

MEASUREMENT OF MORBIDITY

To describe morbidity, two general types of rates are available: incidence and prevalence rates. They are defined as follows:

$$\frac{\text{Incidence rate}}{\text{per 1,000}} = \frac{\begin{array}{l}\text{Number of new cases of a disease occurring in}\\ \text{the population during a specified period of time}\end{array}}{\begin{array}{l}\text{Number of persons exposed to risk of developing}\\ \text{the disease during that period of time}\end{array}} \times 1{,}000$$

$$\frac{\text{Prevalence rate}}{\text{per 1,000}} = \frac{\begin{array}{l}\text{Number of cases of disease present in}\\ \text{the population at a specified period of time}\end{array}}{\begin{array}{l}\text{Number of persons at risk of having}\\ \text{the disease at that specified time}\end{array}} \times 1{,}000$$

The **incidence rate** is a direct estimate of the probability, or risk, of developing a disease during a specified period of time. This contrasts with the **prevalence rate,** which measures the number of cases that are present at, or during, a specified period of time. The prevalence rate (P) equals the incidence rate (I) multiplied by the average duration of the disease (D) or $P = I \times D$. For example, if the average duration of a disease is three years and its incidence rate is 10 cases per 1,000 persons per year, the prevalence rate would be 30 cases per 1,000 persons, i.e., $P = 3 \times 10$. The duration of disease is usually measured from the time of diagnosis to death. Although it would be highly desirable to measure the duration from the time of onset of a disease, it is usually difficult, if not impossible, to ascertain this for most diseases. The constant of 1,000 in the above rates was arbitrarily selected. One could use 1,000,000 instead of 1,000. For example, an incidence rate of 3,000 cases per 1,000,000 population per year is equivalent to an incidence rate of 3 cases per 1,000 population per year.

The two types of prevalence rates that are used by investigators are *point prevalence* and *period prevalence*. Point prevalence refers to the number of cases present at a specified moment of time; period prevalence refers to the number of cases that occur during a specified period of time—for example, a year. Period prevalence consists of the point prevalence at the beginning of a specified period of time plus all new cases that occur during that period. The distinction between these measures of prevalence (Figure 6–2) developed from practical considerations since it usually takes a period of time to conduct a prevalence survey and to ascertain all of the cases. Even if a survey does require some time for its execution, however, it is generally possible to estimate point prevalence.

The cases of disease that would be counted in an incidence rate during the annual period in Figure 6–2 would include case numbers 3, 4, 5, and 8. For measuring point prevalence as of January 1, case numbers 1, 2, and 7 would be included, and for point prevalence on December 31, one would include case numbers 1, 3, 5, and 8. Period prevalence from January 1 to December 31, 1992, would include case numbers 1, 2, 3, 4, 5, 7 and 8.

Clearly, the rates can vary depending upon the measure of morbidity that is used. In evaluating published data, it is important to keep in mind the measure used by the investigator (the two terms are often used erroneously in published reports). For example, the term ''incidence'' has been applied to data when prevalence is actually being measured. This creates some difficulties when rates from two different reports are compared.

The epidemiologist generally prefers to use incidence rates when comparing the development of disease in different population groups or attempting to determine whether a relationship exists between a possible etiological factor and a disease. This is because the incidence rate directly estimates the probability of developing a disease during a specified period of time. It permits the epidemiologist to determine whether the probability of developing a disease differs in

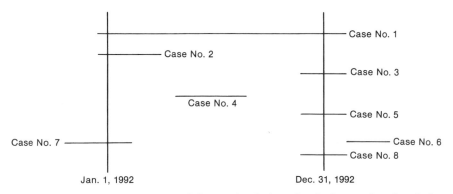

Figure 6–2. Number of cases of disease beginning, developing, and ending during a period of time, January 1, 1992–December 31, 1992. Length of each line corresponds to the duration of each case.

different populations or time periods or in relationship to suspected etiologic factors.

All forms of morbidity rates, including incidence, attack, and prevalence rates, can be made specific for age, gender, or any other personal characteristics that might be important and of interest. They also can be standardized in the same manner as mortality rates. It is important to distinguish between incidence and prevalence rates in comparing different population groups or different time periods. The incidence rates of a disease may be the same in these comparisons, but the prevalence rates may vary with the availability of curative medical services that influence duration of the disease. Thus, a higher prevalence rate does not necessarily reflect an increased probability of developing a disease but rather may reflect the lesser availability or efficacy of medical intervention.

Prevalence rates of disease are useful to the health service administrator in planning medical care services. In the absence of incidence rates, differences in prevalence rates between populations have also been useful in stimulating further epidemiologic studies. In some instances, they may be the only rates that are available for studying a particular disease. In persons with inflammatory bowel disease (Crohn's disease and ulcerative colitis), for instance, it is very difficult to determine accurately when the disorder began; often there are many years between the onset of symptoms and the time that a diagnosis is made.

A special form of incidence or attack rate, initially developed by C. V. Chapin to measure the spread of infection within a family or household following exposure to the first or primary case in the family, is the secondary attack rate (Frost, 1941). It is defined as follows:

$$\text{Secondary attack rate (percent)} = \frac{\begin{array}{c}\text{Number of exposed persons developing the disease}\\ \text{within the range of the incubation period}\end{array}}{\text{Total number of persons exposed to the primary case}} \times 100$$

This rate attempts to measure the degree of spread of a disease within a group that has been exposed to an agent by contact with a case. The numerator can be expressed in terms of clinical disease or any measurable component of the gradient of disease (such as those persons with rising antibody titers), providing the technical means are available to measure this component. The denominator consists of all persons who are exposed to (in contact with) the case. This can be more specifically defined to include those who are susceptible to the specific agent (if means are available to distinguish the immune from the susceptible persons). If the incubation period of a specific disease is unknown, the numerator can be expressed in terms of a specified time period. The primary case is excluded from both the numerator and denominator.

The secondary attack rate is usually applied to biological or social groups such as families, households, friends, or classmates, but it can be used with any closed aggregate of persons who have had contact with a case of disease. Meyer, for example, studied the occurrence of mumps in 170 families, each of which had at least two cases of the disease (Meyer, unpublished). Figure 6–3, taken from this study, presents the distribution of intervals between the day of onset of the first case in the family (designated as day ''0'') and that of one or more subsequent cases. The secondary cases are those occurring during the interval between 7–8 days and 29–30 days, which would approximate the range of the incubation period and, therefore, represents those cases developing as a result of contact with the first case. The cases that occur after this period are usually called ''tertiary'' cases and, for the most part, result from contact with secondary cases. They may also be produced by contact with cases outside the family. When the number of secondary cases has been determined and the total number of persons in the household is established, a secondary attack rate can be computed.

The secondary attack rate serves other purposes in addition to reflecting the degree of transmissibility of the agent, for instance, in evaluating the efficacy of a prophylactic agent. A study of an outbreak of infectious hepatitis among households in a municipal housing project illustrates this application (Lilienfeld et al., 1953). In this outbreak, some household members had received gamma globulin for prophylaxis at the city hospital nearby, and some had not. The gamma globulin was not administered to the household members in a systematic manner; as there was no formal protocol, its administration varied with the hospital staff member

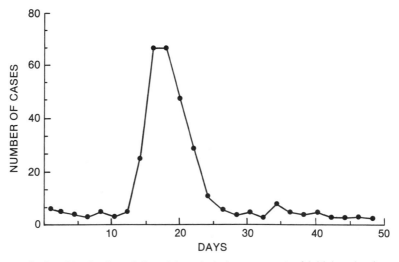

Figure 6–3. Distribution of time intervals between onset of initial and subsequent cases of mumps in 170 families with two or more cases. *Source:* Meyer (unpublished).

Table 6–5.   Age-Specific Secondary Attack Rates of Infectious Hepatitis among Total Number of Persons Exposed to a Case in a Household and among Those Receiving Gamma Globulin

AGE (YEARS)	NUMBER OF PERSONS EXPOSED TO A CASE	CASES OF HEPATITIS	
		NUMBER	PERCENT (SECONDARY ATTACK RATE)
Did Not Receive Gamma Globulin			
0–4	42	2	4.8
5–9	45	5	11.1
10–14	32	6	18.8
15–19	26	3	11.5
20+	83	4	4.8
Received Gamma Globulin			
0–4	17	1	6.0
5–9	21	0	0
10–14	13	0	0
15–19	3	0	0
20+	17	1	1.4

Source: Lilienfeld, Bross, and Sartwell (1953).

on duty. From the available data, it was possible to compute secondary attack rates for the household contacts of the primary case, according to whether or not they had received gamma globulin. Table 6–5 shows that the attack rates were lower among those contacts who had received gamma globulin than among those who had not.

Secondary rates are also used to determine whether a disease of unknown etiology is communicable and thus may indicate the possible etiological role of a transmissible agent. For example, they have been used by Beral and her colleagues to explore the hypothesis that Kaposi's sarcoma, a rare cancer associated with AIDS, may be a sexually transmitted disease (Beral et al., 1990). First, these investigators noted that the risk for Kaposi's sarcoma was ten times higher among homosexual and bisexual men with AIDS than in other HIV transmission groups (Beral et al., 1990). They then observed that the risk of this malignancy among AIDS patients in Britain was higher among those who had sexual partners from the United States or Africa (a secondary attack rate) than among those with partners from Britain or other areas (Beral et al., 1991). Further investigation of the specific behaviors associated with transmission are currently in progress. The agent, however, has not yet been isolated.

MORBIDITY STATISTICS—SOME ISSUES AND PROBLEMS

Although there are several advantages in obtaining information on illnesses from a specific population either by interview or examination, inaccuracy and variability of the information presents problems. These difficulties must be considered in assessing the findings from morbidity surveys, for they influence the methods used by epidemiologists in obtaining data and the inferences they derive from those data.

Validity of Interview Surveys

Several studies have addressed the issue of the validity or accuracy of the information obtained by interview about the presence of illness or about other characteristics (Jabine, 1987; Harlow and Linet, 1989). Generally, these investigations have compared interview-obtained information with that from a prepaid health insurance plan. Such studies have been undertaken in cooperation with the Health Insurance Plan of Greater New York (HIP) (in 1958), the Kaiser-Permanente Foundation Health Plan (KP) (in 1962–1963) and an unnamed plan in Michigan (in 1968) (Marquis et al., 1971; Woolsey et al., 1962; National Center for Health Statistics, 1968; Madow, 1967, 1973). The results of these studies, summarized in Table 6–6, show a consistent underreporting of conditions; in the HIP and KP studies, there was also significant overreporting of some conditions. Both underreported conditions and overreported conditions varied among the studies, and

Table 6–6. Estimates of the Underreporting and Overreporting of Conditions in Three Health Interview Surveys

	PERCENTAGE OF PHYSICIAN-REPORTED CONDITIONS NOT REPORTED IN SURVEY (UNDERREPORTING)	PERCENTAGE OF SURVEY-IDENTIFIED CONDITIONS NOT CONFIRMED BY PHYSICIAN REPORTS (OVERREPORTING)
Survey		
HIP (1958)	68.1	60.4
KP (1962–1963)	46.7	40.4
Michigan (1968)		
(Educational Level)		
≤11 years	35.1	7.9
12+ years	44.7	12.4

Source: Jabine (1987).

both have been found in smaller, more recent investigations, as reviewed by Harlow and Linet (1989). Some illnesses, such as chronic bronchitis or allergies, are less likely to be noted on the medical record than to be reported at interview, while other conditions, such as diabetes or heart disease, are more likely to be accurately reported at interview. Comparable results have been obtained in populations outside the United States as well (Alderson, 1984).

An investigation in the eastern and midwestern parts of the United States was carried out by the National Center for Health Statistics to determine whether a history of hospitalization was accurately reported (United States National Health Survey, 1961). Each of 1,505 persons who had been hospitalized during the previous year was asked to report hospitalizations for the year prior to the Sunday night of the week of the interview. The degree of underreporting of hospitalization is shown in Figure 6–4. It varied with the length of time between hospitalization

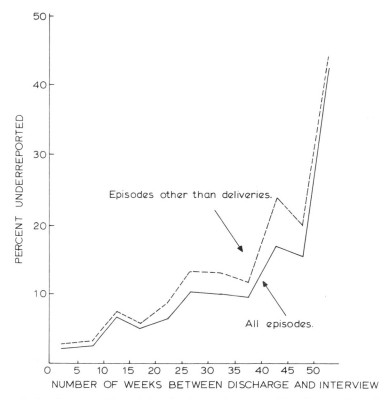

Figure 6–4.   Percent of hospital episodes underreported by the number of weeks between the hospital discharge and interview, including and excluding deliveries. *Source:* United States National Health Survey (1961).

and interview; the longer the interval, the greater the degree of underreporting, ranging from 10 percent at about six months after hospitalization to about 35–45 percent at one year. Underreporting also varied with the length of stay in the hospital, the reason for hospitalization (whether for a delivery or a surgical or nonsurgical procedure), and other factors. Similar findings have been obtained outside the United States (Office of Population Censuses and Surveys, 1973).

Another method of validating interview surveys is to compare the information obtained by interview with that obtained by physical examination. Such comparisons were made in studies conducted in a rural and an urban area by the Commission on Chronic Illness (Commission on Chronic Illness, 1957, 1959).

The rural study was conducted during 1951–1955 in Hunterdon County, New Jersey. A sample of 13,113 persons (about 25 percent of the population) was interviewed. Of these, 1,202 persons were categorized into different strata, according to conditions reported on interview, and were invited to a medical center for a complete physical examination, including any indicated laboratory or diagnostic procedures. Seventy-two percent of those who were invited accepted. The proportions of match between interview-reported and clinically evaluated conditions are shown in Table 6–7 for both disabling and nondisabling

Table 6–7. Proportions of Match between Selected Interview-Reported Conditions and Clinically Evaluated Conditions

| | PERCENT MATCHING INTERVIEW-REPORTED CONDITIONS | |
DISEASE CLASSIFICATION	DISABLING	NONDISABLING
All conditions present during interview year	24	18
Infective; parasitic	22	8
Neoplasms (benign and malignant)	15	7
Allergic	57	12
Diabetes mellitus	63	100
Heart	38	54
Obesity	6	2
Anemias; other blood conditions	52	0
Mental, psychoneurotic, personality disorders	21	30
Nervous system	39	26
Injuries; poisonings	22	46
Genitourinary	7	16
Skin; cellular tissue	36	3
Dental; buccal cavity, and esophageal	15	2
Digestive, other than buccal cavity, and esophageal	23	64

Source: Adapted from Commission on Chronic Illness (1959).

conditions. The interview method clearly resulted in underreporting of clinically evaluated conditions. The degree of underreporting varied with the condition and was quite substantial for several disorders, such as neoplasms, obesity, and genitourinary conditions. On the other hand, many important conditions reported on interview were validated by clinical evaluation; for example, 80 percent of the reports of a heart condition and 85 percent of reported diabetes cases were validated. But for some conditions, such as gastrointestinal disorders, only 48 percent of the reports were clinically confirmed; some of these conditions, however, are not easily subject to clinical confirmation, conditions such as "spastic colitis" or "heartburn." It was of interest that gender and age did not influence the degree of difference. Those with less education and lower family incomes had a higher proportion of validated reports than those in the higher educational and income group. The urban study was conducted in Baltimore in a similar manner, with similar findings (Commission on Chronic Illness, 1957; Krueger, 1957). In both studies, approximately two-thirds of the interview-reported conditions were confirmed during physical examination and two-thirds of the conditions found during the examination were reported during the interview.

It can be seen that there are grounds for skepticism as to the accuracy of certain types of information obtained by interview (Alderson and Dowie, 1979; Alderson, 1984; Harlow and Linet, 1989; Jabine, 1987; Sanders, 1962). This issue is especially relevant in epidemiology, as the search for etiological factors often requires information concerning events that occurred many years in the past. The attempt to determine whether a relationship exists between alcohol consumption and esophageal cancer, for example, may involve interviewing esophageal cancer patients and controls who are mostly over 50 years old. They are asked about their alcohol consumption over a period of years. Thus, it is reasonable to question the validity of the information that is obtained. All this emphasizes the need to validate information obtained by interview with past medical or other records when conducting epidemiologic studies.

Accuracy and Reproducibility of Examinations

The uncertainty of information obtained by interview has stimulated a desire to use more objective methods of examination, laboratory tests, skin tests, or other markers of disease in measuring morbidity whenever possible. The procedure selected depends on the component of the disease spectrum (see Chapter 3) that the investigator is studying. Two aspects of these "objective" tests are important in epidemiology: (a) accuracy or validity, and (b) variability, reproducibility, or precision.

Assessment of accuracy or validity

Two indices are used to evaluate the accuracy of a test—**sensitivity** and **specificity.** These indices are usually determined by administering the test to one group of persons who have the disease and to another group who do not and then comparing the results. As indicated in Table 6–8, those who test positive and have the disease are called "true positives"; those who test positive but actually do not have the disease are called "false positives"; those who test negative and have the disease are called "false negatives"; and those who test negative and do not have the disease are called "true negatives." Using this terminology:

$$\text{Sensitivity} = \frac{\text{True positives}}{\text{True positives plus false negatives}} = \frac{\text{True positives}}{\text{All those with the disease}}$$

$$\text{Specificity} = \frac{\text{True negatives}}{\text{True negatives plus false positives}} = \frac{\text{True negatives}}{\text{All those without the disease}}$$

Sensitivity and specificity are not absolute values. The results of many laboratory tests, such as systolic blood pressure or serum lipoprotein concentrations, cannot be sharply categorized because they form a continuous spectrum. Figure

Table 6–8.   Indices to Evaluate the Accuracy of a Test or Diagnostic Examination: Sensitivity and Specificity

TEST OR EXAMINATION	DISEASE PRESENT	DISEASE ABSENT
Positive (indicating disease is probably present)	A (true positives)	B (false positives)
Negative (indicating disease is probably absent)	C (false negatives)	D (true negatives)
Totals	A + C	B + D

Sensitivity is defined as the percent of those who have the disease, and are so indicated by the test. Thus,

$$\text{Sensitivity (in percent)} = \frac{A}{(A + C)} \times 100$$

Specificity is defined as the percent of those who do *not* have the disease and are so indicated by the test. Thus,

$$\text{Specificity (in percent)} = \frac{D}{(B + D)} \times 100$$

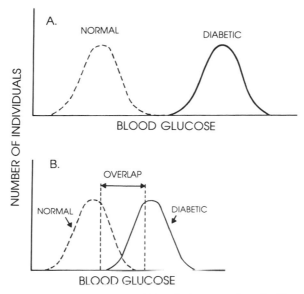

Figure 6–5. Hypothetical distribution of blood glucose values in (A) normal and diabetic population without any overlap and in (B) normal and diabetic populations with overlapping values.

6–5, for example, shows the hypothetical overlap between a normal and a diabetic population in the distribution of blood glucose levels. Table 6–9 presents data obtained from a two-hour postprandial blood test for glucose in a group of 63 true diabetics and 340 true nondiabetics (Wadena Health Study Group, unpublished). The percentage of diabetics so identified (sensitivity) and the percentage of nondiabetics so identified (specificity) are shown for varying levels of fasting blood glucose. An investigator who decides to use a blood sugar level of 5.6 mM as a division point for diabetes, for example, would identify 98.4 percent of the true diabetics and 63.2 percent of the true nondiabetics. In Table 6–10, these results are classified into the four categories of Table 6–8. The results are diagramatically presented in Figure 6–6, which also illustrates the effects of setting different limits of normal on blood glucose level. If the limit is set low, the blood glucose level becomes a very sensitive test, i.e., all diabetics have positive tests. However, this is done at the expense of mistakenly identifying many normal subjects as diabetic. If the limit is set high, the blood glucose level becomes a highly specific test for diabetes. However, many diabetics are erroneously diagnosed as nondiabetics. The intermediate choice minimizes both types of error—false positive and false negative.

Table 6–9. Sensitivity and Specificity of a Two-Hour Postprandial Blood Test for Glucose for 63 True Diabetics and 340 True Nondiabetics at Different Levels of Blood Glucose

REFERENCE VALUE (mg/dl)	BLOOD GLUCOSE (mM)	SENSITIVITY[1] (%)	SPECIFICITY[1] (%)
80	4.4	100.0 (63/63)	0.6 (2/340)
	5.0	100.0 (63/63)	19.7 (67/340)
	5.6	98.4 (62/63)	63.2 (215/340)
	6.1	95.2 (60/63)	93.5 (318/340)
115	6.4	95.2 (60/63)	97.4 (331/340)
	6.7	84.1 (53/63)	100.0 (335/340)
	7.2	74.6 (47/63)	100.0 (340/340)
140	7.8	66.7 (42/63)	100.0 (340/340)
	8.3	55.6 (35/63)	100.0 (340/340)
	8.9	44.4 (28/63)	100.0 (340/340)
	9.4	36.5 (23/63)	100.0 (340/340)
	10.0	33.3 (21/63)	100.0 (340/340)
	10.6	30.2 (19/63)	100.0 (340/340)
200	11.1	23.8 (15/63)	100.0 (340/340)

[1]Figures in parentheses are the number of diabetics with a two-hour postprandial blood glucose level at or above the specified level.

Source: Wadena City Health Study (unpublished).

Table 6–10. Sensitivity and Specificity of a Blood Glucose Level of 5.6 mM for Presumptive Determination of Diabetes Status

BLOOD GLUCOSE LEVEL (mM)	TRUE DISEASE STATUS	
	DIABETICS	NONDIABETICS
All those with level over 5.6 mM are classified as diabetics	62 (98.4 percent) (true positives)	215 (36.8 percent) (false positives)
All those with level under 5.6 mM are classified as nondiabetics	1 (1.6 percent) (false negatives)	125 (63.2 percent) (true negatives)
Total	63 (100.0 percent)	340 (100.0 percent)

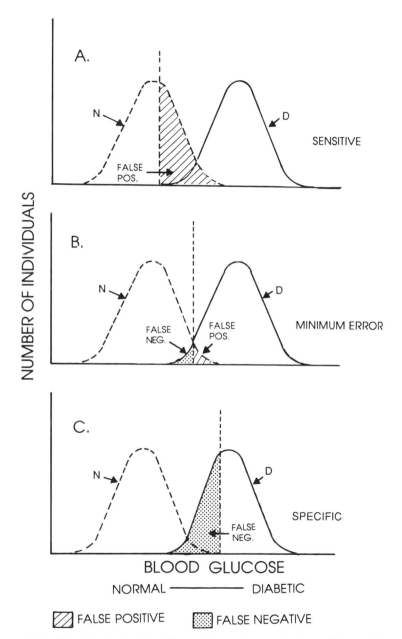

Figure 6–6. The effect of setting different blood glucose levels on false positives and false negatives: (A) a low limit results in a more sensitive test; (B) intermediate limit results in minimum total error; (C) a high limit results in a more specific test.

Predictive value

Although sensitivity and specificity provide information about the accuracy of a test, they do not provide information about the meaning of a positive or negative test result. The probability of the disease being present given a positive test result is the **positive predictive value:**

$$\text{Positive predictive value} = \frac{\text{True positives}}{\text{True positives plus}} = \frac{\text{True positives}}{\text{All those with a positive}}$$
$$\text{false positives} \qquad \text{test result}$$

Negative predictive value is the probability of no disease being present given a negative test result:

$$\text{Negative predictive value} = \frac{\text{True negatives}}{\text{True negatives plus}} = \frac{\text{True negatives}}{\text{All those with a negative}}$$
$$\text{false negatives} \qquad \text{test result}$$

For the data in Table 6–10, the positive predictive value is 22.3 percent (62/(62 + 215)), and the negative predictive value is 99.2 percent (125/(125 + 1)). See Table 6–11.

Unlike sensitivity and specificity, the positive and negative predictive values of a test depend on the prevalence rate of disease in the population. In Table 6–11, for example, the prevalence rate is 15.6 cases per 100 persons. Using the same test, if the prevalence rate were 45 cases per 100, then the positive predictive value would be 68.5 percent and the negative predictive value would be 97.9

Table 6–11.   Positive and Negative Predictive Values of a Blood Glucose Level of 5.6 mM for Presumptive Determination of Diabetes Status with a Prevalence of 15.6 Cases per 100 Persons

BLOOD GLUCOSE LEVEL (mM)	TRUE DISEASE STATUS		TOTAL
	DIABETICS	NONDIABETICS	
All those with level over 5.6 mM are classified as diabetics	62 (22.3 percent) (true positives)	215 (77.7 percent) (false positives)	277 (100 percent) (all positive test results)
All those with level under 5.6 mM are classified as nondiabetics	1 (0.8 percent) (false negatives)	125 (99.2 percent) (true negatives)	126 (100 percent) (all negative test results)

percent (Table 6–12). For a test of given sensitivity and specificity, the higher the prevalence of the disease, the greater the positive predictive value and the lower the negative predictive value (Table 6–13).

In setting a test level at the point desired to identify those with a specific disease and to omit those without it, one must judge the relative costs of classifying persons as false negatives and false positives. The prevalence of the disease in the community, the cost of additional examinations that may be necessary, and the purpose for using the test must also be considered (Morrison, 1992).

Assessment of variability or precision

The problem of variability was initially brought into focus by Yerushalmy (1947) in his studies of the interpretation of chest X-ray films in the diagnosis of tuberculosis. He found two types of variability in interpretation:

1. *Interobserver* variability represents inconsistency of interpretation among different readers of the X-ray films.
2. *Intraobserver* variability reflects the failure of a reader to be consistent with himself in independent interpretations of the same set of films.

Both types of variability are illustrated by drawing on the results of an evaluation of cytologic diagnosis of human papillomavirus (HPV) infection. In this study, 87 cervicovaginal smears seen at a private cytology laboratory in Connecticut between 1973 and 1981 were examined for the presence or absence of HPV infection by two expert pathologists (Horn et al., 1985). A sample of 24 cytology specimens was then independently reexamined by these pathologists. The results show a 74 percent agreement among diagnoses between the two path-

Table 6–12. Positive and Negative Predictive Values of a Blood Glucose Level of 5.6 mM for Presumptive Determination of Diabetes Status with a Prevalence of 45 Cases per 100 Persons

BLOOD GLUCOSE LEVEL (mM)	TRUE DISEASE STATUS		TOTAL
	DIABETICS	NONDIABETICS	
All those with level over 5.6 mM are classified as diabetics	178 (68.5 percent) (true positives)	82 (31.5 percent) (false positives)	260 (100 percent) (all positive test results)
All those with level under 5.6 mM are classified as nondiabetics	3 (2.1 percent) (false negatives)	140 (97.9 percent) (true negatives)	143 (100 percent) (all negative test results)

Table 6–13. Relation between the Prevalence of Disease in a Population and the Positive and Negative Predictive Value of a Test[1]

POPULATION PREVALENCE RATE (PER 100 PERSONS)	POSITIVE PREDICTIVE VALUE (PERCENT)	NEGATIVE PREDICTIVE VALUE (PERCENT)
15.6	22.3	99.2
30.0	53.4	98.8
45.0	68.5	97.9
60.0	80.2	97.1
75.0	89.0	94.1

[1]Test sensitivity = 98.4 percent and specificity = 63.2 percent

ologists (see Table 6–14). Pathologist A's diagnoses were more reproducible than were Pathologist B's.

It is possible that some proportion of the degree of agreement could have arisen by chance. In order to minimize the degree to which chance agreements affect the interpretation of such data, a measure of agreement has been developed that is known as **kappa, κ** (Cohen, 1960). Kappa represents the difference between the observed degree of agreement plus the degree of agreement expected to occur by chance, relative to the degree of agreement that would occur by chance alone (see the Appendix [p. 329] for a more detailed discussion of κ and its calculation). The interpretation of various values of κ is given in Table 6–15. Positive values of κ suggest agreement beyond what would be expected by chance, while negative values indicate that there is little agreement beyond what would occur by chance.

For the results shown in Table 6–14, the values of κ suggest that there was only fair agreement between the two pathologists' diagnoses. On the other hand, this level of agreement is greater than what would be expected by chance alone.

Table 6–14. Reliability of the Cytologic Diagnosis of HPV Infection Made from Cervicovaginal Smears

TYPE OF RELIABILITY	NUMBER OF SLIDES	PERCENT AGREEMENT	κ (KAPPA)
Interobserver (Pathologist A vs. Pathologist B)	87	74	0.38
Intraobserver			
Pathologist A	23	96	0.89
Pathologist B	24	79	0.40

Source: Horn et al. (1985).

Table 6–15.   Interpretation of Various Values of κ

κ	INTERPRETATION
<0	No agreement
0–0.19	Poor agreement
0.20–0.39	Fair agreement
0.40–0.59	Moderate agreement
0.60–0.79	Substantial agreement
0.80–1.00	Almost perfect agreement

Source: Landis and Koch (1977).

Not surprisingly, the measures for the reproducibility of each pathologist's own diagnoses reveal a greater agreement in diagnosis; for Pathologist Λ, a much higher level of agreement. These data suggest that while there are differences among pathologists in the cytological diagnosis of HPV infection, there is diagnostic agreement for many specimens. Similar results have been found for many diagnostic tests.

RECORD LINKAGE

Information on the characteristics of individuals from birth to death exists in the records of many institutions and agencies, private as well as governmental. At birth, a birth certificate is filled out and, when a person is hospitalized, a medical record of the hospitalization is initiated and usually maintained. A record in the Social Security system is filed at the beginning of employment; personnel records are maintained at the place of employment, school records are kept, including health as well as scholastic information; and at the time of death, a death certificate is completed. In Sweden and many other countries, employment censuses are conducted. Also, national medical insurance provides records of pharmaceutical and other medical therapeutics use in many countries.

Some of these records are combined on an *ad hoc* basis in many epidemiologic studies. The basis for this approach, known as record linkage, was stated by Dunn in 1946: "Each person in the world creates a book of life. This book starts with birth and ends with death. Its pages are made up of the records of the principal events in life. Record linkage is the name given to the process of assembling the pages of this book into a volume." A good example of the value of record linkage is the combined use of pharmaceutical and hospitalization billing records to investigate the role of nonsteroidal antiinflammatory drugs (NSAIDs) in the development of upper gastrointestinal hemorrhage (Strom, 1989). These studies found a strong relationship between the use of these agents and subsequent upper gastrointestinal bleeding.

Since the advent of the computer, it has become feasible to develop a systematic method of integrating all these records. This integration can be useful not only for epidemiologic research but also for genetic studies, the planning of medical care facilities, and determining the pattern of patient referrals to medical care in a community. A pioneering effort in record linkage was made by Newcombe (1969, 1974) in British Columbia for both population and genetic studies. He suggested that such a system could be valuable in the study of environmental carcinogenesis.

In 1962, the Oxford Record Linkage Study was initiated in Oxford, England, to determine the feasibility, cost, and methods of medical record linkage for an entire community. This system links morbidity and mortality information and provides the knowledge necessary for planning the allocation of various types of medical facilities as well as for facilitating clinical and epidemiological studies (Acheson, 1967). It is possible to use the system for a variety of inquiries into the etiology and natural history of different diseases. For instance, one of the first Oxford Record Linkage Study investigations focused on the relationship between prenatal events and respiratory morbidity during the first year of life (McCall and Acheson, 1968). Acheson (1987) has recently reviewed the results of this successful medical record linkage effort.

Other record linkage efforts have built upon the Oxford Record Linkage Study. For instance, all Scottish birth, death, hospitalization, cancer incidence, school medical examination, and handicapped children's records are linked (Heasman and Clarke, 1979). Similarly, the Office of Population Censuses and Surveys is conducting a longitudinal survey of one percent of the population of England and Wales alive in 1971, with linkage to cancer registration and mortality records (Office of Population Censuses and Surveys, 1978; Fox, 1981). Similar efforts have been initiated in the United States by the National Center for Health Statistics using data from the NHANES II survey (Jekel, 1984; Kovar, 1989; Feinleib, 1983). In many countries, medical billing data have been linked to hospitalization and other medical record datasets (Strom, 1989). Given the ease with which records can be linked by computers, it is likely that medical record linkage studies will be conducted with increasing frequency.

SUMMARY

Morbidity statistics provide information on the risk of developing disease (incidence) or of having disease (prevalence). Disease incidence is described by the incidence rate, the number of new cases of disease that occur in a population during a given time period divided by the number of persons in that population during that time period who were at risk of becoming a new case. A special type of incidence rate is the secondary attack rate, which is the incidence of disease among those persons exposed to a given case (the index case). Secondary attack rates are useful in studies of transmissibility of the causal agent and can also be used to evaluate the efficacy of a prophylactic agent.

Disease prevalence is described by the prevalence rate. For a given disease, the prevalence rate equals the incidence rate multiplied by the average duration of the disease. The prevalence rate can provide information about the frequency of disease in the community at a specified time (known as point prevalence) or during a period of time (period prevalence). Such data are available from a variety of sources, including the government, insurance companies, health care providers, and dedicated surveys of health status and disease occurrence. Undetected cases of disease can be discovered through screening programs designed to find asymptomatic but treatable individuals.

One means of obtaining morbidity statistics is through a surveillance system. Surveillance systems allow for the routine collection, analysis, and dissemination of information on disease occurrence in the community. If an increase in disease frequency is found, the health authorities are notified so that appropriate disease control activities can be implemented. Active surveillance relies upon routine review of health care records to ascertain new cases of disease. Passive surveillance depends upon reports of disease occurrence to ascertain incident cases. In sentinel surveillance, the occurrence of events indicative of specific health problems in the population is ascertained.

Cross-sectional studies provide information on the frequency of disease in a population. Repeated cross-sectional studies of the same population form a morbidity survey. These surveys are conducted to provide information on both disease occurrence and the correlates of disease in the community on a periodic or continuing basis. Such surveys are now conducted on a regular basis (usually annually) in a number of countries. Information on disease incidence and prevalence is usually gathered, depending on the type of survey. One must remember that the availability of morbidity survey data does not mean that the information itself is valid. Studies of validity suggest that these data must be viewed with some caution.

In order to provide a basis for understanding the validity of laboratory and other measures of health and disease, epidemiologists determine the sensitivity and specificity of a given test. Sensitivity measures the proportion of diseased persons detected by the test; specificity measures the proportion of those without the disease ascertained by the test. Positive predictive value measures the probability that someone with a positive test result actually has the disease, and negative predictive value, the probability that someone with a negative test result does not have the disease. The sensitivity and specificity of a test do not change from population to population. However, the predictive values of a test will vary among populations to the degree that the prevalence of disease varies. As prevalence increases, the positive predictive value increases and the negative predictive value decreases.

Another aspect of understanding such measures of disease is the variability inherent in their use. In X-ray readings, cytology examinations, physical examination findings, and other measures requiring judgment, such variability is present. This variability has two components, intraobserver and interobserver. A measure of of the degree of agreement for each component is κ, kappa. If κ is ≤ 0.0, then no more agreement is present than would be expected by chance. The closer κ is to 1.0, the stronger the agreement is compared with what would be expected by chance.

One approach to the assembly and use of morbidity information is the merger of various health records and personal identifiers into a single comprehensive record (record linkage). Such a unified record can be used for epidemiologic investigations and also benefits a patient who presents to a health care facility for diagnosis and treatment by providing a compilation of all examinations, laboratory findings, and therapeutics prescribed for the patient.

STUDY PROBLEMS

1. Why might clinical health care professionals find positive and negative predictive values more useful than sensitivity and specificity in evaluating a test?
2. The serologic test for past exposure to HIV is very sensitive and also very specific. In the early 1980s, during the first phase of the HIV epidemic, it was suggested that everyone in the United States be screened for past exposure to HIV. Why was this policy not followed?
3. What are the potential strengths and weaknesses of operating a registry for a disease in a community?
4. A colleague informs the local epidemiologist of a new screening test for the early detection of lung cancer. How might the test be assessed before it is used by the general medical community?
5. The World Health Organization MONICA project has established myocardial infarction registries around the world. What problems might attend the establishment of such registries?
6. Many academic medical centers maintain tumor registries. In what ways might such data be used by the epidemiologist? What are the limitations of such data?

7. A health officer has found that in a community of 100,000 persons, there are 250 new cases of osteoarthritis each year. The disease is present, on average, for 10 years. In planning for needed arthritis health care resources, one needs to know the prevalence of the disease. What is it?

8. The secondary attack rate was originally developed as a measure of the extent of familial aggregation of infectious diseases. Give at least four explanations for the observation of familial aggregation in a disease of unknown etiology.

9. Under what circumstances would it be desirable to minimize the percentage of individuals with false negative results on a test? Or with false positive results?

REFERENCES

Acheson, E. D. 1967. *Medical Record Linkage.* London: Oxford University Press.

———. 1987. "Introduction." In *Textbook of Medical Record Linkage.* J. A. Baldwin, E. D. Acheson, and W. J. Graham, eds. Oxford: Oxford University Press.

Adams, P. F., and Benson, V. 1990. "Current estimates from the National Health Interview Survey, 1989." National Center for Health Statistics. *Vital Health Stat* 10:176.

Alderson, M., and Dowie, R. 1979. *Health Surveys and Related Studies.* Oxford: Pergammon Press.

Alderson, M. R. 1984. "Health information resources: United Kingdom—health and social factors." In *Oxford Textbook of Public Health.* W. W. Holland, R. Detels, and G. Knox, eds. Oxford: Oxford University Press, pp. 21–51.

———. 1988. *Mortality, Morbidity and Health Statistics.* New York: Stockton Press.

Alter, M. J., Mares, A., Hadler, S. C., and Maynard, J. E. 1987. "The effects of underreporting on the apparent incidence and epidemiology of acute viral hepatitis." *Am. J. Epidemiol.* 125:133–139.

Bahn, A. K., Gorwitz, K., Klee, G. D., Kramer, M., and Tuerk, I. 1965. "Services received by Maryland residents in facilities directed by a psychiatrist." *Pub. Health Rep.* 80: 405–416.

Beral, V., Bull, D., Jaffe, H., Evan, B., Gill, N., Tillet, H., and Swerdlow, A. J. 1991. "Is risk of Kaposi's sarcoma in AIDS patients in Britain increased if sexual partners came from United States or Africa?" *BMJ* 302:624–625.

Beral, V., Peterman, T. A., Berkelman, R. L., Jaffe, H. W. 1990. "Kaposi's sarcoma among persons with AIDS: a sexually transmitted infection?" *Lancet* 335:123–128.

Brachott, D., and Mosley, J. W. 1972. "Viral hepatitis in Israel: the effect of canvassing physicians on notifications and the apparent epidemiological pattern." *Bull. World Health Org.* 46:457–464.

Chyba, M. M., and Washington, L. R. 1990. "Questionnaires from the National Health Interview Survey, 1980–84." National Center for Health Statistics. *Vital Health Stat* 1:24.

Cohen, J. 1960. "A coefficient of agreement for nominal scales." *Educ. Psych. Meas.* 20: 37–46.

Colsher, P. L., and Wallace, R. B. 1991. "Epidemiologic considerations in studies of cognitive function in the elderly: methodology and nondementing acquired dysfunction." *Epid. Rev.* 13:1–27.

Commission on Chronic Illness. 1957. *Chronic Illness in the United States Vol. IV, Chronic Illness in a Large City: The Baltimore Study.* Cambridge, Mass.: Harvard University Press.

———. 1959. *Chronic Illness in the United States Vol. III, Chronic Illness in a Rural Area: The Hunterdon Study.* Reported by R. E. Trussell and J. Elinson. Cambridge, Mass.: Harvard University Press.

Davis, J. P., and Vergeront, J. M., 1982. "The effect of publicity on the reporting of Toxic-Shock Syndrome in Wisconsin." *J. Infect. Dis.* 145:449–457.

Dunn, H. L. 1946. "Record linkage." *Am. J. Pub. Health* 36:1412–1416.

Eylenbosch, W. J., and Noah, N. D. 1988. *Surveillance in Health and Disease.* Oxford: Oxford University Press.

Feinleib, M. 1983. "Data bases, data banks and data dredging: the agony and the ectasy." *J. Chron. Dis.* 37:783–790.

Fox, J. P. 1981. "Record linkage and occupational mortality." In *Recent Advances in Occupational Health.* J. Corbett McDonald, ed. Edinburgh: Livingstone.

Fraser, P., Beral, V., and Chilvers, C. 1978. "Monitoring disease in England and Wales: methods applicable to routine data-collecting systems." *J. Epid. Com. Health* 32: 294–302.

Frost, W. H. 1941. "The familial aggregation of infectious diseases." In *The Papers of Wade Hampton Frost, M.D.,* K. F. Maxcy, ed. New York: The Commonwealth Fund, pp. 543–552.

Gillum, R. F. 1978. "Community surveillance for cardiovascular disease: methods, problems, applications—a review." *J. Chron. Dis.* 31:87–94.

Gordis, L., Lilienfeld, A. M., and Rodriguez, R. 1969. "An evaluation of the Maryland Rheumatic Fever Registry." *Pub. Health Rep.* 84:333–339.

Halperin, W., and Baker, E. L., eds. 1992. *Public Health Surveillance.* New York: Van Nostrand Reinhold.

Harlow, S. D., and Linet, M. S. 1989. "Agreement between questionnaire data and medical records: the evidence for accuracy of recall." *Am. J. Epidemiol.* 129:233–248.

Heaseman, M. A., and Clarke, J. A. 1979. "Medical record linkage in Scotland." *Health Bull.* 37:97–103.

Heston, J. F., Kelly, J.A.B., Meigs, J. W., and Flannery, J. T. 1986. *Forty-five Years of Cancer Incidence in Connecticut.* NCI Monograph No. 70., Washington, D.C.: U.S. Government Printing Office.

Hinds, M. W., Skaggs, J. W., and Bergeisen, G. H. 1985. "Benefit-cost analysis of active surveillance of primary care physicians for hepatitis A." *Am. J. Pub. Health* 75:176–177.

Horn, P. L., Lowell, D. M., LiVolsi, V. A., and Boyle, C. A. 1985. "Reproducibility of the cytologic diagnosis of human papilloma virus infection." *Acta Cytologica* 29: 692–694.

Jabine, T. 1987. "Reporting chronic conditions in the National Health Interview Survey. A review of tendencies from evaluation studies and methodological test." National Center for Health Statistics. *Vital Health Stat.* 2:105.

Jekel, J. F. 1984. "The Rainbow Reviews: publications of the National Center for Health Statistics." *J. Chron. Dis.* 37:681–688.

Kovar, M. G. 1989. "Data Systems of the National Center for Health Statistics." National Center for Health Statistics. *Vital Health Stat.* 1:23.

Krueger, D. E. 1957. "Measurement of prevalence of chronic disease by household interviews and clinical evaluations." *Am. J. Pub. Health* 47:953–960.

Landis, J. R., and Koch, G. G. 1977. "The measurement of observer agreement for categorical data." *Biometrics* 33:159–174.

Langmuir, A. D. 1963. "The surveillance of communicable diseases of national importance." *N. Engl. J. Med.* 268:182–192.

————. 1971. "Evolution of the concept of surveillance in the United States." *Proc. R. Soc. Med.* 64:681–689.

Lerner, P. R. 1974. "Social Security Disability Applicant Statistics, 1970." United States Department of Health, Education, and Welfare, Social Security Administration, Office of Research and Statistics Pub No. (SSA) 75-11911, Washington, D.C.: U.S. Government Printing Office.

Lilienfeld, A. M., Parkhurst, E., Patton, R., and Schlessinger, E. R. 1951. "Accuracy of supplemental medical information on birth certificates." *Pub. Health Rep.* 66:191–198.

Lilienfeld, A. M., Bross, I.D.J., and Sartwell, P. E. 1953. "Observations on an outbreak of infectious hepatitis in Baltimore during 1951." *Amer. J. Publ. Health* 43:1085–1096.

Madow, W. G. 1967. "Interview data on chronic conditions compared with information derived from medical records." National Center for Health Statistics. *Vital Health Stat.* 2:23.

————. 1973. "Net differences in interview data on chronic conditions and information derived from medical records." National Center for Health Statistics. *Vital Health Stat.* 2:57.

Marier, R. 1977. "The reporting of communicable diseases." *Am. J. Epidemiol.* 105: 587–90.

Marquis, K. H., Cannell, C. F., and Laurent, A. 1971. "Reporting health events in household interviews, effects of reinforcement, question length, and reinterviews." National Center for Health Statistics. *Vital Health Stat.* 2:45.

McCall, M. G., and Acheson, E. D. 1968. "Respiratory disease in infancy." *J. Chron. Dis.* 21:349–59.

McDonald, G. W., Fisher, G. F., and Pentz, P. C. 1966. "Diabetes screening activities, July 1958 to June 1963." In *Chronic Diseases and Public Health,* A. M. Lilienfeld and A. J. Gifford, eds. Baltimore: The Johns Hopkins Press, pp. 652–662.

Milham, S. 1963. "Underreporting of incidence of cleft lip and palate." *Amer. J. Dis. Child.* 106:185–188.

Morrison, A. S. 1992. *Screening in Chronic Disease,* 2nd ed. New York: Oxford University Press.

Most, A. S., and Peterson, D. R. 1969. "Myocardial infarction surveillance in a metropolitan community." *JAMA* 208:2433–2438.

Muir, C., Waterhouse, J., Mack, T., Powell, J., Whelan, S., eds. 1987. *Cancer Incidence in Five Continents, Volume V.* Lyon: IARC.

National Center for Health Statistics. 1963. *Origin, Program, and Operation of the U.S. National Health Survey.* PHS Pub. No. 100, Series 1, No. 1, United States Department of Health, Education, and Welfare, Washington, D.C.: U.S. Government Printing Office.

National Center for Health Statistics. 1968. "Design and methodology for a national survey of nursing homes." National Center for Health Statistics. *Vital Health Stat.* 2:7.

Nelson, L. M., Longstreth Jr, W. T., Koepsell, T. D., and van Belle, G. 1990. "Proxy respondents in epidemiologic research." *Epid. Rev.* 12:71–86.

Newcombe, H. B. 1969. "The use of medical record linkage for population and genetic studies." *Methods Inf. Med.* 8:7–11.

———. 1974. "Record linkage for studies of environmental carcinogenesis." In *Proceedings Tenth Canadian Cancer Conference, 1973.* Toronto: University of Toronto Press.

Office of Population Censuses and Surveys. 1973. *General Household Survey: introductory report.* London: HMSO.

———. 1978. "Household mortality from the longitudinal study." *Population Trends, No. 14.* London: HMSO.

Rutstein, D. D., Berenberg, W., Chalmers, T. C., Child, C. G., Fishman, A. P., and Perrin, E. B. 1976. "Measuring the quality of medical care: a clinical method." *N. Engl. J. Med.* 294:582–588.

Rutstein, D. D., Mullan, R. J., Frazier, T. M., Halperin, W. E., Melius, J. M., and Sestito, J. P. 1983. "Sentinel health events (occupational): a basis for physician recognition and public health surveillance." *Am. J. Pub. Health* 73:1054–1062.

Sanders, B. S. 1962. "Have morbidity surveys been oversold?" *Am. J. Pub. Health* 52: 1648–1659.

Schaffner, W., Scoot, H. D., Rosenstein, B. J., and Byrne, E. B. 1971. "Innovative communicable disease reporting." *HSMHA Health Reps.* 86:431–436.

Sherman, I. L., and Langmuir, A. D. 1952. "Usefulness of communicable disease reports." *Pub. Health Rep.* 67:1249–1257.

Soda, T. A. 1965. "A nation-wide simple morbidity survey in Japan." In *Trends in the Study of Morbidity and Mortality.* Geneva: World Health Organization, pp. 181–196.

Soda, T. A., and Kosaki, N. 1975. *Twenty Years of the Japanese National Committee on Vital Statistics.* Geneva: World Health Organization.

Spiegelman, M. 1968. *Introduction to Demography.* Rev. ed. Cambridge, Mass.: Harvard University Press.

Strom, B. L., ed. 1989. *Pharmacoepidemiology.* New York: Churchill, Livingstone.

Sydenstricker, E. 1974. "Statistics of morbidity." In *The Challenge of Facts, Selected Public Health Papers of Edgar Sydenstricker,* R. V. Kasius, ed. New York: Milbank Memorial Fund, Prodist, pp. 228–245.

Thacker, S. B., and Berkelman, R. L. 1988. "Public health surveillance in the United States." *Epid. Rev.* 10:164–190.

Thacker, S. B., Redmond, S., and Rothenberg, R. M. 1986. "A controlled trial of disease surveillance strategies." *Am. J. Prev. Med.* 2:345–350.

United States National Health Survey. 1961. *Reporting of Hospitalization in the Health Interview Survey.* Health Statistics Series D, No. 4, U.S. Department of Health, Education and Welfare, Washington, D.C.: Public Health Service.

Vogt, R. L., LaRue, D., Klaucke, D. N., and Jillson, D. A. 1983. "Comparison of an active and passive surveillance system of primary care providers for hepatitis, measles, rubella, and salmonellosis in Vermont." *Am. J. Pub. Health* 73:795–797.

Woolsey, T. D., Lawrence, P. S., and Balamuth, E. 1962. "An evaluation of chronic disease prevalence data from the Health Interview Survey." *Am. J. Pub. Health* 52: 1631–1637.

World Health Organization. 1985. *Report of the expanded programme on immunization.* WHO, Geneva (EPI/GEN/85/1).

————. 1988. *Report of the expanded programme on immunization.* WHO, Geneva (EPI/GEN/88/Wp. 4).

Yerushalmy, J. 1947. "Statistical problems in assessing methods of medical diagnosis, with special reference to X-ray techniques." *Pub. Health Rep.* 62:1432–1449.

7

MORBIDITY STUDIES

As with mortality, epidemiologists are interested in the occurrence of morbidity by **time, place and persons.** The reasoning processes used in interpreting morbidity data are similar to those applied to mortality statistics, but such data are not bound by the limitations of death certificates. One can therefore use more personal characteristics for analysis. In addition, epidemiologists often conduct their own morbidity studies, **cross-sectional surveys,** in selected communities and thus obtain information that is particularly relevant to the etiological hypotheses for the specific disease under consideration.

TIME

One aspect of the distribution of an illness in time was considered in the discussion of incubation periods in Chapter 3; basically, these periods represent the time distribution of the onset of disease after exposure to an etiological agent. Much of the discussion of time trends of mortality in Chapter 5 applies equally well to trends in the incidence and prevalence of disease.

An aspect of time distribution that has not been discussed previously is the seasonal trend of disease. Many diseases, particularly the infectious ones, occur more frequently at particular times of the year. In some instances, there are clear-cut explanations for the seasonality; many arthropod-borne diseases, such as Lyme disease, occur more frequently during the summer months because the arthropod vectors of the disease are present then (Figure 7–1) (Ciesielski et al., 1989). The seasonal distribution of asthma attacks is quite different, showing an

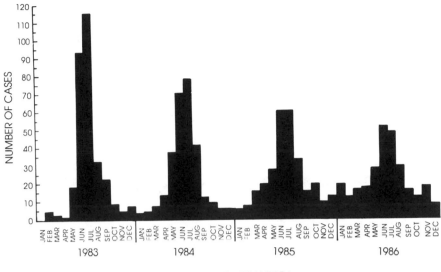

Figure 7-1. Reported number of Lyme disease cases in the United States, by onset month, 1983–1986. *Source:* Ciesielski et al. (1989).

increase in the early fall and reaching its highest levels in the late fall (Figure 7–2). Weiss (1990) examined the seasonality of hospitalization for asthma in the United States between 1982 and 1986 among persons aged less than 35 years, 35 to 64 years, and 65 years and older (Figure 7–3). He observed a distinct peak in asthma hospitalizations among persons 5 to 34 years of age during the fall months, while the pattern for older adults tended to peak in the winter and spring. The pattern for the younger age group probably reflects seasonal changes in the environmental allergen ''triggers'' of the disease. The patterns among the older adults

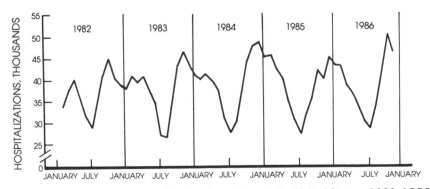

Figure 7-2. Number of hospitalizations for asthma in the United States, 1982–1986, by month. *Source:* Weiss (1990).

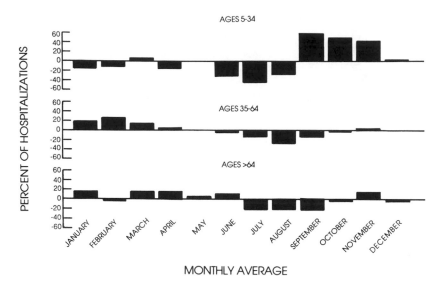

Figure 7–3. Deviation from the average monthly number of hospitalizations for asthma in the United States during 1982–1986, in the stated month, for three different age groups. *Source:* Weiss (1990).

resemble those for bronchitis, influenza, and pneumonia. In older adults, asthma occurrence may therefore be related to co-morbidity with an infectious agent. For instance, a bronchitic infection in an older adult might trigger the asthmatic attack.

The seasonal occurrence of a disease has been used to differentiate between diseases. In his classic study of endemic typhus fever conducted at a time when many investigators thought that endemic typhus in the United States was identical to epidemic typhus fever in Europe, Maxcy (1926) noted that the two diseases differed in their seasonal distribution (Figure 7–4). Together with other epidemiologic evidence (to be discussed below), this observation indicated that these were two distinct diseases with different modes of transmission.

PLACE

The same issues that have been considered in interpreting the occurrence of mortality by place also apply to morbidity. Morbidity data, however, make it possible to analyze disease distribution in smaller geographic areas than do mortality data, as morbidity data are usually derived from surveys in which living respondents can be interviewed. Therefore, one can consider very specific factors that influence morbidity distributions and more specific and definitive etiological hypotheses can be developed.

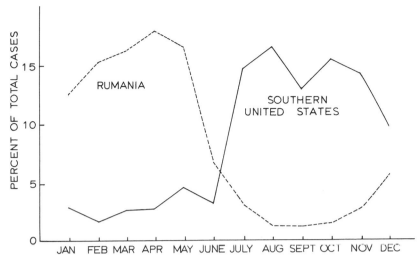

Figure 7–4. Percent distribution of cases of endemic typhus fever by month, Southern United States (Alabama and Savannah, Ga.), 1922–1925 and epidemic typhus fever in Rumania, 1922–1924. *Source:* Maxcy (1926).

A classic example of the use of place in deriving etiological inferences is the above-mentioned study of endemic typhus fever (Maxcy, 1926). At the time of that study, it was known that Old World (epidemic) typhus fever was transmitted from person to person by the louse. From clinical, serological, and experimental evidence, many investigators considered the two diseases to be similar and therefore inferred that endemic typhus was also louse-borne.

Maxcy observed the focal distribution of the disease in certain areas, among them Montgomery, Alabama. Using a "spot map," he analyzed the distribution of cases of disease by place of residence (Figure 7–5) and found no distinct localization of cases. Considering the question of contact, however, he felt that an employed person would be exposed to an even greater number of contacts at his place of occupation than at home and, therefore, he distributed the cases according to place of employment (Figure 7–6). This suggested a focal center of the disease in the heart of the business district. A more detailed analysis of the places of employment indicated a high attack rate among those working at food depots, groceries, feed stores, and restaurants. This led Maxcy to suggest a rodent reservoir of the disease—rats or mice—and transmission by fleas, mites, or louse in terms of the differences in the cases' seasonal distribution (Figure 7–4), their distribution by place of employment (Figures 7–5 and 7–6), and the lack of evidence of communicability from person to person. His inferences were subsequently shown to be correct in an investigation by Dyer that incriminated the rat as the reservoir and the rat flea as the insect vector of *Rickettsia Mooseri (R. Typhi)* (Woodward, 1970).

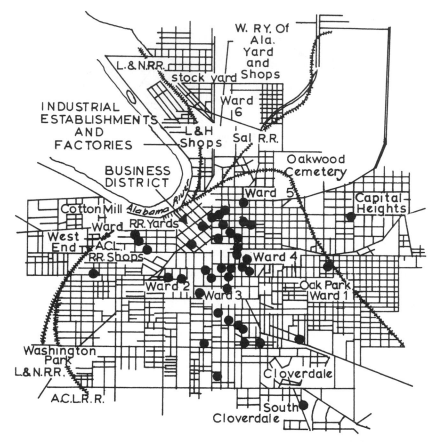

Figure 7–5. Distribution of cases of endemic typhus fever by residence, Montgomery, Alabama, 1922–1925. *Source:* Maxcy (1926).

A more recent example of the use of place in epidemiologic investigations is Gordis's study of rheumatic fever in Baltimore, Maryland. Between 1960–1964 and 1968–1970, he found that the incidence of rheumatic fever among black children in Baltimore, Maryland, had declined by 35.4 percent while the rates for white children had remained essentially unchanged (Figure 7–7) (Gordis, 1973, 1985). One explanation for this observation was the effectiveness of inner-city comprehensive-care programs in Baltimore in providing prompt and efficacious treatment of streptococcal infections. Eligibility for these programs was based on residence in specified census tracts. Gordis compared the annual incidence rate of rheumatic fever among inner-city black children in Baltimore resident in census

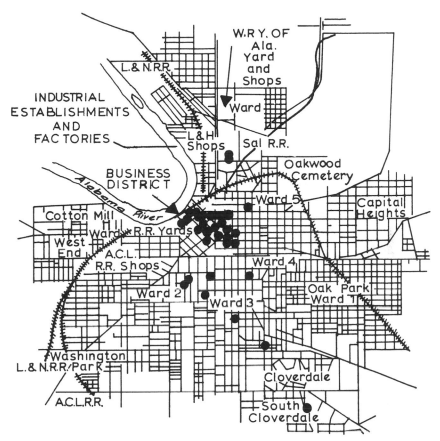

Figure 7–6. Distribution of cases of endemic typhus fever by place of employment or, if unemployed, by place of residence, Montgomery, Alabama, 1922–1925. *Source:* Maxcy (1926).

tracts eligible for treatment in the comprehensive-care programs with the rate of those resident in census tracts not eligible for care (Figure 7–8). The results showed a decline in the incidence of rheumatic fever among children resident in the areas eligible for comprehensive care but not among those who were not eligible for such care. This finding suggested that the programs had altered the natural history of streptococcal infection and thus reduced the occurrence of subsequent rheumatic fever.

The direct influence of place on the occurrence of a disease is illustrated by Lyme disease, caused by a spirochete, *Borrelia burgdorferi,* and spread by

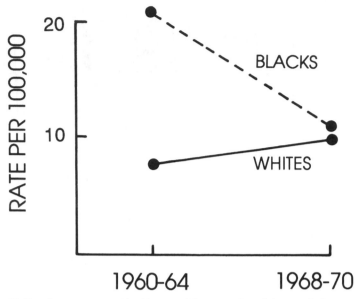

Figure 7–7. Average annual incidence of first attacks of rheumatic fever, ages 5 to 19 years, by race, Baltimore, Maryland, 1960–1970. *Source:* Gordis (1985).

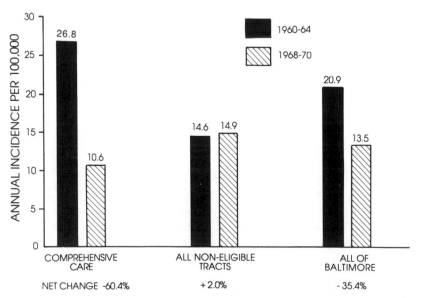

Figure 7–8. Comprehensive care and changes in rheumatic fever incidence 1960–1964 and 1968–1979, Baltimore, black population, ages 5 to 14 years. *Source:* Gordis (1985).

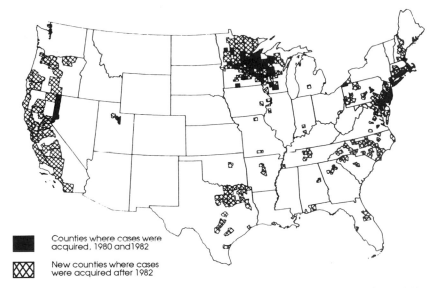

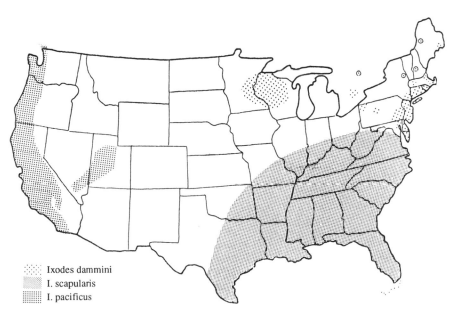

Figure 7–9. Cases of Lyme disease in the United States, by county of acquisition, 1980–1986 (excluding 1981). *Source:* Ciesielski (1989).

Figure 7–10. Geographic distribution in the United States of tick species carrying *B. burgdorferi. Source:* Anderson (1989).

infected Ixodid ticks. Figure 7–9 shows the counties of the United States in which cases of Lyme disease occurred during 1980–1986 (excluding 1981) (Ciesielski et al., 1989). The four regions of the country in which the disease has been reported correspond to the distribution of the three Ixodid tick species that carry the disease (Figure 7–10) (Anderson, 1989). The temporal spread of the disease by the various tick species can be seen in Figure 7–9. No cases developed in counties in which none of the three Ixodid species were present.

These studies illustrate the various ways in which place influences the occurrence of disease. In one instance, endemic typhus, the important place was that of employment, where a disease reservoir was present. In another, place represented an intervention that altered the natural history of streptococcal infection. In the last example, Lyme disease, place represented the presence of the tick species necessary for the continued spread of the etiological agent.

TIME AND SPACE CLUSTERS

A term that has been used increasingly in recent years to describe the distribution of disease in time or place, or both, is "cluster." A clustering of cases in time might indicate that certain etiological factors were introduced into the environment at that time, for example, an infectious agent, a drug, or an environmental pollutant (Centers for Disease Control, 1990; Rothenberg et al., 1990). The food-poisoning outbreak discussed in Chapter 1 was a clustering of cases of gastroenteritis due to exposure to contaminated food. The increase in mortality among asthmatics discussed in Chapter 5 also represented a temporal clustering that resulted from the introduction of a particular "therapeutic" agent. In these instances, it was possible to compute either attack rates or mortality rates when analyzing the data. Clustering of cases in space in Maxcy's spot maps showed the focal distribution of endemic typhus, thus providing the evidence that finally incriminated an animal reservoir and mode of infection.

Space-time clustering data were valuable in unraveling the etiology of infectious diseases, so it is not surprising that interest has now developed in studying the clustering of cases of diseases of unknown etiology to determine whether they may have an infectious origin. For example, there have been many studies of clusters of cases of leukemia and other forms of cancer where an infectious agent is considered to be a possible etiological factor (Caldwell, 1990; Grufferman and Delzell, 1984). These studies have resulted in the development of a variety of complex statistical techniques to determine whether or not these "clusters" could have arisen by chance alone. The advantages and disadvantages of the various statistical techniques utilized is a controversial area of epidemiology (Smith,

1982; Tango, 1984; Shaw et al., 1988; Raubertas, 1988; Centers for Disease Control, 1990).

A major problem in many of these studies is that they deal only with clusters of cases and generally do not take into consideration the varying concentrations of the population in the communities where the cases appear. The occurrence of a cluster should be viewed as only a lead to the possible common exposure of a segment of the population to an etiological agent that may possibly be infectious or toxic. If the search for an infectious or toxic agent is of major interest, these studies should be followed by epidemiologic studies comparing population groups such as families, neighborhoods, and schools whose members have been exposed. Secondary attack rates can then be computed and compared, as has been done most recently for multiple sclerosis (Kurtzke and Hyllested, 1986, 1988; Kurtzke et al., 1988). If the clusters are limited to families, it becomes necessary to consider the possible influence of genetic factors as well as environmental factors that are common to family members.

PERSONS

Epidemiologists are interested in variables that may influence morbidity such as age, gender, ethnicity, and social status. The number of personal characteristics available for study is not as limited as in analyses of mortality data, where the information must often be obtained from death certificates. Routinely collected morbidity statistics share some of the limitations of mortality data, but the variables included in the National Health Survey or in disease registers are generally more extensive than those on death certificates.

An epidemiologist who wishes to determine the incidence or prevalence of a disease entity in a community by means of a morbidity survey can include any factor thought relevant to the investigation, such as demographic, physiological, biochemical, or immunological characteristics and personal living habits. This would permit the analysis of the relationship of these factors to the disease within the surveyed population in terms of individual characteristics (see Chapter 1, p. 12). However, the epidemiologist is also interested in the distribution of the relevant factors in the community as a whole. Consistency in the distribution of a set of these factors with that of morbidity in the population clearly strengthens the evidence upon which an etiological inference is based; this will be discussed in Chapter 12.

The few personal characteristics already reviewed in Chapter 5 in the context of mortality statistics are also pertinent to morbidity studies. These will be discussed together with several additional factors.

Age

Many infectious diseases such as measles and chickenpox are considered child-hood diseases; that is, their highest frequency of occurrence is in the younger age groups. Before the widespread use of measles vaccination in the United States, the incidence rate of measles increased sharply from about one to four years of age, probably as a result of the increasing early socialization of the child and thus increasing exposure to the causative virus (Figure 7–11). This age group also had a low proportion of immune individuals because they had not previously been exposed to the virus. After age four, the incidence rate gradually decreased until it approached zero at about 12–15 years of age. Since an attack of measles conferred life-long immunity, the increasing incidence rate up to age four resulted in a high proportion of immune individuals in the age group from four to about thirteen years and few susceptibles who remained to be infected.

One aspect of age that we have not yet considered is the relationship of maternal age at the time of birth to disorders in the offspring. The relationship of maternal age to infant mortality and prematurity has been known for years, although there have been no widely accepted biological explanations. Perhaps the most consistently observed relationship between maternal age and disease in the offspring is the markedly increased incidence of Trisomy 21 (Down's Syndrome) with increasing maternal age (Figure 7–12) (Harlap, 1974; Hook and Lindjso, 1978).

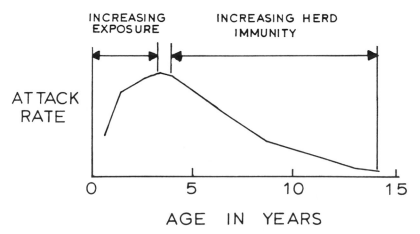

Figure 7–11. Measles age-specific incidence.

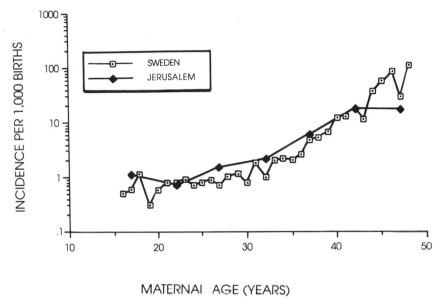

Figure 7–12. Incidence rate of Trisomy 21 (Down's Syndrome) by maternal age in Jerusalem, Israel, 1964–1970, and Sweden, 1968–1970. *Source:* Hook and Linksjo (1978) and Harlap (1974).

Gender

As with mortality, one observes differences in morbidity that are gender-related. Biological and behavioral factors related to gender contribute to differences in the prevalence or incidence of a variety of conditions including heart disease, accident-related disabilities, and autoimmune diseases. The initial observation in the AIDS outbreak that the disease occurred only among men provided one of the clues to the means of disease transmission. Men still have a higher prevalence of HIV infection; the nature of disease transmission, the source of the outbreak, and the behavior of a subgroup of men account for this gender difference.

In the epidemiology of kuru, a neurologic disorder endemic in the New Guinea highlands, it was noted that women were at much greater risk of developing the disease than were men (Gajdusek, 1977). Subsequent investigations revealed that the disease was caused by a ''slow'' virus transmitted during a cannibalistic ritual in which the brains of the deceased were consumed. Since the women were usually given the task of preparing the body for funeral, they often consumed the uncooked brains. In this instance, the epidemiologic characterization of the disease provided an important insight into the etiology of the condition.

Race and Ethnicity

As discussed in Chapter 5, variables such as race, ethnicity, and religion may be associated with some genetic traits such as sickle-cell anemia or Tay-Sach's disease but can also be associated with a wide range of life-style characteristics, such as diet, smoking, alcohol consumption, and childbearing patterns, all of which can be related to health outcomes. Furthermore, race and ethnicity are often associated with socioeconomic status, which may be related to educational level, access to health care, occupation, and other variables that may affect health.

An example was a small epidemic of tapeworm infestation due to *D. latum* among Jewish housewives in the 1940s. Knowing the ethnic group and its eating habits, the investigators were able to trace the epidemic to contaminated fish; housewives became infected by sampling uncooked gefilte fish as they tasted its seasoning (Desowitz, 1978).

SUMMARY

Demographic studies of morbidity concern the classic epidemiologic triad of time, place, and person. **Time** may be viewed from the perspective of temporal trends, whether of morbidity or mortality. And it can also be viewed in terms of the seasonality of a disease. Some diseases characteristically occur in the fall or winter; others in the spring or summer. Whatever the seasonal pattern is, it carries important epidemiologic information about the etiology and natural history of the disease.

Place also conveys information about the etiology and natural history of a disease. If clusters of the disease exist, they may reflect a common exposure to the etiologic agent (such clusters can also occur by chance). Spot maps, in which a geographical feature of cases of the disease (e.g., residence, place of employment) is placed on a map, can provide insight into the etiology or transmission of the agent for a disease.

The characteristics of those **persons** who have developed a disease (in comparison with those who have not developed it) provide further information about the epidemiologic profile or pattern of the disease. Variation in the risk of disease with age may suggest endogenous and exogenous influences on the development of the condition. Gender, ethnicity, religion, and other personal characteristics may help identify those at high risk for a disease, leading to etiologic hypotheses and screening programs.

STUDY PROBLEMS

1. In the United States, St. Louis encephalitis, eastern equine encephalitis, and western equine encephalitis show similar seasonal incidence patterns, with a peak in the summer and early autumn, and few cases developing at other times of the year. Explain this pattern.
2. In the 1930s and the 1940s, the most common agent of hospital-acquired (nosocomial) infections was the staphlococcus bacteria. In the 1950s, it was the streptococcus bacteria. During the 1960s and 1970s, the most common agents were gram negative bacteria. What reasons might explain this changing etiology of nosocomial infections?
3. What factors might be responsible for the reemergence of tuberculosis in the late 1980s and early 1990s as a major cause of morbidity in the United States?
4. In the United States National Health Interview Survey, information was obtained from a sample of households on whether or not anyone in the household had diabetes. Additional information was also obtained regarding several aspects of diabetes, such as treatment and disability, for the periods July 1964–June 1965 and during 1973. The prevalence rate per 1,000 population obtained at these two times by age group and sex are shown in the following table.

AGE (YEARS)	1964–1965		AGE (YEARS)	1973	
	MALE	FEMALE		MALE	FEMALE
All ages	10.5	13.8	All ages	16.3	24.1
<25	1.2	1.3	<17	1.1	1.6
25–44	6.2	6.2	17–44	6.9	10.8
45–54	15.4	20.0 ⎤	45–64	40.6	44.4
55–64	32.0	41.4 ⎦			
65–74	47.1	60.6 ⎤	65+	60.3	91.3
75+	47.0	50.8 ⎦			

(a) What inferences would you derive from these data?
(b) Would you desire any additional information? If so, what?
(c) List a few types of studies that are suggested by the data.

5. The Third National Cancer Survey was conducted in seven metropolitan areas and two entire states of the United States during the three-year period 1969–1971 to obtain information on the incidence of different forms of cancer according to a variety of population characteristics. For all areas combined, the following average annual age-specific incidence rates (per 100,000 population) for cancer of the esophagus as a primary site were observed in white and black males. Discuss possible reasons for the difference in rates between the two groups.

AGE (YEARS)	WHITES	BLACKS
35–39	0.3	1.8
40–44	0.7	8.8
45–49	2.6	22.6
50–54	6.0	40.3
55–59	12.2	59.5
60–64	18.4	59.0
65–69	22.6	66.1
70–74	24.1	108.2
75–79	34.2	57.7
80–84	37.6	46.7
85+	32.1	43.4

6. On St. Lawrence Island, in the Bering Sea, an epidemic of mumps occurred in 1956. A survey demonstrated the following age-specific incidence rates, which were compared with those observed among families in Baltimore during an epidemic in 1959–60. What are the reasons for the difference in age-specific incidence rates between these two areas?

AGE (YEARS)	INCIDENCE RATE PER 100 EXPOSED SUSCEPTIBLES	
	ST. LAWRENCE ISLAND	BALTIMORE
<1	17	12
1–4	56	60
5–9	86	54
10–19	82	18
20–49	68	19
50+	21	0

REFERENCES

Anderson, J. F. 1989. "Epizootiology of *Borrelia* in *Ixodes* tick vectors and reservoir hosts." *Rev. Inf. Dis.* 11(Suppl 6):S1451–S1459.

Caldwell, G. G. 1990. "Twenty-two years of cancer cluster investigations at the Centers for Disease Control." *Am. J. Epidemiol.* 132(Supplement):S43–S47.

Centers for Disease Control. 1990. "Guidelines for investigating clusters of health events." *MMWR* 39(No. RR-11):1–23.

Ciesielski, C. A., Markowitz, L. E., Horsley, R., Hightower, A. W., Russell, H., and Broome, C. V. 1989. "Lyme disease surveillance in the United States, 1983–1986." *Rev. Inf. Dis.* 11(Suppl 6):S1435–1441.

Desowitz, R. S. 1978. "On New Guinea tapeworms and Jewish grandmothers." *Natural History* 85:22–27.

Gajdusek, D. C. 1977. "Unconventional viruses and the origin and disappearance of kuru." *Science* 197:943–960.

Gordis, L. 1973. "Effectiveness of comprehensive-care programs in preventing rheumatic fever." *New Engl. J. Med.* 289:331–335.

———. 1985. "The virtual disappearance of rheumatic fever in the United States: lessons in the rise and fall of disease." *Circulation* 72:1155–1162.

Grufferman, S., and Delzell, E. 1984. "Epidemiology of Hodgkin's disease." *Epi. Rev.* 6:76–106.

Harlap, S. 1974. "Down's syndrome in West Jerusalem." *Am. J. Epidemiol.* 97:225–232.

Hook, E. B., and Lindjso, A. 1978. "Down's syndrome in live births by single year maternal age interval in a Swedish study: comparisons with results from a New York State study." *Am. J. Hum. Genet.* 30:19–27.

Kurtzke, J. F., and Hyllested, K. 1986. "Multiple sclerosis in the Faroe Islands: II. clinical update, transmission, and the nature of multiple sclerosis." *Neurology* 36:307–328.

———. 1988. "Validity of epidemics of multiple sclerosis in the Faroe Islands." *Neuroepi.* 7:190–227.

Kurtzke, J. F., Hyllested, K., Arbuckle, J. D., Baerentsen, D. J., Jersild, C., Madden, D. L., Olsen, A., and Sever, J. L. 1988. "Multiple sclerosis in the Faroe Islands: IV. the lack of a relationship between canine distemper and the epidemics of MS." *Acta Neur. Scand.* 78:484–500.

Maxcy, K. F. 1926. "An epidemiological study of endemic typhus (Brill's disease) in the Southeastern United States with special reference to its mode of transmission." *Pub. Health Reps.* 41:2967–2995.

Raubertas, R. F. 1988. "Spatial and temporal analysis of disease occurrence for detection of clustering." *Biometrics* 44:1121–1129.

Rothenberg, R. B., Steinberg, K. K., and Thacker, S. B. 1990. "The public health importance of clusters: a note from the Centers for Disease Control." *Am. J. Epidemiol.* 132(Supplement):S3–S5.

Shaw, G. M., Selvin, S., Swan, S. H., Merrill, D., and Schulman, J. 1988. "An examination of three spatial disease clustering methodologies." *Int. J. Epidemiol.* 17:913–919.

Smith, P. G. 1982. "Spatial and temporal clustering." In *Cancer Epidemiology and Prevention,* D. Schottenfeld and J. F. Fraumeni, eds. Philadelphia: W. B. Saunders.

Tango, T. 1984. "The detection of disease clustering in time." *Biometrics* 40:15–26.

Weiss, K. B. 1990. "Seasonal trends in U.S. asthma hospitalizations and mortality." *JAMA* 263:2323–2328.

Woodward, T. E. 1970. "President's address: Typhus verdict in American history." *Transactions Amer. Clin. Climatol. Assoc.* 82:7–8.

III

EPIDEMIOLOGIC STUDIES

From the demographic studies in a community or population group described in Chapter 4 to 7, the epidemiologist may observe a statistical association between a population characteristic and the occurrence of a disease. Such associations, however, may be subject to an "ecological fallacy," as noted in Chapter 1. Clinical and/or experimental observations may also suggest an association. One attempts to confirm such associations by conducting **epidemiologic studies,** which determine whether these diseases or conditions are more often present in persons with the characteristic of interest than in those without it.

Epidemiologic investigations may be viewed as the application of the scientific method to populations. Just as a biological investigator wishes to observe the effect of a simple modification in the laboratory environment of two identical species, in the epidemiologic study one seeks to compare the effect of an exposure to a single factor on the incidence of disease in two otherwise identical populations.

Epidemiologic studies may be characterized as **experimental** or **observational** (Figure III–1). The major difference between the two is that in an experimental setting, the epidemiologist *controls the conditions* under which the study is to be conducted; in an observational setting, the epidemiologist is *not able* to control these conditions. In experiments, the epidemiologist controls the method of assigning subjects to either the treatment or the comparison groups. A commonly used means of assignment is to randomly allocate similar persons to the treatment or the comparison group; such an experimental study is called a **randomized clinical trial** and is discussed in Chapter 8. Most of the other types of experiments assign treatment to communities as an aggregate and are known as

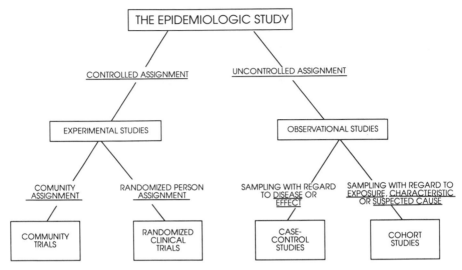

Figure III–1.   The anatomy of the epidemiologic study.

community trials; they are discussed in Chapter 9. Clearly, if there is an alternative between an experimental or an observational study, the former is preferred as the epidemiologist has greater control of the conditions under which the study is carried out. Experiments, however, are not always feasible. For example, consider conducting an experiment on the effects of cigarette smoking; one would have to randomly assign persons either to a group that would be required to smoke or to one that would not be allowed to smoke until the experiment was concluded. Such an experiment would be neither ethical nor practical.

In contrast to experimental epidemiologic studies (in which the epidemiologist assigns the exposure), in observational investigations the epidemiologist observes the associations between exposure and outcome. There are two methods of conducting such investigations: cohort studies and case-control studies. In a **cohort study,** one begins with a group of persons exposed to the factor of interest and a group of persons not exposed. These persons are then followed for the development of various conditions. Such studies are considered in Chapter 10.

Alternatively, in a **case-control study,** one assembles a group of persons with a disease (cases) and a comparison group of persons without the particular disease under investigation (controls); the history of past exposure to the factor of interest is then compared between the cases and the controls. Case-control studies are discussed in Chapter 11.

By its nature an observational study, in which the investigator has no control over exposure assignment, is open to alternative explanations for associations that are excluded in an experimental study. One common alternative explanation is known as **confounding,** in which the association between exposure to a factor and the consequent development of disease is distorted by an additional variable that is itself associated both with the factor and with the disease. An example was given in Chapter 4, in which the confounding effect of age was adjusted for in the comparison of mortality among residents of Alaska and Florida. The control of confounding in observational studies, a major activity of the epidemiologist, is discussed in Chapters 10 and 12 as well as the Appendix.

The synthesis of information provided by epidemiologic studies, together with that from demographic studies and from biology and medicine, is considered in Part IV, ''Using Epidemiologic Data.''

8

EXPERIMENTAL EPIDEMIOLOGY:
I. RANDOMIZED CLINICAL TRIALS

The strength of the experimental method lies in the investigator's direct control over the assignment of subjects (either individually or aggregated) to study groups. In observational studies, by contrast, the investigator essentially accepts the conditions as they are and makes observations about the populations to help answer questions about health and disease.

Broadly considered, there are two forms of epidemiologic experiments: (1) randomized clinical trials and (2) community trials or experiments (the latter are also referred to as *field experiments*). In **randomized clinical trials,** the efficacy of a preventive or therapeutic agent or procedure is tested in *individual subjects.* In **community trials,** as the term implies, a *group of persons as a whole* is used to determine the efficacy of a drug, procedure, or intervention. One example of such a community trial is the evaluation of fluoride in preventing dental caries, discussed in Chapter 1.

DESIGN AND CONDUCT OF THE RANDOMIZED CLINICAL TRIAL

To simplify the discussion, we will consider randomized clinical trials in terms of evaluating the efficacy of a drug in the treatment of a disease. However, such trials can also be used to evaluate a prophylactic agent, such as a vaccine; a public health procedure, such as a screening method; or a medical procedure, such as an operation (e.g., coronary artery bypass graft surgery). Specific conditions of the trial may have to be changed depending upon its purpose, but the general methods and principles, for the most part, remain the same.

The randomized clinical trial is an experiment in which individuals are **randomly** assigned to two (or more) groups, known as the "treatment" and the "comparison" groups. The treatment group is given the drug being tested and the comparison group is given the drug in current use; if no such drug exists, then a placebo, an inert substance such as a sugar pill or saline injection, is used. This approach is directly comparable to that of laboratory experiments.

Randomization

In the randomized clinical trial, the treatment and comparison groups should be comparable in all respects except the one being studied, i.e., the drug being tested (Hill, 1951, 1977; Altman, 1991; Fleiss, 1986; Peto et al., 1976, 1977; Meinert, 1986). The epidemiologist can achieve comparability on factors that are known to have an influence on the outcome, such as age, sex, race, or severity of disease, by *matching* for these factors. But one cannot match persons for factors whose influence is not known or cannot be measured. This problem can be resolved by the random assignment of individuals to the treatment and comparison groups. Randomization helps to ensure that the distribution of *all* factors—known and unknown, measurable and not measurable—except for the therapy being studied, is based on chance and not some factor, such as patient preference, that may lead to a bias in assignment. In addition, randomization is the means by which the investigator avoids introducing conscious or subconscious bias into the process of allocating individuals to the treatment or comparison groups. Preventing biased assignment is important as it permits a more definitive interpretation of the trial results.

Types of Randomized Clinical Trials

Within this basic framework there are several types of randomized clinical trials:

1. **Therapeutic trials,** in which a therapeutic agent or procedure is given in an attempt to cure the disease, *relieve* the symptoms, or prolong the survival of those with the disease.
2. **Intervention trials,** in which the investigator *intervenes* before a disease has developed in individuals with characteristics that increase their risk of developing the disease.
3. **Preventive trials,** in which an attempt is made to determine the efficacy of a *preventive* agent or procedure among those without the disease. These trials are also referred to as **prophylactic trials.**

Table 8–1 provides examples of these three kinds of studies. One should note that a fine line exists between the three types of clinical trials; indeed, intervention studies can be viewed as special types of either a therapeutic or a preventive trial.

If, in a randomized clinical trial of the first type, the therapeutic agent successfully cures the disease, relieves its symptoms, or increases survival, then that agent may be used to treat the disease. One such trial was that of early photocoagulation for persons who have developed diabetic retinopathy (Early Treatment Diabetic Retinopathy Study Research Group, 1991). Those who received this treatment had a 29 percent decrease in the incidence of severe visual loss five years after the therapy. Similarly, in the Beta-Blocker Heart Attack Trial (BHAT), those who received propanolol after a heart attack had 28 percent less mortality during the next 27 months than those who did not receive the drug (β-Blocker Heart Attack Trial Research Group, 1982).

The second type of trial, the treatment of risk factors by intervention, is illustrated by evaluations of drugs intended to reduce hypercholesterolemia and thus decrease the risk of developing coronary heart disease. If, in a randomized controlled trial, a drug successfully lowers serum cholesterol levels and this, in turn, reduces the incidence of coronary heart disease, the utility of the drug has been demonstrated. In addition, a strong link has been added to the chain of evidence showing a causal relationship between elevated serum cholesterol levels and coronary heart disease. An example of this approach is the Coronary Primary Prevention Trial (CPPT). In this randomized trial, individuals who received cholestyramine experienced a 19 percent reduction in coronary heart disease risk compared with persons in the placebo group (Lipid Research Clinics Program, 1984). The **cessation experiment** is also included in this category. Such a study differs from the others in that, instead of the addition of a mode of treatment, an attempt is made to evaluate the termination of a living habit considered to be of etiological importance. One such trial is the Oslo Heart Study, in which 1,232 men at high risk of cardiovascular disease were randomly allocated into two

Table 8–1. Types and Examples of Randomized Clinical Trials

TYPE	EXAMPLE
Therapeutic	AZT treatment for AIDS
	Simple mastectomy for breast cancer
Intervention	AZT treatment of HIV-positive subject without symptoms of AIDS
	Mammography to detect asymptomatic breast cancer
	Cholesterol-lowering drugs to decrease the risk of myocardial infarction
Preventive	Hepatitis B vaccination for hepatitis and hepatocellular carcinoma prevention
	Education in use of condoms to reduce the risk of HIV transmission and infection

groups (Hjerman et al., 1981). One group received nutritional advice on lowering the lipid content of their diets and an educational program on cigarette smoking cessation; the other group received no advice regarding either diet or smoking cessation. After five years, the mean serum cholesterol concentration among those in the intervention group was 13 percent lower than those in the control group; the serum triglyceride concentration was 20 percent lower in the intervention group compared with the control group. Also, average cigarette smoking levels declined by 45 percent more in the intervention group than in the control group. Cessation of a high-cholesterol diet and cigarette smoking (in the intervention group) resulted in a 47 percent decline in myocardial infarction and sudden death risk.

The last type of study, the testing of a preventive agent, is illustrated by the evaluation of a vaccine for a given disease or of some form of chemoprophylaxis, such as aspirin to prevent myocardial infarction or stroke. If a randomized clinical trial shows that the vaccine or chemoprophylactic agent lowers the incidence of the disease, then that vaccine or agent may have value as a preventive measure (Shapiro et al., 1988). An example of such a trial is the Physicians' Health Study, which randomized 22,071 United States physicians to receive either aspirin or a placebo to reduce cardiovascular disease morbidity and mortality (Hennekens and Eberlein, 1985). There was a 39 percent decline in nonfatal myocardial infarction rates in the group that took aspirin compared with the control group (Steering Committee of the Physicians' Health Study Research Group, 1988).

The general principles are essentially the same in conducting clinical trials for infectious and noninfectious diseases, but the spectrum of noninfectious diseases (see Figure 3–9) is more complex. Each stage in the course of a chronic disease usually lasts a number of years, varying with the disease and the individual, and it is often difficult to make the distinctions between the stages. In addition, the etiological agent(s) is often unknown. In many chronic diseases, however, something is usually known about factors that are associated with an increased risk of developing the disease. These "risk factors" include such characteristics as elevation of serum cholesterol (in the case of coronary heart disease) and high blood pressure (in both cerebrovascular disease and coronary heart disease). Thus, in diagramming the natural history of a chronic disease, we can replace "etiological agent" in Figure 3–9 with "risk factor" (Figure 8–1). The stage to which the disease has progressed at the time the trial is started determines the type of trial. The relationship between the risk factor and possible etiological factors for three diseases is shown in Table 8–2.

General Plan of a Clinical Trial

The plan of a clinical trial is formally stated in a **protocol,** which contains the *objectives* and *specific procedures* to be used in the trial. It must be written before

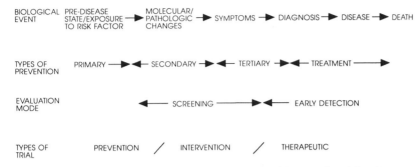

Figure 8–1. Diagrammatic representation of natural history of an infectious or non-infectious disease. *Source:* Meyskens (1988).

the start of the trial and should contain such information as the methods for selecting and then allocating the study groups, details on the performance of any laboratory tests, and the administration of the drug or other therapy. Once the protocol has been written, the epidemiologist compiles a "manual of operations." During the course of the trial, if any questions arise because of a given situation, the manual of operations is referred to as the guide for what the investigator is to do. An outline for a typical protocol is presented in Table 8–3. Bearman's description of how to write such a protocol is an excellent guide (Bearman, 1975). More recently, several textbooks on the subject have appeared (Meinert, 1986; Fleiss, 1986).

Selection of Study Groups

At the beginning of a clinical trial, a decision must be made regarding the characteristics of the population to be studied; that is, what age and sex groups, disease characteristics, etc. are eligible for inclusion in the experiment. For example, in the Hypertension Detection and Follow-Up Project (HDFP), a randomized trial of the efficacy of systematic antihypertensive therapy, the criteria for inclusion in the study population were an age of 30 to 69 years, an average home screening diastolic blood pressure of 95 mmHg or above and a confirmed follow-up average

Table 8–2. Spectrum of Selected Diseases Divided Into Three Categories

	PREDISEASE STATE	
ETIOLOGICAL FACTOR	RISK FACTOR	DISEASE
Diet?	Elevated serum cholesterol ---->Coronary heart disease	
Virus?	Hepatitis B ---------------->Hepatocellular carcinoma	
???	Elevated blood pressure------->Stroke	

Table 8–3.   General Outline of a Protocol for a Clinical Trial

---

1. Rationale and background for study
2. Specific objectives of study
3. Concise statement of the study design (masking, randomization schemes, types and duration of treatments, number of patients)
4. Criteria for including and excluding subjects (including subject recruitment)
5. Outline of treatment procedures
6. Definition of all clinical, laboratory, and other methods
7. Methods of assuring the integrity of the data
8. Major and minor outcomes (e.g., death, myocardial infarction)
9. Provisions for observing and recording side effects
10. Procedures for handling problem cases
11. Procedures for obtaining the informed consent of subjects
12. Procedures for periodic review of trial
13. Procedures for analyzing results
14. Procedures for termination of trial
15. Procedures for communicating results of trial to study subjects and other interested persons
16. Appendices: Forms

Source: Adapted from Bearman (1975).

diastolic blood pressure of 90 mmHg or above, absence of terminal illness, and noninstitutional residence (Davis et al., 1986). In brief, the investigator selects a reference or ''target'' population that may be composed of persons with a certain disease or set of characteristics related to a disease, or persons in specific age groups, geographic areas, or occupations that would suggest their inclusion in the study. The type of reference population selected depends on the purpose of the study as well as the difficulties involved in subject recruitment.

Sample Size

The number of persons (the **sample size**) necessary to detect an effect of a drug or procedure must be computed from various statistical formulae that have been developed (Meinert, 1986; Fleiss, 1986). The importance of having a sufficient number of subjects can be seen in an example.

Suppose that one conducts a randomized trial of the effectiveness of a given drug in treating lung cancer. The epidemiologist hopes to detect a decrease in mortality one year after initiation of the treatment of at least 50 percent compared with the current therapy. There are four possible outcomes of this trial (Table 8–4). If the trial shows that the drug was effective (as defined by the epidemiologist in this example, efficacy would mean that it decreased mortality by at least 50 percent during the year after treatment began) and in reality it is, then the epidemiologist has reached a correct conclusion. The same can be said if the treat-

Table 8–4.   The Possible Outcomes of a Randomized Clinical Trial

		ACTUAL EFFECT	
		TREATMENT EFFECTIVE	TREATMENT NOT EFFECTIVE
Conclusion Resulting from Trial	Treatment Effective	Correct Conclusion	Type I Error ("α-error") (False Positive)
	Treatment Not Effective	Type II Error ("β-error") (False Negative)	Correct Conclusion

ment was in reality not effective and the trial shows this (i.e., it decreased mortality by less than 50 percent).

If the trial result is a false positive one (i.e., the trial result indicates that the treatment is effective but in reality it isn't), then a **Type I error** (also known as an "α-error") has occurred. Alternatively, if the trial conclusion is a false negative one, then a **Type II error** (or "β-error") has taken place. The chances (or probability) of having a Type I error or a Type II error are related. If the epidemiologist reduces the chance of a Type I error, the chance of a Type II error increases, and vice versa. The only ways to simultaneously decrease both Type I and Type II errors are to either (1) increase the sample size or (2) increase the size of the minimum effect that the trial will detect, e.g., to use a decrease in mortality of at least 75 percent instead of 50 percent.

One measure frequently used to characterize the adequacy of the sample size to detect an effect is the **power** of the trial. Power is equal to $1 - P(\text{Type II error})$, where P(Type II) is the chance of a Type II error. Often, the minimum power for a trial is set at 80 percent, but other levels of power and Type I errors are also used by investigators, depending on the circumstances surrounding the trial. Freiman and her colleagues (1978) noted that in many trials in which the treatment was found not to be efficacious, the sample size was inadequate to detect a 25 to 50 percent improvement among those treated. The consequences of an inadequate sample size in a randomized clinical trial extend beyond missing an important therapeutic improvement. In one instance, an outbreak of surgical wound infections was attributed to use of an ineffective prophylactic antibiotic; the sample size of the trial suggesting that the antibiotic was efficacious was, in fact, too small to demonstrate such efficacy (Lilienfeld et al., 1986).

Use of Historical Controls

One type of comparison group should be mentioned because of its frequent use in evaluating preventive and therapeutic agents (Sacks et al., 1982; Ederer, 1975b;

Peto et al., 1976). **Historical controls** are selected from patients who have been treated *in the past* in one way so that their outcome can be compared with that of patients treated with a new method. This term is also used to describe a group of patients having a much broader prior therapeutic experience with a standard form of treatment. Clearly, there was no random assignment of patients to treatment and control group. Such a comparison may provide acceptable evidence if previous experience with a disease indicates that the standard method of treatment had resulted in a very high case-fatality rate, such as 95 percent (i.e., an invariable clinical course), while the new treatment has a marked effect, resulting in, say, a 50 percent fatality rate. This was the case with penicillin. Before its introduction, the case-fatality rate from certain infectious diseases, such as bacterial endocarditis, was almost 100 percent, and this was sharply reduced when these diseases were treated with penicillin. In most instances, however, the difference between new and old treatment methods is not so marked, and the clinical course of the untreated disease is not so fatal.

Incidence, case-fatality, and mortality rates for a given disease may vary with time. Relying on historical experience when assessing the effect of a new therapy may therefore result in a misleading inference. In a classic demonstration of this phenomenon, Pocock (1977) noted that reliance on such an approach would result in marked variability and incorrect conclusions regarding the efficacy of cancer chemotherapeutic agents. Another example of the hazards posed by the use of historical controls is provided by the Coronary Drug Project (1970), a randomized trial comparing the efficacy of several drugs for the long-term therapy of coronary heart disease in middle-aged men with previous myocardial infarction. The observed mortality rate in the control group was 4 percent, 33 percent less than the expected rate of 6 percent that had been previously observed in a group of myocardial infarction patients (Coronary Drug Project Research Group, 1975). Comparison of the mortality rate for any of the treatments with the expected rate might mislead an investigator to conclude that the treatments are more efficacious than they truly are.

Allocation

The subjects, once recruited, are randomly assigned to either the treatment or comparison groups. Simple random allocation can be refined by using such methods as "stratification" (Zelen, 1974; Green and Byar, 1978). This technique takes advantage of some of the factors that are known to influence the disease being studied. For instance, participants are often classified by sex and age, usually in five- or ten-year age groups known as "strata," since matching by individual years of age is impractical. When an individual is of the desired sex and within a certain age stratum, the person is randomly assigned to either the treatment or the comparison group from that stratum. It may also be desirable to stratify by severity of disease as severity generally has an effect on the outcome of the disease. Participants classified by severity of disease can *then* be randomly assigned to treatment or comparison groups by methods assuring approximately equal numbers in both groups within each category of severity. The study group receives the new treatment, preventive agent, or whatever type of intervention is under investigation, and the comparison group receives the usual, accepted treatment.

An example of the recruitment and allocation of study subjects into strata is given in Figure 8–2, from the Hypertension Detection and Follow-up Project (Davis et al., 1986). This trial compared the effect of intensive intervention to control hypertension with that of "usual care." The initial screening served to identify eligible hypertensives, to stratify them by diastolic blood pressure into three groups (90–104 mmHg, 105–114 mm Hg, and 115 mmHg or greater), and then to assign them randomly to either the intensive intervention group or the usual care group. The stratification was necessitated by the strong gradiant of mortality associated with increasing diastolic blood pressure. It allowed the inves-

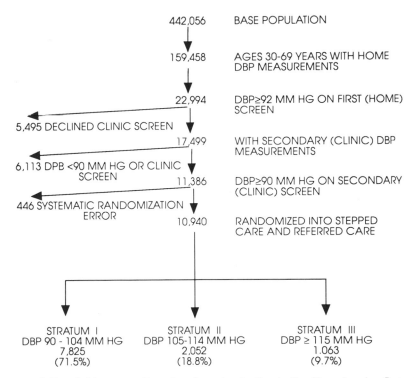

Figure 8–2. Subject recruitment and randomization in the Hypertension Detection and Follow-Up Study. *Source:* Davis et al. (1986).

tigators to examine the effect of intensive intervention not only in those with marked hypertension, i.e., a diastolic blood pressure of 115 mmHg or greater, but also in those with "mild" hypertension, i.e., a diastolic blood pressure of 90–104 mmHg.

Multicenter Comparison Groups

If the study is a multicenter one involving many clinics (which is often necessary to obtain a sufficient number of subjects), a comparison group is needed at each center. Each center represents a separate stratum; one center's comparison group *cannot* serve as a comparison group for the other centers. This is illustrated in Table 8–5, with the results from the two centers in the Swedish Breast Cancer Screening Trial, a randomized clinical trial that attempted to determine the efficacy of low-dose mammography to reduce breast cancer mortality (Tabar et al., 1985). The data in Table 8–5 show the breast cancer death rates among women screened in two counties in Sweden. Although the rates in the comparison groups differ from each other, the proportional decline in the mammography group mortality is the same in both counties (about 33 percent). Without a comparison group at each center, one might have decided that the technique was not effective since the death rate among women having mammography in Kopparberg County was higher than the death rate from breast cancer for comparison subjects in Ostergotland County (131 vs. 124 per 100,000).

Compliance with Treatment

Investigators cannot be certain that a treatment is or is not effective unless they can be assured that the treatment group is actually receiving the treatment; thus, it is necessary to continue to assess compliance with therapy during the trial (Haynes et al., 1978). A common strategy for assessing the compliance of patients in taking their medication, when it is a pill, is to give them more pills than needed for a given time period. They are instructed to return the unused pills, which are then counted. A comparison is made between the number of pills returned and

Table 8–5.   Breast Cancer Mortality per 100,000 Women in the Swedish Breast Cancer Screening Study

	KOPPARBERG COUNTY	OSTERGOTLAND COUNTY
Mammography Group	130.6	92.2
Comparison Group	207.0	123.9

Source: Tabar et al. (1985).

the amount that should have been returned if the patient had taken the proper number.

Other ways of assessing the probability of adherence to assigned therapy have been used. In the previously mentioned Veterans Administration antihypertensive study, patients had to pass certain "reliability" tests before they could be included in the trial. For example, patients unlikely to be compliant with the treatment, such as homeless persons and alcoholics, were excluded from the trial. A biological method of measuring compliance with therapy was used in the Anturane Reinfarction Trial (Anturane Reinfarction Trial Research Group, 1978). Since Anturane has the pharmacologic effect of lowering serum uric acid levels, the investigators determined the serum uric acid levels in both the treatment and comparison groups to assess compliance. Similarly, in the Aspirin Myocardial Infarction Study (AMIS), the urine of participants was examined for salicylates as an indication of compliance (Aspirin Myocardial Infarction Study Research Group, 1980).

Determination of the Effect

The clinical trial requires that observations be made for each participant concerning the effect of the treatment being evaluated. In some situations, the individual participant is essentially the "observer" of the effect, as in the assessment of pain; in other situations a physician must determine if the individual's disease status has been altered or if the disease has been prevented. Unfortunately, knowledge of whether the participant was in the treatment or comparison group can influence the observation or care, resulting in *biased assessment of effect,* either consciously or subconsciously. Of course, if death is the outcome or effect being measured, the potential for bias in assessing outcome is considerably diminished. To remove these sources of bias in the observations, three procedures for making the necessary observations have been developed: single masking, double masking, and triple masking. (Meinert, 1986; Hill, 1951; Ederer, 1975a; Ballentine, 1975; Armitage, 1975). Sometimes, the term "blinding" is used in place of "masking."

Single masking

In a single-masked study, the participants are not given any indication whether they are in the treatment or comparison group. The object of single masking is to *prevent the participant from introducing bias* into the observations; this is often accomplished by means of a placebo. An example of the need for a placebo can be found in the mammary artery coronary bypass surgery trials of the 1950s for the treatment of angina pectoria; the comparison group underwent a sham procedure in which only the skin was cut (Dimond et al., 1958). In one particular trial, 10 of 13 patients who were operated on showed marked reduction in the degree of angina pectoria; however, all five of the patients who had only a skin incision (the mammary artery was not ligated) also reported marked improvement! This suggested that an individual's perception of pain was influenced by the belief that he had received the operation.

Double masking

Double masking seeks to remove biases that occur as a *result of either the subject or the observer of the subject being influenced by knowledge* that the subject is in the comparison or treatment group. The bias due to the subject's knowledge of his or her assignment can be eliminated by single masking, as already described; eliminating the bias that may result from the observer's knowledge requires that the observer also be masked with respect to the subject's allocation. Thus, in a double-masked study, neither the subject nor the observer (or assessor) of the subject has knowledge of the subject's group allocation. Double masking thereby minimizes not only bias in assessment but also any possible bias in the care of the subjects.

When examination of the subjects is not necessary to measure the outcome and an objective test such as an electrocardiogram or laboratory procedure is available, it is a simple matter to assemble the records and have them interpreted by someone not directly involved in the study. In addition, it is desirable to use mortality as the outcome of a study, if possible, since this leaves little room for subjective judgment. Even so, when specific causes of death are used as outcomes, their determination can be biased by knowing in which group the subject belongs. This potential bias in the determination of the cause of death can be prevented by masking the individuals who are assigning cause-of-death codes to deceased study participants.

Triple masking

Triple-masked studies carry the concept of masking one step further than does a double-masked study; *the subject, the observer of the subject, and the person reviewing the data* are all masked with regard to the group to which a specific individual belongs.

An overview of the various types of masking is schematically presented in Table 8–6.

Problems in Randomized Clinical Trials

Volunteers and nonparticipants

In experimental epidemiologic studies, only subjects who consent to participate will enter the study. This limits the inferences that can be derived from their

Table 8–6. Overview of the Various Types of Masking Used in
Randomized Clinical Trials

	TYPE OF MASKING		
	SINGLE	DOUBLE	TRIPLE
Subject	X	X	X
Observer	—	X	X
Data analyst	—	—	X

X = Masked with respect to subject's allocation.

— = May be aware of subject's allocation.

results since it has been shown that volunteers can differ in significant ways from nonparticipants (Crocetti, 1970; Wilhelmsen et al., 1976).

The design of the National Diet-Heart Study, an intervention trial regarding dietary fat intake, made it possible to compare the characteristics of those who volunteered and those who did not (American Heart Association, 1968; Crocetti, 1970). The volunteers were found to be more frequently nonsmokers, concerned about health, members of community organizations, active in community affairs, employed in professional and skilled positions, and they had received more formal education. A larger proportion of volunteers than nonparticipants were Protestants or Jews and lived in households with children. If any of these characteristics were also related to the outcome being measured, the investigator would have to limit the inferences from the study's results and generalize cautiously.

The problem of differences between volunteers and nonparticipants can be dealt with, to some extent, by following the nonparticipants in the same way as the volunteers to determine their outcome. Sampling the nonparticipants often allows for their characterization. Even if such follow-up is limited to mortality data, comparisons between the volunteer and nonparticipant groups provide valuable information on the extent to which the results may be generalized.

Refusals to continue in the study

In any follow-up study, there will be subjects who drop out of the study at some point. In the National Diet-Heart Study, Crocetti found that the long-term participants were more aware of the relationship of diet to heart disease and more active in community organizations than the short-term participants. Similar findings have been reported by Wilhelmsen et al. (1976) in a primary prevention trial of cardiovascular risk factors (hypertension and cigarette smoking). The occurrence of dropouts could bias the results of a study. As with nonparticipants, this problem can be partially solved by obtaining whatever information is available on the characteristics of the dropouts in addition to determining their outcomes.

It may be advisable to select a random sample of dropouts for intensive follow-up depending on their number and the difficulty of obtaining information about them.

Loss to follow-up

The need to keep the proportion of persons lost to follow-up at a minimum will be discussed in the context of cohort studies (see Chapter 10). Attempts should be made to obtain such minimal information on this group as mortality data. It may be necessary to randomly select a sample on which to focus these efforts.

Intervention studies

In the treatment of risk factors and cessation experiments, there is a special problem that reflects the biological features of some chronic, noninfectious diseases. Does a negative result in a risk-factor intervention study indicate that no causal relationship exists between the risk factors that were experimentally modified and the specific disease? The answer is "no," or "not necessarily," since it is quite conceivable that the underlying pathological process could represent the cumulative effect of exposure to the etiological agent over many years and that this process had already reached an irreversible state in those studied. Thus, either type of study may lead to a negative finding from which a negative inference cannot be drawn. There is no general rule for interpreting negative results of cessation and risk-factor treatment studies of chronic disease. The results of each study must be evaluated in terms of the current knowledge of the particular disease.

Integrity of the Data

A frequently overlooked aspect of the design of a clinical trial is maintaining the integrity of the data; this issue is critical to the success of a multicenter trial and is of general importance in any trial (Meinert, 1986; CIOMS, 1960). The epidemiologist must be certain that the data from the trial are accurately recorded, as well as accurately transferred from one data storage medium to another. All research data forms should have clear instructions.

One way of assuring that the integrity of the data has not been violated is to have a group of epidemiologists or biostatisticians not involved in the trial conduct an audit of the data. This was done in the Anturane Reinfarction Trial discussed above. An independent audit of the completed trial found coding errors in less than one percent of the data, a very acceptable rate.

Analysis of the Results

The epidemiologist should first examine the characteristics of the two groups at baseline to assess their comparability, determining whether randomization resulted in the formation of comparable and evenly balanced groups. The British Physicians' Aspirin Trial, an investigation of aspirin as a prophylactic medication to prevent cardiovascular and cerebrovascular disease, offers a good example of this (see Table 8–7) (Peto et al., 1988). Clearly, the two groups were comparable on a large number of characteristics.

After ascertaining the comparability of the treatment and comparison groups, the investigator must determine whether the treatment was effective. The groups are compared and the size of the differences assessed. Statistical tests of significance are used as a guide (and only as a guide) in these comparisons. The data are examined for internal consistency; the researcher assesses the quality of the data and searches for patterns to help interpret and explain the findings. Many of the statistical methods are very specific in their area of application, and new methods are constantly being devised (Peto et al., 1976, 1977; Meinert, 1986; Fleiss, 1986). A discussion of these techniques is beyond the scope of this book.

Table 8–7.   Selected Baseline Characteristics of British Physicians' Aspirin Trial Study Groups at Entry

	ASPIRIN GROUP	COMPARISON GROUP
Number of Participants	3,429	1,710
Age (Years)		
<60	1,604 (46.8%)	804 (47.0%)
60–69	1,349 (39.3%)	658 (38.5%)
70–79	476 (13.9%)	248 (14.5%)
Smoking		
Never	859 (25.1%)	395 (23.1%)
Ex-smoker	1,512 (44.1%)	776 (45.4%)
Current Smoker, cigarettes only		
<20/day	224 (6.5%)	123 (7.2%)
≥20/day	205 (6.0%)	109 (6.4%)
Other, or mixed, current smoker		
	625 (18.2%)	307 (18.0%)
Systolic blood pressure (mmHg)		
<130	816 (23.8%)	473 (27.7%)
130–149	1,235 (36.0%)	584 (34.2%)
>149	612 (17.8%)	288 (16.8%)
Not known	766 (22.3%)	365 (21.3%)

Source: Adapted from Peto et al. (1988).

When analyzing results, it is worthwhile to compare the information obtained early in a study on the dropouts and persons lost to follow-up with that obtained on those who remained in the study, and thus determine whether there are any differences between these groups. To avoid bias, the investigator usually should assume the most conservative outcome (i.e., the outcome that is least favorable for the treatment under evaluation) for those patients who have withdrawn from the study or have been lost to follow-up. A broad estimate of the effect of these groups on the overall findings can be made by calculating the two extremes of a range: one based on assuming the most conservative outcome and the other based on assuming the best possible outcome. Of course, this determination depends on the outcome used in a specific study.

A schematic outline of a clinical trial is given in Figure 8–3. Simply stated, the investigator specifies all aspects of the trial before it starts. One then follows that protocol rigidly. Perhaps the best advice for the conduct of a randomzed experiment is that given by Cornfield (1959): ''Be careful.''

ETHICAL CONSIDERATIONS

Clinical trials are similar in many ways to the observational studies discussed in Chapters 10 and 11. Because of the random assignment of subjects to the treatment and comparison groups, however, certain ethical questions arise. These ethical issues are of increasing concern to investigators, institutions, and sponsoring agencies. A detailed consideration of these issues is beyond the scope of this book. The reader is referred to Hill's (1977) and Chalmers's (1975) discussions of this issue. Hill has aptly stated the dilemma facing the investigator:

> The question at issue, then, is whether it is proper to withhold from any patient a treatment that might, perhaps, give him benefit. The value of the treatment is, clearly, not proven; if it were, there would be no need for a trial. But, on the other hand, there must be some basis for it—whether it be from evidence obtained in test tubes, animals or even in a few patients. There must be some basis to justify a trial at all.

Before a trial can be carried out, the consent of the subjects to participate must be obtained; it is important that the subjects be informed that they may be assigned to *either* the treatment or comparison groups. The risks of having the treatment must be explained; the possible benefits of the treatment must also be explained. If the subjects, provided with this information, still decide to participate in the study, then they are said to have given their **informed consent.** Such consent should be obtained in writing in accordance with regulations of govern-

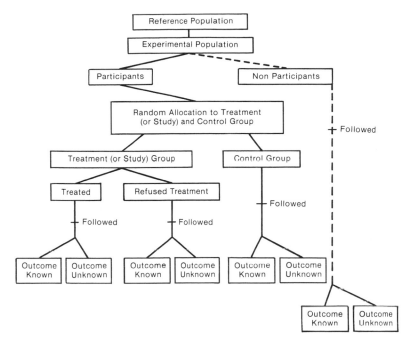

Figure 8–3.   Outline of randomized clinical trial.

mental agencies (in the United States) or of the institution where the trial is to be conducted.

The investigator may, nonetheless, be troubled by the idea of withholding a possibly beneficial treatment from someone who is ill or at the risk of developing a disease. Green's statement is one of the better responses to this problem (Hill, 1977):

> Where the value of a treatment, old and new, is doubtful, there may be a higher moral obligation to test it critically than to continue to prescribe it year-in-year-out with the support merely of custom or wishful thinking.

Hill has provided some general criteria for the ethical conduct of clinical trials (Table 8–8). The investigator must also consider whether it is ethical if *no trial* is conducted.

The demand by persons with AIDS (through organizations representing their interests) that potential therapies be released and licensed for use before thorough scientific testing has led to a reexamination of current U.S. Food and Drug Administration (FDA) governmental regulations. The tension between the desire for early release and the requirement for adequate testing can lead to considerable

Table 8–8.   Ethical Considerations in a Randomized Clinical Trial

---

1. Is the proposed treatment safe for (unlikely to bring harm to) the patient?
2. For the sake of a controlled trial, can a treatment ethically be withheld from any patient in the doctor's care?
3. What patients may be brought into a controlled trial and allocated randomly to any of the different treatments?
4. Is it ethical to use a placebo or dummy treatment?
5. Is it proper for the trial to be in any way masked?

Source: Adapted from Hill (1977).

controversy and conflict, but the scientific "rules of evidence" are bypassed at great peril.

META-ANALYSIS

The completion of many randomized clinical trials of common agents in the past two decades has led to the use of "meta-analysis," in which data from similar studies are pooled in a statistically rigorous manner. The purposes of meta-analysis are four-fold: "(1) to improve the statistical power for primary outcomes for subgroups, (2) to resolve uncertainty when reports disagree, (3) to improve estimates of effect size, and (4) to answer questions not posed at the start of the individual trials" (Sacks et al., 1987). Underlying these aims is the assumption that one has access to all of the relevant data from all randomized clinical trials involving a given agent. Conversely, meta-analysis obscures differences among trials. As Meinert (1989) has noted, there is a tendency in meta-analysis to "knowingly or unwittingly" combine the results of different trials while ignoring the potentially important differences among them.

Dickersin and Berlin (1992) have described the historical development of meta-analysis. The term itself apparently was first used by Glass in 1976 in the context of educational research. Since then, a number of meta-analytic reviews have been published, including a recent one of long-term antiarrythmic therapy after a myocardial infarction (Hine et al., 1989). In this meta-analysis, data from the ten available studies were assembled (Figure 8–4). Although one of the studies had a statistically significant finding indicating an effect for therapy, the others did not. The aggregate effect was nil. The investigators concluded that such therapy is not efficacious and thus is not indicated after a myocardial infarction.

Several registries of randomized trials have been established that assist inves-

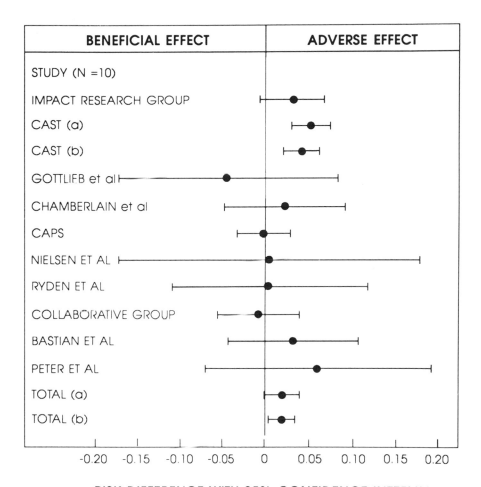

RISK DIFFERENCE WITH 95% CONFIDENCE INTERVAL

Figure 8–4. Mean case-fatality rate differences (and associated 95 percent confidence intervals) in ten randomized clinical trials of antiarrythmic therapy following a myocardial infarction, listed in descending order by quality. *Source:* Hine et al. (1989).

tigators in assembling all of the relevant data for a meta-analysis (Easterbrook, 1992; Dickersin and Berlin, 1992; Boissel, 1986; Simes, 1986; Meinert, 1988). In certain fields, e.g., perinatal medicine, such databases have been operating for some time (Chalmers, 1988). In others, e.g., neurological disorders, such registries need development. For reasons of cost, it is likely that meta-analyses will proliferate in place of large definitive trials; the needed databases should be developed to meet this demand.

For a detailed description of the statistical techniques used in a meta-analysis, the reader is referred to many recent reviews and books (Wolf, 1986; Sacks, et al., 1987; Abramson, 1990; Spector and Thompson, 1991; Louis et al., 1985; Glass et al., 1981; Eddy et al., 1992; DerSimonian and Laird, 1986).

SUMMARY

A randomized clinical trial is an experiment in which all participants are assigned to either the treatment group or the comparison group. These assignments are randomized. The process of randomization, if carried out properly, will provide comparable groups for most factors so that differences in outcomes at the end of the trial can be attributed to the intervention being tested.

There are three types of trials: therapeutic trials (in which the treatment of a disease is evaluated), intervention trials (in which an intervention in persons at elevated risk of developing a disease before the disease develops is evaluated), and preventive trials (in which the efficacy of a preventive agent is evaluated).

In a randomized clinical trial, the study is conducted according to a protocol, which describes in detail the design and rationale for the study. The study population is usually recruited until a predetermined sample size has been met. The sample size is selected to ensure that the study has adequate "statistical power," i.e., so that if the treatment being studied is effective, its efficacy will not be mistakenly missed in the trial. Once the subjects have been recruited, they are randomly assigned to either the treatment or the comparison group. During the course of the trial, a major concern is the compliance of the study population with the study protocol; methods are available to assess the degree of compliance present in a trial. Assessment of an effect from the intervention being tested can be biased if either the subject or the assessor knows the person's group allocation. Masking is used to avoid this bias. It is important to minimize the number of subjects who either drop out or are lost to follow-up in a trial. If possible, the investigator should follow these persons to determine whether their withdrawal from the study introduced an important bias.

The nature of a randomized clinical trial necessitates concern with the ethical basis for its conduct. Often, one is concerned about withholding a possibly beneficial treatment from a patient in order to complete the study. However, one must also be concerned about interrupting a study before the treatment has been demonstrated to be efficacious.

Recently, a new analytic method for pooling the results of randomized clinical trials has been developed: meta-analysis. In this approach, all of the results of randomized trials for a certain issue are assembled and pooled in a statistically rigorous way.

STUDY PROBLEMS

1. Define radomization. List three major objectives in a randomized clinical trial.
2. What types of research on a new agent should be done before using it in a randomized clinical trial?
3. What are the limitations of the randomized clinical trial?
4. A triple-masked multi-center randomized clinical trial of a newly discovered therapeutic drug was conducted recently. Ten centers, all in the same state, participated in the trial; in each center, subjects were randomly assigned to either the experimental or control groups. All observations were sent to a central coordinating center where they were analyzed. The trial indicated that the drug was clearly efficacious (using standard statistical techniques).
   (a) List the various tabulations of the data that would be needed for a proper analysis of the drug's efficacy.
   (b) What inferences can be derived from such a trial?
   (c) List the various problems that could occur during such a trial. How might they be handled?
   (d) What questions should physicians ask themselves about the trial before using the drug in their practices?
5. List several situations in which a randomized clinical trial could be considered unethical. What other methods could be used in these situations? Discuss the limitations of each method.
6. What are the disadvantages of conducting a randomized clinical trial with a small sample size for a new agent when the benefit is small?
7. Can a randomized clinical trial provide useful information about side effects of a new treatment? Suppose that the adverse effects are rare.
8. Surgeons introducing new procedures often use a case series as proof of efficacy. What is the problem with this approach?
9. If one used an α-error value of 0.05 in a randomized clinical trial in which 60 statistical tests were performed, how many of those tests would one expect to be statistically significant even if there were no real difference? How does one deal with the problems posed by this result?

REFERENCES

Abramson, J. H. 1990. ''Meta-analysis: a review of pros and cons.'' *Pub. Health Rev.* 18: 1–47.
Altman, D. G. 1991. ''Randomisation.'' *Br. Med. J.* 302:1481–1482.

American Heart Association. 1968. *The National Diet-Heart Study: Final Report.* American Heart Assoc. Monogr. No. 18, New York: The American Heart Association, Inc.

Anturane Reinfarction Trial Research Group. 1978. "Sulfinpyrazone in the prevention of cardiac death after myocardial infarction." *New Engl. J. Med.* 298:289–295.

Armitage, P. 1975. *Sequential Medical Trials,* 2nd edition. New York: Halsted Press.

Aspirin Myocardial Infarction Study Research Group. 1980. "A randomized, controlled trial of aspirin in persons recovered from myocardial infarction." *J. Am. Med. Assn.* 243:661–669.

Ballentine, E. J. 1975. "Objective measurements and the double masked procedure." *Amer. J. Ophthalmol.* 79:763–767.

Bearman, J. E. 1975. "Writing the protocol for a clinical trial." *Amer. J. Ophthalmol.* 79: 775–778.

B-Blocker Heart Attack Trial Research Group. 1982. "A randomized trial of propranolol in patients with acute myocardial infarction." *J. Am. Med. Assn.* 247:1707–1714.

Boissel, J. 1986. "Registry of multicenter clinical trials: seventh report—1985." *Thromb. Haemost.* 55:282–291.

Chalmers, I. 1988. *Oxford Database of Perinatal Trials.* Oxford, England; Oxford University Press.

Chalmers, T. C. 1975. "Ethical aspects of clinical trials." *Amer. J. Ophthalmol.* 79:753–758.

Cornfield, J. 1959. "Principles of research." *Amer. J. Mental Defic.* 64:240–252.

CIOMS. 1960. *Conference on Controlled Clinical Trials.* Hill, A. B., Chairman. Springfield, Ill.: Charles C Thomas.

Coronary Drug Project Research Group. 1970. "Initial findings leading to modifications of its research protocol." *J. Am. Med. Assn.* 214:1303–1313.

Coronary Drug Project Research Group. 1975. "Clofibrate and niacin in coronary heart disease." *J. Am. Med. Assn.* 231:360–381.

Crocetti, A. F. 1970. "An interview study of volunteers and nonvolunteers in a medical research project." Thesis, Dr.P.H., School of Hygiene and Public Health, The Johns Hopkins University.

Davis, B. R., Ford, C. E., Remington, R. D., Stamler, R., and Hawkins, C. M. 1986. "The Hypertension Detection and Follow-up Program design, methods, and baseline characteristics and blood pressure response of the study population." *Prog. Card. Dis.* 29(3 Suppl 1):11–28.

DerSimonian, R., and Laird, N. 1986. "Meta-analysis in clinical trials." *Controlled Clin. Trials* 7:177–188.

Dickersin, K., and Berlin, J. A. 1992. "Meta-analysis: state-of-the-science." *Epid. Rev.* 14:154–176.

Dimond, E. G., Kittle, C. F., and Crocket, J. E. 1958. "Evaluation of internal mammary artery ligation and sham procedure in angina pectoris (abstract)." *Circulation* 18:712.

Early Treatment Diabetic Retinopathy Study Research Group. 1991. "Early Photocoagulation for diabetic retinopathy." *Ophthalmology* 98:766–785.

Easterbrook, P. J. 1992. "Directory of registries of clinical trials." *Stat. Med.* 11:345–423.

Eddy, D. M., Hasselblad, V., and Shacter, R. D. 1992. *Meta-analysis by the Confidence Profile Method: The Statistical Synthesis of Evidence.* Boston: Academic Press.

Ederer, F. 1975a. "Patient bias, investigator bias, and the double-masked procedure in clinical trials." *Am. J. Med.* 58:295–299.

———. 1975b. "Why do we need controls? Why do we need to randomize?" *Am. J. Ophthalmol.* 79:758–762.

Fleiss, J. L. 1986. *The Design and Analysis of Clinical Experiments.* New York: J. Wiley and Sons.

Freiman, J. A., Chalmers, T. C., Smith Jr., H., and Kuebler, R. R. 1978. "The importance of beta, the Type II Error and sample size in the design and interpretation of the randomized control trial." *New Engl. J. Med.* 299:690–694.

Glass, G. V., McGaw, B., and Smith, M. L. 1981. *Meta-analysis in Social Research.* Beverly Hills, Calif.: Sage Publications.

Glass, G. V. 1976. "Primary, secondary, and meta-analysis of research." *Educ. Res.* 5:3–8.

Green, S. B., and Byar, D. P. 1978. "The effect of stratified randomization on size and power of statistical tests in clinical trials." *J. Chron. Dis.* 31:445–454.

Haynes, R. B., Taylor, D. W., and Sackett, D. L., etc. 1978. *Compliance in Health Care.* Baltimore: The Johns Hopkins University Press.

Hennekens, C. H., and Eberlein, K. 1985. "A randomized trial of aspirin and beta-carotene among U.S. physicians." *Prev. Med.* 14:165–168.

Hill, A. B. 1951. "The clinical trial." *Brit. Med. Bull.* 7:278–282.

———. 1977. *A Short Textbook of Medical Statistics,* 10th ed. Philadelphia: J. B. Lippincott Co.

Hine, L. K., Laird, N. M., Hewitt, P., and Chalmers, T. C. 1989. "Meta-analysis of empirical long-term anti-arrythmic therapy after myocardial infarction." *J. Am. Med. Assn.* 262:3037–3040.

Hjermann, I., Velve Byre, K., Holme, I., and Leren, P. 1981. "Effect of diet and smoking intervention on the incidence of coronary heart disease. Report from the Oslo Study Group of a randomised trial in healthy men." *Lancet* 3:1303–1310.

Lilienfeld, D. E., Vlahov, D., Tenney, J. H., McLaughlin, J. S. 1986. "On antibiotic prophylaxis in cardiac surgery: a risk factor for wound infection." *Ann. Thorac. Surg.* 42:670–674.

Lipid Research Clinics Program. 1984. "The Lipid Research Clinics Coronary Primary Prevention Trial results: II. The reduction in the incidence of coronary heart disease due to cholesterol lowering." *J. Am. Med. Assn.* 251:365–374.

Louis, T. A., Fineberg, H. V., and Mosteller, F. 1985. "Findings for public health from meta-analyses." *Ann. Rev. Public Health* 6:1–20.

Meinert, C. L. 1986. *Clinical Trials.* New York: Oxford University Press.

———. 1988. "Toward prospective registration of clinical trials (editorial)." *Controlled Clin. Trials.* 9:1–5.

———. 1989. "Meta-analysis: Science or religion?" *Controlled Clin. Trials.* 10(45): 257S–263S.

Meyskens Jr, F. L. 1988. "Thinking about Cancer Causality and Chemoprevention." *J. Nat. Cancer Inst.* 80:1278–1281.

Peto, R., Pike, M. C., Armitage, P., Breslow, N. E., Cox, D. R., Howard, S. V., Mantel, N., McPherson, K., Peto, J., and Smith, P. G. 1976. "Design and analysis of randomized clinical trials requiring prolonged observation of each patient: I. Introduction and Design." *Brit. J. Cancer* 34:585–612.

———. 1977. "Design and analysis of randomized clinical trials requiring prolonged observation of each patient: II. Analysis and examples." *Brit. J. Cancer* 35:1–39.

Peto, R., Gray, R., Collins, R., Wheatley, K., Hennekens, C. H., Jamrozik, K., Warlow,

C., Hafner, B., Thompson, E., Norton, S., Gilliland, J., and Doll, R. 1988. "Randomised trial of prophylactic daily aspirin in British male doctors." *Br. Med. J.* 296:313–316.

Pocock S. J. 1977. Letter to the Editor. *Br. Med. J.* 1:1661.

Sacks, H. S., Chalmers, T. C., Smith Jr., H. 1982. "Randomized versus historical controls for clinical trials." *Am. J. Med.* 72:233–240.

Sacks, H. S., Berrier, J., Reitman, D., Ancone-Berk, V. A., and Chalmers, T. C. 1987. "Meta-analysis of randomized controlled trials." *New Engl. J. Med.* 316:450–455.

Shapiro, S., Venet, W., Strax, P., and Venet, L. 1988. *Periodic Screening for Breast Cancer: the Health Insurance Plan Project and Its Sequelae, 1963–1986.* Baltimore: The Johns Hopkins University Press.

Simes, R. J. 1986. "Publication bias: the case for an international registry of clinical trials." *J. Clin. Oncol.* 4:1529–1541.

Spector, T. D., and Thompson, S. G. 1991. "The potential and limitations of meta-analysis." *J. Epid. Com. Health* 45:89–92.

Steering Committee of the Physicians' Health Study Research Group. 1988. "Preliminary report: findings from the aspirin component of the ongoing Physicians' Health Study." *New Engl. J. Med.* 318:262–264.

Tabar, L., Fagerberg, C.J.G., Gad, A., Baldetorp, L., Holmberg, L. H., Grontoft, O., Ljungquist, U., Lundstrom, B., Manson, J. C., Eklund, G., Day, N. E., and Pettersson, F. 1985. "Reduction in mortality from breast cancer after mass screening with mammography." *Lancet* 1:829–833.

Wilhelmsen, L., Ljundberg, S., Wedel, H., and Werko, L. 1976. "A comparison between participants and non-participants in a primary preventive trial." *J. Chron. Dis.* 29:331–339.

Wolf, F. M. 1986. *Meta-analysis: Quantitative Methods for Research Synthesis.* Beverly Hills, Calif.: Sage Publications.

Zelen, M. 1974. "The randomization and stratification of patients to clinical trials." *J. Chron. Dis.* 27:365–375.

9

EXPERIMENTAL EPIDEMIOLOGY:
II. COMMUNITY TRIALS

Experimental epidemiology derives its strength from the investigator's ability to control the conditions under which a study is conducted. One of the principal means of control in a clinical trial is *randomly* allocating individual subjects to the exposed and unexposed groups, as discussed in Chapter 8. Randomized clinical trials are particularly useful when one can identify a high-risk population for which an intervention is available. However, there are situations in experimental epidemiology that do not lend themselves to a randomized clinical trial (Kottke et al., 1985; Puska et al., 1985; Sherwin, 1978).

Experiments that involve communities as a whole are known as "community trials." Such studies have also been called "lifestyle intervention trials," "field trials," and "community-based public health trials" (Fredrickson, 1968; Hulley, 1978; Farquhar, 1978). In a community trial, the group as a whole is collectively studied, while in a randomized clinical trial it is the individual within a group (the experimental or control group) that is studied. If the risk factors for a disease are so prevalent that one cannot easily identify a high-risk group within a population (for which intervention programs could be designed), then an intervention in the community may be needed (Kottke et al., 1985). For example, in the United States, elevated serum cholesterol and cigarette smoking (risk factors for cardiovascular and cerebrovascular disease) are common in the population. Identification of a high-risk group would require extensive screening of people, a process that would be expensive and would require much cooperation from them. Instead, interventions in the general population of the United States to reduce the prevalence of these risk factors (assessed by cross-sectional surveys of the population) may be indicated (Blackburn, 1983). By reducing the prevalence of the risk factors in the population, one seeks to lower the incidence of the disease in the population. Since the incubation period for a noninfectious disease can be years, an intermediate outcome often assessed in a community trial is reduction in the level of the risk factors of interest.

In a community trial, the epidemiologist selects two communities that are similar in as many respects as possible. Community assent for participation in the trial is obtained from various political and other community leaders. A survey is conducted in each community to measure the incidence or prevalence of the disease of interest and the prevalence of the suspected risk factors for which an intervention has been developed. Possible interventions include behavior modification (e.g., health education) or consumption of a preventive agent (e.g., fluoride). The intervention is then carried out in one of the communities (the intervention community); the other community (the comparison community or control community) does not receive it. Then the intervention stops. A survey is again conducted in each community to measure the incidence of the disease of interest and the prevalence of the suspected risk factors. The net difference in the incidence of the disease and in the prevalence of the suspected risk factors between the intervention community and the comparison community is thereby associated with the intervention.

An example of a community trial is the introduction of fluorides into the water supply in order to determine whether this would decrease the frequency of dental caries (see Chapter 1) (Ast and Schlesinger, 1956). Another illustration of the method is Goldberger's demonstration in 1914–1916 of the dietary etiology of pellegra (Golderger et al., 1923; Goldberger, 1964). In both of these instances, however, the interventions were not allocated randomly. Recently, random assignment of the intervention in community trials has become more common.

An example of a randomized community trial is the WHO Collaborative Trial in the Multifactorial Prevention of Coronary Heart Disease (World Health Organization European Collaborative Group, 1980, 1983). In this study, workers in 80 factories in four countries (Belgium, Italy, Poland, and the United Kingdom) were screened between 1971 and 1977 for cigarette smoking, blood pressure, weight, and serum cholesterol level. The 80 factories were arranged into 40 pairs of plants of approximately comparable size, location, and type of industry. Within each pair, one factory was randomly assigned to receive the intervention, which consisted of a health education program for smoking cessation, cholesterol-lowering dietary advice, exercise, weight reduction, and control of hypertension. The use of randomized assignment of the factories reduced the possible bias in the assignment of the intervention that might otherwise be present in the study (Gail et al., 1992; Cornfield, 1978; Buck and Conner, 1982). The results of this trial were that the more overall risk-factor prevalence was reduced, the greater was the net decline in cardiovascular disease incidence and mortality. Strong cultural differences in the degree to which risk-factor prevalence could be reduced by a standardized educational intervention were also identified.

CONDUCT OF A COMMUNITY TRIAL

Community trials have six stages (Table 9–1). Each of these stages relies upon the successful completion of the previous steps.

Development of a Protocol

As in a randomized controlled trial, the development of a formal protocol that states the rationale, procedures, and organization of the community trial is the essential first step. The protocol should also include a detailed description of the methods that will be used in periodic assessment of the progress of the study, as well as the methods of analyzing the results of the trial. In addition, the protocol must provide for such contingencies as adverse reactions to the intervention.

Community Selection and Recruitment

The second stage concerns the selection of the communities (intervention and control) that will be involved in the trial. The number and size of the communities that will be needed for the trial can be determined by using standard statistical formulae (Cornfield, 1978; Buck and Donner, 1982; Donner et al., 1981; Donner, 1987). As in a randomized clinical trial, the investigator must assure that the trial has sufficient power to detect the desired intervention effect. Since community-based interventions are expensive, the number of communities to be studied is often quite small. In the Minnesota Heart-Health Program, for example, a community trial of health education to reduce cardiovascular disease risk-factor prevalence (and ultimately cardiovascular disease occurrence), only six communities were studied (Jacobs et al., 1986). The consequence of a small number of

Table 9–1.   Stages in a Community Trial

1. Development of a protocol
2. Community selection and recruitment
3. Establishment of a baseline and community surveillance
4. Intervention selection and assignment
5. Oversight and data monitoring
6. Evaluation

communities in such trials may be the loss of statistical power to detect a difference between the intervention community (or communities) and the control community (or communities).

Ideally, the selected communities are stable, with little migration, and have self-contained medical care systems (Kessler and Levin, 1972). Five criteria are commonly used in the selection of specific communities: unusual prevalence of the disease, unusual prevalence of suspected risk factors, administrative convenience, favorable community relations, and availability of background demographic information on the communities. Since the administrative convenience with which a study can be managed and favorable community relations are the keys to a successful trial, it is these factors that are most important in the selection of the communities to be studied.

The communities should be similar in as many respects as possible. Their size (populations) should be comparable, as should their economies, the ethnicities of their populations, and so on. If any important factor is dissimilar between the two communities, it is possible that any differences in outcome between the communities could be attributed to that factor and not to the intervention. In the Minnesota Heart Health Program, for example, three different community sizes were selected for study: Two communities were "matched" towns, two were "matched" cities, and two were "matched" suburbs (Jacobs et al., 1986).

After the communities have been selected, they must be recruited to participate in the trial. Such recruitment includes obtaining the assent of local and regional elected officials, community leaders, and the local medical communities (Elder et al., 1986). Sherwin (1978) has noted that it is impossible to obtain informed consent from every member of a community involved in a community trial as the investigator would in a randomized clinical trial. However, aside from the practical issue of the difficulty of conducting surveys in communities in which local leaders have told the investigator that they do not want their localities involved in the study, it would also be unethical to proceed with the trial in those communities without consent from their leadership. Once these persons have agreed to the communities' participation, it is important for the investigator to inform the community members themselves that they will be participating in a study, e.g., through notices in the local newspaper and stories on the local television newscasts.

Establishment of a Baseline and Community Surveillance

The establishment of a baseline or starting point for the outcome(s) of interest in the investigation is the next step in the development of a community trial. The outcome may be relatively easy to assess, such as changes in mortality rates (Puska et al., 1985; Jacobs et al., 1986). Mortality changes can be followed by using death certificates in the participating communities. Incidence of disease can also be used as an outcome; however, many of the problems of ascertainment discussed in Chapter 7 must then be considered (Fortmann et al., 1986; Puska, 1991; Gillum, 1978). An intermediate outcome might also be used, such as changes in risk factors for the disease (e.g., dietary saturated fat consumption or prevalence of cigarette smoking).

Once the outcomes of interest have been selected, the investigator must determine the baseline for those outcomes in each of the communities. The method used for determining the baseline should be the same one that will be used at the end of the investigation to assess the effect of the intervention. It may also be desirable to determine the changes in outcome during the trial. Hence, the surveillance systems used, whether they be vital statistics systems, hospital-based case ascertainment, or community surveys, must be relatively low-cost and sensitive to the outcomes of interest (Puska, 1991).

Community surveillance consists of six steps: development of a protocol, community outreach, establishing diagnostic criteria, ascertainment of cases, validation, and data management (Gillum, 1978). Once the system has been planned in a protocol, the investigator must solicit community support for the trial. Endorsements from the communities' political, social, and medical leaders will facilitate the construction of the needed systems; they may also allow access to systems that communities have already established on their own. The definition of the outcomes must then be specified; for example, what diagnostic criteria apply to a myocardial infarction or to a stroke? The means by which the outcome is ascertained are then selected; a method for validating the ascertainment is also selected. Finally, the data collected during surveillance must be properly processed.

Intervention Selection and Assignment

Once the baseline has been established, the next step is to specify the type of intervention that will be used for the communities in the study. In community trials, the intervention is often education (Farquhar et al., 1977; Farquhar, 1978; Puska et al., 1985). For instance, if the hypothesis to be tested in a community trial is that use of condoms reduces the risk of AIDS, then an educational program might be used to increase the rate of condom use in the intervention community.

The assignment of the intervention to be used in the trial is simple: in a nonrandomized trial, the investigator simply assigns the intervention to one of the communities; in a randomized trial, a coin might be flipped to decide which community receives the intervention. For example, in the Community Intervention Trial for Smoking Cessation (COMMIT) study, a randomized community trial of smoking cessation, eleven pairs of communities were randomly assigned by roulette to either an intensive smoking cessation program (the intervention) or to no program (the comparison) (COMMIT, 1991; Gail et al., 1992). It is always possible that an investigator might unknowingly favor one community over the other one—which is the reason that randomization should be used.

Oversight and Data Monitoring

During the course of a community trial, data are collected and analyzed to determine whether the intervention is having any injurious effect; if such an effect were found, then the trial would have to be stopped. Such data collection and analysis permits surveillance (see Chapter 6, p. 104) of the outcomes that will

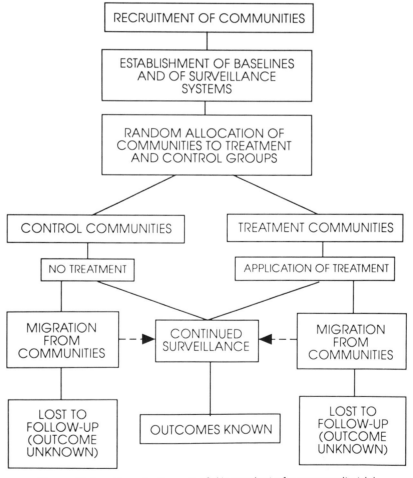

Figure 9–1. Generic diagram of the conduct of a community trial.

be used to assess the effectiveness of the intervention (Gillum, 1978; Puska, 1991). A committee of experts not otherwise associated with the trial may meet regularly to decide whether the trial should continue, from an ethical perspective.

Evaluation

At the conclusion of the trial, the data are analyzed to determine if the intervention was effective. In the first stage of the analysis, no adjustment is made for any potential confounding factors. Since communities as an aggregate, and not as individuals, are compared, however, it is important also to analyze the data with such adjustments.

A major consideration in the evaluation of a trial is the statistical power to validly conclude from the trial that an intervention is effective. The concept of power in a community trial is the same as in a randomized clinical trial (see Chapter 8, p. 161). In the Minnesota Heart-Health Program, for example, the population being studied, about 430,000 persons, is sufficiently large to allow for the detection of a differential 14-percent decline in cardiovascular disease mortality with an Type I error of 5 percent and a power of 85 percent (Jacobs et al., 1986).

A diagram summarizing the conduct of a community trial is shown in Figure 9–1.

NONRANDOMIZED COMMUNITY TRIALS

Two nonrandomized community trials, both started in 1972, provide interesting examples of this type of experimental design. The North Karelia Project developed in response to a community's desire to reduce its high cardiovascular disease rates. It focused on community health education, training of health care providers, increased availability of healthier foods, and the development of community-based health behavior support networks. In contrast, the Stanford Five-City Project focused on community-based health education efforts as the means to reduce cardiovascular morbidity.

The North Karelia Project

The North Karelia Project exemplifies the concepts of a community trial described above. This community trial was launched after the rural Finnish province of North Karelia recognized that it had the highest frequency of cardiovascular disease in the world (Figure 9–2) (Puska et al., 1985). Representatives of North

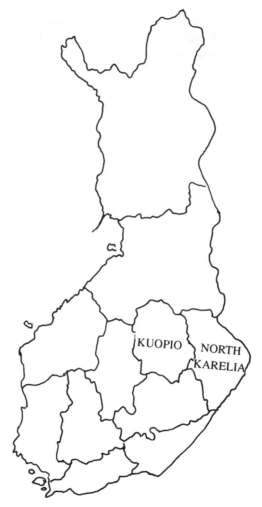

Figure 9–2. Location of North Karelia and Kuopio provinces in Finland. *Source:* Adapted from Salonen et al. (1983).

Karelia petitioned the Finnish government to undertake activities to reduce the occurrence of cardiovascular diseases. Local authorities, in collaboration with scientists and the World Health Organization, developed a protocol for a community trial. The interventions focused on reducing three major risk factors for cardiovascular disease (cigarette smoking, serum cholesterol level, and hypertension) that were known to be quite prevalent within the community as a whole and on improving medical care for those having myocardial infarctions or strokes.

A comparison province, Kuopio, with a population similar to that in North Karelia, was selected (Figure 9–2). Surveys were conducted in both provinces to provide baseline data for these three risk factors. Concurrently, myocardial infarc-

Table 9–2. Prevalence per 100 Population of Smoking among Residents of North Karelia and Kuopio Communities in 1972, 1977, 1982, and 1987, by Gender

| | MEN | | WOMEN | |
YEAR	NORTH KARELIA	KUOPIO	NORTH KARELIA	KUOPIO
1972	52	50	10	11
1977	44	45	10	12
1982	36	42	15	15
1987	36	41	16	15

Source: Vartiainen et al. (1991).

tion and stroke registries were established in both areas. An intervention program was then undertaken in North Karelia, including health education among influential citizens, training for health care providers, community health education, screening for hypertension, and development of needed health care facilities. The program was evaluated in 1977, 1982, and 1987 (Vartiainen et al., 1991). After the first evaluation, efforts were begun to reduce the prevalence of cardiovascular disease risk factors throughout Finland (Puska et al., 1985). Hence, any comparisons between North Karelia and Kuopio after 1977 must take into account the national programs that affected both comparison communities.

The results of the third evaluation of the North Karelia Project are shown in Tables 9–2, 9–3, and 9–4. Notable declines in the three major cardiovascular risk factors in North Karelia can be seen; however, there are also decreases for the comparison community, albeit smaller than for North Karelia. For most of the risk factors examined, the declines were greatest between 1972 and 1982. For the 1982–1987 period, the changes were slight. Ischemic heart disease mortality data for North Karelia and the rest of Finland (including Kuopio) underscore the impact of these declines in risk factors (Table 9–5) (Tuomilehto et al., 1989). Although ischemic heart disease mortality in North Karelia declined for both men and women from the early 1970s through the early 1980s, the death rates have

Table 9–3. Mean Serum Cholesterol Concentrations (mg/dL) among Residents of North Karelia and Kuopio in 1972, 1977, 1982, and 1987, by Gender

| | MEN | | WOMEN | |
YEAR	NORTH KARELIA	KUOPIO	NORTH KARELIA	KUOPIO
1972	274	265	270	264
1977	258	261	254	251
1982	244	242	236	232
1987	242	240	231	227

Source: Vartiainen et al. (1991).

Table 9–4. Mean Diastolic Blood Pressure (mmHg) among Residents of North Karelia and Kuopio in 1972, 1977, 1982, and 1987, by Gender

YEAR	MEN		WOMEN	
	NORTH KARELIA	KUOPIO	NORTH KARELIA	KUOPIO
1972	92.0	93.3	92.4	91.3
1977	88.6	92.6	86.3	88.4
1982	86.7	88.9	84.5	84.8
1987	88.1	89.1	83.2	83.9

Source: Vartiainen et al. (1991).

remained constant during the mid-1980s. This pattern contrasts with that for the rest of Finland, which experienced most of its decline in ischemic heart disease mortality in the late 1970s through the mid-1980s. These changes have been attributed to declines in the prevalence of cardiovascular disease risk factors (Salonen et al., 1989).

The Stanford Five-City Project

Another recent example of a nonrandomized community trial is the Stanford Five-City Project, an attempt to determine whether community health education can decrease the rate of cardiovascular disease (Farquhar et al., 1985; Farquhar et al., 1990). In 1972, the first phase of this trial (the Stanford Three-Community Study) was started in three California communities; it was an attempt to modify the same

Table 9–5. Average Annual Age-Adjusted Ischemic Heart Disease Death Rate per 100,000 Persons in North Karelia and the Rest of Finland from 1969 to 1986, by Gender

PERIOD	MEN		WOMEN	
	NORTH KARELIA	REST OF FINLAND	NORTH KARELIA	REST OF FINLAND
1969–1971	715	491	132	90
1972–1974	637	470	96	87
1975–1977	592	469	89	80
1978–1980	538	417	82	71
1981–1982	501	383	75	63
1983	541	343	56	58
1984	509	343	81	57
1985	526	342	75	58
1986	439	317	93	54

Source: Tuomilehto et al. (1989).

three risk factors (cigarette smoking, elevated serum cholesterol levels, and high blood pressure) by community education (Farquhar et al., 1977). In two of the communities, extensive mass-media campaigns were conducted over a period of two years. In one of these, face-to-face counseling was also provided for a small subgroup of high-risk individuals. The third community served as a comparison.

In each community, people were interviewed and examined before the educational campaign began. One or two years later their knowledge and behavior with respect to diet and smoking were assessed. Physiological indicators of risk—blood pressure, relative weight, and plasma cholesterol—were also measured. The baseline values of the risk factors were remarkably uniform in these communities. After two years of campaigning, the mass media and the combination of mass media plus face-to-face instruction had significant positive effects on all factors except relative weight. The comparison of the treated and control communities yielded an estimated decrease in risk of developing cardiovascular disease of approximately 25 percent (Maccoby et al., 1977). These results were sufficiently encouraging that in 1980 the investigators extended the trial to five communities.

The Stanford Five-City Project involves two intervention communities and three control communities. The education campaign began in 1980 and continued for over five years. The first results of the trial (through 1985) showed small but distinct decreases within the intervention communities in the prevalence of all cardiovascular disease risk factors examined, except for body-mass index (Figure 9–3). Future analyses will deal with both cardiovascular disease and stroke mortality.

RANDOMIZED COMMUNITY TRIALS

Both the North Karelia Project and the Stanford Five-City Project developed in response to local concerns about high cardiovascular disease mortality rates. The use of randomization to assign the intervention to either North Karelia or Kuopio would not have been practical or ethical. The Stanford Five-City Project was an extension of a previous trial, the Stanford Three-Community Study, for which random assignment would also have been problematic, since two of the three communities shared a common television station that was to be used for the intervention. Recent community trials, however, have been started with randomized assignment of the intervention. As in randomized clinical trials, the use of randomized assignment helps to ensure that the distribution of *all* factors—known and unknown, measurable and not measurable—except for the intervention being studied, is based on chance and not some factor, such as investigator preference, that may lead to a bias in assignment. The Aceh Study, a randomized community

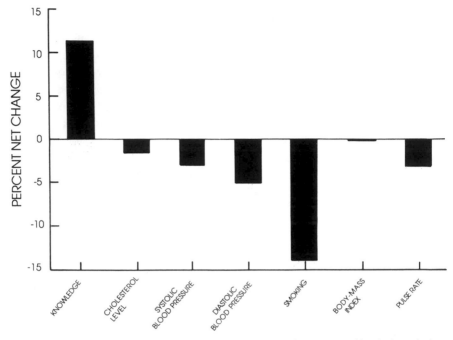

Figure 9–3. Net percentage changes in the intervention communities in knowledge and risk factors for persons 25 to 74 years old in the Stanford Five-City Project. *Source:* Farquhar et al. (1990).

trial of vitamin A supplementation and childhood mortality, illustrates this type of epidemiologic study.

The Aceh Study developed from epidemiologic observations suggesting that children with ophthalmologic indications of mild vitamin A deficiency had elevated death rates as a result of that deficiency (Sommer et al., 1986). Sommer and his colleagues sought to determine whether administration of vitamin A to children with such deficiency would reduce the associated mortality. The residents of an area of Indonesia, the Aceh Province, where xerophthalmia is endemic, were selected as the population to be studied.

Within the province, 2,048 villages in which there was no current or planned vitamin supplementation program were available for the study. From those villages, 450 were systematically selected for inclusion; these villages were then randomly assigned to either intervention (n = 229) or control (n = 221) groups. Some of the communities (18) were found to have started vitamin A supplementation programs before the baseline surveys began; adjacent villages (from among the 2,048) were substituted for them. The study was designed to be large enough to observe a 20-percent decline in mortality in the intervention communities with a Type I error of 5 percent and a power of 80 percent. A baseline survey of all 450 villages was undertaken. All children 0–5 years old were examined for active xerophthalmia; those with the disease were referred for intervention and were excluded from the trial.

The community intervention consisted of a single capsule of 200,000 IU vitamin A and 40 IU vitamin E. These capsules were given to children 1–5 years old by volunteers in the intervention communities about 1–3 months after the baseline survey. Capsules were also distributed six months later in both intervention and control communities during a follow-up examination.

In the trial, 29,236 children were enumerated at baseline; follow-up information was available on 89.0 percent of the treated children and 88.4 percent of the control children. During the follow-up period of six months, 53 children in the intervention villages and 75 children in the control villages died, a reduction in mortality of 34 percent (Figure 9–4). In the intervention villages, xerophthalmia prevalence declined by 85 percent. The investigators concluded that vitamin A supplementation in areas in which vitamin A deficiency is common would likely reduce mortality associated with the deficiency.

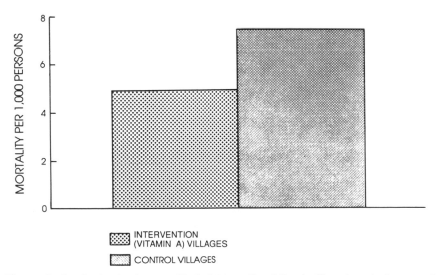

Figure 9–4. Reduction in mortality in intervention (vitamin A) and control groups in the Aceh Study. *Source:* Adapted from Sommer et al. (1986).

LOSS TO FOLLOW-UP

Major concerns in any community trial are that some of the study population (either intervention or control) will be lost to follow-up and that the composition of the study population will change during the course of the trial (Buck and Donner, 1982). Over time, there is movement of persons both into and out of the community. Those who leave the community may be different from those who stay with regard to the factors being studied. The loss of persons from either group can create problems in interpreting the results of the trial. Persons who move into the community after the intervention has been administered, for instance, would not have been exposed to it, yet their health experience would be incorporated with that of the community during the evaluation stage of the trial (Gillum et al., 1980). Also, if there are more persons lost to follow-up in the intervention group than in the control group, the effectiveness of the intervention may be obscured (Farquhar et al., 1990).

COMMUNITY TRIALS VERSUS RANDOMIZED CLINICAL TRIALS

The difference between randomized clinical trials and community trials (randomized or not) is that in the former, the unit of intervention assignment is the individual and in the latter, a community. To help decide which design is more appropriate, four criteria are useful (Blackburn, 1984; Farquhar, 1978; Kottke et al., 1985):

1. *Complexity of the interventions.* If the disease and the intervention are more complex than can be addressed in a randomized clinical trial, a community trial may be more appropriate. For example, smoking cessation as a means of preventing cardiovascular disease and cancer depends in part on minimizing the stimulus to smoke in the smoker's environment. In a randomized clinical trial setting it is often difficult to modify the smoker's environment in this way, while in a community trial it may be less difficult.
2. *Type of factors targeted for intervention.* In randomized clinical trials, intervention for life-style factors, such as use of condoms for AIDS prevention, is often more difficult than for factors amenable to medical intervention, such as hypertension (Syme, 1978). In such situations, a community trial may be more practical.
3. *High prevalence of disease.* If the disease is common in the population, then a community trial may reach a larger group in the population than

would a randomized clinical trial. Hence, the public health impact of the intervention would be more cost-effective. Xerophthalmia in Indonesia and HIV infection among homosexual men in the United States are examples of such high-prevalence conditions.

4. *Health policy formulation.* If a local or regional health care system is inadequate to provide the needed intervention, then a community trial may be necessary to provide the scientific basis for public health policy.

The choice between a randomized clinical trial and a community trial essentially depends on the size of the population to be studied. The larger that population is, the more desirable a community trial becomes (Kottke et al., 1985). This is a matter of cost. For instance, hypercholesterolemia is prevalent in many communities in the United States. Screening and intervention for all persons with elevated serum cholesterol levels in these communities would consume many health care resources. Suppose that an educational program had been developed that purported to lower dietary cholesterol intake. Use of such a program, if effective, would likely consume fewer resources than screening and treating the entire population of those communities. Yet only a community trial could demonstrate its efficacy.

SUMMARY

A community trial is an experimental epidemiologic study design in which entire communities are assigned to either intervention or control groups. This approach is useful when the outcome of interest is so common that it is difficult to identify a high-risk group. It is an alternative to a randomized clinical trial.

The first step in the conduct of a community trial is the development of a protocol in which all of the procedures, definitions, and justifications for the conduct of the trial are stated. The next step is the recruitment of the communities that will be studied. Baselines for the factors targeted for intervention and the outcomes of interest are then established. Surveillance procedures to monitor changes in the factors and the outcomes are also implemented at this time. The intervention is then implemented. Data monitoring continues throughout the conduct of the trial. At the trial's conclusion, the data are analyzed to determine if the intervention had the desired effect. Until recently, intervention assignment in a community trial was not randomized. This was partly the result of the small numbers of communities studied. Recent trials with larger sample sizes, however, have used randomized assignment to reduce the possibility of bias in the results of a study.

STUDY PROBLEMS

1. What is the major difference between randomized clinical trials and community trials? Between natural experiments and human community trials?
2. List the different reasons for conducting community trials.
3. What are the limitations, if any, on the inferences that can be derived from the Stanford Five-City Project regarding the effects of community education in the control of cardiovascular diseases?
4. In previous chapters, the problem of ecological fallacy was discussed. You will recall that it arose from deriving inferences from observations of groups, such as communities, or geographical or political units, rather than of individuals as in a clinical trial or an observational study. Are community trials subject to the ecological fallacy? Explain.
5. In Chapter 8 the use of historical controls in clinical trials was discussed. If historical controls are used in community trials, what factors must be taken into consideration in interpreting the results of such a study?
6. It is generally accepted that the design of a randomized clinical trial is more important than the analysis of its results. Why? Is this also true of a community trial? Explain.
7. List some situations in which it would be preferable to conduct a community trial rather than a randomized clinical trial.
8. The housefly feeds on typhoid bacilli–infected excreta in the sickroom or privy and is able to carry such excreta from the sick to the healthy. In a city with a stable population, the privies were often open and accessible to the housefly. In a period of a few months toward the end

MONTH	TYPHOID CASES OCCURRING YEAR BEFORE FLYPROOFING	TYPHOID CASES OCCURRING YEAR AFTER FLYPROOFING
January	8	9
February	0	5
March	4	7
April	6	4
May	41	11
June	41	18
July	109	10
August	82	5
September	14	7
October	15	8
November	7	2
December	2	4
Total	329	90

of the year, the privies were all made flyproof. The number of cases listed on page 194 of typhoid fever occurred in the city the year before and the year after the privies were made flyproof, by month.

(a) What inferences could you derive from these data?

(b) Are there any additional data you would like to have before deriving any inferences? If so, list the kinds of data.

REFERENCES

Ast, D. B., and Schlesinger, E. R. 1956. "The conclusion of a ten-year study of water fluoridation." *Amer. J. Pub. Health* 46:265–271.

Blackburn, H. 1983. "Research and demonstration projects in community cardiovascular disease prevention." *J. Pub. Health Pol.* 4:398–421.

————. 1984. "Commentary: observation versus experiment." *Stat. Med.* 3:401–403.

Buck, C., and Donner, A. 1982. "The design of controlled experiments in the evaluation of non-therapeutic interventions." *J. Chron. Dis.* 35:531–538.

COMMIT Research Group. 1991. "Community Intervention Trial for Smoking Cessation (COMMIT): summary of design and intervention." *J. Nat. Cancer Inst.* 83:1620–1628.

Cornfield, J. 1978. "Randomization by group: A formal analysis." *Am. J. Epidemiol.* 108:100–102.

Donner, A., Birkett, N., and Buck, C. 1981. "Randomization by cluster: sample size requirements and analysis." *Am. J. Epidemiol.* 114:906–914.

Donner, A. 1987. "Statistical methodology for paired cluster designs." *Am. J. Epidemiol.* 126:972–979.

Elder, J. P., McGraw, S. A., Abrams, D. B., Ferreira, A., Lasater, T. M., Lonpre, H., Peterson, G. S., Schwertfeger, R., and Carleton, R. A. 1986. "Organizational and community approaches to communitywide prevention of heart disease: the first two years of the Pawtucket Heart Health Program." *Prev. Med.* 15:107–117.

Farquhar, J. W., Wood, P. D., Breitrose, H., Haskell, W. L., Meyer, A. J., Maccoby, N., Alexander, J. K., Brown Jr., B. W., McAlister, A. L., Nash, J. D., and Stern, M. P. 1977. "Community education for cardiovascular health." *Lancet* 1:1192–1195.

Farquhar, J. W. 1978. "The community-based model of life style intervention trials." *Am. J. Epidemiol.* 108:103–111.

Farquhar, J. W., Fortmann, S. P., Maccoby, N., Haskell, W. L., Williams, P. T., Flora, J. A., Taylor, C. B., Brown Jr., B. W., Solomon, D. S., and Hulley, S. B. 1985. "The Stanford Five-City Project: design and methods." *Am. J. Epidemiol.* 122:323–334.

Farquhar, J. W., Fortmann, S. P., Flora, J. A., Taylor, C. B., Haskell, W. L., Williams, P. T., Maccoby, N., and Wood, P. D. 1990. "Effects of communitywide education on cardiovascular disease risk factors. The Stanford Five-City Project." *J. Am. Med. Assn.* 264:359–365.

Fortmann, S. P., Haskell, W. L., Williams, P. T., Varady, A. N., Hulley, S. B., and Farquhar, J. W. 1986. "Community surveillance of cardiovascular diseases in the Stanford Five-City Project. Methods and initial experience." *Am. J. Epidemiol.* 123:656–669.

Fredrickson, D. S. 1968. "The field trial: some thoughts on the indispensible ordeal." *Bull. N.Y. Acad. Med.* 44:985–993.

Gail, M. H., Byar, D. P., Pechacek, T. F., and Corle, D. K. 1992. "Aspects of statistical design for the Community Intervention Trial for Smoking Cessation (COMMIT)." *Controlled Clin. Trials* 13:6–21.

Gillum, R. F. 1978. "Community surveillance for cardiovascular disease: methods, problems, applications—a review." *J. Chron. Dis.* 31:87–94.

Gillum, R. F., Williams, P. T., and Sondik, E. 1980. "Some considerations for the planning of the total community prevention trials—when is sample size adequate?" *Community Health* 5:270–278.

Goldberger, J., Waring, C. H., and Tanner, W. F. 1923. "Pellagra prevention by diet among institutional inmates." *Pub. Health Reps.* 38:2361–2368.

Goldberger, J. 1964. *Goldberger on Pellagra.* M. Terris, ed. Baton Rouge: Louisiana State University Press.

Hulley, S. B. 1978. "Symposium on CHD prevention trials: design issues in testing life style intervention." *Am. J. epidemiol.* 108:85–86.

Jacobs Jr., D. R., Luepker, R. V., Mittelmark, M. B., Folsom, A. R., Pirie, P. L., Mascioli, S. R., Hannan, P. J., Pechacek, T. F., Bracht, N. F., Carlaw, R. W., Kline, F. G., and Blackburn, H. 1986. "Communitywide prevention strategies: evaluation design of the Minnesota Heart Health Program." *J. Chron. Dis.* 39:775–788.

Kessler, I. I., and Levin, M. L., eds. 1972. *The Community as an Epidemiological Laboratory.* Baltimore: Johns Hopkins University Press.

Kottke, T. E., Puska, P., Salonen, J. T., Tuomilehto, J., and Nissinen, A. 1985. "Projected effects of high-risk versus population-based prevention strategies in coronary heart disease." *Am. J. Epidemiol.* 121:697–704.

Maccoby, N., Farquhar, J. W., Wood, P. D., and Alexander, J. 1977. "Reducing the risk of cardiovascular disease: effects of a community-based campaign on knowledge and risk." *J. Community Health* 3:100–114.

Puska, P., Nissinen, A., Tuomilehto, J., Salonen, J. T., Koskela, K., McAlister, A., Kottke, T. E., Maccoby, N., and Farquhar, J. W. 1985. "The community-based strategy to prevent coronary heart disease: conclusions from the ten years of the North Karelia Project." *Ann. Rev. Public Health* 6:147–193.

Puska, P. 1991. "Intervention and experimental studies." In *Oxford Textbook of Public Health,* 2nd ed. Holland, W. W., Detels, R., Knox, G., eds.). Oxford: Oxford University Press.

Salonen, J. T., Puska, P., Kottke, T. E., Tuomilehto, J., and Nissinen, A. 1983. "Decline in mortality from coronary heart disease in Finland from 1969 to 1979." *BMJ* 286: 1857–1860.

Salonen, J. T., Tuomilehto, J., Nissinen, A., Kaplan, G. A., Puska, P. 1989. "Contribution of risk factor changes to the decline in coronary incidence during the North Karelia Project: a within-community approach." *Int. J. Epid.* 18:595–601.

Sherwin, R. 1978. "Controlled trials of the diet-heart hypothesis: some comments on the experimental unit." *Am. J. Epidemiol.* 108:92–102.

Sommer, A., Tarwotjo, E., Djunaedi, E., West Jr., K. P., Loeden, A. A., Tilden, R., and Mele, L. 1986. "The Aceh Study Group. Impact of vitamin A supplementation on childhood mortality. A randomised controlled community trial." *Lancet* 1:1169–1173.

Syme, S. L. 1978. "Life style intervention in clinic-based trials." *Am. J. Epidemiol.* 108: 87–91.

Tuomilehto, J., Puska, P., Korhonen, K., Mustaniemi, H., Vartiainen, E., Nissinen, A., Kuulasmaa, K., Niemensivu, H., and Salonen, J. T. 1989. "Trends and determinants of ischemic heart disease mortality in Finland: with special reference to a possible leveling off in the early 1980s." *Int. J. Epid.* 18(Suppl 1):S109–S117.

Vartiainen, R., Korhonen, H. J., Pietinen, P., Tuomilehto, J., Kartovaara, L., Nissinen, A., and Puska, P. 1991. "Fifteen-year trends in coronary risk factors in Finland, with special reference to North Karelia." *Int. J. Epid.* 20:651–662.

World Health Organization European Collaborative Group. 1980. "Multifactorial trial in the prevention of coronary heart disease: 1. recruitment and initial findings." *Eur. Heart J.* 1:73–80.

———. 1982. "Multifactorial trial in the prevention of coronary heart disease: 3. incidence and mortality results." *Eur. Heart J.* 4:141–147.

10

OBSERVATIONAL STUDIES:
I. COHORT STUDIES

In the experimental method, an investigator studies the effect of a change in the genetic composition or environment of a cell, an organ, or an organism and makes a comparison with a similar cell, organ, or organism that has not been subjected to that change. This ideal is the basis of both experimental and observational epidemiologic studies. In an experimental epidemiologic study, the investigator assigns the treatment; however, in the observational study, the investigator can only *observe* the outcomes associated with the individual exposures experienced by participants in the study. The investigator does not control the assignment of that exposure experience.

The data collected in an observational study can be tabulated in the form of a fourfold table, as shown in Table 10–1. If two similar groups can be identified that differ only by being exposed to a given environmental factor, e.g., oral contraceptives, or by possessing a particular characteristic, e.g., a specific blood group, the epidemiologist can follow these two groups and observe the incidence of disease in each. This type of investigation is known as a ''cohort'' study and is the subject of this chapter. In many situations, however, it is impractical for the epidemiologist to identify groups of individuals based upon their exposure histories or characteristics. One can more readily identify those individuals who have (''cases'') or do not have (''controls'') the disease of interest; the individuals' histories of past exposure to the factor or characteristic of interest can then be obtained and compared. This type of investigation is known as a ''case-control'' study, and will be discussed in Chapter 11.

The general concept of a cohort study is relatively simple, although such studies can be conducted in several ways. A sample of the population is selected and information is obtained to determine which persons either have a particular

Table 10–1.   The Distinction between Cohort and Case-Control Studies

ETIOLOGICAL CHARACTERISTIC OR EXPOSURE	CASE–CONTROL STUDY ↓	
	DISEASED GROUP (CASES)	NONDISEASED GROUP (CONTROLS)
COHORT STUDY → Present (exposed) Absent (not exposed)		

characteristic (such as a behavior or physiological trait) that is suspected of being related to the development of the disease being investigated, or have been exposed to a possible etiological agent. These individuals are then followed for a period of time to observe who develops and/or dies from that disease or physiological condition (such as decline in a pulmonary function test). The necessary data for assessing the development of the disease can be obtained either directly (by periodic examinations of everyone in the sample) or indirectly (by reviewing physician and hospital records, disease registration forms, and death certificates). Incidence or death rates for the disease are then calculated, and the rates are compared for those with the characteristic of interest and those without it. If the rates are different (either absolutely or relatively), an association can be said to exist between the characteristic and the disease. It is important to obtain information on other general characteristics of the study groups, such as age, gender, ethnicity, and occupation, in addition to the specific characteristic of interest, in order to account for the influence of any factors that are known to be related to the disease. Statistical methods are available for such analyses (Breslow and Day, 1987; Kelsey et al., 1986; Kahn and Sempos, 1989; Fleiss, 1981).

This type of study has been described by a variety of terms: "prospective," "incidence," "longitudinal," "forward-looking," and "follow-up," but "cohort study" will be used in this book. A distinction should be noted between cohort studies, described in this chapter, and cohort analyses, discussed in Chapter 5. In cohort studies individuals are followed or traced, whereas in cohort analyses there is no actual follow-up of persons; the follow-up is *artificially constructed* by the analysis of mortality (or morbidity) in successive age groups over a series of time periods (see p. 94).

MEASURING ASSOCIATION IN COHORT STUDIES

The data collected in a cohort study consist of information about the exposure status of the individual and whether, after that exposure occurred, the individual developed a given disease. These data may be tabulated into a 2 × 2 table (Table

Table 10–2.   Framework of a Cohort Study

ETIOLOGICAL CHARACTERISTIC OR EXPOSURE	DEVELOPED DISEASE	DID NOT DEVELOP DISEASE	TOTAL
Present (exposed)	a	b	a+b
Absent (not exposed)	c	d	c+d

10–2). The incidence rate among those persons exposed to the factor being investigated is a/(a + b), while the rate for those not so exposed is c/(c + d). The epidemiologist is interested, then, in determining whether the incidence rate for those exposed is greater than the rate for individuals not exposed, i.e., is a/(a + b) greater than c/(c + d)? If it is, then an association is said to exist between the factor and the subsequent development of disease. The question then asked by the epidemiologist is: How strong is the association?

Relative Risk

The **relative risk** ("RR") is used to measure the strength of an association in an observational study (Cornfield, 1951):

$$\text{Relative Risk (RR)} = \frac{\text{Incidence rate of disease in exposed group}}{\text{Incidence rate of disease in unexposed group}}$$

The variance, confidence limits, and statistical tests for the relative risk may be found in the Appendix (p. 317). In a cohort study, if the incidence of myocardial infarction among cigarette smokers was 3 per 1,000 and that for nonsmokers was 1 per 1,000, then the relative risk of myocardial infarction for smokers compared to nonsmokers would be:

$$RR = \frac{(3/1,000)}{(1/1,000)} = 3.0$$

This value of the relative risk means that a cigarette smoker is three times as likely to develop a myocardial infarction as is a nonsmoker.

The magnitude of the relative risk reflects the strength of the association; i.e., the greater the relative risk, the stronger the association. A relative risk of 3.0 or more indicates a strong association; for cigarette smoking and lung cancer, for instance, it is greater than 10.0, signifying a very strong relation (United States Surgeon General, 1982). In contrast, the relative risk for a family history of breast cancer (sister or mother) and female breast cancer is about 2.0, indicating a moderate association (Kelsey, 1979). A relative risk between 1.0 and 1.5 indicates a weak association.

Relative risks may also be less than 1.0 in value, suggesting a protective effect from exposure to a factor. For example, in a cohort study in Mali of meningococcal vaccine efficacy conducted during an epidemic of meningococcal meningitis, Binken and Bond (1982) found that the incidence rate of the disease among those vaccinated was 0.7 per 10,000 persons and among those not vaccinated 4.7 per 10,000 persons over the 5-week period following the vaccination campaign. Hence, the relative risk of meningitis for those vaccinated compared to those not vaccinated was 0.15, meaning that the risk of developing meningitis for someone who was vaccinated is only 15 percent of that for someone who was not vaccinated. This relative risk suggests a strong association between vaccination and protection from developing the disease.

Inferences about the association between a disease and exposure to a factor are considerably strengthened if information is available to support a gradient in the relationship between the degree of exposure (or "dose") to the factor and the disease. Relative risks can be calculated for each dose of the factor. The general approach is to treat the data as a series of 2×2 tables, comparing those exposed at various levels of the factor with those not exposed at all. An example of this type of analysis is the study by Vessey and his colleagues (1989) of the relationship between oral contraceptive use and ovarian cancer.

In the early 1970s, the possibility of a relation between oral contraceptive use and gynecologic cancer occurrence was suggested. During the period 1968–1974, 17,032 white married women, aged 25 to 39 years, were recruited at the Oxford Family Planning Association clinics in England and Scotland (Vessey et al., 1976). Of those enrolled, 6,838 were parous women who used oral contraceptives and 3,154 were parous women who used an intrauterine device (IUD). Some of these women were followed for up to 20 years (from 1968) and deaths were recorded by specific cause. The risk of mortality from ovarian cancer for different duration levels of oral contraceptive use are shown in Table 10–3 compared with those who had no exposure, i.e., women who used an IUD. The relative risks of death from ovarian cancer for oral contraceptive users relative to nonusers were:

RR (less than 48 months of oral contraceptive use) $= 12.1/9.2 = 1.32$

RR (48–95 months of oral contraceptive use) $= 1.8/9.2 = 0.20$

RR (more than 96 months of oral contraceptive use) $= 1.5/9.2 = 0.16$

Table 10–3. Mortality Rates per 100,000 Women-Years and Relative
Risk of Ovarian Cancer by Duration of Use of Oral Contraceptives

TOTAL DURATION OF USE	OVARIAN CANCER MORTALITY RATE	RELATIVE RISK[a] OF OVARIAN CANCER
Never[b]	9.2	1.00
≤ 47 months	12.1	1.32
48–95 months	1.8	0.20
96+ months	1.5	0.16

[a]Compared to "Never" users
[b]Intra-uterine device users
Source: Vessey et al. (1989).

This pattern of declining relative risk of ovarian cancer with increased duration of oral contraceptive use suggests that these pharmaceuticals might protect against this disease. A statistical significance test to determine whether such relative risks are different from 1.0 was developed by Cochran (1954), and a method for calculating an overall (pooled) relative risk for all categories was developed by Mantel and Haenszel (1959) (see Appendix, p. 320). If several studies of the same epidemiologic problem have been carried out at different times and in different places, it may be useful to scrutinize the estimates and then determine whether they are similar (Breslow and Day, 1987; Greenland, 1987; Kahn and Sempos, 1989).

Attributable Fraction

A measure of association that is influenced by the frequency of a characteristic in a population is the **attributable fraction** (also known as the "attributable risk"). Levin (1953) originally defined it in terms of lung cancer and smoking as the "maximum proportion of lung cancer attributable to cigarette smoking." Attributable fraction can also be defined as the maximum proportion of a disease in a population that can be attributed to a characteristic or etiologic factor. Another way of using this concept is to think of it as the proportional decrease in the incidence of a disease if the entire population were no longer exposed to the suspected etiological agent. Although we are discussing attributable fraction in the context of cohort studies, this measure of association is also useful in the interpretation of case-control investigations (see Chapter 11).

   As an example of the calculation of the attributable fraction, suppose that the incidence of lung cancer in the overall population is 120 cases per 100,000 persons; among nonsmokers in that population, it is 30 cases per 100,000 persons;

and among smokers, it is 330 cases per 100,000 persons. The relative risk of lung cancer among smokers compared to nonsmokers would then be 11.0 (330 per 100,000 / 30 per 100,000). Also assume that 30 percent of the population smokes. If the 30 percent of the population that smokes were to stop, then the incidence of lung cancer in that group would be reduced from 330 cases per 100,000 persons to 30 cases per 100,000 persons. The attributable fraction of lung cancer for cigarette smoking would then be:

$$
\begin{aligned}
\text{Attributable Fraction (AF)} &= \frac{0.3\ (330\ \text{per}\ 100,000\ -\ 30\ \text{per}\ 100,000)}{120\ \text{per}\ 100,000} \\
&= \frac{0.3\ (300\ \text{per}\ 100,000)}{120\ \text{per}\ 100,000} \\
&= \frac{90\ \text{per}\ 100,000}{120\ \text{per}\ 100,000} \\
&= 75\%
\end{aligned}
$$

An alternative way to calculate the attributable fraction is:

$$
\text{Attributable Fraction (AF)} = \frac{P\ (RR\ -\ 1)}{P\ (RR\ -\ 1)\ +\ 1} \times 100\%
$$

where RR = the relative risk and P = proportion of the total population that has the characteristic; the derivation of this formula can be found in the Appendix (p. 319). In the lung cancer example, P is 30 percent and RR is 11.0. The attributable fraction would therefore be:

$$
\text{AF} = \frac{0.3\ (11.0\ -\ 1)}{0.3\ (11.0\ -\ 1)\ +\ 1} = \frac{3.0}{3.0\ +\ 1} = \frac{3.0}{4.0} = 75\%
$$

Standard error and confidence limits have been derived for the attributable fraction by Walter (1975, 1976) (see Appendix).

The effect of various values of the relative risk (RR) and various proportions of those with a characteristic in the population (P) on the values of the attributable fraction is shown in Table 10–4. When the frequency of a characteristic in a population is low (e.g., 10 percent) and the relative risk for that characteristic in a given disease is also low (e.g., 2), only a small proportion (9 percent) of the cases of disease can be attributed to that characteristic (Adams et al., 1989). However, with a high relative risk (e.g., 10) and a high proportion of the population having the characteristic (e.g., 90 percent), a much larger percentage (89

Table 10–4.   Attributable Fractions* as a Proportion for Selected Values of Relative
Risk and Population Proportion with the Characteristic

P = PROPORTION OF POPULATION WITH CHARACTERISTIC (%)	RR = RELATIVE RISK			
	2	4	10	12
10	.09	.23	.47	.52
30	.23	.47	.73	.77
50	.33	.60	.82	.84
70	.41	.67	.86	.89
90	.47	.73	.89	.91
95	.49	.74	.90	.92

*Attributable fraction $= \dfrac{P(RR - 1)}{P(RR - 1) + 1}$

percent) of cases can be attributed to it. In these calculations, it is assumed that
other etiological factors are equally distributed among those with and without the
characteristic.

The measurement of attributable fraction is particularly useful in planning
disease control programs (Walter, 1975, 1976; Stellman and Garfinkel, 1989). It
enables health administrators to estimate the extent to which a particular disease
is due to a specific factor and to predict the effectiveness of a control program in
reducing the disease by eliminating exposure to the factor. For example, epidemiologic studies have suggested that throughout the world, the hepatitis B virus
is the etiologic agent for 75 percent to 90 percent of primary hepatocellular cancer
(Beasley, 1988). A global hepatitis B vaccination campaign could therefore
greatly reduce the occurrence of this cancer.

Computations of attributable fraction are also helpful in developing strategies for epidemiologic research, particularly if there are multiple factors. In the
United States, for example, it is estimated that in certain age groups, 80 to 85
percent of lung cancer can be attributed to cigarette smoking. Other etiological
factors apparently play a relatively minor role, and the investigator interested in
ascertaining these factors may decide to limit further studies to nonsmoking lung
cancer patients. In general, if close to 100 percent of a disease is attributable to
one or more factors, a search for additional etiological factors may not be profitable unless one is interested in studying other characteristics that influence those
already exposed to a high-risk factor.

Exposure Assessment

A crucial aspect of the design of cohort studies concerns the categorization of
subjects into "exposed" and "unexposed" groups that can be compared with

respect to disease incidence. If subjects cannot be correctly categorized, a cohort study is not feasible. An example of this inability to correctly classify exposure arose when epidemiologists at the Centers for Disease Control attempted to plan a cohort study of Vietnam veterans in regard to their exposure to Agent Orange, a defoliant that contained the toxic contaminant dioxin (Lilienfeld and Gallo, 1989; Centers for Disease Control Veterans Health Study, 1988). It was hoped that by learning about troop locations each day and comparing them to areas where the defoliant was sprayed the same day, an exposure score could be computed for each subject. However, when this score was compared with serum dioxin levels in a sample of such persons, it was clear that the exposure score would not be valid. Thus, the correct classification of exposure was problematic. The cancellation of the cohort study led to great protest by veterans' organizations who felt that their possible health risks were being ignored. However, conducting a cohort study with this high potential for misclassification might have led to results that underestimated the health risks of exposure to Agent Orange, if such risks actually exist.

Exposure assessment is important in all cohort studies, not only in those of occupational exposures. For example, the possible role of cardiovascular risk factors, such as hypertension and hypercholesterolemia, in pediatric atherosclerosis and adult cardiovascular disease is currently being studied in a cohort study of several thousand children in Bogalusa, Louisiana (Berenson and McMahon, 1980; Berenson, 1986). The exposure to these factors during childhood can be assessed directly, rather than trying to do so later in life.

TYPES OF COHORT STUDIES

Cohort studies can be classified as follows:

1. Concurrent studies
   (a) General population sample
   (b) Select groups of the population
       (i) Special groups—professional, veteran, etc.
       (ii) Exposed groups—occupational, etc.
2. Nonconcurrent studies
   (a) Population census taken in the past—usually special and unofficial
   (b) Select groups of the population
       (i) Special groups—professional, veteran, etc.
       (ii) Exposed groups—occupational, etc.

Concurrent and nonconcurrent cohort studies are contrasted in Figure 10–1. In a **concurrent study,** those with and without the characteristic or exposure are

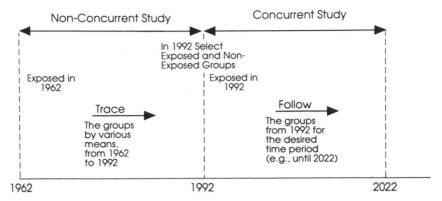

Figure 10–1. Diagrammatic representation of concurrent and nonconcurrent cohort studies.

selected at the start of the study (1992 in Figure 10–1) and *followed* over a number of years by a variety of methods. In a **nonconcurrent study,** the investigator goes back in time (to 1962 in Figure 10–1), selects his or her study groups, and *traces* them over time, usually to the present, by a variety of methods. These two types of cohort studies must be distinguished because they involve different methodological problems.

A simple example of a nonconcurrent cohort study would be an investigation of the safety of silicone breast implants. The epidemiologist might locate a group of plastic surgeons, each of whom used only one brand of silicone breast implant. The patient records of these surgeons would be reviewed for patients who had an implant placed two or three decades ago. Alternatively, if the epidemiologist identified a group of community hospitals in which silicone breast implant procedures were conducted, the medical records of the hospitals could be reviewed to provide information on the patients and the brand of implant used for each procedure. Regardless of the means by which the patients were identified, they would be followed up to the present time by contacting either the patient or the patient's family. For each brand of implant, the morbidity and mortality experience of the patient group would then be compared with that of the general population.

Concurrent Studies

In concurrent studies, the investigator begins with a group of individuals and follows them for a number of years. This was the approach used in the American Cancer Society's Cancer Prevention Study I (CPS I) of the health effects of cigarette smoking (Hammond, 1966; Garfinkel, 1985). The design of this study was similar to that of an earlier, smaller study (Hammond and Horn, 1958). For this investigation, 68,116 volunteers were recruited between October 1, 1959 and February 15, 1960. Each volunteer was asked to enroll families in which at least one person was 45 years of age or older. All persons in each household were asked to complete forms detailing their smoking histories, family history, medical history, occupational history, and various health habits. Follow-up was conducted every year (through the volunteers), and every two years subjects were asked to complete a follow-up questionnaire. Death certificates were obtained for each reported death. About 1,045,000 completed forms were received from persons residing in 1,121 counties in 25 states. Through September 30, 1962, 97.4 percent of the participants were successfully traced; 971,362 were reported to be alive, 46,212 had died, and 27,513 could not be traced. Age- and cause-specific and age-standardized mortality rates by history of tobacco use were computed from the collected data. Since tobacco use differed so markedly between men and women, the data were analyzed separately by gender. Figures 10–2 and 10–3 illustrate some of the findings for men in this classic study.

Figure 10–2 shows an increasing risk of mortality from bronchogenic (or lung) cancer with increasing number of cigarettes smoked and lower mortality rates among ex-smokers than among current smokers. Figure 10–3 shows that the mortality rates among ex-smokers decrease as the period of time since they had stopped increases, except for those who had stopped smoking within a year of entry into the study. This exception may reflect the fact that some of the men gave up smoking because they had already been diagnosed as having lung cancer. Such findings (the outcomes associated with cessation of exposure) are important

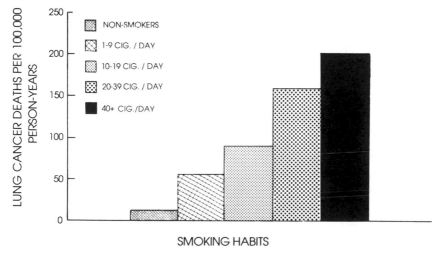

Figure 10–2. Age-adjusted death rates from malignant neoplasm of lung for men by amount of cigarette smoking at beginning of cohort study in 1959–1960. *Source:* Hammond (1966).

208   Epidemiologic Studies

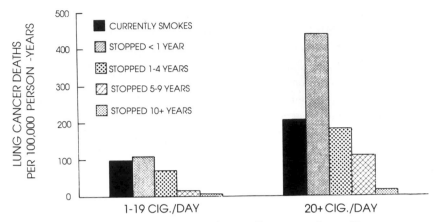

Figure 10–3. Age-adjusted death rates from malignant neoplasm of lung among men who had never smoked, who had stopped smoking, and who were still smoking at beginning of cohort study in 1959–60. *Source:* Hammond (1966).

in deriving etiological inferences from cohort studies (a subject that will be discussed in detail in Chapter 12). The groups in the CPS I study were not probability samples of the general population, which would have been preferable, but a probability sample of the required size would have been impossible to obtain. A similar study, known as the Cancer Prevention Study II, was started by the American Cancer Society in the late 1970s in order to examine more recent exposures of persons who may have been too young to participate in the CPS I study. Data collected in this ongoing investigation are now being analyzed.

A similar approach was used by Hirayama (1981a, b) in his pioneering study of passive smoking and lung cancer. He had collected information on the smoking habits of spouses of 91,540 nonsmoking wives and 20,289 nonsmoking husbands in six prefectures in Japan in 1965. The mortality of these men and women was assessed from death certificates during the 14 years of follow-up. Nonsmoking spouses of smokers had an elevated risk of lung cancer compared with that for nonsmoking couples (Figure 10–4). For nonsmoking men whose wives smoked 20 or more cigarettes daily, the risk was more than twice that of nonsmoking men married to nonsmoking women.

In some situations a cohort study can be conducted in a population selected from a well-defined geographical, political, or administrative area. This is particularly feasible when the disease or cause of death is fairly frequent in the population and does not require recruitment of a large number of persons for the study. The Framingham Heart Study is a good example of this type of cohort study (Dawber, 1980). It was initiated in 1948 by the United States Public Health Service to study the relationship of a variety of factors to the subsequent development

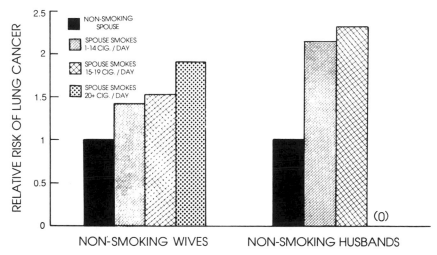

Figure 10–4.   Age-adjusted relative risk of lung cancer among nonsmoking husbands and wives, by the smoking habits of their spouses. *Source:* Adapted from Hirayama (1981a).

of heart disease. The town of Framingham, Massachusetts, was chosen for its population stability, cooperation with previous community studies, presence of a local community hospital, and proximity to a large medical center. The initial population sample was a group of persons 30 to 62 years old that, when followed over a period of twenty years, would result in enough new cases or deaths from cardiovascular disease to ensure statistically reliable findings. The town's population in this age group was approximately 10,000. A sample of 6,507 men and women was selected. About 98 percent of the 4,469 respondents were free of coronary heart disease at the initial examination (Feinleib, 1985). Another 740 volunteers were also included in the cohort as part of a community outreach effort to ensure the continued participation in the study by each cohort member. After the first examination, each person was reexamined at two-year intervals for a thirty-year period. Information was obtained on several factors that could be related to heart disease, such as serum cholesterol level, blood pressure, weight, and history of cigarette smoking. Table 10–5 presents the incidence rates of coronary heart disease (CHD) among men and women during the first thirty years of follow-up by initial systolic blood pressure, gender, and age (Stokes et al., 1989). There is an increasing risk of CHD with increasing initial systolic blood pressure in the 35- to 64-year-old age group, a gradient of CHD disease which is slightly steeper in the older male age group and slightly less steep for the women.

The Framingham Heart Study also illustrates a strength of the cohort study:

Table 10–5.   Average Annual Incidence per 1,000 Persons of Coronary Heart Diseae in Framingham, Massachusetts, 30-Year Follow-Up, by Systolic Blood Pressure and Gender

SYSTOLIC BLOOD	AGE 35–64		AGE 65–94	
PRESSURE (mmHg)	MEN	WOMEN	MEN	WOMEN
<120	7	3	11	10
120–139	11	4	19	13
140–159	16	7	27	16
160–179	23	9	34	35
>180	22	15	49	31

Source: Stokes et al. (1989).

investigating a variety of outcomes associated with a given exposure. For example, in addition to investigating the association between systolic blood pressure and CHD, for example, the Framingham investigators explored the relation between systolic blood pressure and stroke; a strong relationship between increased systolic blood pressure and elevated stroke risk was found.

The Framingham Heart Study became a prototype for similar studies in Tecumseh, Michigan, and other areas (Keys, 1970; McGee and Gordon, 1976; Napier et al., 1970). However, the difficulties in selecting general population samples for such studies tend to make investigators utilize a special group that for one reason or another can be followed more easily; certain professional groups, people enrolled in medical care programs, veterans, and others. In Doll and Hill's (1964) classic cohort study of cigarette smoking and lung cancer, for instance, a questionnaire was sent to all physicians on the British Medical Register who were living in the United Kingdom (see Chap. 1, p. 9). Follow-up was simplified because the subjects were physicians and therefore maintained contact with several professional organizations. Information from death certificates that listed "physician" as occupation was obtained from the Registrar General's Office. Lists were also obtained from the General Medical Council or the British Medical Association for deaths that had occurred abroad or in the military service.

A more recent example of the use of a unique population is the Oral Contraception Study of the Royal College of General Practitioners (1974) in England (Kay, 1984). Between May 1968 and July 1969, 23,000 oral contraceptive users and an equal number of nonusers, matched only for age and marital status, were recruited by physicians from among their patients. The oral contraceptive users selected were the first two women in each calendar month for whom the physicians wrote a prescription for an oral contraceptive. A nonuser was selected by the following procedure: starting with the user's record, returned to its correct place in the doctor's file, each subsequent record was examined in alphabetical order until the next record was found for a woman whose year of birth was within three years either side of that of the user and who had never used an oral contraceptive. Both the user and the nonuser had to be either married or known to be "living as married." These 46,000 women were followed with regard to their morbidity and mortality experience. In 1974, 1977, 1978, 1981, and 1988, progress reports were issued, showing associations between oral contraceptive use and (1) deep venous thrombosis, (2) acute myocardial infarction, and (3) subarachnoid hemorrhage (Table 10–6).

A similar approach was used by Hennekens and his colleagues (1979) in the Nurses' Health Study. These investigators sent questionnaires on possible risk factors (e.g., oral contraceptive use, smoking habits) to 121,700 nurses in 1976. Follow-up questionnaires were sent every two years thereafter to update risk factor information and to ascertain newly diagnosed conditions. Such data allow the epidemiologist to determine the effect of changes in risk factors on subsequent health events.

Concurrent cohort studies are not limited to noninfectious diseases. An example of the application of this method to infectious diseases is the study by Beasley et al. (1981, 1988) implicating the hepatitis B virus in the etiology of primary hepatocellular cancer. These investigators recruited 21,227 male Taiwanese government civil servants between November 1975 and June 1978, and 1,480 from a cohort study of risk factors for cardiovascular disease. Of these 22,707 men, 3,454 were hepatitis B surface antigen (HBsAg) positive, indicating past infection with the hepatitis B virus. By the end of 1986, 161 participants had developed primary hepatocellular cancer. The HBsAg positive group had a significantly higher rate of the disease than did the HbsAg negative group (Table 10–7). The relative risk of death from primary hepatocellular carcinoma among those who were HBsAg positive compared with that for those who were negative

Table 10–6.   Age-Adjusted Relative Risks of Oral Contraceptive Users Compared to Nonusers

DISEASE (ICD–9 CATEGORY)	RELATIVE RISK (ORAL CONTRACEPTIVE USER TO NONUSER)
Nonrheumatic heart disease and hypertension (400–429)	5.6
Ischemic heart disease (410–414)	3.9
Subarachnoid hemorrhage (430)	4.0
Cerebrovascular accident (431–433)	2.1
Deep thrombosis of the leg, pulmonary embolism (450–453)	(*)

Source: Adapted from Layde et al. (1981).

*Rate for nonusers was 0.0; no relative risk could be calculated.

Table 10–7. Relation between HBsAg Antibody Status on Entrance to Study and Subsequent Development of Primary Hepatocellular Carcinoma through December 31, 1986

HBSAg STATUS	NUMBER	CASES OF PRIMARY HEPATOCELLULAR CARCINOMA	AVERAGE ANNUAL[1] INCIDENCE RATE OF PRIMARY HEPATOCELLULAR CARCINOMA PER 100,000 POPULATION
Positive	3,454	152	494.5
Negative	19,253	9	5.3

Relative risk of death from primary hepatocellular carcinoma among those who are HBsAg positive compared with those who are negative is (494.5/100,000)/(5.3/100,000) = 98.4.

[1]For 8.9 years of follow-up.
Source: Beasley (1988).

was 98.4, indicating a very strong association between HBsAg status and primary hepatocellular carcinoma.

The concurrent cohort study is particularly useful when the investigator does not know what the specific agent is when the study begins. In early 1984, for example, before the human immunodeficiency virus (HIV–1) had been identified as the etiologic agent for the acquired immunodeficiency syndrome (AIDS), the Multicenter AIDS Cohort Study (MACS) was begun to investigate the etiology and natural history of the disease (Kaslow et al., 1987). In Baltimore, Chicago, Los Angeles, and Pittsburgh, 4,955 homosexual men were recruited between April, 1984 and March, 1985. Each recruit provided blood, urine, feces, saliva, and semen specimens, which were stored for future analyses. The study population is reexamined every six months to determine if the participants have antibodies to the HIV–1 virus and, if so, what AIDS manifestations, if any, have developed. As hypotheses concerning the various manifestations of AIDS are developed, these specimen banks will be used to test those hypotheses.

In the concurrent cohort studies discussed so far, the study population was divided into those with and those without one or more possible etiological factors. The groups were sometimes classified according to different degrees of exposure or to levels of a characteristic such as the presence of the hepatitis B surface antigen. The incidence and mortality rates of these subgroups were then compared. The study groups were selected because they offered particular advantages for follow-up and information about a specific factor was obtainable from them. In a different type of concurrent study, a specific group that has been exposed to a possible etiological factor is selected and followed to determine the effects of this exposure as compared with the experience of a population not exposed to that substance. This method has been especially useful in studies of the effects of exposure to substances in occupational environments. The elucidation of the relation between occupational exposure to asbestos and lung cancer provides an example of this strategy.

In 1955, Doll reported that the relative risk of lung cancer in a group of asbestos factory workers compared to the general population was 10. In 1963, Selikoff and his co-workers began a cohort study of 370 members of the International Association of Health and Frost Insulators and Asbestos Workers (IAHFIAW) (Selikoff et al., 1968). Follow-up of this cohort continued until 1967, when the investigation ended. The study findings suggested that there was an interaction between asbestos exposure and cigarette smoking in the development of respiratory cancer. These investigators initiated a study in 1967 of all U.S. and Canadian members of the IAHFIAW (Selikoff, 1979). The union provided the investigators with a membership list for 1966. Each member was mailed a questionnaire in which he was questioned about his smoking habits and the use of a mask while working. Some 17,800 men were followed from January 1, 1967 until December 31, 1976; 2,271 men died during the nine-year period. A control group, which had not been exposed to asbestos, was selected from the roster of 1,045,000 persons enrolled by the American Cancer Society in 1959 for the CPS I study described earlier. The control group, selected to be similar to the exposed group except for the exposure to asbestos, consisted of "men, not a farmer, no more than a high school education, a history of occupational exposure to dust, fumes, vapors, gases, chemicals, or radiation, and alive as of January 1, 1967." This group numbered 73,763 such persons. Follow-up of the nonexposed individuals was conducted in September, 1972. Official mortality statistics were used to extrapolate the observed mortality through 1976.

One of the major findings of this study is the positive interaction between both cigarette smoking and asbestos in markedly elevating the risk of lung cancer (Table 10–8). This type of relation is indicated by the fact that the death rate for

Table 10–8. Age-Adjusted Lung Cancer Death Rates per 100,000 Man-Years, by Cigarette Smoking Status and Occupational Exposure to Asbestos Dust

	NONSMOKERS	CIGARETTE SMOKERS
Not exposed to asbestos dust	11.3	122.6
	(1.0)*	(10.9)
Exposed to asbestos dust	58.4	601.6
	(5.2)	(53.2)

*Figure in parentheses is relative risk of lung cancer mortality compared with that for nonsmoking persons not exposed to asbestos dust.

Source: Hammond et al. (1979).

the combination of cigarette smoking and asbestos exposure was five times that of arette smokers without asbestos exposure and ten times that of nonsmoking persons with asbestos exposure. One might expect the relative risk for smoking workers to be about 15 if no positive interaction were present; however, it was 53, indicating such an interaction.

Nonconcurrent Studies

In nonconcurrent cohort studies, the period of observation starts from some date in the past, as illustrated in Figure 10–1; aside from the observation period, however, all other aspects of a nonconcurrent cohort study are the same as for a concurrent cohort investigation. These studies cannot be conducted with samples of the general population unless the investigator has access to a census of a community, usually unofficial, which was conducted in the past. Samples of the population covered by the census can then be selected and traced from the time of the census (Comstock, Abbey, and Lundin, 1970).

Nonconcurrent studies usually involve specially exposed groups or industrial populations because past census information is often unavailable and employment, medical, or other types of records usually are available. This is illustrated by the study of the relation between polycythemia vera (PV) and leukemia, which had been clinically observed since 1905 (Modan and Lilienfeld, 1965). The increased medical use of radiation treatment for PV and the observations of the leukemogenic effect of ionizing radiation in various studies raised the question as to whether the development of leukemia in patients with PV was part of the disease's natural history or a result of treatment with X-ray and/or P^{32}, a radioactive isotope. A study was undertaken to estimate the risk of developing leukemia among patients with PV and to determine whether it was increased as a result of P^{32} and/or X-ray treatment. Medical records of patients with PV who had been seen during 1947–1955 in seven medical centers were obtained at the same time as those of two comparison groups: (a) patients with polycythemia secondary to lung disease and (b) patients with questionable polycythemia. These groups were then classified by method of treatment into four categories: (1) no radiation treatment, (2) X-ray alone, (3) P^{32} only, and (4) a combination of X-ray and P^{32}. The patients were traced through December 31, 1961. Leukemia occurred predominantly in patients who had received some form of radiation, either X-ray, P^{32}, or a combination of the two (Figure 10–5). This finding has since been confirmed in a randomized clinical trial (Berk et al., 1981).

Nonconcurrent cohort studies of industrial exposures to possible etiological agents of disease can only be carried out by using company records of past and present employees that include information on the date that they begin their employment, age at hiring, the date of departure, and whether they are living or

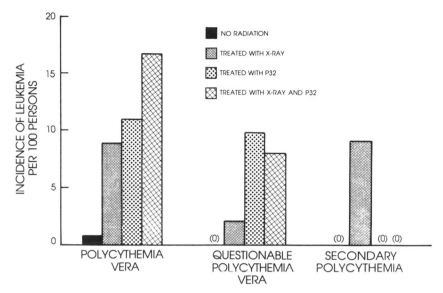

Figure 10–5.   Incidence of leukemia among persons with polycythemia vera, questionable polycythemia vera, and secondary polycythemia vera. *Source:* Modan and Lilienfeld (1965).

dead. The mortality experience can be determined and compared with that of another industry, or with the mortality rate of the state where the industry is located, or of the country as a whole. This approach was used by Rinsky and his colleagues (1987) in a study of the relationship between exposure to benzene and leukemia mortality.

The study population consisted of all 1,165 nonsalaried white men employed in a rubber hydrochloride department of any of three plants in Ohio engaged in the manufacture of this natural rubber film for at least one day between January 1, 1940 and December 31, 1965. The cohort was assembled by using company personnel records. The cohort was traced through December 31, 1981, using vital status data from the Social Security Administration, the Ohio Bureau of Motor Vehicles, and a commercial tracing service. Death certificates were obtained for all deceased members. At the same time, an industrial hygienist used company records of benzene exposure to estimate the cumulative occupational exposure to benzene of each person in the cohort. At the time these exposure estimates were developed, the industrial hygienist did not know which of the cohort members had died from leukemia or from other causes.

The observed mortality from leukemia (nine deaths) was then compared with that expected if the cohort had had the same mortality experience as the United States population during the same time period. The results, shown in Figure 10–6, indicated a striking relationship between cumulative occupational exposure to benzene and leukemia mortality.

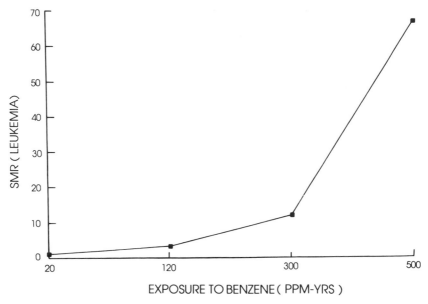

Figure 10–6.   Standardized mortality ratio for 1,165 white men with at least one day of exposure to benzene from January 1, 1940 through December 31, 1965, according to cumulative exposure (parts of benzene per million particles × years of exposure). *Source:* Adapted from Rinsky et al. (1987).

STUDY PROCEDURES

A major source of difficulty in carrying out cohort studies is maintaining follow-up of the selected groups of persons. This is least troublesome in concurrent cohort studies for obvious reasons. At the very start of such studies, methods can be adopted for keeping in contact with the population on an annual basis, including periodic home visits, telephone calls, and mailed questionnaires, or even all three. The names and addresses of several friends and relatives can be obtained at the beginning of a study so that they may be contacted if the person moves out of the community. (Geographic mobility of people, particularly in the United States, can pose a problem.) To minimize the difficulties posed by tracing a cohort, cohort studies are often conducted in a health maintenance organization, in which the study population can be relatively easily followed. Another approach is to use a health or disability (for morbidity) or life (for mortality) insurer's clientele, as there is an economic incentive for the study population to inform the insurance company of the outcomes of interest. For deaths in the United States that have occurred since 1979, the National Death Index (administered by the National Center for Health Statistics) will inform investigators of the year and place of death for a given person (User's Manual, National Death Index, 1981).

In many countries, national or regional registries for cancer and other diseases can be used to follow up subjects in a cohort study.

Despite the best efforts, a certain number of individuals will likely be lost to follow-up. Even for this group, information on mortality status can often be obtained from state vital statistics bureaus. Their mortality experience can then be compared with that of the individuals not "lost to follow-up" to determine if there are any differences between the two groups. In addition, the successfully traced group can be compared to the "lost" group with respect to several known characteristics. To the extent that they show similar frequencies of a variety of characteristics of interest in the study, one's confidence is increased that no bias has been introduced into the findings by the lost group.

In a nonconcurrent cohort study, when one goes back perhaps twenty or thirty years to select a study group, the problem of tracing becomes more difficult. Every available source of information about subjects in the study should be used. Table 10–9 presents the various means used by Modan (1966) in determining the survivorship status of patients in his study of polycythemia vera and leukemia. In all cohort studies, it is desirable to trace as high a percentage of the study group as possible. Questions are frequently raised about the possibility of bias in the results if the degree of follow-up is less than 95 percent. This issue has been considered in several studies. Modan and Lilienfeld (1965) found that a very good estimate of the total mortality rate was obtained from the first 77 percent of the patients traced, although the group that was reached first had a somewhat higher leukemia mortality rate than those traced later. In a study of the outcome of neurosis, on the other hand, Sims (1973) found considerable differences

Table 10–9. Distribution of Sources of Information on Patient's Survivorship Status in the Study of Polycythemia Vera and Leukemia

SOURCE OF INFORMATION	NUMBER OF PATIENTS	PERCENT
Patient	158	12.9
Local physician	201	16.4
Relative	103	8.4
Hospital	540	44.2
Neighbors	49	4.0
Postmaster	18	1.5
Town-County clerk	20	1.6
Health department	89	7.3
Other	24	2.0
Untraced	20	1.6
Total	1,222	100.0

Source: Modan (1966).

between the patients who were easily contacted and those who were traced with more effort. Only three deaths had occurred among the first 110 patients traced (59 percent of the study group), but eighteen additional deaths were discovered in the sixty-six patients (36 percent of the study group) who were found by more intensive tracing. Rimm and his colleagues (1990) have noted that even the type of mail service used during follow-up can affect response rates. Thus, it appears that the pattern varies in different studies and, perhaps, with different diseases, so that a general rule cannot be established about the degree of follow-up necessary to ensure unbiased conclusions. The safest course is to attempt to achieve as complete a follow-up as possible.

ANALYSIS OF RESULTS

General Strategy

It has already been made clear that the results of cohort studies are preferably analyzed in terms of relative risks, which provide a relatively simple expression of the relation between mortality rates from different diseases in the groups being compared. This is particularly true if the follow-up observations are made in the same period for all the study groups.

Many cohort studies, however, whether concurrent or nonconcurrent, involve lengthy and varying periods of observations. Persons are lost to follow-up or die at different times during the course of the study, and consequently they are under observation for different time periods. In some studies, persons are enlisted or enter the study at different times and, if the follow-up is terminated at a specific time, they will have been observed for different lengths of time. Two related methods are available for analyzing the results of such studies:

1. The calculation of person-years or months of observation as the denominator for the computation of incidence or mortality rate.
2. Actuarial, life table, or survivorship analysis (also known as cumulative incidence or mortality analysis).

Person-years of observation are often used as denominators in the computation of rates in cohort studies, as in the Royal College of General Practitioner's Oral Contraceptives Study. They are particularly useful when several factors, such as age, sex, and varying periods of observation (which result from persons entering and leaving the study at different ages and times), make the computation of an actuarial life table difficult or impossible. This analytic approach takes into consideration both the number of persons who were followed and the duration of

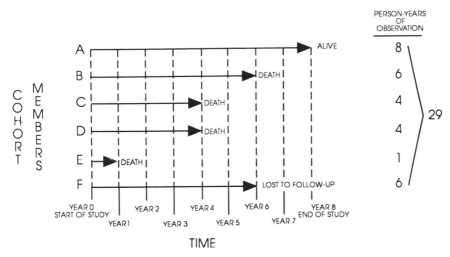

Figure 10–7. Diagrammatic illustration of contribution of person-years observed in a hypothetical eight-year cohort study of six persons (A,B,C,D,E, and F).

observation. In Figure 10–7, six persons are followed during an eight-year concurrent cohort study. Four of these persons (B, C, D, and E) die during the course of the follow-up. One person (A) is alive at the end of the study, and one person (F) is lost to follow-up after six years. The total number of person-years of observation (during which the cohort members were at risk of dying) is 29 years. The death rate in this study is therefore 4 deaths/29 person-years of observation (13.8 per 100 person-years of observation).

The use of person-years of observation makes it possible to express in one figure the time period when a varying number of persons is exposed to the risk of an event such as death or the development of disease. In addition, the age distribution of the groups under observation changes as a study progresses, as do the mortality and morbidity rates over time (Matanoski et al., 1975). The use of person-years is limited by the assumption that the risk of occurrence of an event per unit time is constant during the period of observation for the individual and that that risk is the same among similar persons in the cohort (Sheps, 1966; Breslow and Day, 1987). The overall effect of these limitations is modest and usually acceptable in most cohort studies.

Many regard using life tables (also known as survivorship methods) as the preferred method of analyzing data from cohort studies (see Appendix) (Chiang, 1961; Kahn and Sempos, 1989; Breslow and Day, 1987). They provide direct estimates of the probability of developing or dying from a disease for a given time period, and relative risks can be computed as the ratio of these probabilities. Life table methods can be used when the assumptions for person-years cannot be satisfied.

Latency

Regardless of the technique used to estimate the relative risk of developing a disease, one must also examine the possible effect of different latency or incubation periods. For instance, if a malignancy does not develop for at least a decade after the exposure to the suspected carcinogen began, then persons in the cohort would not be at risk for developing the disease until at least a decade had passed since their first exposure. Only after that decade had passed would those persons begin to accrue person-years of observation or be included in a life table (in the first interval); likewise, only if the disease developed after that first decade would that event be included in the analysis.

Adjustment for Age and Other Factors

The relative risks that are calculated by using either person-years or life table methods are unadjusted for age or other possible **confounding** factors. A confounding factor is one that is related both to the disease of interest and to another factor that is itself associated with the disease. For example, suppose that an epidemiologist conducted a cohort study of cigarette smoking and lung cancer. Many factors related to cigarette smoking (e.g., age, gender, and race) are independently associated with lung cancer. Hence, to measure the true relative risk between lung cancer and cigarette smoking, the epidemiologist would need to adjust the observed relative risk for these and other possible confounding factors. If adjustment for these factors does not change the relative risk, then little or no confounding is said to be present.

The epidemiologist may use two different approaches to adjust (or "control") for possible confounding factors:

1. Stratify the data by the possible confounding factors into multiple 2×2 tables to calculate the stratum-specific relative risk. An adjusted relative risk may then be calculated with Mantel-Haenszel techniques.
2. Use statistical techniques to mathematically model the risk of developing the disease, adjusted for the effects of the possible confounding factors. Examples include the logistic, the log-linear, and the proportional hazards models.

Where the entire study groups was exposed, however, it is necessary to use an external comparison or control group. If none is available, the mortality (or, if such data are available, the morbidity) experience of the exposed group is usually compared with that of the entire population living in the same geographical area as the exposed group, with statistical adjustments for age, sex, and calendar time of exposure and follow-up. For mortality, the number of deaths in the exposed group is compared with the expected number, based on the appropriate death rates for that geographical area. This comparison is then expressed as a Standardized Mortality Ratio (SMR) (see Chapter 4). This approach is frequently used in epidemiologic studies of occupational exposures (Monson, 1990). The previously described benzene-leukemia study by Rinsky et al. (1987) provides an example of this type of data analysis (see p. 215).

SUMMARY

In a cohort study, the investigator assembles a group of persons exposed to a possible etiologic factor and another, comparable group not exposed to that factor. These two groups are followed for the development of diseases. The investigator then calculates the incidence rate for a given condition in the exposed and unexposed groups, and a relative risk of developing the disease is calculated from those incidence rates. The stronger the association, the larger the relative risk; relative risks of 3.0 to 4.0 or more are usually indicative of strong associations between the factor and the disease. The proportion of disease in a population that is associated with that factor (assuming an etiologic relation) is the attributable fraction. The larger the attributable fraction of a disease for a given factor, the more difficult it becomes to study other possible agents of that disease.

There are two types of cohort studies: concurrent and nonconcurrent. In a concurrent study, the investigator assembles the exposed and nonexposed groups at the same time that the study is being conducted; these groups are then followed concurrently with the conduct of the study. In a nonconcurrent study the investigator reconstructs the groups in their entirety at some time in the past. This may be done with any set of records that provides information on all members of the population regarding their exposure at the same time in the past. Both groups are then followed to the present for the development of disease.

The process of following up the cohort of persons exposed and not exposed poses the greatest challenge to the epidemiologist in this study design. Inadequate follow-up can result in biased data and either spurious associations or missed relationships. It is also possible that the follow-up conducted in the early phases of a study may provide information on a portion of the cohort that is not reflective of the entire group. Analysis of the data at such a stage might result in different inferences than if one waited until both groups had been followed up completely.

Two methods are available for the analysis of cohort studies: (1) the calculation of incidence rates among those exposed and those not exposed using person-years of observation, and (2) the calculation of life-tables to provide interval-specific incidence rates of disease among those exposed and those not exposed.

The use of person-years assumes that the risk of developing the disease is the same in each time period of follow-up and also that the risk of developing disease for each member of the cohort is the same. The incidence rates for those exposed and those not exposed are then compared by calculating the relative risk of disease, a measure of the strength of the association between the exposure and the disease. The magnitude of the relative risk may be affected by the presence of confounding factors, which may be related to the exposure, to the disease, or both. The effects of confounding may be adjusted for by stratification (calculating stratum-specific relative risks) or by constructing a statistical model of the data. If the entire cohort was exposed to the factor (e.g., an occupational study), an SMR-based analysis may be used to control for possible confounding factors, such as age and gender.

STUDY PROBLEMS

1. It has often been stated that the Standardized Mortality Ratio (SMR) and the relative risk are equivalent. Are they? Why might such a statement be made?
2. How useful is the attributable fraction to the epidemiologist?
3. A certain virus V is suspected of being the cause of infectious disease D. Design a cohort study to elucidate the relationship between V and D. How does the design change if V is a ''slow virus'' or if D is currently viewed as a noninfectious disease?
4. Internationally, several medical billing data bases are being developed by health maintenance organizations (HMOs) and national health care systems. How can these systems be used to conduct both concurrent and nonconcurrent cohort studies?
5. A few surgeons seek your advice (as the local epidemiologist) concerning a study they would like to conduct to determine the effect of tonsillectomy on subsequent mortality. What might you recommend?

REFERENCES

Adams, M. J., Khoury, M. J., and James, L. M. 1989. ''The use of attributable fraction in the design and interpretation of epidemiologic studies.'' *J. Clin. Epid.* 42:659–662.

Beasley, R. P., Hwang, L.-Y., Lin, C.-C., and Chien, C.-S. 1981. ''Hepatocellular carcinoma and hepatitis B virus.'' *Lancet* 2:1129–1133.

Beasley, R. P. 1988. ''Hepatitis B virus. The major etiology of hepatocellular carcinoma.'' *Cancer* 61:1942–1956.

Berenson, G. S. 1986. "Bogalusa Heart Study." In *Causation of Cardiovascular Risk Factors in Children: Perspectives on Cardiovascular Risk in Early Life.* G. S. Berenson, ed. New York: Raven Press.

Berenson, G. S., and McMahon, G. A., eds. 1980. *Cardiovascular Risk Factors in Children: The Early Natural History of Atherosclerosis and Essential Hypertension.* New York: Oxford University Press.

Berk, P. D., Goldberg, J. D., Silverstein, M. N., Weinfeld, A., Donovan, P. B., Ellis, J. T., Landau, S. A., Laszlo, J., Njean, Y., Pisciotta, A. V., and Wasserman, L. R. 1981. "Increased incidence of acute leukemia in polycythemia vera associated with chlorambucil therapy." *New Engl. J. Med.* 304:441–447.

Binken, N., and Bond, J. 1982. "Epidemic of meningococcal meningitis in Bamako, Mali: epidemiological features and analysis of vaccine efficacy." *Lancet* 2:315–317.

Breslow, N. E., and Day, N. E. 1987. *Statistical Methods in Cancer Research, Vol. 2. The Design and Analysis of Cohort Studies.* Lyon: International Agency for Research on Cancer.

Centers for Disease Control Veterans Health Study. 1988. "Serum 2,3,7,8-tetrachlorodibenzo-p-dioxin levels in U.S. Army Vietnam-era veterans." *JAMA* 260:1249–1254.

Chiang, C. L. 1961. "A stochastic study of the life table and its applications. III. The follow-up study with the consideration of competing risks." *Biometrics* 17:57–78.

Cochran, W. G. 1954. "Some methods of strengthening the common χ^2 tests." *Biometrics* 10:417–451.

Comstock, G. W., Abbey, H., and Lundin, F. E., Jr. 1970. "The nonofficial census as a basic tool for epidemiologic observations in Washington County, Maryland." In *The Community as an Epidemiologic Laboratory: A Casebook of Community Studies.* I. I. Kessler and M. L. Levin, eds. Baltimore, Md.: The Johns Hopkins Press, pp. 73–99.

Cornfield, J. 1951. "A method of estimating comparative rates from clinical data. Applications to cancer of the lung, breast, and cervix." *J. Nat. Cancer Inst.* 11:1269–1275.

Dawber, T. R. 1980. *The Framingham Study: the Epidemiology of Atherosclerotic Disease.* Cambridge, Mass.: Harvard University Press.

Doll, R., and Hill, A. B. 1964. "Mortality in relation to smoking: Ten years' observation of British doctors." *BMJ* 1:1399–1410; 1460–1467.

Doll, R. 1955. "Mortality from lung cancer in asbestos workers." *Br. J. Ind. Med.* 12:81–86.

Feinleib, M. 1985. "The Framingham Study: sample selection, follow-up, and methods of analysis." In *Selection, Follow-up, and Analysis in Prospective Studies: A Workshop.* Garfinkel, L., Ochs, O., Mushinski, M., eds. NCI Monograph No. 67. Washington, D.C.: U.S. Government Printing Office.

Fleiss, J. 1981. *Statistical Methods for Rates and Proportions,* 2nd ed. New York: J. Wiley and Sons.

Garfinkel, L. 1985. "Selection, follow-up, and analysis in the American Cancer Society Prospective Studies." In *Selection, Follow-up, and Analysis in Prospective Studies: A Workshop.* Garfinkel, L., Ochs, O., Mushinski, M., eds. NCI Monograph No. 67. Washington, D.C.: U.S. Government Printing Office.

Greenland, S. 1987. "Quantitative methods in the review of epidemiologic literature." *Epi. Rev.* 9:1–30.

Hammond, E. C. 1966. "Smoking in relation to the death rates of one million men and women.'' In *Epidemiological Studies of Cancer and Other Chronic Diseases*. NCI Monograph 19, pp. 127–204.

Hammond, E. C., and Horn, D. 1958. ''Smoking and death rates—Report on forty-four months of follow-up of 187,783 men. Part I. Total mortality. Part II. Death rates by cause.'' *JAMA* 166:1159–1172; 1294–1308.

Hammond, E. C., Selikoff, I. J., Seidman, H. 1979. ''Asbestos exposure, cigarette smoking, and death rates.'' *Ann. N.Y. Acad. Sci.* 330:473–490.

Hennekens, C. H., Speizer, F. E., Rosner, B., Bain, C. J., Belanger, C., and Peto, R. 1979. ''Use of permanent hair dyes and cancer among registered nurses.'' *Lancet* 1:1390–1393.

Hirayama, T. 1981a. ''Non-smoking wives of heavy smokers have a higher risk of lung cancer: a study from Japan.'' *BMJ* 282:183–185.

———. 1981b. ''Non-smoking wives of heavy smokers have a higher risk of lung cancer'' (letter). *BMJ* 283:1466.

Kahn, H. A., and Sempos, C. T. 1989. *Statistical Methods in Epidemiology*. New York: Oxford University Press.

Kaslow, R. A., Ostrow, D. G., Detels, R., Phair, J. P., Polk, B. F., Rinaldo Jr., C. R. 1987. ''The Multicenter AIDS Cohort Study: rationale, organization, and selected characteristics of the participants.'' *Am. J. Epidemiol.* 126:310–318.

Kay, C. R. 1984. ''The Royal College of General Practitioners' Oral Contraception Study: some recent observations.'' *Clinic. Obs. Gyn.* 11:759–781.

Kelsey, J. L. 1979. ''A review of the epidemiology of human breast cancer.'' *Epi. Rev.* 1: 74–109.

Kelsey, J. L., Thompson, W. D., and Evans, A. S. 1986. *Methods in Observational Epidemiology*. New York: Oxford University Press.

Keys, A., ed. 1970. *Coronary Heart Disease in Seven Countries*. Amer. Heart Assoc. Monog. No. 29. New York: The American Heart Association.

Layde, P. M., Beral, V., and Kay, C. R. 1981. ''Further analyses of mortality in oral contraceptive users. Royal College of General Practitioners' Oral Contraception Study.'' *Lancet* 1:541–546.

Levin, M. L. 1953. ''The occurrence of lung cancer in man.'' *Acta Unio In Contra Cancrum* 9:531–541.

Lilienfeld, D.E., and Gallo, M. 1989. ''2,4–D, 2, 4, 5–T, and 2, 3, 7, 8–TCDD: an overview.'' *Epi. Rev.* 11:28–58.

Mantel, N., and Haenszel, W. 1959. ''Statistical aspects of the analysis of data from retrospective studies of disease.'' *J. Nat. Cancer Inst.* 22:719–748.

Matanoski, G. M., Selter, R., Sartwell, P. E., Diamond, E. L., and Elliott, E. A. 1975. ''The current mortality rates of radiologists and other physician specialists: deaths from all causes and from cancer.'' *Am. J. Epidemiol.* 101:188–198.

McGee, D., and Gordon, T. 1976. *The Framingham Study: The Results of the Framingham Study Applied to Four Other U.S.-Based Epidemiologic Studies of Cardiovascular Disease*. Washington, D.C.: U.S. Government Printing Office.

Modan, B. 1966. ''Some methodological aspects of a retrospective follow-up study.'' *Am. J. Epidemiol.* 82:297–304.

Modan, B., and Lilienfeld, A. M. 1965. ''Polycythemia vera and leukemia—the role of radiation treatment.'' *Medicine* 44:305–344.

Monson, R. 1990. *Occupational Epidemiology,* 2nd edition. Boca Raton, Florida: CRC Press.

Napier, J. A., Johnson, B. C., and Epstein, F. H. 1970. "The Tecumseh, Michigan Community Health Study." In *The Community as an Epidemiologic Laboratory: A Casebook of Community Studies.* I. I. Kessler and M. L. Levin, eds. Baltimore, Md: The Johns Hopkins University Press, pp. 25–46.

Rimm, E. B., Stampfer, M. J., Colditz, G. A., Giovannucci, E., and Willett, W. C. 1990. "Effectiveness of various mailing strategies among nonrespondents in a prospective cohort study." *Am. J. Epidemiol.* 131:1068–1071.

Rinsky, R. A., Smith, A. B., Filloon, T. G., Young, R. J., Okun, A. H., and Landrigan, P. J. 1987. "Benzene and leukemia: An epidemiologic risk assessment." *New Engl. J. Med.* 316:1044–1050.

Selikoff, I. J., Hammond, E. C., and Churg, J. 1968. "Asbestos exposure, smoking, and neoplasia." *JAMA* 204:106–112.

———, ———, and Seidman, H. 1979. "Mortality experience of insulation workers in the United States, 1943–1976." *Ann. N.Y. Acad. Sci.* 330:91–116.

Sheps, M. C. 1966. "On the person-years concept in epidemiology and demography." *Milbank Mem. Fund Q.* 44:69–91.

Sims, A.C.P. 1973. "Importance of a high tracing-rate in long-term medical follow-up studies." *Lancet* 2:433–435.

Stellman, S. D., and Garfinkel, L. 1989. "Proportions of cancer deaths attributable to cigarette smoking in women." *Women Health* 15(2):1–29.

Stokes III, J., Kannel, W. B., Wolf, P. A., D'Agostino, R. B., and Cupples, L. A. 1989. "Blood pressure as a risk factor for cardiovascular disease." *Hypertension* 13 (Supplement 1):I13–I18.

User's Manual: The National Death Index. 1981. U.S. Department of Health and Human Services Publication (PHS)81-1148. Hyattsville, Maryland: National Center for Health Statistics.

United States Surgeon General. 1982. *The Health Consequences of Smoking. Cancer.* Washington, D.C.: U.S. Government Printing Office.

Vessey, M. P., Doll, R., Peto, R., Johnson, B., and Wiggins, P. 1976. "A long-term follow-up study of women using different methods of contraception. An interim report." *J. Biosocial Sci.* 8:373–427.

Vessey, M. P., Villard-Mackintosh, L., McPherson, K., and Yeates, D. 1989. "Mortality among oral contraceptive users: 20-year follow-up of women in a cohort study." *Brit. Med. J.* 299:1487–1491.

Walter, S. D. 1975. "The distribution of Levin's measure of attributable risk." *Biometrika* 62:371–374.

———. 1976. "The estimation and interpretation of attributable risk in health research." *Biometrics* 32:829–849.

11

OBSERVATIONAL STUDIES:
II. CASE-CONTROL STUDIES

In case-control studies, comparisons are made between a group of persons that have the disease under investigation and a group that do not. Usually those with the disease are called "cases" and those without the disease are called "controls." Indeed, case-control studies may be viewed as an extension of the case series that a health professional might assemble from his or her practice but with an important addition—the *control group allows for a comparison* to be made with regard to exposure history. Since the exposure history is assessed for some period in the past, case-control studies are also called "retrospective studies."

Whether the characteristic or factor of interest is (or was) present in the two groups is usually determined by interview, review of records, or biological assay. The proportion of cases exposed to the agent or possessing the characteristic (or factor) of etiological interest is compared to the corresponding proportion in the control group. If a higher frequency of individuals with the characteristic is found among the cases than among the controls, an association between the disease and the characteristic may be inferred.

When interested in determining whether prior exposure to an environmental factor is etiologically important, the epidemiologist will attempt to obtain a history of such exposure by interviewing the cases and controls. In practice, information on both current and past characteristics is usually obtained. One must constantly be aware that the derivation of inferences depends upon the temporal sequence between the characteristic and the disease.

The data for a case-control study are generally tabulated in the form of a four-fold table, as shown in Table 11–1. Such a table allows for the comparison

Table 11–1. Framework of a Case-Control Study

	NUMBER OF INDIVIDUALS		
	WITH DISEASE	WITHOUT DISEASE	
CHARACTERISTIC	(CASES)	(CONTROLS)	TOTAL
With	a	b	a + b
Without	c	d	c + d
Total	a + c	b + d	a + b + c + d = N

of the prevalence of exposure among the cases, $a/(a + c)$, with that for the controls, $b/(b + d)$.

In a case-control study the odds ratio is an estimate of relative risk calculated as the cross-product of the entries in Table 11–1, ad/bc (see Appendix). Two assumptions are necessary in making this estimate: (a) the frequency of the disease in the population must be small, and (b) the study cases should be representative of the cases in the population and the controls representative of the noncases in the population. This cross-product estimate can be made with either actual numbers or percentages (Cornfield, 1951). The relative risk (or odds ratio) stays the same whatever the frequency of the exposure in a population. For example, whether smoking is highly prevalent or not, for a mother who smokes, the odds ratio describes her increased risk of delivering a low-birth-weight baby.

A study by Hurwitz and his colleagues (1987) of the relationship between the use of various medications and Reye's syndrome shows how the case-control approach can be used to investigate an etiological hypothesis and how the data can be analyzed with a four-fold table. Reye's syndrome is a rare, acute, and often fatal encephalopathy marked by brain swelling, low blood sugar, and fatty infiltration of the liver. Observations from case-series studies, case reports, and smaller case-control studies had implicated aspirin (salicylate) ingestion during viral illness as a possible cause of this disease of children. Cases deemed eligible for the Hurwitz study had to have received a diagnosis of Reye's syndrome from a physician, reported an antecedent respiratory or gastrointestinal illness or chicken pox within the three weeks before hospitalization, and experienced stage II or deeper encephalopathy. The control group consisted of children who did not have Reye's syndrome but did have chicken pox or a respiratory or gastrointestinal illness within a period of a few weeks before selection for the study. In this study there were four types of controls: emergency room patients (ER controls), inpatients (hospital controls), school children at the same school as the patient (school controls), and children located by the use of random-digit telephone dialing (community controls). The controls were matched to the cases on three patient characteristics: age, race, and the presence of an antecedent illness. The key data from the study are shown in Table 11–2. The percentage of salicylate users among

Table 11–2.   Number of Hospitalized Reye's Patients and Number of Pooled Controls
with a History of Salicylate Use in Three-Week Period

	CASES OF REYE'S SYNDROME	CONTROLS (POOLED)
Used salicylates	26	53
Did *not* use salicylates	1	87
Total	27	140

Source: Hurwitz et al., 1987.

the cases was 96.3% (26/27) as compared to 37.9% (53/140) among the controls, and the odds ratio (the estimate of relative risk) was calculated as follows:

$$\frac{ad}{bc} = \frac{26 \times 87}{53 \times 1} = \frac{2262}{53} = 42.7$$

The variance, standard error, confidence limits, and significance test for the odds ratio can be computed by the procedures presented in the Appendix.

Children with viral illnesses (chicken pox, upper respiratory, or gastrointestinal) who used salicylates during the illness were 42.7 times more likely to develop Reye's syndrome than were children with the same viral illness who did not use salicylates. Thus, aspirin use during viral illness appeared to be strongly associated with the development of Reye's syndrome, increasing the risk over forty-fold.

While these data provide an estimate of risk, they do not allow one to estimate the incidence of Reye's syndrome in the population of children at risk. To estimate the incidence one would need to know the number of all cases of Reye's syndrome among children (for the numerator) and the number of children who experienced respiratory or gastrointestinal illnesses or chicken pox (the denominator). Most case-control studies do not allow one to estimate incidence because denominator data are not available and numerator data may be incomplete.

THE SELECTION OF CASES AND CONTROLS

Various methods have been used to select cases and controls for case-control studies (Table 11–3) Sometimes investigators select cases from one source and controls from a variety of sources, permitting comparisons with different control groups as in the Reye's syndrome study (see Table 11–4). Consistency of results among studies using different types of control groups increases the validity of inferences that may be derived from the findings.

How many controls should be obtained for each case? Appropriate controls are often scarce or limited. In comparing workers at a factory who were or were not exposed to a substance, for instance, one would be limited to the finite set of workers who worked at the factory. In other situations, appropriate controls are readily available, as when studying normal birth outcomes compared to undesirable birth outcomes. Even when controls are abundant, it may be costly and time-consuming to enroll and interview controls; one would want to include only as many as are needed. In studies of rare diseases the number of cases may be so small that the study has insufficient power to detect meaningful differences in exposure. An increased number of controls—up to four per case—may give the study more power (Gail et al., 1976). When the number of cases is large and the power is greater than 0.9 with only one control per case, additional controls cannot add very much to the power.

In selecting cases one may often use all cases occurring in a defined time

Table 11–3.   Some Sources of Cases and Controls in Case-Control Studies*

CASES	CONTROLS
All cases diagnosed in the community (in hospitals, other medical facilities including physicians' offices)	Probability sample of general population in a community obtained by various methods including random-digit dialing
All cases diagnosed in a sample of the general population	Noncases in a sample of the general population or subgroup of a sample of general population (e.g., random-digit dialing)
All cases diagnosed in all hospitals in the community	Sample of patients in all hospitals in the community who do not have the diseases being studied
All cases diagnosed in a single hospital	Sample of patients in same hospital where cases were selected
All cases diagnosed in one or more hospitals	Sample of individuals who are residents in same block or neighborhood of cases
Cases selected by any of the above methods	Spouses, siblings, or associates (schoolmates or workmates) of cases Accident victims

*Various combinations of sources are possible.

Table 11–4. Comparison of Salicylate Exposure among Reye's Patients and Four Types of Controls

| | | CONTROLS | | | |
	CASES	EMERGENCY ROOM	INPATIENT	SCHOOL	COMMUNITY
Exposed to aspirin (%)	96	40	27	44	34
Total N	27	30	22	45	43
Odds ratios	—	39	66	33	44

Source: Hurwitz et al., 1987.

period or geographic area. The researcher then has an idea about the age, race, and gender of the cases, as well as other characteristics. To ensure comparability of cases and controls one may **restrict** the controls to the same age range, race, and gender (or other characteristic) as the cases, or one may **group match** (also known as **frequency match**). For example, the cases can be stratified into different ten-year age groups. The control group can then be similarly stratified. Comparisons can then be made at each factor level between cases and controls with the usual statistical significance tests (Cochran, 1954; Mantel and Haenszel, 1959).

As an alternative to group matching, individual cases and controls can be **pair-matched** for various characteristics so that each case has a pairmate. Ideally, these pairmates should be chosen to be alike on all characteristics except for the particular one under investigation. In practice, if many characteristics are chosen for matching, or if many levels are chosen for each characteristic, it becomes difficult to find matching controls for each of the cases. In epidemiologic studies, there are usually a small number of cases and a large number of potential controls to select (or sample) from. Each case is then classified by characteristics that are not of primary interest, and a search is made for a control with the same set of characteristics. If the factors are not too numerous and there is a large reservoir of persons from which the controls can be chosen, case-control pair matching may be readily carried out. However, if several characteristics or levels are considered and there are not many more potential controls than cases, matching can be difficult. It is quite likely that for some cases, no control will be found; indeed, it may be necessary to either eliminate some of the characteristics from consideration or reduce the number of levels for some of them. With age matching, for example, it is often unlikely that pairs can be formed using one-year age intervals, but five- or ten-year age groups may make matching feasible.

The number of characteristics or levels for which matching is desirable and practical is actually rather small. It is usually sensible to match cases and controls only for characteristics such as age and gender whose association with the disease under study is already known or has been observed in available mortality statistics, morbidity surveys, or other sources. In addition, when cases and controls are matched on any selected characteristic, the influence of that characteristic on the disease can no longer be studied. Hence, caution should be exercised in determining the number of variables selected for matching, even when feasible. If the effect of a characteristic is in doubt, the preferable strategy is not to match but to adjust for these characteristics in the statistical analysis.

POTENTIAL SOURCES OF BIAS

Selection Bias

A method commonly used in conducting case-control studies is to select the cases of the disease under study from one or more hospitals. The control groups usually consist of patients admitted to the same hospital, with diseases other than the one under study. This is a popular method for the initial studies that explore a suspected relation because the data can generally be obtained quickly, easily, and inexpensively. But several assumptions and sources of bias must be considered in analyzing the findings from such studies.

Selection bias is one of the major methodological problems encountered when hospital patients are used in case-control studies. W. A. Guy (see Chapter 2) was the first to suggest that a spurious association between diseases or between a characteristic and a disease could arise because of the different probabilities of admission to a hospital for those with the disease, without the disease, and with the characteristic of interest (Guy, 1856). This possibility was then demonstrated mathematically by Berkson (1946).

The influence of these differences on the study group in the hospital can be illustrated with a hypothetical example.

Let X = Etiological factor or characteristic

A = Disease group designated as cases

B = Disease group designated as controls

Assume that there is no real association between disease A and X in the group population, as indicated in Table 11–5; that is, the percentage of those with A who have X and the percentage of those with B who have X is equal. Assume also that there are different rates or probabilities of admission to the hospital for persons with X, A, and B, each of which acts independently, as follows: X = 50

Table 11–5.   Frequency of Characteristic X in Disease
Groups A and B in the General Population

	NUMBER OF INDIVIDUALS IN DISEASE GROUPS	
	A	B
CHARACTERISTIC	(CASES)	(CONTROLS)
With X	200	200
Without X	800	800
Total	1,000	1,000
Percent of total with X	20	20

percent; A = 10 percent; B = 70 percent. Now consider the actual numbers of people in these groups who are admitted to the hospital:

(a) *For those with A and X:*
    10 percent of the 200 in this category are admitted because
    they have A   = 20
    50 percent of the remaining 180 in this category are admitted
    because they have X   = 90

    Total admitted   = $\overline{110}$

(b) *For those with A and without X:*
    10 percent of the 800 in this category are admitted because
    they have A   = 80

(c) *For those with B and X:*
    70 percent of the 200 in this category are admitted because
    they have B   = 140
    50 percent of the remaining 60 in this category with B are
    admitted because they have X   = 30

    Total admitted   = $\overline{170}$

(d) *For those with B and without X:*
    70 percent of the 800 in this category are admitted because
    they have B   = 560

These numbers are then inserted into the four cells of Table 11–5, allowing a comparison of disease A (cases) and disease B (controls) with respect to those who do and do not have the characteristic in our hypothetically constructed hospital population, as shown in Table 11–6. The result is that 58 percent of those with disease A have X as compared to 23 percent of those with disease B. This indicates that an association exists between A and X, even though this association

Table 11–6. A Hypothetical Hospital Population
Based on Differential Rates of Hospital Admission

CHARACTERISTIC	NUMBER OF INDIVIDUALS IN DISEASE GROUPS	
	A (CASES)	B (CONTROLS)
With X	110	170
Without X	80	560
Total	190	730
Percent of total with X	58	23

is not present in the general population (the source of the hospital population). This spurious association results from the different rates of admission to the hospital for people with the different diseases and X. However, spurious associations such as this will not arise if either (Kraus, 1954):

1. X does not affect hospitalization, that is, no person is hospitalized simply because of X; or
2. the rate of admission to the hospital for those persons with A is equal to those with B.

One can never be absolutely certain that the first condition is met in any given study. For example, if X represents eye color, it might be assumed that this would not influence the probability of hospitalization. It is possible, however, that persons with a particular eye color belong to an ethnic group whose members are mainly of a specific social class, which, in turn, may influence the probability of their hospitalization. The likelihood of a spurious association is greater if the factor under investigation (i.e., X) is another disease rather than a characteristic or an attribute. The second condition is, of course, the exception rather than the rule since persons with different diseases usually have different probabilities of hospitalization. In any event, one cannot assume that these differences do not exist unless it is demonstrated that there are no differences in the hospitalization rates for individuals regardless of the disease.

In hospital studies, the same factors that may produce a spurious association, also termed "Berksonian" or "selection" bias, can have the reverse effect. The differences in hospital admission rates may conceal an association in a study and fail to detect one that actually exists in the population.

Selection bias is not limited to the analysis of hospital patients. It may be present in any situation or type of population where persons with different diseases or characteristics enter a study group at different rates or probabilities. For example, in studying an autopsy series from a specified hospital population where the autopsy rates differ for the diseases and characteristics being studied in the manner described above, the inferred associations will be biased and may result in a spurious association or mask a real association (McMahan, 1962; Mainland, 1953; Waife et al., 1952).

Selection biases, however, do not necessarily invalidate study findings. This issue should be resolved on its own merits for any particular investigation, and the following means are available to increase the likelihood that an observed association is real:

1. The strength of the association can be evaluated to see if it could result from the type of selection bias described above. A strong association is less likely to result from selection bias than a weak one.

2. Depending on the disease and the personal characteristic (such as serum cholesterol level) or the possible etiological factor (such as cigarette smoking), it may be possible to classify the characteristic or factor into a gradient from low to high levels. If the degree of association between the disease and the characteristic or factor consistently increases or decreases with increasing levels of the characteristic or factor, this "dose-response relationship" reduces the likelihood that the association is a result of selection bias. For selection bias to occur, it would be necessary to hypothesize the very unlikely occurrence of a similar gradient of rates of entry into the study group or of hospitalization in a study of hospitalized patients for the characteristic and the disease. This can be illustrated with some data from a recent study of oral contraceptive use and breast cancer among women 45 years old and younger in England (McPherson, et al., 1987). Information was obtained on past oral contraceptive use by women with breast cancer in six London hospitals and two Oxford hospitals during 1980–1984. The same information was obtained from a similarly aged control group (female

Table 11–7. Duration of Oral Contraceptive Use before
First Term Pregnancy among Female Breast Cancer
Patients and Hospital Controls 45 Years Old and Younger

DURATION OF ORAL CONTRACEPTIVE USE	CASES (%)	CONTROLS (%)
No Use	235 (67%)	273 (78%)
≤ 1 Year	27 (8%)	26 (7%)
1–4 Years	43 (12%)	29 (8%)
> 4 Years	46 (13%)	23 (7%)
Total	351 (100%)	351 (7%)

Source: McPherson et al., 1987.

patients in these hospitals admitted for conditions not related to contraceptive use) during this time period. Table 11–7 presents the results of a comparison of breast cancer patients and controls according to the duration of oral contraceptive use before the first pregnancy. Not only is there a higher proportion of oral contraceptive users among the breast cancer patients than the controls, but the breast cancer patients tended to use oral contraceptives for a longer time period than the control patients. A gradient showing an increase in oral contraceptive use among the cases compared with the controls is evident. Another illustration is provided by Antunes and his colleagues (1979), who examined the possible relationship between estrogen use and endometrial cancer with a case-control research design. Their findings are shown in Figure 11–1. A gradient of duration of postmenopausal estrogen use and endometrial cancer is evident.

3. As a precaution against the influence of selection biases, one may draw controls from a variety of sources. Should the frequency of the study characteristic be similar in each control group and differ from the case group, selection bias would not be a likely explanation for the observed association. The study of Reye's syndrome used controls from an emergency room, in patients, school children, and the community and found consistent results for each group (Table 11–4). In their classic study of lung cancer and smoking Doll and Hill (1952) demonstrated the importance of multiple control groups. They obtained infor-

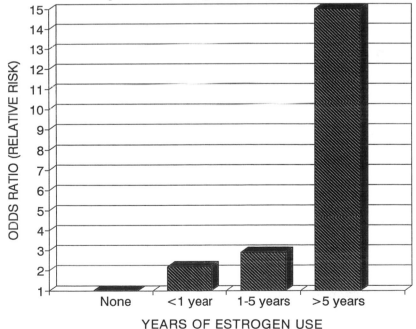

Figure 11–1. Odds ratios for endometrial cancer cases and controls according to duration of use of postmenopausal estrogen. *Source:* Adapted from Antunes, et al. (1979).

mation on the smoking habits of a sample of the general population from a social survey that was conducted in Great Britain during 1951. The smoking habits of patients in their control group were compared with those of persons in the social survey who were residents of Greater London, after adjusting for the age differences between the two groups. Table 11–8 shows the distribution of smoking habits among males in these two groups. The smaller proportion of nonsmokers and the higher proportion of heavy smokers among the controls than in the general population may result from the fact that patients in the control group had diseases that were also related to smoking habits. Thus, the degree of relationship between smoking and lung cancer shown in Table 11–8 was actually underestimated by the use of hospital controls in that investigation.

Representativeness

When cases are drawn from death certificate data bases or centralized registries, it is possible to select a representative sample of cases. This applies to case-control studies of various causes of death or of cancer or other registered illnesses. When cases are drawn from a limited, well-defined population it is also fairly easy to identify all cases. Thus, a case-control study of diarrhea in a day-care center can be designed to interview the parents of every child in the day-care center, or even to examine every child.

Many times it is not easy to identify all the cases of a disease. Even if one canvasses physicians, laboratories, and hospitals to find cases of an illness, there may be people with the illness who are not being treated or who are unaware of their condition. An example might be early miscarriage; a proportion of miscarriages may occur in women who are not aware that they are pregnant (and thus not aware that they miscarried), or women who have not yet been to a physician

Table 11–8. Comparison between Smoking Habits of Male Patients without Cancer of the Lung (Control Group) and of Those Interviewed in the Social Survey: London, 1951

SUBJECT	PERCENTAGE OF NONSMOKERS	PERCENT SMOKING DAILY AVERAGE OF CIGARETTES				NUMBER INTERVIEWED
		1–4	5–14	15–24	25+	
Patient with diseases other than lung cancer	7.0	4.2	43.3	32.1	13.4	1,390
General population sample (Social Survey)	12.1	7.0	44.2	28.1	8.5	199

Source: Doll and Hill (1952).

to begin prenatal care. There is probably no easy way to ensure obtaining a representative sample of women having early miscarriages. Cases of miscarriage drawn from a population of female physicians, for example, would probably select higher educated, higher social class women who are more likely to seek prenatal care earlier in pregnancy. In a study of life style and miscarriages this might introduce a bias, especially if the controls were selected from the general population.

Bias in Obtaining Information

Another bias that may distort the findings from case-control studies develops from the interviewer's awareness of the identity of cases and controls. This knowledge may influence the structure of the questions and the interviewer's manner, which in turn may influence the response. Whenever possible, interviews should be conducted without prior knowledge of the identify of cases and controls, although administrative constraints often prevent such "blind" interviews. In special circumstances, hospital patients may be interviewed at the time of admission so that information of epidemiologic interest is obtained before the patient is seen by a physician and thus before a diagnosis is made establishing the identity of cases and controls. This requires a comprehensive, general-purpose interview routinely administered to all patients admitted. Several epidemiologic studies have utilized a unique set of data from the Roswell Park Memorial Institute, where such a procedure is used (Bross, 1968; Bross and Tidings, 1973; Levin et al., 1950; Levin et al., 1955; Lilienfeld, 1956; Solomon et al., 1968; Winkelstein et al., 1958). Comparing their results with those of studies that depend on more conventional sources of controls provides a means for evaluating possible interviewer bias. A similar approach is used by the Slone Epidemiology Unit which routinely obtains drug histories from patients entering hospitals in the Boston region and other cities.

Patients interviewed as diagnosed cases in studies occasionally have had their diagnoses changed later. If data obtained from the erroneously diagnosed group resemble data from the control rather than the case series, interviewer bias can be discounted (Table 11–9).

The association of a factor and a disease may often be restricted to a specific histologic type or other component of the disease spectrum, as determined by objective means. For example, the fact that oat cell pulmonary carcinoma is more positively related to a history of exposure to bis-chloromethyl ether (BCME) than adenocarcinoma of the lung more firmly established the relationship between the two (Pasternak, et al., 1977). When such diagnostic details and their significance are unknown to the interviewer, another check on possible interviewer bias is provided.

The subjects' responses to an interview can also be directly validated by

Table 11–9.   The Smoking Habits of Patients in Different Disease Groups, 45–74 Years of Age, Standardized According to the Age Distribution of the Population of England and Wales as of June 30, 1950

		PERCENT SMOKING DAILY AVERAGE OF CIGARETTES				
DISEASE GROUP	PERCENTAGE OF NONSMOKERS	<5	5–14	15–24	25+	NUMBER INTERVIEWED
Males						
Cancer of lung	0.3	4.6	55.9	35.0	24.3	1,224
Patients incorrectly thought to have cancer of lung	5.3	9.9	35.5	37.8	11.4	102
Other respiratory diseases	1.9	9.9	38.3	38.7	11.2	301
Other cancers	4.6	9.4	47.2	26.0	12.8	473
Other diseases	5.6	9.0	44.8	26.9	13.7	875
Females						
Cancer of lung	40.6	13.7	22.0	9.5	14.2	90
Patients incorrectly thought to have cancer of lung	66.9	16.4	12.7	4.2	0.0	45
Other respiratory diseases	66.5	22.4	0.0	11.1	0.0	25
Other cancers	68.4	14.3	11.0	5.0	1.2	294
Other diseases	55.9	22.1	17.5	3.6	0.9	157

Source: Doll and Hill (1952).

comparison with other records. This was shown in a study of the accuracy of recall of the history of contraceptive use. Case-control studies of the relation between oral contraceptive use and a variety of diseases assumed that women recalled their use of oral contraceptives with reasonable accuracy (Collaborative Group for the Study of Stroke in Young Women, 1973; Mann et al., 1975; Thomas, 1972; Vessey and Doll, 1968). This assumption was tested by comparing oral contraceptive histories of seventy-five women attending family planning clinics with information available in the clinic records. It was found that the type of information obtained in the case-control studies was likely to be remembered with reasonable accuracy (Glass et al., 1974). This finding has been confirmed by Stolley et al. (1978).

Most investigators take great pains to prevent bias by rigorously training study interviewers in proper interview methods. Moreover, it is possible to check the interviewers' technique by video-taping the interview or reinterviewing a sample of the subjects to detect information bias at an early stage of a study when corrective measures are possible.

ANALYZING CASE-CONTROL STUDIES

We described the odds ratio in the beginning of this chapter. The comparison of exposure among cases and controls and the calculation of the odds ratio are the unique features in analyzing data from case-control studies. Odds ratios can be calculated for different amounts of exposure, or for subgroups stratified by other risk factors. Analysis of matched pairs is a special case when each pair is a separate strata. Multivariate methods can be used to estimate the effect of several variables on the odds ratio, and one can consider each variable while controlling for the others.

Odds Ratio for Multiple Levels of Exposure

Inferences about the association between a disease and a factor are considerably strengthened if information is available to support a gradient between the degree of exposure (or "dose") to a characteristic and the disease in question. Odds ratios can be computed for each dose of the characteristic. The general approach is to treat the data as a series of 2×2 tables, comparing controls and cases at different levels of exposure, and then calculating the risk at each level. The data from Table 11–7 are presented in Table 11–10, together with the computed odds ratios. The users with different durations of oral contraceptive use are compared with the nonusers, whose risk of breast cancer is set at 1.0. The odds ratios (OR) for users relative to nonusers are:

$$\text{OR } (\leq 1 \text{ year's use}) = \frac{27 \times 273}{26 \times 235} = \frac{7,371}{6,110} = 1.2$$

$$\text{OR } (1\text{–}4 \text{ years' use}) = \frac{43 \times 273}{29 \times 235} = \frac{11,739}{6,815} = 1.7$$

$$\text{OR } (>4 \text{ years' use}) = \frac{46 \times 273}{23 \times 235} = \frac{12,558}{5,405} = 2.3$$

It is possible to employ statistical tests of significance to determine whether or not the obtained relative risks differ from "unity" or 1.0. These tests can be applied to the summary relative risk (Cochran's test) or to all the categories (the Mantel-Haenzel test) (Cochran, 1954; Mantel and Haenszel, 1959) (see Appendix).

Table 11–10.   Relative Risk of Breast Cancer for Smokers and Nonsmokers, by
Duration of Oral Contraceptive Use (Data from Table 11–7)

DURATION OF ORAL CONTRACEPTIVE USE	BREAST CANCER CASES	HOSPITAL CONTROLS	ODDS RATIO (ESTIMATED RELATIVE RISK)
No use	235	273	1.0
≤ 1 Year	27	26	1.2
1–4 Years	43	29	1.7
> 4 Years	46	23	2.3

Source: McPherson et al., 1987.

Matched Cases and Controls

When cases and controls are matched in pairs in order to make the two groups comparable with regard to one or more factors, the fourfold (2 × 2) table takes a form different from that shown in Table 11–1. The status of the cases with regard to the presence or absence of the characteristic is compared with its presence or absence in their respective controls (Table 11–11). The cell in the upper left-hand corner of Table 11–11 contains r number of pairs in which both cases and controls possess the characteristic of interest. The marginal totals (a, b, c, d) represent the entries in the cells of Table 11–11 and the total for the entire table is $\frac{1}{2}N$ pairs where N represents the total number of paired individuals. The calculation of the odds ratio for this table is simple (Kraus, 1958): OR = s/t (provided t is not 0). Both a test of significance and a method of calculating the standard error are presented in the Appendix.

An example of the method of analysis for matched pairs in a case-control study comes from the work of Chow et al. (1990) on the relation between past exposure to *Chlamydia trachomatis* and ectopic pregnancy. Prior *Chlamydia trachomatis* infection had been associated with both tubal infertility and pelvic inflammatory disease, conditions associated with ectopic pregnancy. Chow and

Table 11–11.   Symbolic Representation of Matched Cases and
Controls with and without the Exposure of Interest

	CONTROLS		
	EXPOSED	UNEXPOSED	TOTAL
Exposed	r	s	a*
Unexposed	t	u	c*
Total	b*	d*	½ N

*a, b, c, and d correspond to the cells of Table 11–1.

Table 11–12. Matched Pair Analysis of a Case-Control Study of the Association between *Chlamydia trachomatis* and Ectopic Pregnancy

| | | CONTROLS | |
		PAST EXPOSURE TO *C. TRACHOMATIS*	NO EXPOSURE TO *C. TRACHOMATIS*
Cases	Past exposure to *C. trachomatis*	72	109
	No exposure to *C. trachomatis*	36	40

Source: Chow, 1990, personal communication.

her colleagues recruited the cases of ectopic pregnancies from admissions and the controls from prenatal clinics. The case-control pairs were matched for age (± 1 year), ethnicity, hospital, and restricted to women whose pregnancy was of 12 to 24 weeks duration. Cases with previous bilateral tubal ligation, ectopic pregnancy, or an intrauterine device present at the time of conception were excluded from the study. A total of 257 matched case-control pairs were assembled and each pair was categorized as to past exposure to *Chlamydia trachomatis* (assessed by antibody titer of $\geq 1:64$). Based on Table 11–11, each pair could be categorized in one of four ways:

    r. Case exposed and control exposed $(++)$ = 72
    s. Case exposed and control not exposed $(+-)$ = 109
    t. Case not exposed and control exposed $(-+)$ = 36
    u. Case not exposed and control not exposed $(--)$ = 40

Group s is the group where cases were exposed and controls were not $(+-)$; group t is the group where cases were not exposed, but controls were exposed $(-+)$. As in the above formula, the odds ratio is estimated as s/t or 109/36 = 3.0 (see Table 11–12). The calculation considers only the discordant pairs, and this can be explained intuitively: One can see that pairs where both were exposed or where both were unexposed would give no information about the relationship of exposure to disease. For example, one could not measure the effect of fluoride on cavities in a group of pairs that had all received fluoride, or that had all been unexposed to fluoride (Schlesselman, 1982).

Interrelationships between Risk Factors

Odds ratios can also be used to determine whether interrelationships exist between various characteristics or risk factors. A case-control study of lung cancer, cigarette smoking, and asbestos exposure among workers in southern Norway exposed to multiple risk factors provides an example of this (Kjuus et al. 1986). In two neighboring counties in the southern part of Norway, all cases of lung cancer in males during 1979–1983 were ascertained. For each case, a similarly aged control was selected from among the patients in the same geographical area as the case. All men with conditions that would have precluded possible employment in heavy industry were excluded from the study. The 176 cases and 176 controls were interviewed about their history of exposure to asbestos and their smoking habits. The histories were then coded into four categories according to the level of asbestos exposure the person had reported (no exposure, light or sporadic exposure, moderate exposure between 1 and 10 years duration or heavy exposure less than 1 year in duration, and more than 10 years of moderate exposure or more than 1 year of heavy exposure). The relative risks for each category of asbestos exposure and smoking habit are shown in Table 11–13. From these data, it appears that the relative risk increases with an increase in either smoking or asbestos exposure. When the factors are considered together, the odds ratio rises sharply. This suggests that these factors modify and increase each other's effect on the disease.

Effect of Misclassification

Misclassification of both disease and exposure can occur in any type of study. In a case-control study, misclassification of disease would lead to some of the selection biases already discussed; it would alter a person's probability of entering the study. Assuming that selection bias has been dealt with, misclassification of exposure must be addressed in a case-control study. Exposure status usually cannot be measured directly by the researcher in such a study. Instead, the researcher relies on records (e.g., employment records describing work assignments and possible occupational exposures), recall (e.g. employment, residential, smoking, pharmaceutical histories), or even the recall of a close friend or relative, usually a spouse (e.g. diet, smoking, alcohol consumption, exercise). There are two types of misclassification that can occur: (1) differential—where the amount or direction of misclassification is different in the cases and controls, and (2) nondifferential—where the amount and direction of misclassification is the same in cases and controls. Misclassification error can occur in one direction for cases and controls; for example, everyone may underreport their own or their spouse's habitual alcohol consumption. Misclassification can occur in opposite directions; spouses of cirrhosis patients might overreport alcohol consumption, while spouses of other patients might continue to underreport alcohol use. People typically may misreport their abortion histories, smoking histories, number of sexual partners, and income, and this may be all in one direction or not. People may also misreport information because they can't remember their typical breakfast 10 years ago, the number of cigarettes their husbands used to smoke, the length of their menstrual

Table 11–13. Odds Ratio Estimates of the Relative Risks of Lung Cancer for
Combined Exposure to Asbestos and Smoking

| CIGARETTES | ASBESTOS EXPOSURE | | | |
SMOKED DAILY	NONE	LITTLE	MODERATE	HEAVY
0–4	1.0	1.2	2.7	4.1
5–9	2.9	1.2	7.8	11.9
10–19	9.1	1.9	24.6	37.3
20–29	16.5	19.8	44.6	67.7
≥30	90.3	108.4	243.8	370.2

Source: adapted from Kjuus et al. (1986).

cycle during each decade of life, or how many hours a day they were exposed to silica dust during each year of employment.

Differential misclassification (because the exposure status of cases is more or less likely to be miscategorized than that of the controls) can produce bias in either direction, raising or lowering the estimate of risk (Schlesselman, 1982). Nondifferential misclassification (randomly distributed among cases and controls) generally shifts the odds ratio toward the null hypothesis (OR = 1.0), but exceptions to this can occur (Dosemeci et al., 1990). The effect of misclassification may also depend on how exposure is defined, as a continuous or categorical variable, and if categorical, as a two-level or multilevel variable.

These effects of misclassification emphasize the need to verify the information obtained in a study by every feasible means. Information with respect to previous exposures or characteristics of study individuals may be verified by obtaining records from independent sources (such as hospitals, physicians, schools, military services, and employment records) on either all or a sample of individuals in the study. Disease diagnoses should be verified whenever possible by independent review of medical records, histological slides, electrocardiograms, etc. The degree of verification possible depends upon the factors or characteristics and the diseases being studied. For example, verification of alcohol consumption or of the content of an individual's diet over a period of time poses serious problems of verification. Alternatively, in a health maintenance organization, for instance, records of prior illness or drug prescriptions may be available, eliminating the possibility of misclassification. Another approach is to use antibody titers as an index of past exposure to an infectious agent. This method has been used in case-control studies of hepatitis B infection and primary liver cancer (Szmuness, 1978). Recently, biological markers for some other exposures have been developed. For example, the presence of cotinine, a metabolite of nicotine, in the blood, urine, or saliva can serve as a biomarker of exposure to cigarette smoking; a high level would indicate active smoking, and a low level, exposure to environmental tobacco smoke.

Attributable Fraction

Another measure of association, influenced by the frequency of a characteristic in the population, is the attributable fraction. As noted in Chapter 10, this is the proportion of a disease that can be attributed to an etiological factor; alternatively, it is considered the proportional decrease in the incidence of a disease if the entire population were no longer exposed to the suspected etiological agent. As in cohort studies, the attributable fraction may be estimated in case-control studies as follows:

$$\text{Attributable Fraction (AF)} = \frac{P(OR - 1)}{P(OR - 1) + 1} \times 100\%,$$

where OR = the odds ratio and P = proportion of the total population classified as having the characteristic. The derivation of this formula can be found in the Appendix. Standard errors and confidence limits have been derived for the attributable fraction by Walter (1975, 1978) (see Appendix).

Computations of attributable fraction are also helpful in developing strategies for epidemiologic research, particularly if there are multiple etiological factors (Walter, 1975). In the study of past *Chlamydia trachomatis* infection and ectopic pregnancy, for example, the attributable fraction for past chlamydial infection was 47 percent, while that for douching (an independent risk factor) was 45 percent (Chow et al., 1990). These data suggest the need for further investigation of douching practices in relation to ectopic pregnancy occurrence, while underscoring the need for control of chlamydial infections to prevent ectopic pregnancies.

Regression Models and Adjustment for Confounding Variables

In a case-control study, several variables may be studied as potential risk factors, variables thought to influence the outcome (occurrence of disease). As will be discussed in Chapter 12, it is always possible that these variables may be **confounded** with one another. For example, in a case-control study of lung cancer, exposures of interest may include cigarette smoking, exposure to asbestos, and use of alcohol. Which of these exposures are associated with lung cancer and which are not (but are associated with one another)? The epidemiologist can deal with this problem by using **multivariate analysis,** a set of techniques for studying the effects of several factors simultaneously (Kleinbaum et al., 1982). These techniques range from simple cross-classification and adjustment to more complex methods of statistical regression analysis.

Various models have been used by epidemiologists, such as "multiple logistic," "log-linear," "multiple linear," and "simple linear" regression. These techniques permit the investigator to determine which of the variables has an independent association with the outcome, to determine which variables interact among themselves, and to quantify the relative contribution of each variable or combination of variables to the risk of the disease. Multivariate analysis does not necessarily distinguish causal from noncausal associations, but it may give indications about the relative strengths of the independent and joint effects of multiple exposures.

ADVANTAGES AND DISADVANTAGES OF CASE-CONTROL STUDIES

Advantages

The case-control study can be used to test hypotheses concerned with the long-term effects of an exposure on a disease, and the study can often be completed quickly. For example, in one to two years data can be collected about 20 or 30 years of exposure to an environmental or occupational hazard.

The case-control study can also be used to test hypotheses about rare diseases or diseases that have long latency periods. The first case-control study estimating the association between diethylstilbestrol (DES) and adenocarcinoma of the vagina in young women used only 8 cases and 32 controls (Herbst et al., 1971). The disease was very rare (about 10 cases in 10 million young women) and 15 to 20 years elapsed between exposure and disease, but the case-control study identified the risk factor and estimated the relative risk. In Table 11–14 one may see how the rareness of disease influences the number of subjects needed in cohort or case-control studies and the advantage of a case-control study for studying rare conditions.

The case-control study is well suited to the study of adverse effects of a drug or treatment, or of a new disease where efficient identification of a risk factor can lead to prompt public health intervention.

The case-control study can be relatively inexpensive because it may use fewer study subjects and take a shorter period of time than some other designs. It also allows examination of several risk factors for a single disease.

Disadvantages

It is sometimes difficult to find an appropriate control group, for theoretical or practical reasons. For example, what is the appropriate control group for auto accident victims? What is the appropriate control group for tennis players with a particular injury? Will there be enough subjects available for a control group?

It is sometimes difficult to decide if the exposure preceded the disease. In

Table 11–14.   Sample Size Requirements for Cohort and Case-Control Studies*

DISEASE INCIDENCE IN UNEXPOSED GROUP	FREQUENCY OF ATTRIBUTE DETECTABLE IN POPULATION (%)	RELATIVE RISK	SAMPLE SIZE NEEDED IN EACH GROUP	
			COHORT STUDY	CASE-CONTROL STUDY
1/1,000	50	1.2	576,732	2,535
		2.0	31,443	177
		4.0	5,815	48
1/100	50	1.2	57,100	2,535
		2.0	3,100	177
		4.0	567	48
1/10	50	1.2	5,137	2,535
		2.0	266	177
		4.0	42	48

*Power = 90%; alpha = 5%.
Source: Kahn and Sempos (1989).

studying diarrhea among breast-fed or formula-fed babies, one would want to know if diarrhea led to cessation of breast feeding, or if cessation of breast feeding led to an episode of diarrhea. Similarly, in a study of heart disease among letter carriers, one would like to know whether healthy people choose to become letter carriers or whether letter carrying (and walking each day) leads to healthier cardiovascular systems.

Case-control studies are subject to a number of biases, especially survival biases, selection biases, recall biases, and misclassification. Well-designed studies can sometimes minimize the introduction of biases, but the potential for biases must be considered for each study question. Case-control studies frequently rely on information collected from living cases of the disease of interest. If the deceased cases are different from the surviving cases, a bias may be introduced into the study.

Case-control studies do not actually measure incidence of disease in the population at risk, although estimates can sometimes be made (when all cases of the disease are known, and the population at risk is known).

SUMMARY

In a case-control study, the investigator compares the history of past exposure to a factor or presence of a characteristic among those persons with a given disease or condition (cases) and among those who do not have the disease or condition (controls). The proportion of those exposed among the cases is compared with that among the controls. If these proportions are different, then an association exists between the factor and the disease. Cases can be ascertained from hospitals, clinics, disease registries, or during a prevalence or incidence survey in a population. Controls can likewise be sampled from hospitals, clinics, or a random sample of the population. Care must be exercised in the case and control selection methods, because selection biases can lead to spurious associations. An alternative approach to control selection is to match each control to each case, based on factors thought to be related to the exposure of interest and the disease. In the process of matching, the investigator loses representativeness, i.e., the ability to generalize the findings to the general population, but gains greater comparability among the cases and controls. Unbiased collection of data from both cases and controls is necessary. Biases can occur in recalling past exposures.

The measure of the strength of an association in a case-control study is the odds ratio estimate of the relative risk of developing the disease for those who have been exposed compared with that for those not exposed. Odds ratios can be calculated for both matched and unmatched designs. Misclassification of either the presence or absence of disease, or of exposure status, can affect the estimate of the relative risk. Confounding factors can also affect the estimate of the relative risk. Techniques such as the Mantel-Haenszel test and logistic regression can be used to adjust for confounding factors in the data analysis. However, such statistical techniques cannot make up for errors in study design or data collection. Another measure of association is the attributable fraction, which measures the proportion of disease occurrence that is associated with the factor of interest.

Case-control studies have many advantages and disadvantages compared with cohort studies (Table 11–15). Among the advantages are their lower costs, shorter time to completion, and the ability to examine the association of many

Table 11–15.   Advantages and Disadvantages of Case-Control Studies

---

Advantages
1. Generally a short study period.
2. One may study rare diseases.
3. Inexpensive.
4. One may study several risk factors for a single disease.
5. Useful for studying adverse drug reactions or new diseases.

Disadvantages

1. Sometimes difficult to choose appropriate control.
2. Sometimes difficult to determine if exposure preceded the disease.
3. Prone to biases in selection and information.
4. One is usually unable to calculate incidence rates.

---

factors with a given disease. Among their disadvantages are the potential for bias in case and control selection, the potential for recall bias during data collection, and the possible bias associated with investigating survivors of a disease.

STUDY PROBLEMS

1. What would be an appropriate control group (or groups) for the following conditions (mention possible exclusions):
   (a) Babies born at very low birth weight (≤ 1500 grams).
   (b) Infants with chronic ear infections.
   (c) Transplant patients who reject a transplant.
   (d) Russian roulette suicide victims.

2. Marzuk et al. (1992) conducted a case-control study of cocaine and alcohol use as risk factors for suicide by Russian roulette. The controls were handgun suicides. Toxicological analyses were performed and the data below were obtained. The authors did not calculate an odds ratio, but you can. Calculate the odds ratios and write one sentence for each odds ratio explaining its meaning.

(a)	DRUGS OR ALCOHOL PRESENT IN BLOOD	NO DRUGS OR ALCOHOL IN BLOOD	TOTAL
Russian roulette suicide victims	11	3	14
Handgun suicide victims	33	21	54
Total	44	24	68

(b)	COCAINE DETECTED IN BLOOD	NO COCAINE DETECTED IN BLOOD	TOTAL
Russian roulette suicide victims	9	5	14
Handgun suicide victims	19	35	54
Total	28	40	68

3. Name an advantage and a disadvantage of using a case-control study design to test the hypothesis that cocaine use increases the probability of death from Russian roulette.

4. The recent controversy over silicone breast implants began with the observation of breast cancer among women with the implants.
   (a) What is the advantage in using a case-control study to test the hypothesis that silicone breast implants are associated with breast cancer?
   (b) Who should be the cases in such a study?
   (c) What groups would make appropriate controls?
   (d) What variables might one use to select the control group?
   (e) What variables might be useful in group or pair matching?
   (f) What would be the problem in choosing many variables for matching?
   (g) How could one collect information about women's silicone breast implants?
   (h) What problems arise in collecting the women's medical histories?

REFERENCES

Antunes, C.M.F., Stolley, P. D., Rosensheim, N. B., Davies, J. L., Tonascia, J. A., Brown, C., Burnett, L., Rutledge, A., Pokempner, M. and Garcia, R. 1979. "Endometrial cancer and estrogen use." *New Engl. J. Med.* 300:9–13.

Berkson, J. 1946. "Limitations of the application of fourfold table analysis to hospital data." *Biometrics* 2:47–53.

Bross, I.D.J., and Tidings, J. 1973. "Another look at coffee drinking and cancer of the urinary bladder." *Prev. Med.* 2:445–451.

Bross, I.D.J. 1968. "Effect of filter cigarettes on the risk of lung cancer." *Nat. Cancer Inst. Monogr.* 28:35–40.

Cancer and Steroid Hormone Study of the Centers for Disease Control and the National Institute of Child Health and Human Development. 1987. "The reduction in risk of ovarian cancer associated with oral contraceptive use." *NEJM* 316:650–655.

Chow, J. M., Yonekura, M. L., Richwald, G. A., Greenland, S., Sweet, R. L., Schachter, J. 1990. "The association between *Chlamydia trachomatis* and ectopic pregnancy." *JAMA* 263(23):3164–3167.

Cochran, W. G. 1954. "Some methods of strengthening the common χ^2 tests." *Biometrics* 10:417–451.

Collaborative Group for the Study of Stroke in Young Women. 1973. "Oral contraception and increased risk of cerebral ischemia or thrombosis." *New Engl. J. Med.* 288:871–878.

Cornfield, J. 1951. "A method of estimating comparative rates from clinical data. Applications to cancer of the lung, breast and cervix." *J. Natl. Cancer Inst.* 11:1269–1275.

Doll, R. and Hill, A. B. 1952. "A study of the aetiology of carcinoma of the lung." *Brit. Med. J.* 2:1271–1286.

Dosemeci, M., Wacholder, S. and Lubin, J. H. 1990. "Does nondifferential misclassification of exposure always bias a true effect toward the null value?" *Am. J. Epidemiol.* 132(4):746–748.

Gail, M., Williams, R., Byar, D. P., and Brown, C. 1976. "How many controls?" *J. of Chronic Disease* 29:723–731.

Glass, R., Johnson, B., and Vessey, M. 1974. "Accuracy of recall of histories of oral contraceptive use." *Brit. J. Prev. Med.* 28:273–275.

Guy, W. A. 1856. "On the nature and extent of the benefits conferred by hospitals on the working classes and the poor." *J. Roy. Stat. Soc.* 19:12–27.

Herbst, A. L., Ulfelder, H. and Poskanzer, D. C. 1971. "Association of maternal stilbestrol therapy with tumor appearance in young women." *NEJM* 284(16):878–881.

Hurwitz, E. S., Barrett, M. J., Bregman, D., et al. 1987. "Public health service study of Reye's Syndrome and medications: Report of the main study." *JAMA* 257(14):1905–1911.

Kahn, H. A. and Sempos, C. T. 1989. *Statistical Methods in Epidemiology*. New York: Oxford University Press.

Kjuus, H., Skjaerven, R., Langard, S., Lien, J. T., Aamodt, T. 1986. "A case-referent study of lung cancer, occupational exposures and smoking. II: Role of asbestos exposure." *Scand. J. Work Environ. Health* 12:203–209.

Kleinbaum, D. G., Kupper, L. L., Morgenstern, H. 1982. *Epidemiologic Research*. Belmont, Calif.: Lifetime Learning Publications.

Kraus, A. S. 1954. "The use of hospital data in studying the association between a characteristic and a disease." *Pub. Health Rep.* 69:1211–1214.

———. 1958. "The Use of Family Members as Controls in the Study of the Possible Etiologic Factors of a Disease." Sc.D. Thesis, Graduate School of Public Health, University of Pittsburgh.

Levin, M. I., Goldstein, H., and Gerhardt, P. R. 1950. "Cancer and tobacco smoking: A preliminary report." *JAMA* 143:336–338.

Levin, M. I., Kraus, A. S., Goldberg, I. D., and Gerhardt, P. R. 1955. "Problems in the study of occupation and smoking in relation to lung cancer." *Cancer* 8:932–936.

Lilienfeld, A. M. 1956. "The relationship of cancer of the female breast to artificial menopause and marital status." *Cancer* 9:927–934.

Mainland, D. 1953. "Risk of fallacious conclusions from autopsy data on incidence of disease with applications to heart disease." *Amer. Heart J.* 45:644–654.

Mann, J. I., Vessey, M. P., Thorogood, M., and Doll, R. 1975. "Myocardial infarction in young women with special reference to oral contraceptive practice." *Brit. Med. J.* 2: 241–245.

Mantel, N., and Haenszel, W. E. 1959. "Statistical aspects of the analysis of data from retrospective studies of disease." *J. Natl. Cancer Inst.* 22:719–748.

Marzuk, P. M., Tardiff, K., Smyth, D., Stajic, M., Leon, A. C. 1992. "Cocaine use, risk taking and fatal Russian Roulette." *JAMA* 267(19):2635–2637.

McMahan, C. A. 1962. "Age-sex distribution of selected groups of human autopsied cases." *Arch. Path.* 73:40–47.

McPherson, K., Vessey, M. P., Neil, A., Doll, R., Jones, L., Roberts, M. 1987. "Early oral contraceptive use and breast cancer: results of another case-control study." *Br. J. Cancer* 56:653–660.

Pasternak, B., Shore, R. E., Albert, R. E. 1977. "Occupational exposure to chloromethyl ethers." *J. Occupational Medicine* 19:741–746.

Schlesselman, J. J. 1982. *Case-Control Studies: Design, Conduct, Analysis*. New York: Oxford University Press.

Snedecor, G. W., and Cochran, W. G. 1967. *Statistical Methods* 6th ed. Ames, Iowa: The Iowa State University Press.

Solomon, H. A., Priore, R. I., and Bross, I.D.J. 1968. "Cigarette smoking and periodontal disease." *J. Amer. Dent. Assoc.* 77:1081–1084.

Stolley, P. D., Tonascia, J. A., Sartwell, P. E., Tockman, M. S., Tonascia, S., Rutledge, A., and Schinnar, R. 1978. "Agreement rates between oral contraceptive users and prescribers in relation to drug use histories." *Am. J. Epid.* 107:226–235.

Szmuness, W. 1978. "Hepatocellular carcinoma and the hepatitis B virus: Evidence for a causal association." *Prog. Med. Virol.* 24:40–69.

Thomas, D. B. 1972. "Relationship of oral contraceptives to cervical carcinogenesis." *Obstet. Gynec.* 40:508–518.

Vessey, M. P., and Doll, R. 1968. "Investigation of relation between use of oral contraceptives and thromboembolic disease." *Brit. Med. J.* 2:199–205.

Waife, S. O., Lucchesi, P. F., and Sigmond, B. 1952. "Significance of mortality statistics in medical research: Analysis of 1,000 deaths at Philadelphia General Hospital." *Ann. Intern. Med.* 37:332–337.

Walter, S. D. 1975. "The distribution of Levin's measure of attributable risk." *Biometrics* 62:371–374.

―――. 1978. "Calculation of attributable risk from epidemiological data." *Int. J. Epid.* 7:175–182.

Winkelstein Jr., W., Stenchever, M. A., and Lilienfeld, A. M. 1958. "Occurrence of pregnancy, abortion, and artificial menopause among women with coronary artery disease: A preliminary study." *J. Chron. Dis.* 7:273–286.

IV

USING EPIDEMIOLOGIC DATA

This final section deals with the use of epidemiologic data. The means by which the results of epidemiologic studies, demographic studies, and toxicological and clinical findings are assembled into a consistent biological inference are discussed in Chapter 12. It is important to recognize that the aggregate of available data on the relationship between a factor and a disease must be integrated before a biological inference is derived. This means that the epidemiologist often must venture into other scientific disciplines. It also means that the process of deriving a biological inference may be a subjective one in which the evidence is weighed in order to determine whether a causal relationship exists. The process of epidemiologic reasoning to achieve this purpose is considered in Chapter 12.

The clinical uses of epidemiologic data are discussed in Chapter 13. The application of decision analysis to clinical medicine and policy-making is illustrated. We try to show how epidemiology can help physicians and other health care providers review reports in the clinical literature critically and we provide a checklist for this purpose. Finally, the use of epidemiologic methods in describing the full spectrum and natural history of disease and in studying disease etiology is briefly outlined.

12

DERIVING BIOLOGICAL INFERENCES FROM EPIDEMIOLOGIC STUDIES

> I cannot give any scientist of any age any better advice
> than this: The intensity of the conviction that a hypothesis
> is true has no bearing on whether it is true or not.
> Sir Peter Medawar, 1979

The demonstration of a statistical relationship between a disease and a biological or psychosocial characteristic is but the first step in the epidemiologic analysis of its etiology and/or natural history. The second step is to ascertain the meaning of the relationship. This chapter will deal with the inferences about a disease's etiology that can be derived from epidemiologic observations and the reasoning by which epidemiologists select the most plausible one. Several elements in this process have been discussed previously, but here they are brought together into a whole. Broadly speaking, a series of reported statistical associations can be explained as:

1. Artifactual (spurious).
2. Due to association of interrelated but non-causal variables.
3. Due to uncontrolled confounding.
4. Causal or etiological.

ARTIFACTUAL ASSOCIATIONS

The possibility that an observed association represents a statistical artifact has been pointed out repeatedly in this book. As indicated in Chapter 11, an artifactual association can result from biased methods of selecting cases and controls. This point can be illustrated by the objections raised to certain case-control studies of exogenous estrogens and endometrial cancer. It was argued that the users of exogenous estrogen, having had to see a physician for their prescriptions, would

255

be more closely observed than the controls and therefore would be more likely to have endometrial cancer diagnosed than those who did not use estrogen. (This turned out not to be the case.) A spurious association may also arise from biased methods of recording observations or obtaining information by interview. This is illustrated in its simplest form by a fictional example. Suppose that in a case-control study of the possible relationship between automobile driving and "slipped discs" (herniated lumbar vertebral discs), an investigator with a preconceived notion that automobile driving is of etiological importance asks the patients, "You frequently drive an automobile, don't you?" and the controls, "You don't drive an automobile frequently, do you?" This difference in phrasing the question could lead to a difference in the responses of cases and controls, resulting in an artifactual statistical association between automobile driving and slipped discs.

Errors in the conduct or design of a study can also introduce artifactual errors through nonrepresentative study groups, misclassification of exposure or disease, measurement errors, nonresponse or loss to follow-up, and observer biases. Well-designed studies can avoid most of these problems or even measure the effect of misclassification and of loss to follow-up.

ASSOCIATIONS DUE TO INTERRELATED BUT NON-CAUSAL VARIABLES

An association between two or more variables can be observed and still be non-causal because many variables can occur together without being a part of the causal chain. For example, currently in the United States, cigarette smoking is associated with lower educational status, "blue-collar" occupational status, and relative poverty. But only cigarette smoking is truly causal of lung cancer; the associations with cigarette smoking just mentioned will be detected with an epidemiologic study of the etiology of lung cancer but are interrelated with smoking rather than a cause of the tumor. Examination of these interrelated associations is useful as they may suggest ways to reduce exposure to the causal variable, in this case, smoking.

CONFOUNDING

If any factor either increasing or decreasing the risk of a disease besides the characteristic or exposure under study is unequally distributed in the groups that are being compared with regard to the disease, this itself will give rise to differences in disease frequency in the compared groups. Such distortion, termed *con-*

founding, leads to an invalid comparison. The extraneous variable resulting in a confounded comparison is a **confounding variable** (confounding factor) or a "confounder."

The relationship between the confounding factor (CF), the etiological factor (E), and the disease or outcome of interest (D) is shown in Figure 12–1. The confounding variable is associated with both the etiological factor and the disease. For simplicity, this illustration uses only one confounding factor and one etiological factor, but there may be many confounding variables and etiological factors. The above discussion can be extended to such multivariate situations. However, a complete discussion of such situations is beyond the scope of this book; several references for dealing with more than one confounding variable and/or etiological factor are given in the Appendix.

An example of a confounded comparison is provided by consumption of alcoholic beverages, cigarette smoking, and lung cancer. Cigarette smoking is an etiological factor for lung cancer. Persons who smoke cigarettes also tend to drink more alcoholic beverages than those who do not smoke; and those who smoke more cigarettes tend to drink more than those who smoke fewer cigarettes. Hence, cigarette smoking might be a confounding variable in a study of the relationship between alcohol consumption and lung cancer.

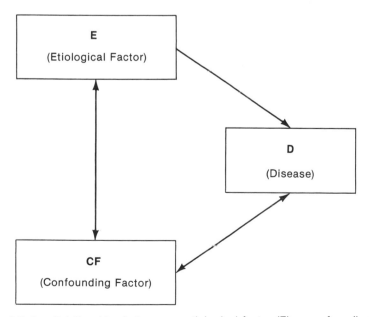

Figure 12–1. Relationships between an etiological factor (E), a confounding factor (CF), and a disease (D).

Another example was given in Chapter 4, in the comparison of mortality among residents of Florida and Alaska. In that instance, age (C) was a confounding variable in evaluating the effect of place of residence (E) on mortality (D). The possible presence of confounding must be considered when conducting an epidemiologic study, particularly during its design and the analysis of its data, and when assessing the results of an epidemiologic study reported in the literature.

Three methods can be used to address the issue of confounding in an epidemiologic study: (1) the study can be restricted to a specific population group, minimizing the presence of potential confounding variables; (2) the study participants can be *matched* for the potential confounding variable or (3) information can be collected on that variable during the study and the analysis adjusted for its possible effect. Reports in the literature can often be useful in determining what the potential confounding variables might be in a given study so that data on them can be collected. If no data about a possible confounding variable are collected, then the epidemiologist may not be able to disentangle the possibly distorting effects of the confounding.

In analyzing the data collected during a study, one must determine whether

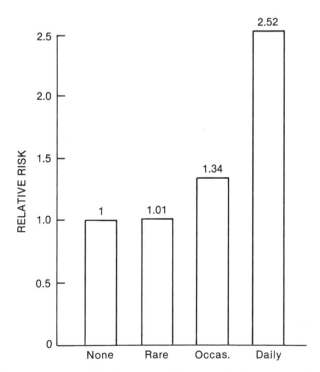

Figure 12–2. Relative risks for lung cancer in women by frequency of alcohol consumption. *Source:* Hirayama (1990).

or not a variable is a confounder in the study data set. If the variable is a confounder, then the distortion of effect created by its presence must be controlled
statistically in the analysis. The statistical approach to the assessment of confounding is to measure the overall association (using either odds radios or relative
risks) between exposure and disease and the change in this value after control for
a variable (Miettinen, 1974; Kleinbaum et al., 1982; Schlesselman, 1982).

In stratified analyses, data are broken down into levels of one or more variables and analyzed by level; summary statistics then can be used. One common
technique for estimating a summary relative risk across strata is the Mantel-Haenszel approach (Mantel and Haenszel, 1959, 1960; Kahn and Sempos, 1989). In
this method, each stratum is assigned an appropriate weight. These weights are
then used to calculate the summary relative risk. Multivariate analysis techniques
incude both multiple and logistic regression and log-linear models. In these
approaches, the epidemiologist mathematically models the occurrence of disease
based upon the presence or absence of possible risk factors and confounders.
These techniques allow several independent variables (potential confounders) to
be in the model simultaneously. In general, control for confounding is technical

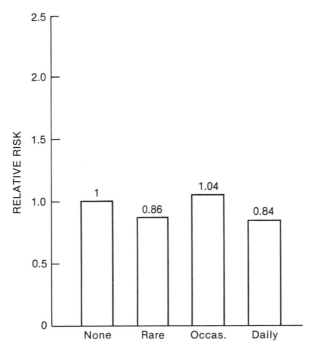

Figure 12–3.   Relative risks for lung cancer in women by frequency of alcohol consumption, adjusted for cigarette smoking. *Source:* Hirayama (1990).

but straightforward; more difficult is deciding which variables are to be considered potential confounders.

An example of the analysis of data to reveal confounding comes from a cohort study by Hirayama (1990). He found that the relative risk for lung cancer in women who consume alcoholic beverages increased with ascending consumption (Figure 12–2). This indicates that consumption of alcoholic beverages is associated with the risk of developing lung cancer. However, when the data were adjusted for differences in cigarette smoking patterns among those persons in the different alcohol consumption categories, the association between alcohol consumption and lung cancer disappeared (Figure 12–3). In this instance, cigarette smoking was a confounding variable. Its presence misled the investigators about the role of alcohol in the development of lung cancer until they unravelled the confounding.

Concerns about confounding also arise when interpreting the results of epidemiologic studies reported in the literature. One must ask whether studies showing a relationship between a risk factor and a disease have controlled for potential confounders in their design or analysis. If the study did not adequately control for the presence of confounding variables, the inferences drawn from the results may not be well founded. A study examining a new risk factor for lung cancer, for instance, would have to show that differences in smoking do not explain the relationship between the new risk factor and lung cancer. Studies in which there was inadequate control of all known confounders may be criticized on those grounds; their results may be explained by an unequal distribution of extraneous variables in the study groups and not by the effect of exposure on disease.

It is possible that risk factors may interact in their biological effect. For example, exposures to asbestos fibers and cigarette smoking interact to cause lung cancer at a greater rate than either would individually. Some epidemiologists refer to this phenomenon as "effect modification." Such interactions must be distinguished from confounding, as was illustrated with the associations between cigarette smoking, alcohol consumption, and lung cancer (Figures 12–2 and 12–3). Since there was no relationship between alcohol consumption and lung cancer *after* controlling for the effect of cigarette smoking, there was *no* interaction between cigarette smoking and alcohol consumption to produce lung cancer. Hence, cigarette smoking *confounded* the relationship between alcohol consumption and lung cancer, that is, created the appearance of a causal relationship where none existed. Since there is no causal relationship, there can be no interaction between these two variables (alcohol consumption and cigarette smoking).

As with confounding, there is much debate about the appropriate way to assess and analyze interaction. When interaction is found in a data set, it should be described. One may point out that men and women showed different responses to a treatment or that children in a particular age group were especially prone to accidents.

CAUSAL ASSOCIATIONS

The Evolution of Causal Thinking in Epidemiology

Some investigators have held the view that a factor must be both necessary and sufficient for the occurrence of a disease before it be considered the cause of that disease. This is the logician's definition of "cause." As one might intuitively guess, *necessary* refers to the fact that the factor must be present for the disease to occur, while *sufficient* means that the factor alone can lead to the disease (but the factor's presence does not *always* result in the disease's occurrence). The concept of "necessary *and* sufficient" implies that there must be a one-to-one relationship between the factor and the disease; that is, whenever the factor is present, the disease must occur, and whenever the disease occurs, the factor must be present. Even in infectious diseases, however, a microorganism is not necessary and sufficient for the development of disease; many environmental and host factors are also involved. For example, the tubercle bacillus is a necessary but not a sufficient factor in the development of tuberculosis; additional factors usually included under the term "susceptibility" are also important.

The classical rules for determining whether a microorganism can be regarded as a causal agent of an infectious disease are collectively known as the "Henle-Koch postulates." Although the wording of these postulates varies, they can be simply stated as follows:

1. The organism must be found in all cases of the disease in question.
2. It must be possible to isolate the organism from patients with the disease and to grow it in pure culture.
3. When the pure culture is inoculated into susceptible animals or humans, it must reproduce the disease.

To be considered a causal agent under these requirements, a microorganism must be a necessary condition for the occurrence of disease in humans but need not be sufficient.

An example of sufficient cause for the development of disease is given in Figure 12–4. Each of the factors A_1, A_2, A_3, and so on is sufficient to induce the cellular events (B) resulting in the development of disease (C). None of these factors, however, is necessary for the development of the disease since any of

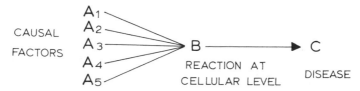

Figure 12-4. Diagrammatic representation of a causal relationship with multiple independent (sufficient) etiological factors.

them is sufficient to produce the cellular changes. In Figure 12–5, all three causal factors (A_1, A_2, and A_3) are necessary for the induction of the cellular reactions (B) that result in disease (C). None of these three factors is sufficient for the development of the disease as all three must be present to initiate the cellular reactions.

Evans (1976) has developed a unified concept of causation that parallels the Henle-Koch postulates and is generally applicable to both infectious and noninfectious diseases.

1. The prevalence of the disease should be significantly higher in those exposed to the hyothesized cause than in controls not so exposed (the cause may be present in the external environment or as a defect in host responses).
2. Exposure to the hypothesized cause should be more frequent among those with the disease than in controls without the disease when all other risk factors are held constant.
3. Incidence of the disease should be significantly higher in those exposed to the cause than in those not so exposed, as shown by prospective studies.
4. Temporally, the disease should follow exposure to the hypothesized cause.
5. A spectrum of host responses should follow exposure to the hypothesized agent along a logical biologic gradient from mild to severe.
6. A measurable host response following exposure to the hypothesized cause should have a high probability of appearing in those lacking the response before exposure (e.g., antibody, cancer cells), or should

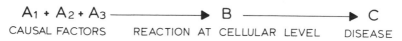

Figure 12-5. Diagrammatic representation of a causal relationship with three cumulative (necessary) causal factors.

increase in magnitude if present before exposure; this response pattern should occur infrequently in persons not so exposed.

7. Experimental reproduction of the disease should occur more frequently in animals or humans appropriately exposed to the hypothesized cause than in those not so exposed; this exposure may be deliberate in volunteers, experimentally induced in the laboratory, or demonstrated in a controlled regulation of natural exposure.

8. Elimination or modification of the hypothesized cause or of the vector carrying it should decrease the incidence of the disease (e.g., control of polluted water, removal of tar from cigarettes).

9. Prevention or modification of the host's response on exposure to the hypothesized cause should decrease or eliminate the disease (e.g., immunization).

10. All of the relationships and findings should make biologic and epidemiologic sense.

Assessing Causality

The epidemiologist applies criteria of causality to the research before recommending clinical or public health actions. These criteria need not be satisfied in every way before causality can be inferred. Rather, they provide a framework for deriving a biological inference from epidemiologic and other scientific data. In practice, *a relationship is considered causal whenever evidence indicates that the factors form part of the complex of circumstances which increases the probability of the occurrence of disease and that a diminution of one or more of these factors decreases the frequency of the disease.* The etiologic factor need not be the only cause of the disease, and it may have effects on other diseases.

The following concepts are used by epidemiologists in making a causal inference:

- Strength of association
- Consistency of the observed association
- Specificity of the association
- Temporal sequence of events
- Dose-response relationship
- Biological plausibility of the observed association
- Experimental evidence

Strength of association

The strength of association is measured by the relative risk (or odds ratio estimate of the relative risk). A strong association between exposure and outcome gives support to a causal hypothesis. When a weak association is found (for example, a relative risk of 1.2 to 1.5), other information is needed to support causality. Repeated findings of a weak association in well-conducted studies can still lead to effective public health action. When an exposure affects many people and the outcome is extremely adverse, a small increase in risk can be of major concern to public health officials. Action may be taken to lower the exposure and reduce the risk for large segments of the population. Strength of association supports a hypothesis of causality, but weak associations supported by other evidence of causality are sometimes equally important.

Consistency of the observed association

Confirmation by repeated findings of an association in case-control and cohort studies in different population groups and different settings strengthens the inference of a causal connection. Finding such consistency is logically equivalent to the replication of results in laboratory experiments under a variety of environmental or biological conditions.

Consistency of association can be illustrated by data from many studies of the relationship of oral contraceptives to cardiovascular disease. Many cohort and case-control studies have shown an increased risk of cardiovascular disease associated with oral contraceptive use in a variety of settings and population groups (Vessey, 1978).

Specificity of the association

It was formerly thought that to be causal, a one-to-one relationship should exist between the exposure and the disease; one exposure should cause one disease, and no other exposures should cause the disease. This has its roots in the bacteriological model where one microorganism is associated with one disease. In the study of chronic diseases, less emphasis has been given to specificity as a criterion of causality. The development of cancer is associated with a number of exposures, many of which are accepted as causal. Conversely, exposures such as smoking are associated with a number of adverse outcomes from cancer and cardiovascular disease to birth problems, and these associations are accepted as causal by the medical and public health communities. Specificity of a relationship between exposure and outcome strengthens confidence in a causal inference, but lack of specificity does not rule out causality.

Temporal sequence of events

It seems obvious that in order for an exposure to cause an event (disease), it must precede and not follow the disease. In many cases, the temporal sequence of events is clear-cut. One example is the study of prenatal exposures and malformations; it is usually easy to document that an exposure precedes the birth of the malformed baby. However, for many other associations the temporal relationship is subject to debate.

In studying the relationship between age when breast-feeding ceases and infections of the baby, for instance, some researchers claim that longer duration of breast-feeding leads to fewer infections, but others claim that illness of the child leads to a cessation of breast-feeding. Which came first, the illness or the weaning? A cohort study design can resolve the issue of temporality, but for many study questions prospective studies are difficult or impossible to carry out.

Dose-response relationships

If a factor is of causal importance in the occurrence of a disease, then the risk of developing the disease shoud be related to the degree of exposure to the factor, i.e., a dose-response relationship should exist. The dose-response relationship between serum cholesterol level and the risk of coronary heart disease is an example. Another example is the relationship between duration of estrogen use and risk of endometrial cancer. Several studies also suggest that low-dose estrogen contraceptives carry a lower risk of venous thromboembolism than do higher dose estrogens.

An observed dose-response relationship strengthens a causal hypothesis. Unfortunately, it is sometimes difficult to quantify an exposure in terms of a dosage or gradient. Dosage and duration of exposure are often interchanged in study designs, and both may cause a gradient in disease frequencies. Dosage can refer to the amount of a given exposure in a given time period, as in the number of cigarettes smoked per day, the amount of a hazardous chemical or particle in the work environment, or the amount of a drug taken each day. Information on actual dosage is often not available, so duration of exposure is substituted, as in years of cigarette smoking, years working in a given occupational environment, or length of time using a drug. Use of duration as a proxy for dosage necessitates an analysis that accounts for time; people with longer exposure times may have a greater time period in which to develop or discover the disease.

Biological plausibility of the observed association

A causal hypothesis must be viewed in the light of its biological plausibility. A causal association between ingrown toenails and leukemia, to take an absurd example, would be highly improbable. On the other hand, an association that does not appear biologically credible at one time may eventually prove to be so; indeed, the observation of a seemingly implausible association may actually represent the beginning of an extension of our knowledge. The established statistical association between circulatory diseases and oral contraceptive use is an excellent example of this. At first, there was no known physiological mechanism by which hormones could so profoundly affect the circulatory system. Yet, the statistical association was present, and possible physiological mechanisms were later discovered, such as alteration of the clotting cascade, increased platelet adhesiveness, and direct effects on the arterial wall. It becomes important, therefore, to further investigate associations even if they are initially thought to be biologically implausible. The cigarette smoking–lung cancer relationship was initially considered biologically implausible by some, but carcinogens in cigarettes were identified, which lent biological plausibility to the observed association.

The ability to produce a particular disease in animals by exposing them to possible etiologic agents considerably enhances the causal hypothesis. Though one must be cautious in generalizing from the results of animal experiments to the human condition, this may be a relatively minor problem if the results of both animal experiments and epidemiologic studies in human populations are consistent. Animal experiments can also be valuable in determining the intermediate biological mechanisms that are involved in a disease, thereby providing the basis for seeking similar mechanisms in humans. Darwin's signal contribution to biological thinking was that the human species is not so unique a biological phenomenon as we may like to think; modern molecular biology confirms the unity of human and other animal species.

Experimental evidence

The randomized clinical trial (RCT) is the closest approximation in epidemiology to an experiment, and a well-run trial may confirm a causal relationship between an exposure and an outcome. The "exposure" is generally a drug, treatment, or procedure, and the outcome is reduction of disease or mortality. The Lipid Research Clinics Trial demonstrated that a pharmacological reduction in serum cholesterol led to lower heart disease, and other clinical trials have shown that pharmacologic lowering of blood pressure also reduces heart disease. Similar comments apply to the results of community trials. Ethics prevent the conduct of a trial of an exposure that is thought to have deleterious effects, and thus the randomized clinical trial and the community trial are limited to a subset of study questions related to potentially beneficial effects of an exposure.

Some situations approximate an experiment without the benefit of randomized, concurrent controls. The efficacy of inner-city comprehensive-care programs in reducing the incidence of rheumatic fever was demonstrated by comparing neighborhoods in a city that were simlar to one another except for their eligibility for the programs, but the populations may have differed in ways not known or documented in the study (Gordis, 1973). Conversely, removal or reduction of an exposure may result in a decrease in disease. The decrease in smoking among physicians led to a decrease in lung cancer among physicians while rates in the general population continued to rise. The decline in the use of isoprenaline in England in the 1960s led to a decline in asthma-related deaths.

SUMMARY

One of the foremost biometricians of the twentieth century, A. Bradford Hill (1937), noted the importance of common sense in developing inferences. He summarized the questions that should guide a consideration of causality as follows: "Is there any other way of explaining the set of facts before us, is there any other answer more likely than cause and effect?" An association between exposure and outcome can be evaluated within the context of epidemiologic criteria of causality; with common sense, reasonable inferences may be made and actions taken.

Epidemiologic inferences lead to action, to changes in clinical practice, public policy, legislation, health education, or new research directions. Health care providers no longer prescribe diethylstilbestrol (DES) to prevent miscarriages, they now use blood pressure–lowering agents to treat patients with moderate hypertension, and they now have evidence that regular sigmoidoscopic examinations can lower colon cancer mortality.

An example of the role of epidemiologic data in the development of public policy is the recent legislation in the United States regulating where people may smoke to protect citizens from exposure to environmental tobacco smoke. Health education efforts emphasize the use of condoms in preventing the spread of AIDS, the need to reduce alcohol intake during pregnancy to prevent fetal-alcohol syndrome, the use of seat belts to reduce auto accident injuries, and the role of low-fat diets in reducing heart disease.

Experimentation and the determination of biological mechanisms provide the most direct evidence of a causal relationship between a factor and a disease. Epidemiologic studies can provide very strong support for hypotheses of either a causal or an indirect association. However, inferences from such studies are not made in isolation; they must take into account all relevant biological information. Epidemiologic and other evidence can accumulate to the point where a causal hypothesis becomes highly probable. Unfortunately, it is not yet possible to quantitate the degree of probability achieved by all the evidence for a specific hypothesis about the cause of a disease, so an element of subjectivity remains. Nevertheless, a causal hypothesis can be sufficiently probable to provide a reasonable basis for successful preventive and public health action, as the history of public health amply demonstrates.

STUDY PROBLEMS

1. Name two important ways to control for confounding when designing a study.
2. What options are there for controlling confounding in the analysis stage?

3. What is the difference between biological significance and statistical significance?

4. Name three concepts that are useful in assessing causality.

REFERENCES

Evans, A. S. 1976. "Causation and disease: The Henle-Koch postulates revisited." *Yale J. Biol. Med.* 49:175–195.

Gordis, L. 1973. "Effectiveness of comprehensive-care programs in preventing rheumatic fever." *New Engl. J. Med.* 289:331–335.

Hill, A. B. 1971. Statistical Evidence and Inference. In *Principles of Medical Statistics.* New York: Oxford University Press, 309–323.

Hirayama, T. 1990. *Life-style and mortality: a large-scale census-based cohort study in Japan.* Basel: S. Karger.

Kahn, H. A., and Sempos, C. T. 1989. *Statistical Methods in Epidemiology.* New York: Oxford University Press.

Kleinbaum, D. G., Kupper, L. L., and Morgenstern, H. 1982. *Epidemiologic Research.* Belmont, Calif.: Lifetime Learning Publications.

Mantel, N., Haenszel, W. 1959. Statistical aspects of the analysis of data from retrospective studies of disease. *Journal of the National Cancer Institute* 22:719–748.

Miettinen, O. 1974. "Confounding and effect modification." *Am. J. Epidemiol.* 100:350–353.

Schlesselman, J. J. 1982. *Case-Control Studies.* New York: Oxford University Press.

Vessey, M. P., and Mann, J. I. 1978. "Female sex hormones and thrombosis: Epidemiological aspects." *Brit. Med. Bull.* 34:157–162.

13

EPIDEMIOLOGY IN CLINICAL PRACTICE

with the Assistance of Tamar Lasky, Ph.D., M.S.P.H.

Clinicians apply the principles of epidemiology to everyday practice in three main ways: (1) clinical decision making, (2) reading and interpreting medical literature, (3) describing and understanding the etiology of disease.

In the first category are the decisions to order diagnostic tests or procedures, assign a diagnosis, and recommend a treatment. Second, physicians who can intelligently and efficiently read the literature will make the best use of new information in providing optimal care to their patients. Finally, clinicians with an understanding of epidemiology are better able to identify disease entities, suggest etiologic hypotheses, monitor and evaluate the safety of drugs and other therapies, find the causes of local epidemics and institute preventive measures, and participate in collaborative research. These related concerns are the domain of what is sometimes called clinical epidemiology, though not its exclusive domain (Fletcher et al., 1988; Sackett et al., 1991; Schuman, 1986; Weiss, 1986).

CLINICAL DECISION MAKING

In all aspects of medical practice, the physician faces a series of choices—choices that are made in a specific context for a particular patient. Despite the intention to provide well-reasoned care, however, patterns of diagnosis and treatment are sometimes less than optimal.

One classical example is that of the diagnosis of tonsillitis and referral for tonsillectomy and adenoidectomy (Bakwin, 1945). Three groups of pediatricians had an opportunity to screen a group of children for tonsillectomy. The first group referred 174 out of 389 children (45 percent) for tonsillectomy. The "healthy" remaining 215 children were examined by the second group of physicians. They recommended tonsillectomy for 99 of these children (46 percent). The third group of physicians examined the remaining 116 children and referred 51 (44 percent) of them for tonsillectomy. The pediatricians referred approximately the same proportion of children for tonsillectomy, which perhaps reflected habit, expectations, carelessness, and a lack of objective and validated criteria for surgery (Figure 13–1).

Sackett et al. (1991) compared university hospital physicians with family physicians treating the same group of 230 hypertensive patients. All the patients were recommended for treatment by the university group, but only two-thirds of the family physicians started the patients on antihypertensive drug regimens. Three factors predicted the decision of family physicians to prescribe antihypertensives. First and third were the patient's diastolic blood pressure (as it should

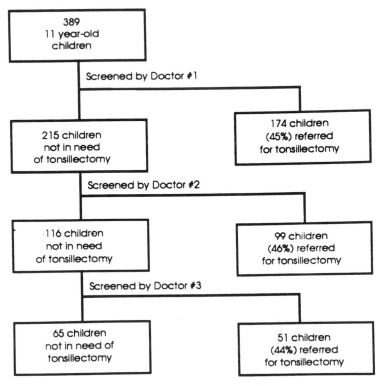

Figure 13–1. Patterns of tonsillectomy referrals in three groups of pediatricians. *Source:* Bakwin (1945).

have been) and evidence of target organ damage, but second was the physician's year of graduation from medical school. More recent graduates were more likely to treat for hypertension, reflecting advances in research findings and teaching. This study illustrates the well-known problem of keeping up to date in medicine and perhaps other factors.

Epidemiologic research can be used to analyze decision-making behavior (factors influencing a clinician's decision to use a test, procedure, or treatment), and it helps clinicians improve their decision-making skills. After reviewing the literature, a clinician may wish to apply research findings to an individual patient; however, information about a study population is sometimes difficult to use in this way. The decision to order a diagnostic test may vary with the patient's characteristics (e.g., age, other medical conditions), the availability of treatment options, and the risks of injury or side effects associated with a procedure. Similarly, the decision to order a treatment must be weighed against the probability that the treatment works, that side effects are likely or unlikely, and that the patient will comply with the course of treatment. This decision-making process has both objective and subjective aspects. The probability that the procedure will work or that the patient will die in surgery, for instance, can be derived from the literature. But what value does the patient assign to the risks and benefits of a diagnostic test, procedure, or treatment? Thus, there is also a "subjective" aspect to clinical decision-making.

Decision Analysis

Decision analysis is an approach that can help the clinician deal with such situations, weighing the probabilities of various outcomes with the subjective value accorded to them by the patient. The selection and interpretation of diagnostic tests involves the application of probability theory, whether applied consciously or unconsciously. When a test is ordered for a patient, the physician has some sense of the probability that the results will be positive and thus help establish the correct diagnosis. If that probability (on a scale of 0.0 to 1.0) were close to 0.0, there would usually be little point in performing the test. Similarly, if the clinician is so sure of the diagnosis that the test has a 1.0 probability of being positive, again there would be little point to ordering the test as the diagnosis is established without benefit of the test. It is between these extremes of expecting a surely negative or surely positive test result that most clinical decision-making lies, and in these situations decision analysis may be helpful.

Descriptions of decision analysis include variations on the following steps as adapted from Sackett et al., (1991) and Pauker (1991).

1. *Frame the question in terms of specific choices that are mutually exclusive and exhaustive.* This means that a physician should consider all treatments, the possibility of no treatment, and, if appropriate, the possibility of combined treatments. Decision analysis forces one to think through, and define, the full range of choices.

2. *Create a decision tree.* One must structure the problem by diagramming the decision tree for the specific clinical question, showing the clinical options and the possible outcomes of each option. The decision tree for a question about ordering a diagnostic test will have different branches than the decision tree for a question about treatment.

3. *Assign probabilities to the outcomes.* Here one relies on the literature and one's experience to estimate probabilities for branches and points of the decision tree. In deciding on the probability of various outcomes, a clinician may use information about the prevalence of a disease, the sensitivity and specificity of a diagnostic test, the probability of side effects of a procedure or treatment, the probability that a treatment will cure or prevent a disease, etc.

4. *Assign utilities to the outcomes.* The outcomes can include loss of life, complete recovery, and the risks of side effects. The utilities (relative values) are subjective and any scale can be used (e.g., years of survival, dollars spent, or an arbitrary scale of 0 to 100). It is usually easy to assign the lowest value to death and the highest value to complete healthy recovery, but it is not always easy to place intermediate outcomes on the scale. The risks and side effects of procedures and treatments have different meanings for different people. Sometimes the patient can help assign values to intermediate outcomes in discussions with his or her physician or in response to direct questions such as, ''On a scale of 0 to 100, how would you rate the following side effect to a treatment for your condition?'' The patient has to live with one of the outcomes and knows how he or she feels about them. Of course, the physician can consult with other physicians, social workers, or groups of patients in developing values for outcomes. As shown below, the subjectivity and variability in assigning values makes decision analysis adaptable for different contexts.

5. *Calculate the expected utility.* One calculates back from the outcomes to the first choices on the decision tree. The probability of an outcome is multiplied by the value (subjectively assigned) and then averaged with the product calculated for other outcomes in the same decision branch (see example below).

6. *Perform sensitivity analysis.* Depending on the specifics of a decision tree, one might do the analysis again under different assumptions. For example, one might vary the values assigned to outcomes to see how one's subjective judgment changes the overall analysis. This helps clarify the contribution of different factors to the ultimate decision.

An Example of Decision Analysis

We present an example of decision analysis below, following the steps just described.

1. *Frame the question.* In this example, we ask the question, "Should antihypertensive treatment be given to prevent stroke in patients over 60 with no symptoms other than isolated systolic hypertension (ISH—systolic blood pressure 160–219 mm Hg and diastolic blood pressure less than 90 mm Hg)?" This question arose from reading the results of a multicenter, randomized, controlled clinical trial which showed that treated patients aged 60 and over had a reduced risk of stroke compared to untreated patients (SHEP Cooperative Research Group, 1991). The authors stated that the trial demonstrated the efficacy of active antihypertensive drug treatment in preventing stroke in persons aged 60 and older with ISH, but they did not say whether a clinician should prescribe the treatment regimen (a combination plan of chlorthalidone and atenolol or reserpine) to all patients similar to those in the trial. One physician may be enthusiastic about treating this group, but another physician may be reluctant to prescribe long-term medication to a fairly healthy group of patients. Is there an objective way to decide this clinical question?

2. *Create a decision tree.* The decision tree in Figure 13–2 shows the two choices facing the clinician who diagnoses ISH in a patient. The physician can treat the hypertension with drugs or decide not to treat. This decision is controlled by the clinician (and the patient) and is represented by a square. In this example we have identified three possible outcomes for patients. They can suffer a stroke, they can experience intolerable symptoms (some of which may be associated with the treatment), or they can live free of stroke and intolerable symptoms.

3. *Assign probabilities to the possible outcomes.* In this case probabilities are derived from the paper that presented the results of the trial. The authors reported that 5.2 percent of the treated group experienced a stroke, compared to 8.2 percent of the placebo group. This is expressed as a probability of .052 of stroke if treated and .082 if not treated. The authors also reported the prevalence of symptoms characterized as intolerable by the patients. These symptoms included faintness, loss of consciousness, chest pain, trouble with memory, problems with sexual function, and nausea or vomiting. In the treatment group, 28.1 percent experienced intolerable symptoms compared to 20.8 percent in the placebo group. These prevalence data can be used to represent the probability of experiencing intolerable symptoms. We assigned a probability of .281 to the treated group and .208 to the untreated group. The people who did not experience stroke or intolerable symptoms were considered to be healthy and symptom-free

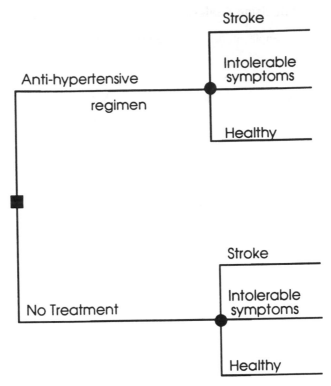

Figure 13–2. A decision tree.

in this analysis. The probability of being healthy and symptom free was 1.00 minus the probability of stroke and the probability of intolerable symptoms, or .667 in the treatment group and .710 in the untreated group.

4. *Assign a utility to each possible outcome.* In this example, we assigned the value of 0 to stroke and 100 to a healthy, symptom-free condition. How does one assign a value to having intolerable symptoms? Some of the symptoms described could greatly reduce the quality of life, necessitating job and activity changes (less driving, less eating out, etc.), so we assigned a value of 50 to these symptoms.

5. *Calculate the expected utilities.* In the group of patients receiving anti-hypertensive treatment, the probabilities of each outcome were as follows: .052 for stroke, .281 for intolerable symptoms, and .667 for a healthy symptom-free status. Each probability is multiplied by its utility as follow:

Stroke	.052 (0) = 0
Intolerable symptoms	.281 (50) = 14.05
Healthy, symptom-free	.667 (100) = 66.70

One then sums the three products (80.75) and averages them. In this case one divides by three, even though one product is zero, and the expected utility is 26.92 for treating with antihypertensives (Figure 13–3). Similar calculations for not treating yield an expected utility of 27.13, slightly higher than treating. This suggests that it is a toss-up whether to treat or not.

6. *Perform sensitivity analysis.* We can do the analysis again assigning a value of 75 to the outcome of intolerable symptoms (Figure 13–4). The expected utilities are then 29.26 for treatment and 28.87 for no treatment. It is again very close, confirming the previous analysis that the decision to treat is a toss-up.

In our example we did not separate stroke resulting in death from nonfatal stroke, consider nonstroke fatal events or heart disease, or include the economic cost of treatment. We simplified the options in order to illustrate the principle, but more complex anlayses are possible. Even this simplified decision analysis of the SHEP study helped put the authors' findings in clinical perspective. That

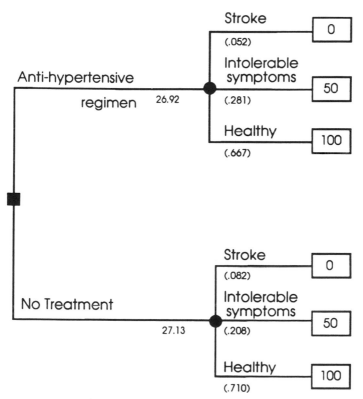

Figure 13–3.   A decision tree with probabilities, values, and calculated utilities.

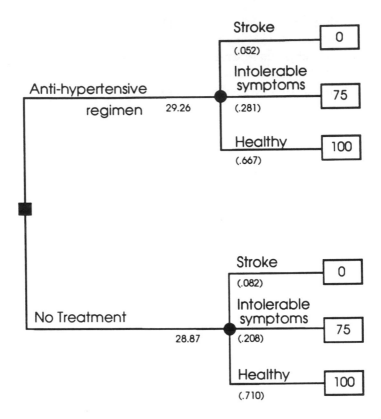

Figure 13–4. A decision tree with different values than Figure 13–3, and recalculated utilities.

is, after a clinical trial has been conducted among many patients, the results of the clinical trial can be used in decision analysis to decide an individual's course of treatment. The medical risks and benefits of treatment can be balanced against cost and the patient's personal preferences. The significant finding of a reduced risk of stroke does not necessarily mean that physicians should place all their healthy elderly patients with isolated systolic hypertension on treatment. Our analysis suggests that the choice of treatment can be viewed as an option for physicians and patients and depends on the circumstances and the patient's preferences.

Decision analysis can be a cumbersome tool. It is limited by our ability to describe outcomes and probabilities and to assign subjective values to outcomes. It can help a physician, researcher, or policymaker think through a decision, gain understanding of the factors affecting a decision, and place the clinical decision in a broader context. Researchers can use this tool to develop guidelines for clinicians to follow, and policymakers can use it in making recommendations.

READING AND INTERPRETING SCIENTIFIC LITERATURE

The epidemiologic principles presented in this book can contribute to a critical reading of clinical research literature (Stolley and Davies, 1980; Sackett et al., 1991). Whether one wishes to learn more about the value of a diagnostic test, evaluate a new therapy, or determine the etiology of a disease, epidemiologic principles can be of clinical use. The suggestions that follow may be helpful in reading or writing clinical and epidemiological research papers.

Identifying the Study Problem

The title, abstract, and introductory paragraph should state the study's objectives. The reader may ask, "What is the study hypothesis? What is the main exposure of interest? What is the disease or condition being studied?" "Exposure" can refer to beneficial or detrimental factors, behavioral patterns, treatments, procedures, or drugs suspected of causing adverse effects. Many studies focus on more than one risk factor or disease, and the paper should identify them.

In Chapters 4, 5, 6, and 7 we discussed the variety of disease outcomes studied by epidemiologists and the difference between morbidity and mortality as endpoints in a study. A reader should be able to identify the illness or cause of death that is the focus of the study and the criteria for categorizing patients into disease categories. For example, a report of a study of hypertension should describe the blood pressure levels used to determine which patients were considered hypertensive. Similarly, a report of a study whose major focus is a reduction in blood pressure should specify the exact amount or percent decline that was considered a meaningful decrease in blood pressure.

Describing the Study Design

In Chapter 8, 9, 10, and 11 we described the study designs used in epidemiologic studies. Each study design—randomized clinical trial, community trial, cohort study, and case-control study—has its value and is appropriate for particular types of study questions. The randomized clinical trial is usually the best design to supply the information needed to determine the efficacy of a treatment. More and more, screening measures and diagnostic tests are also being evaluated by clinical trials to determine whether early detection of a condition (e.g., breast cancer by mammography) leads to an improvement in morbidity or mortality. Case-control studies are a cost-efficient way to investigate a new disease, an increase in a known disease, or a suspected adverse reaction to a drug or procedure because the researcher may examine several suspected risk factors and test hypotheses about their causal association with the disease of interest. Community trials are well suited to the testing of interventions that affect a community at large, such as changes in driving, drinking, or gun control laws, public education campaigns, or changes in pollutant emissions.

Cohort studies, reconstructed from records or conducted prospectively, are often useful in understanding the etiology of disease or the consequences of certain suspect exposures. The reader of a report describing a cohort study knows that certain selection biases have been avoided; incidence rates may be calculated, and a description of more than one health outcome is possible. Cohort studies are particularly suited to the investigation of etiology because exposure to suspected agents can be documented and then tracked over time to determine the "disease destiny" of the exposed and unexposed populations. The control of potential confounders and the investigation of possible biases can often be more thoroughly handled in a cohort study than is possible with other observational designs. It is particularly easy to study cohorts of pregnant women or infants to observe birth or childhood outcomes because patients are available and the follow-up time period is relatively short. The cohort design can also be used in occupational studies, nutritional studies, studies of the elderly, and many other areas.

Describing the Study Sample

Many questions may be raised about the sample described in an article. In general, the reader wishes to know if the sample has been chosen in a way that minimizes bias, if results can be generalized to other patients, and if the sample is large enough to allow the appropriate statistical analyses and to provide adequate statistical power to answer the question posed. A critical reader should look for descriptions of the sample selection process, the characteristics of the study sample (age, gender, ethnicity, etc.) and the sample size calculations.

Throughout this book we have stressed the importance of sample selection, whether in studies relying on routinely collected data such as death certificates or in studies that actively recruit subjects. If the researchers used death certificates to identify cases, did they address the possibility of any coding changes that took place during the study period or in the geographic areas where the study was conducted? If the researchers identified patients in prenatal clinics for a cohort study, did they consider the characteristics of pregnant women not attending those clinics? Did the researchers describe the eligibility criteria, the people who were excluded from the study, and the nonrespondents?

A good description of the study sample will allow a reader to consider the possible introduction of bias, and it will also allow the critical reader to decide what generalizations can be made from the data. Reports of most studies provide information about the age and gender of the study subjects, but more information is often useful. In a study of mammography screening among older women, it might be useful to know if the patients were using replacement estrogens, had a family history of breast cancer, or were smokers. Such specific information allows the reader to apply the study findings to the appropriate population of patients.

Many researchers do not report their sample size calculations; that is, they do not describe the sample sizes needed to detect a given difference with a specified probability that the observed difference is not due to chance, and they do not describe the probability that an observation of no difference is not due to too small a sample (alpha and beta). This is particularly relevant when reading articles about drug safety. Studies with small sample sizes will often conclude that a new drug is as safe as a previously used drug although the study may be too small to detect clinically meaningful differences in safety between the new and old drugs.

Data Analysis

A general reader may be reluctant to critique the data analysis, but some simple questions can help the reader sift out the studies that employ appropriate statistical techniques. Epidemiologists prefer to use relative measures of effect or association such as relative risk or the odds ratio. Many researchers do not calculate such a measure. Authors often include the necessary data for the reader who wishes to calculate a relative risk or an odds ratio, but the authors should carry out the analysis. Confidence intervals allow a reader to know if the measure of effect may be attributed to chance variation or if an association is likely or unlikely to be due to chance. The authors should address the subject of confounding by describing the variables that are generally thought to be confounders, their efforts to collect data on possible confounders, and the results of analyses of confounding variables.

Inferences

The researchers' conclusions may not be justified by the study results. A common example is the finding of a trend which is not statistically significant and which the authors interpret as supporting a particular point of view. In the discussion, authors often address issues of bias or confounding and their possible effects on the study findings. The reader may or may not be convinced by the authors' arguments and conclusions. When the reseachers' conclusions go beyond the study findings, the reader may apply the criteria of causality to their argument. Does the study show an association that is strong? Is it consistent with other studies? Is the temporal sequence logical? Are the results biologically plausible? Can the association be explained by bias in study design or by confounding?

Most often a study will be conducted in a specific population characterized by age, gender, social class, or medical condition, and the reader may wonder whether the findings can be applied to patients who differ from the study sample. The authors should address this issue and describe how widely the inferences from their study can be justifiably applied. An author may suggest, for example, that a screening test will be useful for patients five years younger than the patients in the study group and may then explain the reasoning behind this recommendation. A reader should sort out the firm conclusions from the suggested possibilities and keep in mind the applications to his or her clinical practice. Table 13–1 provides a useful checklist for the reader of medical papers.

Table 13–1.   Guide to Reading the Literature

Identify the study problem

What is the study hypothesis?
What is the exposure (risk factor, treatment, cause)?
What is the outcome (physiologic measurement, disease, death)?

Describe the study design

What design was used (clinical trial, case-control study, etc.)?
Is the design appropriate to the study question?

Describe the study sample

How was the sample selected?
Are inclusion and exclusion criteria described?
Do the authors describe those that refused to participate or were lost to follow-up?
What size samples were used?
Do the authors discuss the sample size calculations?

Data analysis

Do the authors calculate a measure of effect (OR, RR or other)? What was it?
Do they calculate confidence intervals for the measure of effect? What was it?
Does the analysis assess and control for confounding? What were the results?

Inferences

What are the study results (what do the numbers say)?
What are the authors' conclusions (do they differ from what the numbers say)?
Does their discussion convince the reader to accept their conclusions?
Are the authors' conclusions supported by the criteria of causality?
Can the results be generalized beyond the study group? To which groups?
To what group of your patients can you apply the study results?
What changes would you make in your practice as a result of the study?

DESCRIBING AND UNDERSTANDING THE ETIOLOGY OF DISEASE

It is a humbling experience to read older textbooks of medicine. Statements that are now known to be incorrect were often written with great certainty and authority. One wonders which of today's certainties will be overturned tomorrow. Consider the following example from the early 1960s.

The 11th edition of *Cecil-Loeb Textbook of Medicine* contains this description of the migraine sufferer:

> Patients with migraine headaches are anxious, striving, perfectionistic, order-loving, rigid persons, who, during periods of threat or conflict, become progressively more tense, resentful and fatigued. . . . The person with migraine attempts to gain approval by doing more and better work than his fellows by "application" and "hard work," and to gain security by holding to a stable environment (Beeson and McDermott, 1963).

This description of the "typical" migraine patient was derived from the experience of the author, Harold Wolff, a well-known neurologist, in examining and treating patients who attended his headache clinic in New York City. The headache sufferers who elected to go to a specialty clinic at a large medical center may have been a highly selected sample of all migrainous individuals. They may have represented those hard-driving and compulsive people who hate to lose a day of work from headaches.

Several community surveys of migraine have been conducted since Harold Wolff wrote the above passage, and they do not support the generalizations he drew from the skewed sample attending his clinic (Linet and Stewart, 1984). Instead, they reveal migraine to be a common disorder affecting about 10 to 15 percent of the population and all sorts of personality types; indeed, no particular personality type can be identified as being at special risk of migraine.

If we learn the cause of a disease, or the risk factors, we are usually in a better position to treat or prevent it. An apparently new disease was identified in 1989 and was labeled the eosinophilia-myalgia syndrome (EMS). In the first cluster of cases in New Mexico, a striking eosinophilia and severe muscle aching (myalgia) were noted. Many of the patients were women 30 to 60 years old, and the diagnosis of trichinosis was excluded during the course of the clinical investigation. Some patients experienced skin rashes, peripheral edema, various neuropathies, and respiratory symptoms. Quickly organized case-control studies revealed that all the patients had taken the food supplement L-tryptophan, an amino acid sold in health food stores for the relief of insomnia and depression; few of the controls consumed L-tryptophan (Eidson et al., 1990). Further investigations showed that the L-tryptophan implicated in the disease all came from a single Japanese manufacturer (Slutsker et al, 1990; Belongia et al., 1990). The eosinophilia-myalgia syndrome was due to an as yet unidentified contaminant.

The story of subacute myelo-optic neuropathy (SMON) is another example of an epidemiologic investigation that had immediate relevance to clinical practice. During the years 1956 to 1970, over 10,000 cases of this new syndrome were described in Japan. The patients showed peripheral neuropathy and myelopathy, ranging from minimal dysesthesia to death and including optic atrophy (Oakley, 1973).

The disease occurred most frequently in the summer. Because of its seasonal pattern, some scientists concluded that the epidemic was caused by a virus. It took a decade of multidisciplinary investigation to identify halogenated hydroxyquinolines as the causal agent. These drugs had been sold over the counter for the treatment of intestinal amebiasis and diarrhea. The sales of hydroxyquinolines increased with the seasonal increase in diarrhea, producing a seasonal increase in the incidence of SMON. After the halogenated hydroxyquinolines were removed from the market, the incidence of SMON declined sharply (Figure 13–5).

Clinical practitioners can contribute to epidemiologic research. Schuman (1986) has written a useful guide for clinicians who want to relate their observations in the course of practice to the larger world of medical research. Clinicians practicing in university medical centers can easily become involved in collabo-

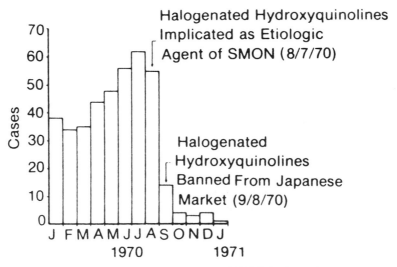

Figure 13–5. Cases of subacute myelo-optic (SMON) in Japan by month reported. *Source:* Oakley, 1973.

rative studies, but physicians in individual practices can also join or start studies. They can initiate research by observing and describing trends in their own practices, consulting with other specialists, and identifying issues to study.

Schuman points out the number of syndromes, diseases, and adverse drug reactions that were first noticed by an alert clinician. For instance, Pittman was first in the United States to recognize optic atrophy in a child treated with diiodohydroxyquin for diarrhea, and his subsequent persistence in identifying cases led to warning labels and the eventual withdrawal of the drug from the market (Pittman and Westphal, 1974). Schuman himself identified a previously unnoticed osteosarcomal malformation syndrome (now called Schuman-Burton syndrome) based on observations he made in a home visit with a physician in training. The history of epidemiology is filled with examples of observant physicians whose curiosity and persistence led to the discovery of important associations, such as Gregg's discovery in 1941 of the association between rubella exposure during pregnancy and congenital malformations, and the association between smoking and lung cancer about which Wynder published his landmark paper while still a medical student (Wynder and Graham, 1950).

In clinical practice a physician may notice trends in patient compliance, new patient characteristics, adverse drug reactions, and associations between exposures and diseases. Reporting such observations may lead to further studies and produce information that is useful to the medical community at large.

SUMMARY

Epidemiologic principles can be applied by the clinician in clinical decision making, in clinical research, and in reading and interpreting the literature. Ideally, a critical reading of the literature should inform practice, and clinical experience can in turn lead to research questions. The interrelationship between practice and research can improve the quality of care and increase the probability that clinical decisions will benefit and not harm the patient. An alert physician can add to medical knowledge by identifying unknown diseases, syndromes, or previously unsuspected associations and by identifying possible causal factors.

STUDY PROBLEMS

1. Describe a way in which decision analysis can be applied to clinical practice.
2. Decision analysis can be useful in many situations, but it also has a number of limitations. Name one of the limitations.

3. When reading the literature, a critical reader should look for information about the study reported. Name three things that should be described in the report of a study.
4. Why is a discussion of bias essential to any article describing a study and its results?
5. Name two ways that a clinician can participate in epidemiologic research.

REFERENCES

Bakwin, H. 1945. "Pseudodoxia pediatrica." *NEJM* 232:691–697.

Beeson, P. B. and McDermott, W., eds. 1963. *Cecil-Loeb Textbook of Medicine,* 11th edition. Philadelphia: W.B. Saunders.

Belongia, E. A., Hedberg, C. W., Gleich, G. J., et al. 1990. "An investigation of the cause of eosinophilia-myalgia syndrome associated with tryptophan use." *NEJM* 323:357–365.

Eidson, M., Philen, R. M., Sewell, C. M., Voorhees, R. and Kilbourne, E. M. 1990. "L-tryptophan and eosinophilia-myalgia syndrome in New Mexico." *Lancet* 355:645–648.

Fletcher, R. H., Fletcher, S. W. and Wagner, E. 1988. *Clinical Epidemiology: The Essentials.* Baltimore: Williams & Wilkins.

Gregg, N. W. 1941. "Congenital cataract following German Measles in the mother." *Trans. Ophthalmol. Soc. Aust.* 3:35.

Linet, M. S. and Stewart, W. F. 1984. "Migraine headache: epidemiologic perspectives." *Epidemiologic Reviews* Vol. 6:107–139.

Oakley, Jr., G. P. 1973. "The neurotoxicity of the halogenated hydroxyquinolines." *JAMA* 225(4):395–397.

Pauker, S. G. Clinical Decision Making. In: Wyngaarden, J. B., Lloyd, H., Smith, J., Bennett, J. C., ed. Cecil Textbook of Medicine. 19th ed. Philadelphia: W.B. Saunders Company, 1992: vol 1: pp. 68–73.

Pittman, F. E. and Westphal, M. C. 1974. "Optic atrophy following treatment with di-iodohydroxyquin." *Pediatrics* 54:81–83.

Sackett, D. L., Haynes, R. B., and Tugwell, P. 1991. *Clinical Epidemiology: A Basic Science for Clinical Medicine,* 2nd edition. Boston: Little, Brown & Co.

Schuman, S. H. 1986. *Practice-Based Epidemiology.* New York: Gordon and Breach Science Publications.

SHEP Cooperative Research Group. 1991. "Prevention of stroke by antihypertensive drug treatment in older persons with isolated systolic hypertension." *JAMA* 265(24):3255–3264.

Slutsker, L., Hoesly, F. C., Miller, L., Williams, L. P., Watson, J. C., Fleming, D. W. 1990. "Eosinophilia-myalgia syndrome associated with exposure to tryptophan from a single manufacturer." *JAMA* 264:213–217.

Stolley, P. D., Davies, J. L. 1980. "Reading the Medical Literature." In *The Physician's*

Practice, Eisenberg, J. M., and Williams, S. V., with Smith, E. S., eds. New York: John Wiley & Sons.

Weiss, Noel S. 1986. *Clinical Epidemiology: The Study of the Outcome of Illness.* New York: Oxford University Press.

Wynder, E. L. and Graham, E. A. 1950. "Tobacco smoking as a possible etiologic factor in bronchiogenic carcinoma." *JAMA* 143:329–336.

Appendix

SELECTED STATISTICAL PROCEDURES

This appendix describes some of the statistical tools and concepts that epidemiologists use. The methods selected are limited to those that can be applied to most studies and that do not require elaborate computing devices. The discussion is condensed and certain technical aspects have been omitted or only briefly described. More detailed expositions of these methods can be found in many textbooks of biostatistics.

SAMPLING OF A POPULATION

Some General Considerations

In most epidemiologic studies, it is necessary to deal with a sample of the population or a subgroup of a population about whose members certain information is desired. The population may be an entire community, the male members of the community, or another subgroup of the community that has a certain characteristic such as gender, race, or religion. Hospital inpatients can also be regarded as a population from which a sample may be taken. The sample does not have to be individuals, but may consist of households, families, or blocks in a city.

When a list of all members of the population is available, the selection of a representative sample is relatively simple. However, it is important to make certain that any available list of names, households, or addresses is indeed complete. The investigator should determine how the list was obtained and maintained, to make sure that duplicates and mistaken entries were removed and that necessary additions were made. Most routinely obtained lists that have not been developed for specific research purposes will reveal one or more deficiencies.

The members of the population list from which a sample is selected will be referred to as the sampling unit. If it is a list of names of individuals, each name is the sampling unit; if of addresses, each address is the sampling unit.

Samples are selected from a population and their characteristics are studied so that one can make inferences from the sample about the population from which it is derived. In other words, the investigator wants the sample to be representative of the population.

Samples may be selected in a variety of ways: the recommended method is known as *probability sampling,* in which each sampling unit has a known probability of being selected. This allows one to derive inferences from the sample about the population with a measurable degree of precision. There are various methods of probability sampling, and they will be discussed below.

Other sampling procedures are of limited or no value in epidemiology since the probability by which a sampling unit enters the sample is not known. Therefore, no statistical assessment can be made of the accuracy of the characteristics of the selected sample in representing the population. Also, unlike probability sampling, there is no objective assurance that potential biases have not entered into the method of selecting the sample. The following are some examples of these sampling procedures:

1. The sample is chosen haphazardly, as in many laboratory experiments where experimental animals are chosen as the investigator can catch and remove them from a cage.
2. An investigator may select individuals who, in his opinion, are typical of the population being studied. The disadvantage of this method is that one really does not know if there are differences between these ''typical'' or ''representative'' individuals and the population, so that generalizations made from the sample may be incorrect.
3. The sample consists of self-selected individuals such as those who have volunteered for an experiment, series of measurements, or interview.

Such methods may be used in exploratory epidemiologic studies to obtain a ''quick and dirty'' look at the problem being investigated. They could provide some information about the population, serving as a basis for planning more adequate studies.

Selecting a Probability Sample

For probability sampling it is necessary to have a complete list of the sampling units of the total population, whether the units are individual persons, households, addresses, blocks, etc. as the specific study requires. If some type of list is available, it may have to be revised; if not available, it is necessary to prepare a list and this usually requires ingenuity and work.

The simplest form of probability sampling is simple random sampling in which each unit in the population list has an equal probability of being selected for the sample. To select a simple random sample the investigator (1) makes a numbered list of the units in the population that he wants to sample; (2) decides on the size of the sample, a matter which is beyond the scope of this book but is discussed in most texts on statistics and sampling, e.g., Cochran (1977); and (3) selects the required number of sampling units using a table of random numbers. Such tables of random numbers are found in most books of statistical tables or texts on statistics. Table A–1 is a table of 1,000 random digits from Snedecor and Cochran (1967) for illustrative purposes.

If such a table is not available and the size of the population to be sampled is not too large, one can write the numbers 1 to N on small cards, place them in a bowl, and mix them thoroughly. If the size of the sample to be selected is n, the cards are selected from the bowl in succession until n cards are drawn. These cards are not returned to the bowl after being drawn. The different numbers are

Table A–1.   One Thousand Random Digits

	00–04	05–09	10–14	15–19	20–24	25–29	30–34	35–39	40–44	45–49
00	54463	22662	65905	70639	79365	67382	29085	69831	47058	08186
01	15389	85205	18850	39226	42249	90669	96325	23248	60933	26927
02	85941	40756	82414	02015	13858	78030	16269	65978	01385	15345
03	61149	69440	11286	88218	58925	03638	52862	62733	33451	77455
04	05219	81619	10651	67079	92511	59888	84502	72095	83463	75577
05	41417	98326	87719	92294	46614	50948	64886	20002	97365	30976
06	28357	94070	20652	35774	16249	75019	21145	05217	47286	76305
07	17783	00015	10806	83091	91530	36466	39981	62481	49177	75779
08	40950	84820	29881	85966	62800	70326	84740	62660	77379	90279
09	82995	64157	66164	41180	10089	41757	78258	96488	88629	37231
10	96754	17676	55659	44105	47361	34833	86679	23930	53249	27083
11	34357	88040	53364	71726	45690	66334	60332	22554	90600	71113
12	06318	37403	49927	57715	50423	67372	63116	48888	21505	80182
13	62111	52820	07243	79931	89292	84767	85693	73947	22278	11551
14	47534	09243	67879	00544	23410	12740	02540	54440	32949	13491
15	98614	75993	84460	62846	59844	14922	48730	73443	48167	34770
16	24856	03648	44898	09351	98795	18644	39765	71058	90368	44104
17	96887	12479	80621	66223	86085	78285	02432	53342	42846	94771
18	90801	21472	42815	77408	37390	76766	52615	32141	30268	18106
19	55165	77312	83666	36028	28420	70219	81369	41943	47366	41067

Source: Snedecor and Cochran (1967). Reprinted by permission from *Statistical Methods* by George W. Snedecor and William G. Cochran, 6th ed. © 1967 by The Iowa State University Press, South State Avenue, Ames, Iowa 50010.

recorded and the correspondingly numbered sampling units in the population are then selected. Mixing the cards provides equal probability of selection and assures randomness. However, since mixing and selection may not be done properly, it is better to use a table of random numbers.

To illustrate the use of these tables, assume that the investigator has a population of 900 case records and a simple random sample of 250 records is desired for a study. The records are numbered from 1 to 900, and a table such as A–1 is entered in a variety of ways, either from the beginning, or by arbitrarily placing a pencil at any number in the table, or by selecting certain columns. Since $N = 900$, it is only necessary to select random numbers composed of three digits. The investigator can go down columns 15–17, for instance, selecting the numbers between 001 and 900 until 250 have been selected. Any number greater than 900 is discarded, as well as any number that is repeated. Since these three columns will not provide all the 250 numbers, another set of three columns, e.g., 30–32, can be used to repeat the procedure. If large sample sizes are required, the most practical method is to use a larger table and select all eligible numbers. The Rand Corporation (1955) has published a table of one million digits, and Kendall and Smith (1938) one of 100,000 digits. Books with smaller tables usually provide instructions as to the most convenient method of using the table.

Simple random sampling may become tedious if the sample and population are large. Suppose an investigator has a list of 250,000 inhabitants or file cards and wants to choose a sample of 1,000. A method of sampling that is used more frequently than simple random sampling in such cases is systematic sampling. To select a systematic sample, two things are needed: a sampling interval and a random start. For example, if $N = 250,000$ and $n = 1,000$, one divides 250,000 by 1,000, which equals 250. Beginning with a random number between 1 and 250 (random start), one selects every 250th number thereafter. Thus if the random number is 125, the next number would be 375, then 625, etc. If n does not divide evenly into N, one selects the nearest whole number. One advantage of systematic sampling is that it spreads the sample more evenly over the population. It is conceivable, however, that the systematic sample may be biased if there is a periodicity or systematic ordering in the population list, e.g., it may always be a corner household.

Certain assumptions must be made about the characteristics of the population to be sampled in order to estimate the sampling error. A full discussion of these problems and their solutions can be found in Cochran (1977).

It should be emphasized that the listings of the population must have the same units as the desired sample, e.g., samples of individuals from lists of persons and samples of households from household lists. If a household list is available to the investigator but a simple random sample of persons is desired, there are additional considerations. If the investigator selects a simple random sample of

n households and interviews or examines one person per household, the resulting sample of n persons will not be a simple random sample since individuals in smaller households will have a greater chance of being selected than those in larger households. Thus, each individual would not have had an equal probability of being selected for the sample. If the factor being studied is related to the size of the household, a biased sample will result. More complex methods can be used to obtain an unbiased sample in such situations and some of these will be mentioned below, but again the interested reader should consult Cochran (1977).

The population to be sampled can be divided into subgroups or *strata* by one or more characteristics, such as age, gender, or severity of disease, and within each stratum a random sample can be selected. This procedure is known as *stratified sampling* and it has several advantages. It reduces sampling variability by eliminating variation with respect to the characteristic by which the strata are constructed and if the strata are more uniform than the total population with respect to other factors. It also has the advantage of allowing one to use different sampling fractions (percent of individuals in the strata that is being selected for the sample) in the different strata since it is possible to obtain larger fractions in strata with a smaller number of units.

Sampling where no population lists exist

In many areas where epidemiologic studies are needed, there is no satisfactory population list of individuals. Frequently, lists of various groupings of individuals are available or can be compiled. These groups are socially or politically defined clusterings of individuals, such as households, addresses of buildings, city blocks, or census enumeration districts. When such lists are available or when they can be readily compiled, two methods may be used to select the desired sample of individuals:

1. A random sample of clusters is selected and all individuals in the cluster are included in the study. This is known as single-stage cluster sampling.

2. A random sample of clusters is selected, a list is made of all the individuals in each cluster, and a random sample of individuals is then selected independently within each cluster. This is known as two-stage cluster sampling with subsampling.

If a list of households is available and a random sample of individual persons is desired, a random sample of households may be selected and all individuals in the household may be interviewed or studied. This is an example of single-stage cluster sampling. If, after selecting the households, a roster of all individuals in each household is made and a random sample of one or more individuals is randomly selected from each roster, one has performed two-stage cluster sampling.

There may be more than two stages of sampling. For example, a list of blocks in a city may be available from the population census. A sample of blocks may be randomly selected. Each of the selected blocks may be canvassed to obtain a list of households. A sample of households may then be selected and for each household a roster of household members compiled. This procedure results in a three-stage sample with subsampling at all stages.

If not available, lists of such clusters can be constructed by the investigator. In addition, aerial photographs or maps can be used to divide a geographical area into smaller areas with definable boundaries and then samples of areas and sub-areas can be selected.

One form of cluster sampling is **random digit dialing** (RDD). In this technique, telephone numbers for households in a specific geographic area are selected at random from clusters of such telephone numbers. The investigator can then sample individuals in households with telephones (Hartge et al., 1984; Waksberg, 1978; Wacholder et al., 1992; Greenberg, 1990). There are many potential problems in random digit dialing, including the inability to include in the sample individuals in households lacking a telephone, the greater likelihood of sampling households with two telephone numbers than those with only one number, and the different numbers of individuals living in each household. Methods have been developed to circumvent these difficulties. The interested reader is referred to the reviews of Greenberg (1990) and Wacholder et al. (1992) for further information.

Cluster sampling is convenient not only when no population lists are available but also when the investigator wants to study people living in a small number of households or villages rather than individuals in more scattered populations.

Cluster multistage samples have larger sampling errors than simple random samples of the same size. A cluster is composed of individuals who are likely to be more similar to each other than those selected at random from the population. For example, individuals in the same household have similar dietary and smoking habits (generally known as "intra-class correlation"). In addition, fewer large clusters will be available for sampling and the sample will be concentrated in a smaller number of clusters. It is therefore preferable to have a large number of small clusters than a small number of large clusters. It should be emphasized that biases can result if a cluster sample of individuals is analyzed as if it were a random sample of individuals. It should also be noted that clusters, like individuals, can be grouped into more homogeneous strata and a certain percentage of clusters selected from within each stratum. Thus, the methods used in analyzing stratified sampling can be applied. Again, the reader is referred to Cochran for a detailed discussion of these methods (1977).

ESTIMATING POPULATION CHARACTERISTICS AND THEIR SAMPLING VARIABILITY

Drawing a sample so that biases of selection are avoided does not guarantee that it will be completely representative of the population from which it was derived. The sampling procedure itself (unless it is a "sample" of 100 percent of the population) will eliminate individuals with certain characteristics. If many different samples are drawn from the same population by random sampling or by one of its variants, different values or estimates will be obtained of the same characteristic from each sample selected. If all the possible samples of a certain size drawn from a population vary considerably, the investigator has less assurance that his particular selection is representative of the population characteristic to be estimated. However, if there is little variation from sample to sample and no biases are present, either in the method of selecting the sample or in the way the population characteristic is estimated, the investigator has more assurance that a particular sample is a representative one.

Estimating Population Characteristics

The selection of the sample from a population allows for the characterization of various features of that population, e.g., serum cholesterol concentration, prevalence of cigarette smoking, etc. Three measures (the mean, the median, and the mode) are used to summarize the characteristics of interest. Each has its advantages and disadvantages in describing the features of a sample and the population from which the sample was drawn. In discussing these three summary measures, we will refer to the systolic blood pressures in a random sample of 63 nulliparous pregnant women measured at the start of their second trimester shown in Table A–2.

The mean

The *mean* is the most frequently used summary measure. Also known as the *arithmetic mean* or the *arithmetic average,* it is symbolized as $\bar{x}$ (termed "x-bar"). The mean is calculated by summing all of the observed values and dividing by the sample size. For the data in Table A–2, the mean is calculated as: $(113 + 114 + 100 + 113 + 115 + \ldots + 102 + 109 + 128)$ mmHg/63, which is equal to 106.38 mmHg. Although there may be considerable variation in the individual

Table A–2. Measurements of Systolic Blood Pressure among 63 Nulliparous Pregnant Women at the Beginning of the Second Trimester

113	114	100	113	115	84	115	119	99	95	113	111	114
128	96	107	88	93	99	103	92	108	122	107	104	99
95	122	97	112	120	105	100	105	111	113	110	121	106
107	114	102	103	99	96	93	103	107	102	105	116	95
118	114	105	111	92	113	97	103	102	109	128		

values of a characteristic in samples from the same population, the means for those samples will tend to be similar in value. This consistency is one advantage of the mean. Another is its use in many statistical tests (described below). However, the mean has one major disadvantage: depending on the simple size, it can be greatly affected by an extreme value, i.e., an observation that differs greatly from the other ones (sometimes referred to as ''outliers''). For example, suppose that in addition to the values in Table A–2, there were a 64th individual in the sample, whose systolic blood pressure was 300 mmHg. Clearly, this value is quite different from the other 63. If it were included in the calculation of the mean, then $\bar{x}$ would be 109.4 mmHg. In order to reduce the effect of one or more outliers on the characterization of a population, some investigators use a different summary measure, the median, which relies only on the ranking of observations in the sample.

The median

The *median* is defined as the observation that corresponds to the 50th percentile of the sample, i.e., the midpoint of the data. One-half of all of the data are greater than the median, and one-half are less than the median. To calculate the median, the observations are ranked in ascending order. Table A–3 shows the data in Table A–2 assembled in ascending order. The median observation is then the 32nd observation (31 observations above the median, 31 observations below the median), 106 mmHg. If there is an even number of observations, the median is the mean of the middle two observations.

The main advantage of the median is the lack of effect of extreme values on it. For instance, if there were a 64th observation of 300 mmHg for the data in Table A–3, the median would be 106.5 (the average of the 32nd and 33rd observations). This benefit contrasts with the disadvantage that the median is not as amenable to statistical testing as the mean. Hence, although the median is sometimes used as a summary measure, it is less often used than the mean.

Table A-3.   Measurements of Systolic Blood Pressure among 63 Nulliparous Pregnant Women, Arranged in Ascending Order

RANK	OBSERVATION	RANK	OBSERVATION	RANK	OBSERVATION
1	84	23	103	45	113
2	88	24	103	46	113
3	92	25	103	47	113
4	92	26	103	48	113
5	93	27	104	49	114
6	93	28	105	50	114
7	95	29	105	51	114
8	95	30	105	52	114
9	95	31	105	53	115
10	96	32	106	54	115
11	96	33	107	55	116
12	97	34	107	56	118
13	97	35	107	57	119
14	99	36	107	58	120
15	99	37	108	59	121
16	99	38	109	60	122
17	99	39	110	61	122
18	100	40	111	62	128
19	100	41	111	63	128
20	102	42	111		
21	102	43	112		
22	102	44	113		

The mode

The third summary measure is the *mode,* which is the most frequently occurring value. For the data in Table A–2, the mode is 113; this is considerably different from both the mean and the median. Frequently, there is no particular value in a sample that occurs more often than all the other values; in this instance, the mode does not exist. Although the mode can summarize some information regarding a characteristic in a sample (and the population from which it was drawn), it does not provide as much information as the mean or the median. For this reason, it is not frequently used by investigators.

Assessing Sampling Variability

Random sampling provides the means of measuring the degree of assurance from the particular sample selected. It can be shown theoretically or by experimental sampling that the amount of variation in the frequency of a characteristic from one sample to another depends upon the amount of variation of the characteristic (whether quantitative or qualitative) in the population. Random sampling allows one to obtain from any selected sample an unbiased estimate of the population variation. This estimate is then used to set limits within which the population value being estimated will lie, with varying degrees of confidence. A numerical value for these degrees of confidence can be calculated by making some assumptions, or preferably by having some knowledge about the distribution of the estimated characteristic in the population.

As already mentioned, when random sampling is used, the variability of samples drawn from a population can be measured in terms of the variability found in the population itself, which can be estimated from the selected sample. For example, if the average age at menarche is estimated from a sample, the variation in the estimate from that sample reflects the variation in the age of menarche in the population, which can be estimated in a randomly selected sample.

Variation of individuals in a population can be measured in several ways. Most frequently it is measured by its variance or the square root of the variance, the standard deviation. The *variance* of a characteristic or measurement is defined as the mean of the sum of squared deviations of individuals from the population's arithmetic mean. The standard deviation of a characteristic is usually denoted by the Greek lowercase letter sigma (σ) and the variance as σ^2. Symbolically, the variance may be defined as:

$$\sigma^2 = \frac{1}{N} [(x_1 - \overline{X})^2 + (x_2 - \overline{X})^2 + \ldots + (x_N - \overline{X})^2]$$

where N is the size of the population, x is the particular characteristic being measured, x_i is the value of the characteristic for the ith individual in the population, and $\overline{X}$ is the arithmetic mean of the xth characteristic in the population.

An equivalent formula which makes the calculation of σ^2 easier is:

$$\sigma^2 = (\Sigma x_i^2 - N\overline{X}^2)/N.$$

If the characteristic being examined is dichotomous (i.e., present or absent) rather than a measurement, the variance reduces to $P(1 - P)$, where P is the proportion of individuals with the characteristic.

It is important to note that the sampling variation depends essentially on two quantities: the variance of the population (σ^2) and the sample size (n). Populations with more variable characteristics of interest require larger sample sizes to compensate for this fact. With a qualitative characteristic, the greatest amount of variation in the population occurs when P, the frequency of the characteristic in the population, equals 0.50. This decreases as P is higher or lower than 0.50. Thus, when sampling from a population where the characteristic occurs 50 percent of the time, much larger samples are necessary to provide the same degree of assurance one has in a population where the characteristic occurs only 10 percent of the time.

Study results are usually assessed in terms of the standard deviation. The formula used to determine the precision of the sample mean or proportion is:

$$\sigma_{\bar{x}} = \frac{\sigma}{\sqrt{n}}.$$

It should be noted that a change in the sample size affects the standard deviation. To reduce the standard deviation by one-half, for example, it is necessary to quadruple the sample size. Thus it is possible to achieve any desired reduction in the standard deviation, but the necessary increase in the sample size may be prohibitively costly.

Rarely does the investigator have knowledge of the variance or standard deviation of the population being studied. When the sample is a probability sample, an estimate of the sampling variation is obtained from the sample itself. For a simple random sample, the estimated variance of a sample mean is:

$$s_{\bar{x}}^2 = \frac{s^2}{n}$$

where s^2 is the sample estimate of the variance defined by:

$$s^2 = \frac{1}{n - 1} [(x_1 - \bar{x})^2 + (x_2 - \bar{x})^2 + \ldots + (x_n - \bar{x})^2],$$

where $x_1, x_2, \ldots, x_n$ are the sample values of the xth characteristic and $\bar{x}$ is the arithmetic mean of the xth characteristic in the sample. An equivalent formula which makes the calculation of s^2 easier is:

$$s^2 = (\Sigma x_i^2 - N\bar{x}^2)/(N - 1).$$

An example of the calculation of s^2, using the data in Table A–2, is shown in Table A–4. The standard error, $S_{\bar{x}}$, is the square root of the variance of the mean.

Table A–4.   Calculation of s^2 for Data in Table A–2

$n = 63$
$\Sigma x = 6{,}702$
$\Sigma x^2 = 718{,}700$
$\bar{x} = \Sigma x/n = 6{,}702/63 = 106.38$
$s^2 = (\Sigma x^2 - n\bar{x}^2)/(n - 1) = (718{,}700 - [63 \cdot (106.38)^2])/62 = 5747.65/62 = 92.70$
$s = \sqrt{s^2} = \sqrt{92.70} = 9.63$
$s_{\bar{x}} = s/\sqrt{n} = 9.63/\sqrt{63} = 1.21$

The estimate of the variance of the sample proportion is:

$$P(1 - P)/N,$$

where P is the proportion of individuals in a sample of size N with the characteristic being studied.

Thus, if a simple random sample of 100 individuals is selected from a large population, among whom 40 persons have a certain characteristic, the estimated proportion of people with this characteristic in the population is $p_0 = \dfrac{40}{100} = 0.40$ (p_0 will be used as the sample estimate of P). The estimated sampling variability is:

$$s = \sqrt{\frac{p_0(1 - p_0)}{n}} = \sqrt{\frac{(.40)(1 - .40)}{100}} = \sqrt{.0024} = .049$$

or approximately .05. This can be interpreted to mean that while the estimated frequency of the characteristic in the population as derived from this sample was 40 percent, other samples of the same size, drawn similarly from the same population, would vary from each other on the average by about 5 percent.

However, the value of .049 was also derived from sample values so that another sample would likely give a different estimate of the precision or standard deviation of the sample. The estimates of precision are not likely to vary as much as the estimated proportions themselves. If only ten (or even ninety) persons had been found to have the characteristic rather than forty, the estimated precision would have changed from 5 to 3 percent.

The formula:

$$s = \sqrt{\frac{P(1 - P)}{n}}$$

is known as the standard error of a proportion. It refers to the variability of a sample proportion p_0 from one sample to another. It is estimated from the sample itself by:

$$s = \sqrt{\frac{p_0(1 - p_0)}{n}}.$$

CONFIDENCE INTERVALS FOR PROPORTIONS

The estimation of variation represents the average amount of sampling variability. Under certain conditions, however, it can be shown that for reasonably large samples [large enough so that $n(1 - p) > 10$], the proportion estimated from approximately 95 percent of samples of a given size will lie within ± 1.96 standard errors of the true population proportion P.

If the value of P is known, it can then be stated that 95 percent of the samples of size n selected from this population have a proportion that will fall in the interval

$$P - 1.96 \sqrt{\frac{P(1 - P)}{n}}, \ P + 1.96 \sqrt{\frac{P(1 - P)}{n}}.$$

If, for example, random samples of size 100 are selected from a population in which 50 percent of the persons have a certain characteristic, 95 percent of the samples will provide estimates of this percentage that will lie between

$$0.50 - 1.96 \sqrt{\frac{0.5(1 - 0.5)}{100}} \text{ and } 0.50 + 1.96 \sqrt{\frac{0.5(1 - 0.5)}{100}}$$

or between 40 and 60 percent (the multiplier 2.0 can be used rather than 1.96 for convenience). Thus, estimates that are less than 40 percent or greater than 60 percent will occur in only 5 percent of the samples of size 100 selected from such a population. It can be further shown that 99 percent of the samples will lie within the interval

$$P - 2.58 \sqrt{\frac{P(1 - P)}{n}} \text{ and } P + 2.58 \sqrt{\frac{P(1 - P)}{n}}.$$

Using data from the above example, 99 percent of the estimates from samples of size 100 will lie between 38 and 62.9 percent.

Then, what can be inferred from any particular random sample of size n that is selected from this population? From the sample, first compute p_0, and then the following expression:

$$p_0 \pm 1.96 \sqrt{\frac{P(1 - P)}{n}},$$

i.e., $\left(p_0 - 1.96 \sqrt{\frac{P(1 - P)}{n}}\right) - \left(p_0 + 1.96 \sqrt{\frac{P(1 - P)}{n}}\right).$

This interval will include P only if p_0 is one of the 95 percent of all possible estimates that fall within the interval

$$P \pm 1.96 \sqrt{\frac{P(1 - P)}{n}}.$$

In the numerical example above, if p_0 were one of the estimates between 0.40 and 0.60, the interval formed by adding and subtracting

$$2 \sqrt{\frac{0.5(1 - 0.5)}{100}} = 0.10$$

will contain the population proportion, 0.50. This interval will not contain 5 percent of the samples that have estimates of p_0 greater than 0.60 or less than 0.40, and therefore will not contain the population proportion, 0.50. Thus, 95 percent of the samples will provide intervals that contain the population percentage, while 5 percent will not. Before selecting a particular sample of size n, the investigator is thus assured in 95 times out of 100 that the interval calculated from his sample will contain the population proportion he is interested in estimating.

The investigator will not know before (or after) selecting the sample whether or not this particular estimate is one of the 95 percent lying within the two standard error range of the true proportion or if it is one of the 5 percent outside this range. If the investigator's sample is one of the latter 5 percent, then the statement that the interval

$$p_0 \pm 2 \sqrt{\frac{P(1 - P)}{n}}$$

contains the population proportion will be wrong; otherwise, it will be a correct statement. For these reasons the interval

$$p_0 \pm 2 \sqrt{\frac{P(1 - P)}{n}}$$

is called a 95 percent confidence interval, the word "confidence" referring to the investigator's assurance that the selected sample is one of 95 percent of all samples that will provide a correct statement based on the interval.

It should be noted that in order to calculate these confidence intervals the unknown population proportion P has been used in the standard error formula. Since the investigator is either attempting to estimate P or to test some hypothesis about it, its value is not known. The obvious solution is to substitute the sample value of p_0 in the formula for the standard error and calculate the interval

$$p_0 \pm 1.96 \sqrt{\frac{p_0(1 - p_0)}{n}} .$$

This increases the variation of the interval since the standard error will vary from sample to sample. Fortunately, as was pointed out earlier, the standard error changes little from sample to sample, even though the sample proportion p_0 might. Thus, the statements that were made using P in the standard error hold fairly well when the sample estimate p_0 is used in place of P.

In summary: If a simple random sample of size n is selected from a population and the sample proportion p_0 is calculated, a 95 percent confidence interval for P, the population proportion, is given by

$$p_0 \pm 1.96 \sqrt{\frac{p_0(1 - p_0)}{n}} .$$

If a 99 percent confidence interval is desired, the multiplier 1.96 is replaced by 2.58. (For most practical applications, 1.96 can be replaced by 2.0 and 2.58 by 2.6 with little loss of accuracy.)

For example, suppose in a simple random sample of 400 persons from a large population of smokers, 80 are found to be "heavy" smokers (smoking more than one pack of cigarettes a day). The proportion of "heavy" smokers in the population can be estimated by the 95 percent confidence interval

$$p_0 \pm 2 \sqrt{\frac{p_0(1 - p_0)}{n}} = \frac{80}{400} \pm 2 \sqrt{\frac{\frac{80}{400}\left(1 - \frac{80}{400}\right)}{400}} = 0.20 \pm .04,$$

or 16 percent to 24 percent. Thus, it can be stated that there is a 95 percent probability that the percentage of "heavy" smokers in the population lies between 16 and 24 percent.

The confidence interval can be made as small as desired by increasing the sample size, but the decrease is proportional to the square root of the increase rather than to the increase itself. In the example, in order to decrease the confidence interval from 16–24 percent to 18–22 percent, the sample size would have to be quadrupled from 400 to 1,600 persons. Thus, beyond a certain level, reductions in the confidence interval can only be achieved at higher cost.

NINETY-FIVE PERCENT CONFIDENCE INTERVAL FOR RARELY OCCURRING EVENTS

We have seen that for a percentage or rate, good approximations for 95 percent confidence intervals are easily computed when the condition $n(1 - p) > 10$ is satisfied. But many diseases, such as cancer, have annual incidence, prevalence, or mortality rates ranging from 1 to 100 per 100,000 population so that sample sizes of 10,000 to 1,000,000 would be necessary before the above calculations of confidence limits could be used safely. In practice, rates must often be estimated from smaller samples.

In calculating confidence intervals for rarely occurring events, different methods must be used. These are based on the Poisson rather than the normal (Gaussian) distribution used earlier. With these methods, unfortunately, it is not possible to use multipliers for the standard error that are analogous to 1.96 and 2.58, which are derived from the normal curve. To simplify matters, a table of 95 percent confidence interval factors* was prepared by Haenszel, Loveland, and Sirken (1962) and is reproduced as Table A–5. The authors tabulated factors necessary to calculate 95 percent confidence limits for standardized mortality ratios (SMRs). The following calculation of 95 percent confidence limits for low incidence rates exemplifies the method used.

If, in a simple random sample of 5,000 adult males, 2 new cases of stomach cancer had occurred during a year of observation, which projects to an incidence rate of 40 per 100,000 population. In order to calculate 95 percent confidence limits, enter Table A–5 at $n = 2$ (observed number of cases on which the estimate is based). A lower limit factor (L) of 0.121 and an upper limit factor (U) of 3.61 are found corresponding to $n = 2$. To convert these numbers to a rate per 100,000, multiply both lower and upper limits by the sample rate per 100,000 (i.e., by 40). Thus, L = 40 × 0.121 = 4.84, and U = 40 × 3.61 = 144.40. The 95 percent confidence interval for the incidence of stomach cancer is therefore 4.84–144.40 cases per 100,000 of population. This interval is wide, reflecting the uncertainties based on estimates involving only two cases.

If, in a sample of any size, no cases are found, an upper 95 percent confidence limit can be estimated by using $n = 3$ as the upper limit. Thus, if in a sample of

---

*These factors facilitate the calculation of a confidence interval for a Poisson-distributed variable.

Table A–5   Tabular Values of 95 Percent Confidence Limit Factors for Estimates of a
Poisson-Distributed Variable

OBSERVED NUMBER ON WHICH ESTIMATE IS BASED (n)	LOWER LIMIT FACTOR (L)	UPPER LIMIT FACTOR (U)	OBSERVED NUMBER ON WHICH ESTIMATE IS BASED (n)	LOWER LIMIT FACTOR (L)	UPPER LIMIT FACTOR (U)	OBSERVED NUMBER ON WHICH ESTIMATE IS BASED (n)	LOWER LIMIT FACTOR (L)	UPPER LIMIT FACTOR (U)
1	0.0253	5.57	21	0.619	1.53	120	0.833	1.200
2	0.121	3.61	22	0.627	1.51	140	0.844	1.184
3	0.206	2.92	23	0.634	1.50	160	0.854	1.171
4	0.272	2.56	24	0.641	1.49	180	0.862	1.160
5	0.324	2.33	25	0.647	1.48	200	0.868	1.151
6	0.367	2.18	26	0.653	1.47	250	0.882	1.134
7	0.401	2.06	27	0.659	1.46	300	0.892	1.121
8	0.431	1.97	28	0.665	1.45	350	0.899	1.112
9	0.458	1.90	29	0.670	1.44	400	0.906	1.104
10	0.480	1.84	30	0.675	1.43	450	0.911	1.098
11	0.499	1.79	35	0.697	1.39	500	0.915	1.093
12	0.517	1.75	40	0.714	1.36	600	0.922	1.084
13	0.532	1.71	45	0.729	1.34	700	0.928	1.078
14	0.546	1.68	50	0.742	1.32	800	0.932	1.072
15	0.560	1.65	60	0.770	1.30	900	0.936	1.068
16	0.572	1.62	70	0.785	1.27	1000	0.939	1.064
17	0.583	1.60	80	0.798	1.25			
18	0.593	1.58	90	0.809	1.24			
19	0.602	1.56	100	0.818	1.22			
20	0.611	1.54						

Source: Haenszel et al. (1962).

10,000 persons, $n = 0$ cases of a disease were found, the upper 95 percent confidence limit would be calculated as 3 per 10,000 cases, or 30 per 100,000.

This method is also applicable to subclasses of the sample population. If
simple random sampling is not used, or if the numerators and denominators of
the rates are not derived from the same survey, then certain complications can
arise from using Table A–5. Some of these complications are discussed by Haenszel et al. (1962).

TESTS OF HYPOTHESES FOR PROPORTIONS

Samples are often selected not only to estimate the frequencies or proportions but
also to test certain hypotheses. It is often desirable to know if an incidence or

prevalence rate for a certain group of the population has decreased or increased over a period of time. The new rate p_0 can be estimated from a simple random sample and the investigator wants to determine ("test the hypothesis") whether the sample with this rate may have come from a population with a certain hypothesized rate. Is the difference between the observed and hypothesized rate large enough to exclude sampling variation as an explanation? For example, it might be known that the yearly survival rate from a certain group of diseases is 30 percent. After a new method of treatment is introduced, it is observed in a random sample of 100 persons with the disease, that 50 have survived one year. Is this difference of 20 percent due to sampling variation or must one hypothesize another explanation of the difference? (This issue is hypothetical since, as discussed in Chapter 8, a randomized clinical trial is the best method for determining whether a new treatment has an effect.)

In the previous section, it was noted that for samples which are large enough $[n(1 - p) > 10]$, the 95 percent confidence interval is

$$p_0 - 2.0 \sqrt{\frac{P(1 - P)}{n}} \leq P \leq p_0 + 2.0 \sqrt{\frac{P(1 - P)}{n}} \, .$$

This relationship would be true for 95 percent of the samples selected from that population. This can be rewritten in the form:

$$|p_0 - P| \leq 2.0 \sqrt{\frac{P(1 - P)}{n}} \, .$$

The vertical strokes on either side of a quantity refer to the absolute value of the quantity regardless of algebraic sign.

Thus, if a sample with a proportion p_0 comes from a population with proportion P, the difference (either in a positive or negative sense) can be expected to exceed twice the standard error *only* 5 percent of the time. If the observed difference does, indeed, exceed twice the standard error, it can be concluded that this sample belongs to that group that occurs infrequently (less than 5 percent of the time), or that it has in fact been derived from some other population. If the latter explanation is accepted, then there is a 5 percent chance of being wrong.

In the hypothetical survival rate problem, $p_0 = \dfrac{50}{100} = .50$, $P = .30$, and

$$\sqrt{\frac{P(1 - P)}{n}} = \sqrt{\frac{(.30)(.70)}{100}} = .046;$$

$1.96(0.46) = .0902$ and $|p_0 - P| = |.50 - .30| = .20$. Since the difference of .20 is greater than .090, one can conclude that either there was no increase in survival and a rather rare event was observed, or that there really was an increase in survivorship, resulting in the observed difference. If the investigator is unwilling to accept the possibility that the study sample is one that occurs rarely, then the difference is said to be statistically significant at the 5 percent probability level. If one is reluctant to accept a sample that occurs less than 5 percent of the time as being rare, a higher level of statistical significance may be specified; for example, by classifying as rare those samples that occur less than 1 percent of the time. It is then necessary that the difference $|p_0 - P|$ exceed

$$2.6 \sqrt{\frac{P(1 - P)}{n}} \; .$$

This will occur less than 1 percent of the time if the hypothesis is true that p_0 was derived from a population with proportion P. If this hypothesis is rejected, there is a 1 percent chance of having rejected a true hypothesis.

The test appears in its simplest form if the following quantity is calculated:

$$\frac{|p_0 - P|}{\sqrt{\dfrac{P(1 - P)}{n}}} = \frac{\text{difference}}{\text{standard error (S.E.)}}$$

If this difference exceeds 2.0, the difference is said to be statistically significant at the 5 percent level; if it exceeds 2.60 the difference is said to be statistically significant at the 1 percent level. The 5 percent and 1 percent levels correspond to α, the chance of a Type I error occurring, that was discussed in Chapter 8 (p. 161).

CONFIDENCE INTERVALS AND TESTS OF HYPOTHESES FOR THE SAMPLE MEAN

There are also 95 percent confidence interval and statistical tests for the mean $(\bar{x})$ of sample data that are "continuous," i.e., not dichotomous. The maternal systolic blood pressure readings given in Table A–2 are examples of such data. The 95 percent confidence interval for the mean of such continuous data $(\bar{X})$ would be

$$\bar{x} - 1.96\sqrt{(\sigma^2/N)}, \ \bar{x} + 1.96\sqrt{(\sigma^2/N)}.$$

(This confidence interval should only be used if the population distribution from which the data were drawn is a normal one or if $N \geq 30$.) For the data given in Table A–2, the mean was 106.38 mmHg. Suppose that the variance (σ^2) were known from previous surveys to be 100.2 mmHg^2. Then the 95 percent confidence interval would be

$$106.38 - 1.96\sqrt{(100.2/63)}, \ 106.38 + 1.96\sqrt{(100.2/63)}$$

or 103.91 mmHg to 108.85 mmHg.

An alternative analysis of these data might use the investigator's knowledge that the average maternal systolic blood pressure in the general population is 110.1 mmHg. The investigator wishes to determine whether the difference between the population value and the mean for the sample is due to sampling variation or whether some other explanation must be sought. The 95 percent confidence interval for $\overline{X}$ is

$$\bar{x} - 1.96\sqrt{(\sigma^2/N)} \leq \overline{X} \leq \bar{x} + 1.96\sqrt{(\sigma^2/N)}.$$

This relationship may be rewritten as

$$|\bar{x} - \overline{X}| \leq 1.96\sqrt{(\sigma^2/N)}.$$

or

$$\frac{|\bar{x} - \overline{X}|}{\sqrt{(\sigma^2/N)}} \leq 1.96.$$

If the left side of this equation is found to be less than 1.96, then the investigator would conclude that there is at least a 5 percent chance that the difference between the sample mean and the known population value resulted from sampling variation; i.e., no other explanation is needed to explain the discrepancy. Alternatively, if the left side of the equation is greater than 1.96, then the probability that this difference results from sampling variation is less than 5 percent; i.e., there are other explanations for the discrepancy. Substituting the sample mean and the population values into this criterion, one finds that

$$\frac{|\bar{x} - \overline{X}|}{\sqrt{(\sigma^2/N)}} = \frac{|106.38 - 110.1| \text{ mmHg}}{\sqrt{(100.2 \text{ mmHg}^2/63)}}$$

$$= (3.72 \text{ mmHg})/(1.26 \text{ mmHg})$$
$$= 2.95.$$

Hence the investigator would conclude that the sample mean is statistically significantly different from the population mean at the 5 percent level.

Suppose that the variance for the data in Table A–2 were not known before the sample was selected. The investigator may still test the hypothesis that the difference between the sample mean and the population mean is attributable to sampling variation, but the formula used differs slightly from that presented above. In particular, since σ^2 must be estimated by s^2, the test criterion is:

$$\frac{|\bar{x} - \overline{X}|}{\sqrt{(s^2/N)}} \leq t_{N-1}.$$

where t_{N-1} is the value of the t-distribution (a statistical frequency distribution) with $N - 1$ "degrees of freedom" (df) for the desired level of significance. Selected values of the t-distribution for various degrees of freedom are given in Table A–6. It is important to recognize that the degrees of freedom depend only on the sample size, not on the magnitude of $\bar{x}$, s, or $\overline{X}$.

Suppose that the investigator wishes to determine if the sample mean of 106.38 mmHg differs significantly from the population value of 110.1 mmHg and does not know the value of σ^2. Using the information in Table A–4, we can see that the test criterion is

$$\frac{|106.38 - 110.1|}{\sqrt{(s^2/63)}} \leq t_{62},$$

$$\frac{3.72}{1.21} \leq t_{62},$$

$$3.07 \leq t_{62}.$$

Since the left side of the equation is greater than the right side, the investigator would conclude that the sample mean is statistically significantly different from the population mean at the 5 percent level; i.e., sampling variation alone cannot explain the difference. For more information on the t-distribution, the reader is referred to Colton (1974) and Snedecor and Cochran (1977).

Table A–6.   Value of the *t*-
Distribution for 5 Percent Statistical
Significance Tests for Various Degrees
of Freedom

DEGREES OF FREEDOM (df)	t_{df}
1	25.45
2	6.21
3	4.18
4	3.50
5	3.16
6	2.97
7	2.84
8	2.75
9	2.69
10	2.63
15	2.49
20	2.42
25	2.39
30	2.36
35	2.34
40	2.33
45	2.32
50	2.31
55	2.30
60	2.30
70	2.29
80	2.28

TESTING HYPOTHESES ABOUT TWO SAMPLE PROPORTIONS

It can be shown that the standard error of the difference between two sample
percentages p_1 and p_2 from the same population will have a standard error of

$$\sqrt{\frac{P(1 - P)}{n_1} + \frac{P(1 - P)}{n_2}}.$$

where P is the proportion of the population with the characteristic, $(1 - P)$ is the
proportion of the population without the characteristic, n_1 is the size of one sample, and n_2 is the size of the other sample. If one wants to test the hypothesis that
the two samples have been independently selected from a population having the
common population proportion P, a ratio is calculated that is similar to the one
given in previous sections, namely,

$$\frac{\text{difference between proportions}}{\text{standard error of difference}} = \frac{|p_1 - p_2|}{\sqrt{\dfrac{P(1-P)}{n_1} + \dfrac{P(1-P)}{n_2}}}.$$

This provides a satisfactory method of testing the hypothesis that there is no difference between p_1 and p_2 at the 5 percent or 1 percent significance level, if an estimate of P and $(1-P)$ is available. Up to this point we have assumed that the values of P and $(1-P)$ were provided or known. The hypothesis to be tested states that the two samples come from a population with a common population proportion without specifying the value of the proportion. Thus, it is necessary to estimate the value of P from the two samples by taking a weighted average of their proportions,

$$\hat{p} = \frac{n_1 p_1 + n_2 p_2}{n_1 + n_2} = \frac{\text{total number in both samples}}{\text{having the characteristic}}{\text{total number of observations}}$$

The test criterion then becomes:

$$\frac{\text{difference between proportions}}{\text{standard error of difference}} = \frac{|p_1 - p_2|}{\sqrt{\dfrac{\hat{p}(1-p)}{n_1} + \dfrac{\hat{p}(1-\hat{p})}{n_2}}}.$$

If this value exceeds 1.96 (or 2.0), then the hypothesis, that the observed difference is due to sampling alone, is rejected at the 5 percent level of statistical significance. If it exceeds 2.58 (or 2.6), the hypothesis is rejected at the 1 percent level.

For a simple example of the procedure, assume that an investigator has observations on the number of patients who have and have not been cured after receiving one of two treatments, A and B, as shown in Table A–7. The hypothesis to be tested is whether the observed cure rate of those who had received treatment A is significantly different from those who had received treatment B. This can be restated as follows: would one frequently observe a difference of .156 (or 15.6 percent) in these cure rates if these two samples being compared were derived from a population with the same cure rate? The estimate of the population cure rate is given by $\hat{p} = \dfrac{75}{200} = .375$.

The statistical test can now be calculated as

$$\frac{.156}{\sqrt{\dfrac{(.375)(.625)}{40} + \dfrac{(.375)(.625)}{160}}} = \frac{.156}{.0866} = 1.8.$$

Table A–7. Determination of Percentage Cured for
Patients Receiving Treatments A and B

| TREATMENT | NUMBER OF PATIENTS | | |
	CURED	NOT CURED	TOTAL
A	10	30	40
B	65	95	160
Total	75	125	200

The cure rate for those receiving treatments A and B are
$p_a = 10/40 = .25$, $p_b = 65/160 = .406$, respectively. The
difference in cure rates is $p_a - p_b = .156$.

Since this value is less than 1.96, it is concluded that either the difference observed
is due to sampling (or chance) variation in the two groups or that the sample
sizes used in this comparison are not large enough to detect differences of this
size.

The test can be put into another form that allows simpler computations. If
the observations in the fourfold table (Table A–7) are expressed in a more general
form, as in Table A–8, it is possible to obtain, after some algebraic manipulation,
the following:

$$\text{(test criterion)}^2 = \frac{N(ad - bc)}{(a + c)(b + d)(a + b)(c + d)} = X^2 \text{ (chi square)}.$$

This last quantity is often given as the computational form when data are
expressed in a fourfold table such as A–7 or A–8. Rather than comparing the
observed value with 1.96 to determine the significance, X^2 is compared with
$(1.96)^2 = 3.84$. If X^2 is greater than 3.84, the difference of the observed proportions is said to be significantly different at a probability level of 0.05. Equiva-
lently, there is said to be a significant association between the method of treatment

Table A–8. Symbolic Representation for Determining Cure
Rates for Receiving Treatments A and B

| TREATMENT | NUMBER OF PATIENTS | | |
	CURED	NOT CURED	TOTAL
A	a	b	a + b
B	c	d	c + d

Total $a + c = n_1$; $b + d = n_2$ $N = a + b + c + d = n_1 + n_2$

and cure of the disease. For a further explanation of X^2 tests and examples of their extension to other situations involving qualitative data, the reader is referred to Hill (1967), Snedecor and Cochran (1977), and Fleiss (1981).

TESTING HYPOTHESES ABOUT TWO SAMPLE MEANS

As was the case with the difference in two sample percentages from the same population, the standard error for the difference in two sample means from the same population is

$$\sqrt{[(n_1 - 1)s_1^2 + (n_2 - 1)s_2^2]/(n_1 + n_2 - 2)},$$

where s_1^2 is the estimated variance for one sample of size n_1 and s_2^2 is the estimated variance of the other sample of size n_2. If one wants to test the hypothesis that the two samples have been selected from the same population, a ratio is calculated similar to the one given in previous sections, namely,

$$\frac{\text{difference between means}}{\text{standard error of difference}} = \frac{|\bar{x}_1 - \bar{x}_2|}{\sqrt{[(n_1 - 1)s_1^2 + (n_2 - 1)s_2^2]/(n_1 + n_2 - 2)}}.$$

The degree of freedom for this ratio is given by $n_1 + n_2 - 2$. If the ratio exceeds the t-statistic in Table A–6 with the corresponding degrees of freedom, then the hypothesis, that the observed difference is due to sampling alone, is rejected at the 5 percent level of statistical significance.

For a simple example of the procedure, assume that an investigator has made observations on the total serum cholesterol levels in 41 men and 41 women. The average total serum cholesterol level for the men is 220 mg/dL (with a standard deviation of 10 mg/dL) and for the women, 198 mg/dL (with a standard deviation of 8 mg/dL). The investigator wishes to determine if the difference in the means of 22 mg/dL can be attributed to random sampling variation alone. This question can be restated as follows: Would one frequently observe a difference of 22 mg/dL in average total serum cholesterol if the two samples being compared were derived from the same population? The standard error of the difference would be

$$\begin{aligned}
\text{S.E.} &= \sqrt{[(n_1 - 1)s_1^2 + (n_2 - 1)s_2^2]/(n_1 + n_2 - 2)} \\
&= \sqrt{[(41 - 1)(10)^2 + (41 - 1)(8)^2]/(41 + 41 - 2)} \\
&= \sqrt{[40(100) + 40(64)]/(80)} \\
&= \sqrt{6560/80} \\
&= 9.1 \text{ mg/dL.}
\end{aligned}$$

The investigator would then calculate the ratio of the difference in the sample means to the standard error of the difference:

$$\frac{\text{difference in sample means}}{\text{standard error of difference}} = \frac{22 \text{ mg/dL}}{9.1 \text{ mg/dL}} = 2.42$$

This ratio is then compared with the t-statistic given in Table A–6 for $(n_1 + n_2 - 2) = 80$ degrees of freedom. Since this ratio is greater than the t-statistic (2.28), the investigator would conclude that random sampling alone cannot explain this large a difference in the sample means if the samples were derived from the same population. Hence, other explanations for the difference in the means must be sought.

CORRELATION AND REGRESSION

The statistical analysis of the relationship between two continuous variables may be considered by either of two approaches: (1) correlation and (2) regression. Although these two methods are related, they remain separate in their range of applications.

Correlation

The assessment of the linear association between two continuous variables is called *correlation*. The degree of such association is measured by the *correlation coefficient, r*, also known as *Pearson's correlation coefficient* or the *product-moment correlation coefficient*. If the ranks of the observations are substituted for the observations themselves, the correlation coefficient is then known as *Spearman's rank correlation coefficient*. For further information about rank correlation, see Colton (1974). For n pairs of observations of the two variables of interest, x and y, the correlation coefficient is

$$r = \frac{\Sigma(x_i - \bar{x})(y_i - \bar{y})}{\sqrt{[\Sigma(x_i - \bar{x})^2][\Sigma(y_i - \bar{y})^2]}} .$$

Computationally, the numerator of r may be calculated as $\Sigma(x_1 y_1) - n\bar{x}\bar{y}$, and the denominator as $\sqrt{[\Sigma(x_i^2 - n\bar{x}^2)\Sigma(y_i^2 - n\bar{y}^2)]}$. An example of the calculation of the correlation coefficient for hypothetical observations of annual per capita tobacco consumption and lung cancer incidence twenty years later is shown in Table A–9.

The correlation coefficient can range from -1 to 1. A value of 1 means that there is a strong positive linear association between the two variables; i.e., when the value of one variable is small, the other variable is small, and when the value of one variable is large, the other variable is large. If r is equal to -1, then there is a strong inverse linear association between the two variables; i.e., when the value of one variable is large, the value of the other variable is small, and vice versa. The closer the value of r is to either 1 or -1, the greater the degree of linear association present between the two variables, with values of .5 or $-.5$

Table A–9. Example of the Calculation of the Correlation Coefficient

ANNUAL PER CAPITA TOBACCO CONSUMPTION (lbs) (x)	AVERAGE AGE-ADJUSTED LUNG CANCER RATE PER 100,000 PERSONS TWENTY YEARS LATER (y)
98	65.2
96	68.7
100	69.5
106	75.2
109	77.3
115	82.4
140	95.4
141	96.7
137	93.6
146	98.9
151	99.3
165	103.3
171	104.4
174	104.7
180	105.3
169	99.4
175	104.3
$n = 17$	$\Sigma x_i y_i = 222,175.1$
$\Sigma x = 2,373; \bar{x} = 139.6$	$\Sigma y = 1543.6; \bar{y} = 90.8$
$\Sigma x^2 = 345,857$	$\Sigma y^2 = 143,455.06$

$$r = \frac{\Sigma(x_i - \bar{x})(y_i - \bar{y})}{\sqrt{[\Sigma(x_i - \bar{x})^2][\Sigma(y_i - \bar{y})^2]}} = \frac{\Sigma(x_i y_i) - n\bar{x}\bar{y}}{\sqrt{[\Sigma(x_i^2 - n\bar{x}^2)][\Sigma(y_i^2 - n\bar{y}^2)]}}$$

$$= \frac{222,175.1 - (17 \times 139.6 \times 90.8)}{\sqrt{[(345,857 - (17 \times 139.6^2)][(143,455.06 - (17 \times 90.8^2)]}}$$

$$= \frac{6706.7}{6940.3} = 0.97$$

indicating moderate association. A value for r of 0 means that there is no linear association between the two variables.

An investigator may want to determine if the value of r observed in a sample can be attributed to sampling variation, i.e., is the value of the correlation coefficient in the population equal to 0? A test statistic for this purpose has been developed and is:

$$r\sqrt{\frac{(n-2)}{1-r^2}},$$

where r is the observed correlation coefficient and n is the number of pairs of the variables of interest. This statistic can then be compared to the entries in Table A–6, using $n-2$ degrees of freedom. For the example in Table A–9, the test statistic is 15.4, which is greater than the corresponding entry in Table A–6 for 15 degrees of freedom. This suggests that the difference between the observed correlation coefficient and zero (indicating no linear association) is not accounted for by sampling variation alone, i.e., the investigator must seek other explanations for this degree of correlation. One explanation is that tobacco use is involved in the etiology of lung cancer and that two decades is necessary for the disease to become clinically apparent.

Correlation is useful for analyzing associations, but it does not provide the investigator with a method to mathematically relate the value of one variable to the value of the other variable. To obtain such a mathematical relationship, the investigator must use regression analysis.

Regression

In *regression analysis,* the mathematical relationship between two variables is examined. One variable, designated x, is known as the *independent variable,* and the other one, designed y, is the *dependent variable.* Using the example of annual per capita tobacco consumption and lung cancer incidence twenty years later, the annual per capita tobacco consumption would be the independent variable and lung cancer incidence twenty years later would be the dependent one.

The relationship between x and y is known as a *model.* It is possible for the model to assume different mathematical forms. In this section, we will discuss the linear model, in which $y = ax + $ b; the investigator then must estimate a and b with the sample data. (Another regression model, the *logistic,* is discussed later in the Appendix, p. 324.) There are different statistical methods for estimating a and b. One of the most frequently used techniques is known as *least squares linear regression.* In this method, the distance between the observed value of y and the estimated value of y based upon the estimates of a and b is minimized.

In least squares linear regression, the estimate of a is

$$a = \frac{\Sigma(x_i - \bar{x})(y_i - \bar{y})}{\Sigma(x_i - \bar{x})^2} .$$

and for b, it is

$$b = \bar{y} - a\bar{x},$$

where $\bar{y}$ is the average of the observations of y and $\bar{x}$ is the mean of the observations of x. An example of the calculation of these two estimates is shown in Table A–10.

Although regression analysis and correlation are two distinct approaches to data analysis, there are certain relationships between the two areas. For example, the correlation coefficient and the least squares estimate of a in the linear model are related:

$$r = a \frac{s_x}{s_y},$$

where s_x is the standard deviation of the x observations and s_y is the standard deviation of the y observations. Accordingly, the statistical test described above

Table A–10. Example of the Calculation of Linear Regression Coefficients (a and b) Using Data from Table A–9

$n = 17 \; \Sigma x_i y_i = 222,175.1$

$\Sigma x = 2,373; \; \bar{x} = 139.6 \; \Sigma y = 1543.6; \; \bar{y} = 90.8$

$\Sigma x^2 = 345,857 \; \Sigma y^2 = 143,455.06$

$$a = \frac{\Sigma(x_i - \bar{x})(y_i - \bar{y})}{\Sigma(x_i - \bar{x})^2} = \frac{\Sigma(x_i y_i) - n\bar{x}\bar{y}}{\Sigma x_i^2 - n\bar{x}^2}$$

$$= \frac{222,175.1 - (17 \times 139.6 \times 90.8)}{345,857 - (17 \times 139.6^2)}$$

$$= \frac{6,706.7}{14,556.3} = 0.46$$

$b = \bar{y} - a\bar{x}$
$\quad = 90.8 - 0.46(139.6)$
$\quad = 90.8 - 64.2$
$\quad = 26.6$

Hence, the least squares linear regression model would be:
$y = 0.46x + 26.6.$

---

for assessing whether r is statistically significantly different from 0 (suggesting that no linear association exists between x and y) is equivalent to the statistical test that a is 0.

THE RELATIVE RISK, THE ODDS RATIO, AND THE ATTRIBUTABLE FRACTION: DERIVATION, STATISTICAL TESTS, VARIANCE, AND CONFIDENCE INTERVALS

Relative Risk

In Chapter 10, the method of calculating the relative risk as a measure of association in cohort studies was presented, and the estimation of the relative risk by the odds ratio in the analysis of data collected in case-control studies was noted in Chapter 11. The reasons for the use of the odds ratio as an approximation of the relative risk may be seen in the derivation of the formula for the relative risk. Using the relationship of cigarette smoking to lung cancer as an example:

Let P = Frequency of lung cancer in population
p_1 = Frequency of smokers among lung cancer patients
$(1 - p_1)$ = Frequency of nonsmokers among lung cancer patients
p_2 = Frequency of smokers among non-lung cancer cases (controls)
$(1 - p_2)$ = Frequency of nonsmokers among non-lung cancer cases (controls).

In a population, the lung cancer cases and controls are distributed by smoking habits according to Table A–11. Therefore:

$$\text{The lung cancer rate among smokers} = \frac{p_1 P}{p_1 P + p_2(1 - P)}$$

$$\text{The lung cancer rate among nonsmokers} = \frac{(1 - p_1)P}{(1 - p_1)P + (1 - p_2)(1 - P)}$$

Table A–11. Distribution of Lung Cancer Patients and Controls by Smoking Habits

	LUNG CANCER PATIENTS	CONTROLS	TOTAL
Smokers	$p_1 P$	$p_2(1 - P)$	$p_1 P + p_2(1 - P)$
Nonsmokers	$(1 - p_1)P$	$(1 - p_2)(1 - P)$	$(1 - p_1)P + (1 - p_2)(1 - P)$
Total	P	$(1 - P)$	1

The Relative Risk is

$$RR = \frac{\text{Lung cancer rate among smokers}}{\text{Lung cancer rate among nonsmokers}} = \frac{\dfrac{p_1 P}{p_1 P + p_2(1-P)}}{\dfrac{(1-p_1)P}{(1-p_1)P + (1-p_2)(1-P)}}$$

$$= \frac{p_1 P}{p_1 P + p_2(1-P)} \times \frac{(1-p_1)P + (1-p_2)(1-P)}{(1-p_1)P}$$

and, *if P is small,* this reduces to $\dfrac{p_1(1-p_2)}{p_2(1-p_1)}$, which is an estimate of the relative risk. In terms of the symbols used in Table 10–1, this expression is equivalent to ad/bc.

Test of Significance, Variance and Confidence Intervals

When the relative risk equals one, then ad/bc as an approximation of the relative risk (RR) is exact. This is the case when the risk of disease for those with and without the characteristic under study is the same (ad/bc = 1 or ad = bc); one can therefore say that the disease and the characteristic are unrelated.

A test of whether or not the observed difference between ad and bc is due to sampling variation is provided by the χ^2 test for fourfold tables:

$$\chi^2 = \frac{\left(|ad - bc| - \dfrac{N}{2}\right)^2 N}{N_1 N_2 M_1 M_2}$$

where $N = a + b + c + d$; $N_1 = a + c$; $N_2 = b + d$; $M_1 = a + b$; $M_2 = c + d$, as shown in Table 10–1, with one degree of freedom. The term N/2, which is subtracted from the difference, is the correction factor that is needed to make the test valid for small sample sizes. If the value of χ^2 is greater than 3.84, one may conclude that it is unlikely that the difference in risk between the group with and the group without the characteristic is a result of chance, at a probability level of 0.05.

A more useful method of testing the hypothesis of equal realtive risks, which at the same time provides an estimate of the confidence limits of the relative risk, is that recommended by Haldane (1956). Confidence limits of the logarithm (to the base e) of a corrected relative risk are computed and the logarithmic confidence intervals are then reconverted to the original scale. The addition of 0.50 to each of the values a, b, c, and d corrects for a bias that can occur with small numbers of observations.

Using the log-relative risk rather than the relative risk itself simplifies calculations of standard errors necessary for computing confidence intervals. If the reconverted confidence interval does not contain the value 1.0, the hypothesis that there is no difference in risk between the two groups (cases and controls) is rejected. The risk of falsely rejecting the hypothesis depends upon the level of confidence interval selected. If, for example, a 95 percent confidence interval is selected, there will be a 5 percent chance of falsely rejecting the hypothesis of equal relative risk. If the hypothesis is rejected, an interval within which the investigator is confident the "true" relative risk lies is then provided.

For an example of the above procedure, consider the data of Breslow et al. (1954) presented in Table A–12.

$$\text{The relative risk of lung cancer of smokers to nonsmokers} = \frac{ad}{bc} = \frac{(499)(56)}{(462)(19)} = 3.18.$$

The χ^2 test of equal risk is:

$$\chi^2 = \frac{\left(|ad - bc| - \dfrac{N}{2}\right)^2 N}{N_1 N_2 M_1 M_2}$$

$$= \frac{\left(|(499)(56) - (462)(19)| - \dfrac{1036}{2}\right)^2 1036}{(518)(518)(961)(75)} = 18.63$$

with one degree of freedom. The value of χ^2 is statistically significant at the 1 percent level, indicating that there is less than one chance in one hundred that such a relative risk could occur by chance alone if the two risks were equal.

While the χ^2 test shows that the risks are significantly different at the 1 percent level of significance, no indication is given of the limits within which the "true" relative risk might lie in the population from which these two sam-

Table A–12. Distribution of Smokers and Nonsmokers Among Lung Cancer Patients and Controls

	LUNG CANCER PATIENTS	CONTROLS	TOTALS
Smokers	a = 499	b = 462	M_1 = 961
Nonsmokers	c = 19	d = 56	M_2 = 75
Total	N_1 = 518	N_2 = 518	N = 1036

Source: Breslow et al. (1954).

ples have been selected. The first step is to calculate $\log_e$ (corrected relative risk):

$$\log_e \frac{(a + 0.50)(d + 0.50)}{(b + 0.50)(c + 0.50)} = \log_e \frac{(499.5)(56.5)}{(462.5)(19.5)}$$

$$= \log_e(3.129)$$
$$= 1.1408.$$

One should note that the correction of 0.50 added to each cell made little difference in the relative risk calculated in this example (3.13 versus 3.18). When the sample size is of the order of 50 rather than 500 in each of the disease groups, the correction will be more important.

The formula given by Haldane for the variance of the $\log_e$ (RR) is

$$\text{Var}(\log_e \text{ RR}) = \frac{1}{(a + \frac{1}{2})} + \frac{1}{(b + \frac{1}{2})} + \frac{1}{(c + \frac{1}{2})} + \frac{1}{(d + \frac{1}{2})}.$$

Using the data in Table A–12:

$$\text{Var}(\log_e \text{ RR}) = \frac{1}{499.5} + \frac{1}{462.5} + \frac{1}{19.5} + \frac{1}{56.5} = .073145.$$

The standard error is the square root of this quantity, 0.2705. A 95 percent confidence interval for the $\log_e$ of the corrected relative risk is calculated as

$$\log_e(\text{corrected RR}) \pm 1.96 \text{ S.E.}(\log_e \text{ RR}) = 1.1408 \pm 1.96(0.2705)$$
$$= 0.6101 \text{ to } 1.6705.$$

Upon reconverting to the original measurement scale by taking antilogs of the upper and lower limits, one finds that the 95 percent confidence interval for the relative risk is 1.8406 to 5.3148, which means that one is approximately 95 percent confident that the risk of developing lung cancer is between 1.84 and 5.31 times as great in smokers as in nonsmokers.

Additional statistical methods for the use of the relative risk in both retrospective and prospective studies may be found in Fleiss (1981), Schlesselman (1982), and Kahn and Sempos (1989).

Attributable Fraction

The calculation of attributable fraction was presented in Chapter 10. It was derived in the following manner by Levin (1953):

Let X = Incidence of a disease in those without the characteristic

RR = Relative risk

(RR)X = Incidence of disease in those with the characteristic

P = Proportion of total population with the characteristic

1 − P = Proportion of total population without the characteristic.

Then:

1. $P(RR)X + X(1 - P)$ = The incidence of disease in the total population and

2. $\dfrac{(RR)X - X}{(RR)X} = \dfrac{X(RR - 1)}{X(RR)} = \dfrac{RR - 1}{RR}$ = The proportion of disease attributable to the characteristic among those with the characteristic

3. $\dfrac{P(RR)X \left(\dfrac{RR - 1}{RR}\right)}{P(RR)X + X(1 - P)} = \dfrac{P(RR - 1)}{P(RR - 1) + 1}$ = The proportion of disease in the population that is attributable to the characteristic, that is, the attributable fraction (AF).

Walter (1975) has derived a formula from which the variance of the attributable fraction can be estimated from a retrospective study. Using the symbols of Table 10–1, the variance of $\log_e(1 - AF)$ is

$$\frac{a}{c(a + c)} + \frac{b}{d(b + d)} .$$

Walter showed that $\log_e(1 - AF)$ is normally distributed, and tests of significance and approximate confidence intervals can therefore be calculated using the normal distribution. Whittemore (1983) extended this work to include situations in which confounding is present.

CONTROLLING EXTRANEOUS FACTORS

We have been assuming that the groups being compared were homogeneous with respect to all characteristics other than the specific ones for which the strength of association was being measured. Thus, when measuring the association between stroke and elevated blood pressure, we assumed that the individuals with stroke and those without the disease were similar in all respects (age, gender, socioeconomic status) except for the factor being studied, namely, their blood pressure levels.

If the samples of diseased and nondiseased persons are randomly selected from the populations of diseased or nondiseased persons, they may be similar with regard to the distribution of some extraneous factors if the populations from which they were derived are similar with respect to these factors. However, any population differences would be reflected in these samples. If, for example, lung cancer patients differ in age and gender from the population from which the controls are selected, the samples will also differ in these characteristics. To avoid biases that can arise from such differences, various methods of selection or analysis are available to the investigator. The adjustment procedure described in Chapter 4 is useful when comparing incidence or mortality rates as well as other sets of data.

It is also possible to make a series of specific comparisons for each level of the extraneous factor; for example, age- and sex specific comparisons of the frequency of stroke in persons with normal blood pressure and persons with elevated blood pressure. One disadvantage with factor-specific comparisons is that they separate the total sample into many segments, and some of these may contain too few observations (or none at all) to make a factor-specific comparison within these segments. Even when a particular segment contains both cases and controls, there may be a large number of cases but only a small number of controls, or vice versa. Generally speaking, the precision of the comparison varies with the factor,

$$\frac{1}{\sqrt{\dfrac{1}{n_1} + \dfrac{1}{n_2}}}$$

where n_1 is the number of cases in a particular segment and n_2 is the number of controls. For a fixed total $n = n_1 + n_2$, the precision will be greater when $n_1 = n_2$. If n_1 happens to be small, an increase in the size of n_2 will not necessarily compensate for this. If a random sample is drawn from both the case and control populations, the factor-specific comparisons will vary in their degrees of precision and the comparisons that have the lowest precision may be in those segments where the greatest interest lies.

Group Matching

One means of assuring equal numbers of disease and control samples for each factor level is to ''group match'' the samples by stratification of one of the groups, using each factor level as a stratum. Usually the cases are self-selected in terms of the disease, with the investigator having no control over the number of cases at each factor level. The investigator then attempts to select controls that have the same characteristics as the cases. If the characteristics of the cases are known in advance, the best method of group matching is to stratify the control population on the levels of the factor to be controlled. Simple random samples of the same size as found in the disease sample at each factor level are then selected independently from the corresponding stratum of the population controls.

If the comparisons are to be made on a factor-specific basis, the percentage with and without the characteristic can be compared at each factor level by the simple binomial test described earlier. However, a useful method of combining the comparisons for each factor level has been developed by Cochran (1954) and modified by Mantel and Haenszel (1959). It takes into account the variation in the number of observations in both cases and controls at each factor level and the variation in the proportion of individuals (cases and controls combined) having the characteristic of interest at each level. The method and its limitations are reviewed by Snedecor and Cochran (1967), Fleiss (1981), Kahn and Sempos (1989), and Schlesselman (1982).

For the ith factor level, let

n_{i1}, n_{i2} = sample sizes of cases and controls, respectively
p_{i1}, p_{i2} = observed proportion with the characteristics of interest in the two groups

$$\hat{p}_i = \text{combined proportion} = \frac{n_{i1}p_{i1} + n_{i2}p_{i2}}{n_{i1} + n_{i2}}$$

$$\hat{q}_i = 1 - \hat{p}_i$$

$$d_i = p_{i1} - p_{i2} = \text{observed difference in proportions}$$

$$w_i = \frac{n_{i1}n_{i2}}{n_{i1} + n_{i2}} \; ; w = \Sigma w_i.$$

The weighted mean difference is first computed:

$$\bar{d} = \frac{\Sigma w_i d_i}{w}$$

which has a standard error of

$$\text{S.E.} = \frac{\sqrt{\Sigma w_i \hat{p}_i \hat{q}_i}}{w}.$$

As in the binomial test, the criterion for testing the hypothesis of no difference in proportions is:

$$\frac{\bar{d}}{\text{S.E.}} = \frac{\Sigma w_i d_i}{\sqrt{\Sigma w_i \hat{p}_i \hat{q}_i}}.$$

(This is referred to in the tables of normal distribution.) If it is greater than 1.96, it is concluded that the overall difference is statistically significant at a probability of 5 percent.

An example of the computations is presented in Tables A–13 and A–14. These are derived from a study of the possible relationship between prenatal and perinatal factors and childhood behavior disorders by Rogers et al. (1959). The cases were those children referred by their teachers as behavior problems and the controls were those not so referred. A factor of interest was the history of previous infant loss prior to the birth of the study children as reported on the birth certificates of the study children among the mothers of case and control children. Since this is influenced by the birth order of the child, and its distribution may vary in the cases and controls, it was necessary to take the birth order into account in comparing the cases and controls. The criterion for the significance test in the

Table A–13. Number and Percent of Mothers with History of Previous Infant Loss among Cases and Controls by Birth Order (Birth Certificate Data)

| BIRTH ORDER | CHILDREN'S STATUS | NO. OF MOTHERS WITH HISTORY OF | | TOTAL | PERCENT WITH HISTORY OF LOSS |
		LOSSES	NO LOSSES		
2	Cases	14	86	$100 = n_{11}$	$14.0 = p_{11}$
	Controls	7	67	$74 = n_{12}$	$9.5 = p_{21}$
	Total	21	153	$174 = n_1$	$12.1 = p_1$
3–4	Cases	22	44	$66 = n_{21}$	$33.3 = p_{21}$
	Controls	7	35	$42 = n_{22}$	$16.7 = p_{22}$
	Total	29	79	$108 = n_2$	$26.9 = p_2$
5+	Cases	22	14	$36 = n_{31}$	$61.1 = p_{31}$
	Controls	10	7	$17 = n_{32}$	$58.8 = p_{32}$
	Total	32	21	$53 = n_3$	$60.3 = p_3$

Source: Rogers et al. (1959).

Table A–14.   Computations for the Combined Test

BIRTH ORDER	d_i	p_i	$p_i q_i$	w_i^*	$w_i d_i$	$w_i p_i q_i$
2	+ 4.5	12.1	1,063.6	42.5	+191.3	45,203.0
3–4	+16.6	26.9	1,996.4	25.7	+426.6	51,307.5
5+	+ 2.3	60.3	2,393.5	11.6	+ 26.68	27,769.2

$$*w_i = \frac{n_{i1} n_{i2}}{n_{i1} + n_{i2}}$$

$\Sigma w_i d_i = 644.6$

$\Sigma w_i p_i q_i = 124{,}279.7$

$$\text{Test Criterion} = \frac{\Sigma w_i d_i}{\sqrt{\Sigma w_i \hat{p}_i \hat{q}_i}} = \frac{644.6}{\sqrt{124{,}279.7}} = 1.83$$

example is 1.83, which is referred to the table of the normal distribution. This indicates a P value of 0.07, which is slightly higher than the usually accepted value of 0.05 for statistical significance. However, one can regard the difference as having borderline significance.

Relative risks can also be calculated for group matching with the method developed by Mantel and Haenszel (1959), and for this reason, the statistical test is generally referred to as the "Mantel-Haenszel test." This and other methods are more fully discussed in Fleiss (1981), Kahn and Sempos (1989), and Schlesselman (1982).

Logistic Regression

Another approach to the calculation of a relative risk adjusted for the effect of extraneous factors uses *logistic regression.* In this technique, a logistic model is fitted by statistical regression to the sample data. For one variable x, the logistic model is

$$\text{Pr(disease)} = \frac{1}{1 + e^{-(a+bx_i)}},$$

where Pr(disease) is the probability of the disease in the ith individual, and the value of variable x in that individual is x_i. The values of a and b are estimated from the sample data. If the relative risk associated with exposure to x is one, then the value of b will be zero; conversely, if the value of b is greater than zero, then the relative risk for x will be greater than one; for negative values of b, the corresponding relative risk is less than one. For further information on logistic regression, see Kahn and Sempos (1989), Schlesselman (1982), and Breslow and Day (1983, 1987).

Individual Case-Control Matching

As an alternative to group matching, individual cases and controls can be matched for various factors so that each case in the study has its own pairmate. Ideally, pairmates should be as much alike as possible in all characteristics except the one being studied. If many factors are selected for matching, it becomes difficult to find matches for each of the cases. In epidemiologic studies there is usually a limited number of cases and a large number of controls. Each case is then classified according to the factor to be controlled, and a search is made for a control with the same characteristics. If the number of factors and their levels are not too great and there is a large enough number of controls from which to select, matching may be carried out with little effort. Matching becomes difficult and time-consuming if a large number of factors and levels are considered and the number of potential controls is of a magnitude similar to the number of cases. It is likely that there will be many cases for which no control can be found. Therefore, it becomes necessary either to eliminate some of the factors or to reduce the number of levels of some factors. If age is a factor, for example, it is unlikely that pairs can be formed readily using six-month or one-year age intervals; but with five- or ten-year age intervals, matching becomes feasible.

While matching is probably desired to reduce biases, the number of factors or levels on which it is practical is rather small. There should be good reasons for including a factor as a matching variable in any study. Matching should usually be limited to a small number of factors, rarely more than four, each consisting of a small number of levels or categories (Ury, 1975).

In addition to eliminating bias, matching also increases the precision of the comparisons by providing more homogeneous groups within which the comparisons are made. The increased precision is largely dependent on the degree of association of the matching factor with the variable of interest. Rather strong associations must exist before substantial increases in precision can be expected. Therefore, the major aim of matching in case-control studies should be to provide comparisons that are relatively free from bias that might arise from the dissimilarities of the case and control populations.

When cases and controls are individually matched, the fourfold table assumes the form presented in Table 11–12. For matched pairs where RR = s/t (Kraus, 1958), (using the symbols in Table 11–12), Fleiss (1981) shows that the estimated variance $= (1 + RR)^2 \left(\dfrac{RR}{s + t}\right)$ and the estimated standard error $=$

$(1 + RR) \sqrt{\dfrac{RR}{(s + t)}}$.

A useful test of significance for matched pairs, when s and t are not small (>3), is the McNemar test:

$$\chi^2 = \frac{(|t - s| - 1)^2}{t + s} ,$$

with one degree of freedom.

In this section we have dealt only with factors that are qualitative and dichotomous. The reader is referred to Fleiss (1981) for a more detailed discussion of these issues, including the use of multiple controls in such studies. When the study characteristics are quantitative, other methods of controlling for extraneous factors are available. Extraneous effects often can be eliminated more efficiently in the analysis of the data by the method of analysis of covariance. This allows the investigator to select simple random samples of case and control groups without first matching pairs for the factors to be controlled. The reader is referred to Snedecor and Cochran (1967) for details of this technique.

LIFE TABLES AND SURVIVORSHIP ANALYSIS

In the previous sections, we discussed analyses of epidemiologic study data in which the time until the occurrence of the event of interest was not a focus of the investigation. However, the time to occurrence of an outcome (whether mortality or a form of morbidity) is often of interest. The statistical analysis of these time periods and their relationship to various factors is known as *survivorship analysis.* The techniques used in survivorship analysis derive from the *life table.*

The Life Table

The life table provides a simple, systematic way of organizing and analyzing survivorship data. Suppose that an investigator has identified 500 Parkinson's disease patients who have started to use a new treatment that stabilizes their condition and wishes to know the probability of these patients having no progression of their disease. Each year, the investigator evaluates each patient to determine if the condition has progressed. The hypothetical data collected after five years of follow-up for each patient are given in Table A–15.

Table A–15. Example of a Life Table for 500 Persons Using a New Therapy for Parkinson's Disease

YEAR (x)	NUMBER OF PERSONS WITH STABLE DISEASE STATUS AT START OF YEAR (Q_x)	NUMBER OF PERSONS WHOSE DISEASE STATUS DECLINED DURING YEAR ($_nd_x$)	PROBABILITY OF DISEASE STATUS DECLINING ($_nq_x$)	PROBABILITY OF DISEASE STATUS REMAINING STABLE ($_np_x$)
1	500	100	0.22	0.78
2	400	100	0.29	0.71
3	300	150	0.67	0.33
4	150	90	0.86	0.14
5	60	38	0.93	0.07

There are two measures of interest for the investigator: the probability of progression in a given year and the probability of an individual's disease remaining stable throughout the five years of follow-up. The probability of declining disease status can be estimated for each year of follow-up using the data in Table A–15. For the time period from x to $x + n$, this probability ($_nq_x$) is equal to,

$$\frac{\text{the number of persons whose disease status declined during the year}}{\text{the mid-year number of persons at risk of declining disease status}}$$

or

$$_nq_x = \frac{_nd_x}{O_x - (_nd_x/2)},$$

where O_x is the number of persons who began the xth year with stable disease status and $_nd_x$ is the number of those persons who began the xth year with stable disease status but whose disease status declined by the end of the $(n + x)$th year. This estimate assumes that the number of persons whose disease status declines is equal in both the first half of the year and in the latter half; if this assumption is incorrect, the number used to divide $_nd_x$ in the denominator would need to be adjusted accordingly.

A second estimate shown in Table A–15, $_np_x$, is the probability of an individual finishing the $(n + x)$th year with stable disease status given that the individual's disease status was stable at the start of the year. The probability of an individual completing the five years with stable disease status can be estimated by multiplying the $_np_x$ for each of the years, i.e.,

$$(0.78)(0.71)(0.33)(0.14)(0.07) = 0.0016.$$

Hence, the probability of completing all five years with stable disease status is 0.00106, or about 1.5 in 1,000 persons using the new therapy for five years.

Further information on life tables and their calculation, including the standard error of the various probabilities estimated in them, may be found in Chiang (1968) and Kahn and Sempos (1989).

The Logrank Test

The logrank test was suggested by Mantel (1966) as a method for comparing two groups with regard to the time until the occurrence of the outcome of interest. In the logrank test, these times are ranked and the ranks are compared using a χ^2 test. For computational details of the logrank test, the reader is referred to Peto et al. (1977) or Kahn and Sempos (1989).

AGE-ADJUSTED MORTALITY RATES: VARIANCE AND STANDARD ERRORS

The direct method of age adjustment of death rates and the standardized mortality ratio (SMR) were described in Chapter 4. It is often useful to calculate the variance and standard error of these rates, and therefore the formulas for these statistics will be presented. For a more detailed discussion, the reader may consult Kahn and Sempos (1989) and Fleiss (1981).

Age Adjustment by the Direct Method

Let r = the age specific death rate in the ith age group
N_i = the number of people in the ith age group of the standard population
n_i = the number of people in the ith age group of the population that is being age-adjusted

The age-adjusted death rate is then $R = \Sigma \left(\dfrac{N_i}{\Sigma N_i} \right) r_i$, the

$$\text{Variance of } R = \Sigma \left(\frac{N_i}{\Sigma N_i}\right)^2 \frac{r_i(1 - r_i)}{n_i} \text{ and the}$$

$$\text{Standard Error } = \sqrt{\Sigma \left(\frac{N_i}{\Sigma N_i}\right)^2 \frac{r_i(1 - r_i)}{n_i}}.$$

Standardized Mortality Ratio (SMR)

The SMR $= \dfrac{\text{O (Observed number of deaths per year)}}{\text{E (Expected number of deaths per year)}} \times 100$, and is usually expressed as a percentage.

Assuming that the standard population from which the expected numbers are calculated is much larger than the population being studied, and that the age-specific death rates in the standard population are small, which is usually the case, the variance of SMR (or O/E) is approximately O/E^2, and the standard error $= \sqrt{O}/E$.

KAPPA AND THE ASSESSMENT OF INTER- AND INTRA-OBSERVER VARIABILITY

The use of the κ (kappa) statistic for an assessment of inter- and intra-observer variability was presented in Chapter 6 (p. 124). Two situations may occur: an individual classifies a set of data twice and the disagreements in classification are analyzed, or two individuals classify the same data and their disagreements are analyzed. In either case, the analysis of the data is the same. κ, developed by Cohen (1960), adjusts for agreement in classification that would occur by chance. Formally stated,

$$\kappa = \frac{\text{Observed frequency of agreement} - \text{Expected frequency of agreement}}{\text{Total observed} - \text{Expected frequency of agreement}}.$$

If there is only chance agreement between two classifications, then the value of κ is zero. If there is perfect agreement, then the value of κ is one. It is possible to use κ for situations involving many different classification categories. In this example, however, we will restrict our consideration to the case of two classification categories.

An example of the calculation of κ may provide insight into its use. The data in Table A–16 from Paganini-Hill and Ross (1982) were cited by Kelsey et al. (1986) in such a description. These data compare a patient's recall of reserpine use with the history of use on the patient's medical chart. The expected frequency

Table A–16.   Example of the Calculation of Kappa: Agreement Between Personal
Interview and Medical Chart Concerning Use of Reserpine Among Control Subjects
from a Case-Control Study of Breast Cancer in Two Retirement Communities

| | | HISTORY OF USE OF RESERPINE ACCORDING TO MEDICAL CHART | | |
		YES	NO	TOTAL
History of use of reserpine	Yes	14	7	21
according to patient's report	No	25	171	196
Total		39	178	217

Source: Paganini-Hill and Ross (1982).

of agreement between the patient's recall of reserpine use and that which was
indicated on the medical chart is the expected frequency of both indicating such
use ((21)(39)/217) and the expected frequency of both indicating no such use
((196)(178)/217), i.e., 164.5. The observed frequency of agreement is 14 + 171,
i.e., 185. Hence,

$$\kappa = \frac{\text{Observed frequency of agreement} - \text{Expected frequency of agreement}}{\text{Total observed} - \text{Expected frequency of agreement}}$$

$$= \frac{185 - 164.5}{217 - 164.5} = \frac{20.5}{52.5} = 0.39.$$

This result suggests that there is only fair agreement between the two sources of
information about a patient's past use of reserpine.

For further information about κ, the reader is referred to Fleiss (1981) and
Kelsey et al. (1986).

REFERENCES

Breslow, L., Hoaglin, L., Rasmussen, G., and Abrams, H. K. 1954. "Occupations and
cigarette smoking as factors in lung cancer." *Amer. J. Public Health* 44:171–181.
Breslow, N. E., and Day, N. E. 1983. *Statistical Methods in Cancer Research, Vol. 1. The
Design and Analysis of Case-Control Studies.* Lyon: International Agency for
Research on Cancer.
———. 1987. *Statistical Methods in Cancer Research, Vol. 2. The Design and Analysis
of Cohort Studies.* Lyon: International Agency for Research on Cancer.

Chiang, C. L. 1968. *Introduction to Stochastic Processes in Biostatistics,* New York: John Wiley and Sons.

Cochran, W. G. 1954. "Some methods of strengthening the common χ^2 tests." *Biometrics* 10:417–451.

———. 1977. *Sampling Techniques.* 3rd ed. New York: John Wiley and Sons.

Cohen, J. 1960. "A coefficient of agreement for nominal scales." *Educ. Psych. Meas.* 20: 37–46.

Colton, T. 1974. *Statistics in Medicine.* Boston: Little, Brown and Company.

Fleiss, J. L. 1981. *Statistical Methods for Rates and Proportions,* 2nd ed. New York: J. Wiley and Sons.

Greenberg, E. R. 1990. "Random digit dialing for control selection. A review and a caution on its use in studies of childhood cancer." *Am. J. Epidemiol.* 131:1–5.

Haenszel, W., Loveland, D., and Sirken, M. G. 1962. "Lung-cancer mortality as related to residence and smoking histories." *J. Natl. Cancer Instit.* 28:947–1001.

Haldane, J.B.S. 1956. "The estimation and significance of the logarithm of a ratio of frequencies." *Ann. Hum. Genet.* 2:309–311.

Hartge, P., Brinton, L. A., Rosenthal, J. F., Cahill, J. I., Hoover, R. N., and Waksberg, J. 1984. "Random digit dialing in selecting a population-based control group." *Am. J. Epidemiol.* 120:825–833.

Hill, A. B. 1977. *A Short Textbook of Medical Statistics.* 10th ed. Philadelphia: J. B. Lippincott.

Kahn, H. A., and Sempos, C. T. 1989. *Statistical Methods in Epidemiology.* NewYork: Oxford University Press.

Kelsey, J. L., Thompson, W. D., and Evans, A. S. 1986. *Methods in Observational Epidemiology.* New York: Oxford University Press.

Kendall, M. G. and Smith, B. B. 1938. "Randomness and random sampling numbers." *J. Roy. Stat. Soc.* 101:147–166.

Kraus, A. S. 1958. "The use of family members as controls in the study of the possible etiologic factors of a disease." Sc.D. Thesis. Graduate School of Public Health, University of Pittsburgh.

Levin, M. L. 1953. "The occurrence of lung cancer in man." *Acta Unio. Internat. Contra Cancrum* 9:531–541.

Mantel, N. 1966. "Evaluation of survival data and two new rank order statistics arising in its consideration." *Cancer Chemother. Reports* 60:163–170.

Mantel, N., and Haenszel, W. 1959. "Statistical aspects of the analysis of data from retrospective studies of disease." *J. Natl. Cancer Inst.* 22:719–748.

Paganini-Hill, A., and Ross, R. K. 1982. "Reliability of recall of drug usage and other health-related information." *Am. J. Epidemiol.* 116:114–122.

Peto, R., Pike, M. C., Armitage, P., Breslow, N. E., Cox, D. R., Howard, S. V., Mantel, N., McPherson, K., Peto, J., and Smith, P. G. 1977. "Design and analysis of randomized clinical trials requiring prolonged observation of each patient: II. Analysis and examples." *Brit. J. Cancer* 35:1–39.

Rand Corporation. 1955. *A Million Random Digits.* Glencoe, Ill.: Free Press.

Rogers, M. E., Lilienfeld, A. M., and Pasamanick, B. 1959. *Prenatal and Paranatal Factors in the Development of Childhood Behavior Disorders.* Baltimore, Md.: The Johns Hopkins University School of Hygiene and Public Health.

Schlesselman, J. J. 1982. *Case-Control Studies.* New York: Oxford University Press.

Snedecor, G. W., and Cochran, W. G. 1967. *Statistical Methods.* 6th ed. Ames, Iowa: Iowa State University Press.

Ury, H. K. 1975. "Efficiency of case-control studies with multiple controls per case: continuous or dichotomous data." *Biometrics* 31:643–649.

Wacholder, A., McLaughlin, J. K., Silverman, D. T., and Mandel, J. S. 1992. "Selection of controls in case-control studies. II. types of controls." *Am. J. Epidemiol.* 135: 1029–1041.

Waksberg, J. 1978. "Sampling methods for random digit dialing." *J. Am. Stat. Assn.* 73: 40–46.

Walter, S. D. 1975. "The distribution of Levin's measure of attributable risk." *Biometrika* 62:371–374.

Whittemore, A. S. 1983. "Estimating attributable risk from case-control studies." *Am. J. Epidemiol.* 117:76–85.

ANSWERS TO PROBLEMS

Chapter 1

1. The epidemiologist views disease from the perspective of its occurrence among persons, in places, and at varying times. Essentially, it is the intersection of time, place, and persons that defines the development of disease in a given population.

2. An ecological fallacy may be operating when an association between a characteristic and a disease is based on the study of group characteristics rather than of characteristics among individuals in the group. For example, an investigation into the relationship between religion and suicide might find that regions of Europe in which Protestants are more prevalent than Catholics have higher suicide rates compared with rates in those areas in which Catholics are more prevalent. The conclusion that Protestantism is associated with suicide would be an ecological fallacy if, in an epidemiologic study, the risk of suicide among Catholics was the same as or higher than that for Protestants.

3. Population-based data, such as mortality rates, provide an initial means by which the epidemiologist can compare populations. Such comparisons seek to develop hypotheses for the pattern of diseases observed among the populations. Caution is needed in using such data since the possibility of an ecological fallacy exists.

4. The major steps in the investigation of a food-borne outbreak are:
   (a) to identify the disease being investigated,
   (b) to define what a case is,

(c) to ascertain cases,

(d) to determine a common event among cases,

(e) to define the population present at the common event,

(f) to develop a questionnaire to assess consumption of food items at the common event,

(g) to administer the questionnaire to all those present at the common event,

(h) to calculate food-specific attack rates to determine which food item was contaminated,

(i) to investigate the preparation of the contaminated food item, including medical examinations of all food handlers involved in such preparation,

(j) to take appropriate public health action to stop the possibility of such outbreaks in the future (e.g., slaughtering of infected flocks producing contaminated eggs).

5. (a)

TYPE OF FOOD	CONSUMED FOOD			DID NOT CONSUME FOOD		
	NUMBER OF INDIVIDUALS	NUMBER III	ATTACK RATE (%)	NUMBER OF INDIVIDUALS	NUMBER III	ATTACK RATE (%)
Tomato Juice	204	47	23	263	21	8
Cantaloupe	290	53	18	177	15	3
Chipped beef with sauce	147	60	41	320	8	3
Potatoes	161	44	27	306	24	8
Eggs	169	39	23	298	29	10
Pastry	204	34	17	263	34	13
Toast	238	46	19	229	22	10
Milk	301	50	17	166	8	1

(b) The chipped beef is the likely culprit since it produced the highest attack rate of all consumed foods (41%). Those who did not consume the chipped beef had a low attack rate (3%).

(c) Additional investigations that could be conducted to determine the source and the likely microorganism include:

1. Using microbiological laboratory methods to culture a pathogen from leftover food.

2. Attempting to isolate and culture pathogens from the stools of victims.

3. Examining food handlers in search of skin lesions that may lead to food contamination, including bacterial culture studies of stools of food handlers. In this epidemic, the disease was caused

by enterotoxin-producing staphylococcal organisms that were found in the food, in the stools of victims, and in a skin lesion ("boil") on the thumb of the cook. The salty and fatty sauce provided a good growth medium for this microorganism.

(d) Proper storage (refrigeration) and cooking (heating) of food has proven more effective than physical examination of food handlers in preventing food-borne disease outbreaks due to bacterial contamination.

Chapter 3

1. The latency period for noninfectious diseases is the time between exposure to a disease-causing agent and the appearance of manifestations of the disease. It varies with the specific disease. In some instances in which the time of exposure to the disease-causing agent is known, the latency period for disorders has been quantified. For example, the latency period for leukemias following the radiation exposure from the explosion of the atomic bomb at Hiroshima is five to six years, while that for female breast cancer from the same exposure is about twenty years.

2. (a) In a common-vehicle, single-exposure outbreak, the epidemic curve is skewed to the right, with a sharp initial rise and a gradual tapering, as in Figure 3–4. (b) In a common-vehicle, continuous-exposure outbreak, the epidemic curve also shows a sharp initial rise with a gradual tapering, but the curve does not taper as fast as the single-exposure curve would and it does not decrease to zero cases. Rather, it becomes a series of peaks and troughs as new cases occur. (c) The curve for an outbreak propagated by serial transfer is a flat line with occasional bumps in the curve as exposures and subsequent cases occur. (d) In an epidemic due to a slow virus, the epidemic curve will be the same as for a common-vehicle, continuous-exposure epidemic, which is, after all, what it is.

3. Herd immunity is important to the public health administrator because it implies that in order to contain or prevent an outbreak of disease, immunization of the entire population is not mandated. Only as large a proportion as required for herd immunity to develop in the population need be immunized to prevent an outbreak of disease.

4. Subclinical cases of both infectious and noninfectious diseases pose several problems for the epidemiologist: (a) the identification of all factors relating to the occurrence of the disease will be limited to those that characterize the clinical cases; (b) the testing of a biological hypothesis will be limited to the clinical cases; and (c) the characteristics of the subclinical cases (particularly those which prevent the clinical manifestation of the disease) cannot be elucidated.

The applicability of these problems to both infectious and noninfectious diseases should underscore the importance of the "spectrum of disease" concept in any epidemiologic investigation. The major impact of subclinical cases concerns the prognosis of a given clinical case. It is only with information about the "spectrum of disease," including both clinical and subclinical cases, that an accurate assessment of prognosis can be made.

5. This observation suggests that the etiologic event was either prenatal or perinatal. It suggests that studies focused on prenatal or perinatal factors would be useful in determining the etiologic agent of Legg-Perthes disease.

6. The sexually transmitted disease epidemic in the United States today is a combination of epidemiologic categories of outbreaks. If a single instance of infection is not treated, it will serve as a continuous source of the agent. Since that individual infection can also serve as a common exposure for others, it would also be a common vehicle.

7. (a)   **NUMBER OF ILL PERSONS**

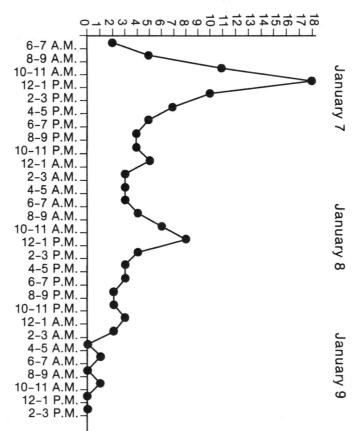

(b) This was a common-vehicle, single-exposure outbreak. Secondary cases occurred as a result of serial transfer from the primary case. The epidemic curve for the secondary cases can be seen as being imposed on that of the primary cases around noon, January 8.

(c) The bimodality is the result of the occurrence of both primary and secondary cases.

(d) The health officer should define the disease that is being investigated. After he or she has defined the disease, the common exposure of the primary cases can be determined. This part of the investigation would be similar to that described in Chapter 1 (pp. 13–18). The health officer should then determine if the secondary cases were the result of serial transfer from the primary ones.

8. The correlations found by Rose suggest that the latency period of coronary heart disease is at least 10 years. Similar correlations should be sought in other population groups.

Chapter 4

1. The numerators are the number of deaths from all accidents occurring in those 5–44 years old in the United States, Alaska, and Florida in 1987. The denominators are the numbers of those 5–44 years old living in the United States, Alaska, and Florida in 1987. The death rates for accidents among those 5–44 years old are:

$$\text{United States} = \frac{50,377}{150,020,000} \times 100,000 = 33.6 \text{ per } 100,000 \text{ per year}$$

$$\text{Alaska} = \frac{242}{368,000} \times 100,000 = 65.8 \text{ per } 100,000 \text{ per year}$$

$$\text{Florida} = \frac{2,584}{6,543,000} \times 100,000 = 39.5 \text{ per } 100,000 \text{ per year}$$

2. The numerators are the number of deaths from all malignant neoplasms occurring in those 65 and over in the United States, Alaska, and Florida in 1987. The denominators are the numbers of people 65 and older living in the United States, Alaska, and Florida in 1987. The death rates for malignant neoplasms among those 65 and older are:

$$\text{United States} = \frac{242,617}{29,840,000} = 100,000 = 813.1 \text{ per } 100,000 \text{ per year}$$

$$\text{Alaska} = \frac{210}{19,000} \times 100,000 = 1105.3 \text{ per } 100,000 \text{ per year}$$

$$\text{Florida} = \frac{21,599}{2,140,000} \times 100,000 = 1009.3 \text{ per } 100,000 \text{ per year}$$

3. The numerators are the total deaths from malignant neoplasms and from accidents in the United States, Alaska, and Florida in 1987. The denominators are the total populations of the United States, Alaska, and Florida in 1987. The overall death rates from malignant neoplasms are:

$$\text{United States} = \frac{363,656}{243,400,000} \times 100,000$$
$$= 149.4 \text{ per } 100,000 \text{ per year}$$

$$\text{Alaska} = \frac{442}{525,000} \times 100,000 = 84.2 \text{ per } 100,000 \text{ per year}$$

$$\text{Florida} = \frac{30,164}{12,023,000} \times 100,000 = 250.9 \text{ per } 100,000 \text{ per year}$$

The overall death rates from all accidents are:

$$\text{United States} = \frac{94,893}{243,400,000} \times 100,000 = 39.0 \text{ per } 100,000 \text{ per year}$$

$$\text{Alaska} = \frac{320}{525,000} \times 100,000 = 61.0 \text{ per } 100,000 \text{ per year}$$

$$\text{Florida} = \frac{5,120}{12,023,000} \times 100,000 = 42.6 \text{ per } 100,000 \text{ per year}$$

4. The expected number of deaths from malignant neoplasms for Alaska and Florida's age distribution are calculated by multiplying the age-specific death rates for each state by the U.S. population in each age group. The expected number of deaths are divided by the total U.S. population (check table in problem 3 to see what the death rate would be if the U.S. had the age structure of Alaska or Florida.

AGE GROUP	EXPECTED NUMBER OF DEATHS	
	ALASKA	FLORIDA
<5	0	548
5–44	24,753	21,153
45–64	124,912	97,628
65+	301,175	329,822
Total	450,840	449,151

$$\text{Mortality rate for Alaska} = \frac{450,840}{243,400,000} \times 100,000$$
$$= 185.2 \text{ deaths per } 100,000$$

$$\text{Mortality rate for Florida} = \frac{449,151}{243,400,000} \times 100,000$$
$$= 184.5 \text{ deaths per } 100,000$$

5. In the indirect method (SMR) the expected number of deaths from accidents for Alaska and Florida is calculated by multiplying the U.S. age- and cause-specific death rates by the populations in each age group for Alaska and Florida. The expected number of deaths is divided by the actual number of deaths and multiplied by 100 to produce the standardized mortality ratio.

AGE GROUP	EXPECTED NUMBER OF DEATHS	
	ALASKA	FLORIDA
<5	13	172
5–44	124	2,198
45–64	27	885
65+	16	1,853
Total	180	5,108
Total observed number of deaths (from table in problem 1)	320	5,120

$$\text{SMR Alaska} = \frac{180}{320} \times 100 = 56.3$$

$$\text{SMR Florida} = \frac{5,108}{5,120} \times 100 = 99.8$$

6. The crude rates show Florida's death rate from malignancies to be three times higher than Alaska's, but age adjustment shows the rates to be more similar (185.2 and 184.5 for Alaska and Florida, respectively).
7. The crude rates show Florida as having a lower rate of deaths from accidents than Alaska. The age-adjusted rates show Alaska's death rate from accidents to be lower than Florida's.
8. Age adjustment is especially useful in these examples because we are comparing two populations with different age structures, because the two populations are of different sizes, and because the diseases are associated with age (death from accidents occurs most frequently in younger people, deaths from malignancies occur mostly in older people).

Chapter 5

1. These are some of the possible explanations of why motor vehicle deaths vary with the day of the week:
   (a) The variation is a result of chance and has no other meaning.
   (b) People do more driving on Fridays, Saturdays, or Sundays.
   (c) Different people (worse drivers) drive on Fridays, Saturdays, or Sundays.
   (d) People are more likely to drink and drive on weekends.
   (e) Hospital care is worse on the weekend and accident victims are more likely to die.
   (f) Day of death is not filled out correctly for accident deaths.
2. (a) Some hypotheses to explain high HIV death rates are:
   - Urban areas are associated with behaviors such as intravenous drug use and needle sharing or unprotected sex with multiple partners that can lead to HIV infection.
   - Urban areas have hospitals that will care for dying HIV patients.
   - Washington, D.C., New Jersey, New York, California, and Florida all have large proportions of age groups that are more likely to engage in behaviors leading to death from HIV.
   - The disease spreads from the two coasts to the rest of the country.
   Some hypotheses to explain low HIV death rates are:
   - Deaths from HIV in South Dakota, North Dakota, Montana, Wyoming, Idaho, and Iowa are coded under another cause.
   - Westerners are resistant to HIV.
   - Persons in the West who are diagnosed with HIV move to another

part of the country to receive care and die where they receive treatment.

- Residents of these states do not engage in behaviors that lead to HIV infection.

  (b) Washington, D.C., is a city, entirely urban, but New York is a state and mixes urban and rural populations, areas with a high and low HIV mortality. A comparison of Washington, D.C., to New York City would probably show more similar rates. Data for Washington, D.C., are summarized separately from other states for political rather than scientific reasons. From an epidemiologic point of view it would be preferable to compare similar geographic units.

3. (a) The trend is steadily downwards over 70 years. The decline in mortality is dramatic; in 1987 it is less than one-tenth of what it was in 1915–1919 for whites, and slightly above one-tenth for blacks. The decline occurred in both whites and blacks.

  (b) Improved birth registration would increase the denominator (live births) and decrease the infant mortality rate.

  (c) Improved death registration would increase the numerator (deaths for infants under 1 year of age) and increase the infant mortality rate.

4. The elimination of many infectious diseases through improved sanitation, sterile techniques, vaccinations, and antibiotics could explain the decline in infant mortality between 1915 and 1960.

5. Between 1960 and 1987 hospital-based technology reduced the mortality for many high-risk infants including those born at low or very low birth weight and those with congenital malformations.

6. Some hypotheses are:

  (a) Black infants have genetically determined lower survival rates.

  (b) Black mothers are less likely to have access to medical care during pregnancy.

  (c) Black mothers are more likely to be of lower socioeconomic class than are white mothers.

  (d) Black infants are more likely to be low birth weight than are white infants.

  (e) Deaths of white infants are less likely to be recorded than deaths of black infants.

  (f) Births of black infants are less likely to be recorded than are births of white infants.

Chapter 6

1. Positive predictive value is the probability of the disease being present given a test result. For the clinical health care provider, this probability

provides a basis for interpreting a positive test result, one which the patient might also understand. The same is true for negative predictive values, negative test results, and the absence of disease. However, neither positive nor negative predictive values provide a basis for evaluating the performance of a test.

2. The number of individuals likely to be identified with the virus in the early 1980s was low, but even with a very specific test, the number of false-positive persons would likely be high (perhaps even greater than the number of true positives identified). The other problem with the proposed policy in the early 1980s was that there were no treatments for HIV infection at that time.

3. The major strength of a registry is that it provides a central place where all cases of a disease in a community can be ascertained. Such data are useful for epidemiologic observational studies (discussed in Chapters 10 and 11) and also for enrolling those with the disease in therapeutic randomized clinical trials (discussed in Chapter 8). Registries provide unique information for characterizing secular trends of a disease. The weakness of registries is their cost. They are generally expensive to operate.

4. The sensitivity and specificity of the test may be characterized and compared with those for other early lung cancer screening tests. Also, a study could be initiated to determine if those who have been screened with the test have greater survivorship than those not screened.

5. Major problems will include different standards used to diagnose cardiovascular disease, different patterns of access to medical care for diagnosis of the disease, and different patterns of migration to and from the communities being monitored. An additional problem is obtaining the support of health care providers in each community where a registry is to be established.

6. Such data provide a basis for assessing diagnostic criteria, survivorship, and referral patterns. A given tumor registry, however, will often lack a defined population. This makes it difficult to calculate rates of disease. Also, since there may be many factors that influence which patients with which diseases present to which hospitals, there may be selection bias.

7. The prevalence of osteoarthritis is 2,500 cases per 100,000 population.

8. The observation may be artifactual, resulting from increased accessibility of health care. It may represent a genetic etiology of the condition. It may result from the common environment of the family, with consequent exposure to the environmental agent of the disease. Or it may result from a combination of genetic and environmental factors (i.e., a genetic susceptibility coupled with exposure to the environmental agent of the disease).

9. It is desirable to minimize the percentage of individuals with false-negative test results if the disease is very serious or fatal and a treatment exists that affects the prognosis of the disease. It is desirable to minimize the percentage of individuals with false-positive results if such a finding has adverse social or economic consequences or if the treatment itself has adverse side effects.

Chapter 7

1. The development of cases in the summer and early autumn reflects the availability of the insect agents responsible for the transmission of the agent to humans, i.e., the mosquito. This means of transmission is much less available during other times of the year, hence the fewer cases observed at other times.

2. Three possible explanations for these changes are (1) changes in the pathogenicity of the different types of bacteria, with staphlococcus and streptococcus bacteria becoming much less pathogenic by the 1960s and 1970s compared with the 1930s, 1940s, and 1950s; (2) the increased use of antibiotics, with consequent change in the availability of pathogenic bacteria to infect a given host; and (3) the increased use of immunosuppressive agents (including those used in cancer chemotherapy), which allows agents such as gram negative bacteria, from which a host is normally protected by a fully functioning immune system, to thrive.

3. The large number of immigrants to the United States from areas of world in which tuberculosis is much more common than the United States (the 1980s saw more immigrants to the United States than in any decade since the 1920s) and the increasing number of AIDS cases (first reported in 1980) in the United States have together resulted in the increasing number of tuberculosis cases observed in the United States.

4. (a) These data indicate that the prevalence rates were higher in 1973 than in 1964–1965 for all age groups among both men and women. The rates among women were greater than among men. From these data, one may conclude that women have a greater prevalence of diabetes than men, that the prevalence increases with ascending age, and that the prevalence of disease may have increased from 1964–1965 to 1973.

   (b) It would be desirable to have validation of the data, including diagnostic criteria, further information on case ascertainment, confirmation of the diagnoses, and information on changes in survivorship of those with the disease.

   (c) The data suggest the need for studies to validate diagnoses in both time periods and for further analysis of secular trends.

5. The differences in rates among whites and blacks may be artifactual, reflecting underascertainment of the black population. Assuming that errors in the population data could not account for the differences, the possibility of different definitions of disease being used by health care providers for blacks and whites must be considered. Lastly, it is possible that these differences result from differences in the incidence of esophageal cancer in both populations. Such differences could be due to genetic or environmental etiological factors being more common in the black population.

6. These differences could be the result of inconsistencies in data collection and analysis between the two areas or of differences in population enumeration. Assuming that such inconsistencies do not exist, it is possible that a herd immunity effect was present among the older population of Baltimore, accounting for the marked decrease in older age groups compared with St. Lawrence Island.

Chapter 8

1. Randomization is the process by which subjects are assigned to groups in an investigation such that each subject has the same chance of being assigned to each of the groups. Randomization performs three functions in a randomized clinical trial. First, it eliminates bias resulting from assignment to either treatment or placebo (or comparison) groups. Second, it assures the comparability of the two groups. Third, randomization facilitates the use of statistical tests of significance (or the calculation of confidence intervals).

2. Before using a new agent in a randomized clinical trial, one would need to determine its toxicology, both in animals and, to the degree possible in a small clinical study, in humans. This knowledge is essential if the clinical trial is to be conducted without bringing avoidable harm to individuals using the agent. Also, pharmacokinetic information is needed for adequate dosing of individuals using the agent.

3. The limitations of the randomized clinical trial are that it is relatively expensive, it is ethically difficult or impossible to conduct for some questions, it is only useful for beneficial outcomes, and poor compliance in either the experimental or the comparison groups is possible.

4. (a) Tabulations that will be needed include center-specific comparisons of the characteristics of the experimental and control groups, center-specific comparisons of the outcomes, and center-specific comparisons of adverse reactions. Aggregate tabulations of these comparisons would also be required to assess the drug's effectiveness.

   (b) The inference that could be derived from this trial is that the drug is effective at a certain dose in treating a certain disease in a specific population.

(c) The problems that may occur during the course of such a study are manifold. An important one is withdrawals, which can be handled by having a sufficiently large sample size to allow for the withdrawals and by following the withdrawals to determine if they are different from those who continue in the study. Other problems are adverse reactions, which may require that the trial be halted, and a treatment that is so efficacious that the continuance of the trial would be unethical.

(d) Physicians must consider several issues before prescribing the drug. Is the patient population studied in the trial comparable to those for whom the drug would be prescribed? What dosages of the drug were used? What adverse reactions accompanied the use of the drug at that dose? What were the definitions of disease used in the trial? Was the trial properly designed? Were the results analyzed properly? These questions would serve as a guide for physicians considering whether or not to prescribe the drug.

5. A randomized clinical trial would be unethical if no alternative treatment existed for the disease and the treatment had some effectiveness, or if the treatment was known to cause major disease or to have some toxicity with an unclear benefit to patients using it. If a randomized clinical trial can not be conducted, observational data could be collected in an epidemiologic study to provide additional insight into the issue. The limitation of the nonrandomized studies are due to the possibility that strong selection biases may be present.

6. The power of the trial may be inadequate to detect the small beneficial effect.

7. The randomized clinical trial can detect adverse reactions, but only if they are common enough to occur in the relatively small sample sizes used in such studies. It is for this reason that so-called postmarketing surveillance studies are conducted after a new drug has been approved by the federal government. It is also for this reason that morbidity and mortality surveys are needed to detect the less common adverse reactions.

8. The problem with this approach is that there is no comparison group against which the treatment's true efficacy can be assessed.

9. Three (60 × 0.05) statistical tests would be expected to be statistically significant even if there were no true difference. The best way to protect against this phenomenon (commonly referred to as "multiple comparisons") is to use statistical tests wisely and not to use them when they are not needed. Statisticians have developed techniques to deal with such

situations; consulting a statistician before using such tests (and during the design of the trial) should protect against this problem.

Chapter 9

1. The major difference between randomized clinical trials and community trials is that in randomized clinical trials the efficacy of a preventive or therapeutic agent or technique is tested in individual subjects, while in community trials it is tested in a group of subjects as a whole. Natural experiments and community trials are quite similar, the major difference being the control that the investigator has over the populations studied.

2. The main reason for conducting a community trial is to test an etiologic hypothesis or preventive procedure in an experimental setting comparable to that which might be used by a local or federal public health department in developing programs to prevent or reduce the incidence of disease in a population. Community trials facilitate the evaluation of such programs, specifically evaluation of their efficacy. If the activity to reduce disease incidence or to prevent disease is community-based, then it must be evaluated in a community trial, not in a randomized clinical trial.

3. These inferences are limited insofar as there may have been considerable differences among the communities studied. There was no randomized assignment of treatment, hence such differences might affect the results of the study. Another limitation was that the follow-up focused on the risk factors for cardiovascular diseases, not the incidence of cardiovascular disease. Although it is reasonable to expect that intervention aimed at the risk factors will result in a decline in cardiovascular disease, without such data from the trial, one cannot assume that such a decline will indeed take place.

4. Community trials are subject to ecological fallacy. The lack of specific information on individuals in community trials provides an opportunity for an ecological fallacy to occur.

5. When using historical controls, the investigator loses some control over the conditions within which the trial is conducted. Since there may be a loss of comparability in the communities studied and there may also be a lack of comparability in the methods used for disease diagnosis or risk factor assessment at different times, the use of historical controls greatly reduces the validity of the study findings.

6. The design of a randomized clinical trial is more important than its analysis because the quality of the data being analyzed is determined by the design of the trial. If the design of the trial is faulty, it is doubtful that the analysis will provide much meaningful information. The same reasoning applies to a community trial. Good study design facilitates proper analysis of the data, regardless of the type of study being discussed.

7. Community trials are conducted in those situations in which an intervention is best undertaken for an entire community, such as health education.

8. (a) These data suggest that making the privies flyproof reduced the occurrence of typhoid fever, presumably by reducing its transmission. However, it is important to note that the comparison data were not collected concurrent with the data on the intervention.

   (b) It would be very important to know what other changes took place in the city. Specifically, did the water supply change? Also of importance would be knowledge of changes in any other risk factor for typhoid fever.

Chapter 10

1. The SMR and the relative risk are not necessarily the same. The relative risk compares the frequency of disease in a given population that was exposed to a factor and the frequency of that disease in a similar population that was not exposed to that factor. In contrast, the numerator of an SMR is the number of cases in a group exposed to a factor. The denominator includes the number of cases that would have occurred in that group if their mortality experience had been the same as that of some comparison population. The comparison population may or may not have been exposed to the factor; alternatively, it might include some individuals who have been exposed to the factor. If no such persons are present in that population, then the SMR is indeed equivalent to the relative risk.

2. The attributable fraction is useful to the epidemiologist as a guide to how many risk factors it is worthwhile to investigate. For example, if a factor F has an attributable fraction of 95 percent for disease D, further investigations into those factors responsible for the other 5 percent of the disease are likely to be very difficult to conduct and unproductive in finding a relationship.

3. The basic design of this study would be:

   (a) Identify a high-risk group for D (such as college students for infectious mononucleosis or homosexual men for AIDS).

   (b) Recruit members of the high-risk group into the study.

   (c) Eliminate from the study any individuals with D.

   (d) Obtain blood or sera from study participants.

   (e) Determine, from the sera, which individuals have been exposed to V.

   (f) Follow all study participants for the development of D.

   (g) Compare the incidence rate of D for those individuals with V in their sera (or a marker for V, such as antibodies) to that for individuals without the virus or the marker in their sera.

This design is unchanged if V is a slow virus. It is also unchanged if D is thought to be noninfectious.

4. These databases may be used to determine exposures in the past, such as operations or pharmaceutical use, and relate it on an individual-by-individual basis to the subsequent development of a disease (which would be noted in the HMO's records for that patient.) Such a study would be nonconcurrent. If the exposure is determined at present with follow-up occurring from the present into the future, then the study would be concurrent.

5. The question that the surgeons have posed is one of exposure (What is the effect of tonsillectomy?). The surgeons could either identify a group of patients at some time in the past and a similar group of surgical patients (perhaps having hernia repairs or appendectomies), and in a nonconcurrent manner, follow up those patients through the National Death Index or some similar means. An alternative approach would be for the surgeons to identify a group of patients currently undergoing tonsillectomies and a similar group not having that operation and following both groups for subsequent mortality. This would be the concurrent approach.

Chapter 11

1. The choice of an appropriate control group may vary with the hypothesis to be tested. Often one chooses more than one type of control. Some possible answers are:

   (a) Babies born at normal birth weight (over 2500 gms), babies born over 1500 gms, or babies with birth defects. Exclude twins since low birth weight is related to twinness.

   (b) Infants with strep throat, infants coming to pediatrician for well baby visits, or infants coming to pediatricians for all causes except ear infections or well baby visits. Exclude infants with tubes in ears since they have a lower likelihood of becoming cases.

   (c) Transplant patients who do not reject transplant.

   (d) All other suicide victims, all other handgun victims (suicide or not), handgun owners, handgun suicide victims, or handgun suicide victims where witnesses were present.

2. (a) The odds ratio is $\dfrac{(11)(21)}{(33)(3)} = 2.33$, suggesting that drug and alcohol use increases the risk of death by Russian roulette compared to handgun suicide.

   (b) The odds ratio is $\dfrac{(9)(35)}{(19)(5)} = 3.31$. Cocaine use may increase by about three-fold the probability of suicide from Russian roulette compared to suicide by handgun.

3. Some advantages of the case-control design in studying this question are:

- Suicide by Russian roulette is a rare event that is most easily studied by the case-control method.
- The study used small sample sizes ($N = 68$) and was relatively inexpensive to conduct.
- The study could look at several risk factors (alcohol and cocaine use).

   Two typical disadvantages of case-control studies do not apply to this study. Exposure (alcohol or cocaine use) clearly preceded the outcome (suicide by handgun), so temporality of events is unquestioned. Cases and controls were easily identified by the Medical Examiner's office, with a low probability of missing cases.
   Some disadvantages are:

- Errors may have occurred in blood measurements of cocaine and alcohol because of different amounts of time elapsing between death and examination. The presence of witnesses may have led to a shorter time lag before blood samples were taken. The presence of witnesses was also associated with Russian roulette suicides.
- Cases and controls might be misclassified if Russian roulette occurred in the absence of witnesses. The authors do not describe how they distinguished a Russian roulette case from other handgun suicides if witnesses were absent. Perhaps the appropriate control group should have been handgun suicides that took place in the presence of witnesses. A high proportion of cocaine and alcohol users might have been found in this group also.
- Incidence rates of suicide by Russian roulette, handgun, or other method among cocaine and noncocaine, alcohol and nonalcohol users cannot be calculated. Although complete numerator data may be available from death certificates, denominator data are not available. The data give no information about the overall risk of suicide by alcohol or drug use.

4. (a) We can collect information about exposure among cases and controls immediately, when the subject arises, and come up with an answer in a short period of time (six months to a year), to inform public decision-making.
   (b) Women with breast cancer diagnosed in a reasonable period of time (i.e., the last two years).
   (c) Women without the disease—women who have recently had exams (for example, mammograms) showing they are free of the disease— or a group of women willing to be screened for the study to show

that they are free of the disease. However, for most diseases that are rare, this is not necessary.

(d) The controls should be restricted to women only, about a certain age (to allow comparable times for the disease to have occurred, and to be the same age as women who would have already had breast implants).

(e) It might be useful to match on socioeconomic status because women who get breast implants (and pay for them privately) are probably wealthier than a representative sample of women. Socioeconomic status might also be associated with other risk factors for the disease.

(f) When many variables are used in matching, it becomes difficult to find controls; one cannot examine the relationship between the matching variables and the disease; one may overmatch, match on a variable that is causally related to the disease, so that the groups or pairs are too similar.

(g) One could ask the women to describe their own histories or ask them to give permission to look at their medical records.

(h) Some women will be more accurate and more informative about their medical histories. Some women will not be willing to share information or give permission for the researchers to obtain medical information. Some women have moved often, or changed caregivers frequently, and this will make it difficult to obtain medical records. Older patients may have received care from physicians who are now retired or dead—again making it difficult to find out about silicone implants. All these variations can affect the classification of women as exposed or not exposed, and can be diffeernt in the cases and controls. This can affect the measure of effect—the odds ratio—reducing or increasing it depending on the particular circumstances.

Chapter 12

1. One must identify potential confounders in the literature and collect data on all potential confounders. One may restrict study subjects to a particular subgroup or match study subjects to controls.

2. One may use stratified analysis, multiple regression, or a combination of both techniques.

3. Biological significance refers to findings that affect many people, explain the cause of a disease, suggest new approaches to treatment or prevention, or suggest new research directions. Statistical significance means that the observed differences are greater than would be expected by chance alone.

4. The following concepts are used in assessing causality:
   - Strength of association
   - Consistency of the observed association
   - Specificity of the association
   - Temporal sequence of events
   - Dose-response relationship
   - Biological plausibility of the observed association
   - Experimental evidence

Chapter 13

1. Decision analysis can be applied to a specific clinical problem in a given patient, or it can be applied in a general way to a problem and can result in a recommendation for a group of patients.
2. Some of the limitations of decision analysis are that (a) information about probabilities of outcomes is not always available; (b) the decision tree can become very complicated, even for what appear to be simple choices; (c) it is hard to assign quantitative values to some outcomes.
3. The paper should describe (a) the study problem, (b) the study design, (c) selection of the study sample, (d) data analysis, and (e) inference and results.
4. All studies are susceptible to biases. Authors should address the ways in which their study may have been affected by bias, and how they dealt with potential biases in the design and analysis.
5. A physician can participate in epidemiologic research by participating in a collaborative study or by initiating an investigation in response to an observation of an outbreak, a new syndrome, or an out-of-the-ordinary occurrence.

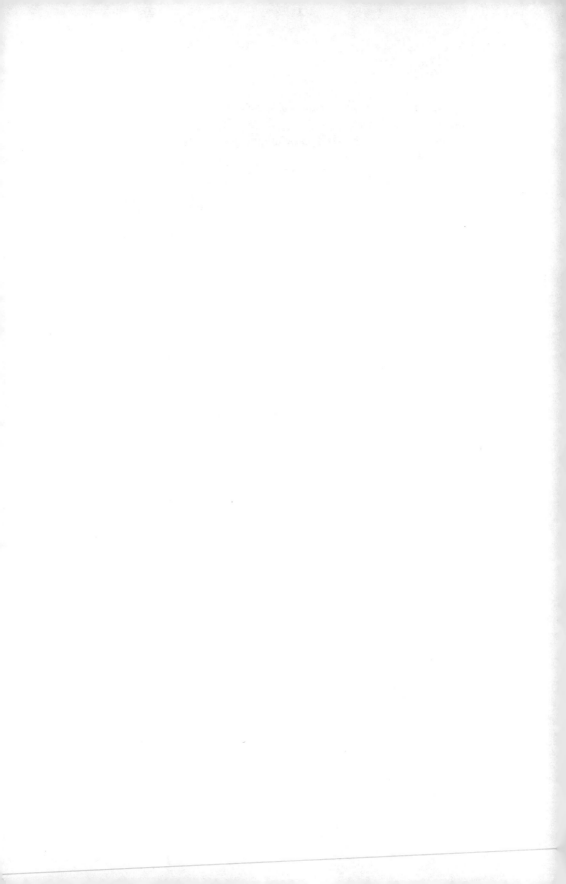

AUTHOR INDEX

SUBJECT INDEX

Essential Law Revision
from Oxford University Press

The perfect pairing for exam success

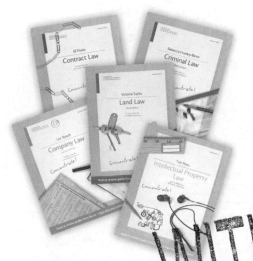

Concentrate!

For students who are serious about exam success, it's time to concentrate!

- ✓ Written by experts
- ✓ Developed with students
- ✓ Designed for success
- ✓ Trusted by lecturers, loved by students

Don't miss the **Law Revision apps!**

Download the apps from the iTunes app store for your iPad, iPhone, or iPod touch. Hundreds of multiple choice questions with feedback, helping you to study, learn and revise, anytime, anywhere.

QUESTIONS & ANSWERS

Keeping you afloat through your exams.

- ✓ Typical exam questions
- ✓ Suggested answers
- ✓ Advice on exam technique and making your answer stand out

'Nothing else compares to such reliable study-aids and revision guides.'

Heather Walkden, law student

'Comprehensive, functional, stylishly innovative; superior to any of its rivals.'

Michael O'Sullivan, law lecturer

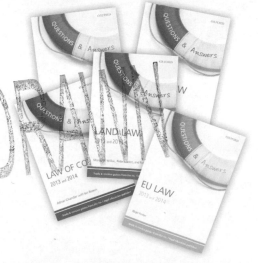

For the ... ... es visit: www.oxfordtextbooks.co.uk/orc/lawrevision/

Study & revision guides from the no. 1 legal education publisher

Todd & Wilson's
Textbook on Trusts

Todd & Wilson's

Textbook on
Trusts

....

Eleventh edition

Sarah Wilson
LLB, MA, PhD

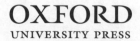
OXFORD
UNIVERSITY PRESS

OXFORD
UNIVERSITY PRESS

Great Clarendon Street, Oxford, OX2 6DP,
United Kingdom

Oxford University Press is a department of the University of Oxford.
It furthers the University's objective of excellence in research, scholarship,
and education by publishing worldwide. Oxford is a registered trade mark of
Oxford University Press in the UK and in certain other countries

British Library Cataloguing in Publication Data

Data available

ISBN 978-0-19-966319-4

Printed in Great Britain by
Ashford Colour Press Ltd, Gosport, Hampshire

In memory of
Alfreda Naylor, 2 March 1911–13 December 2007
Marion Wilson, 20 August 1938–27 February 2012
On my wedding day I was able to give thanks for "two wonderful mothers",
and I will do so for ever more. Rest in peace.

PREFACE

It has become a tradition for this text to state in its Preface that it is continuing in the tradition started by Paul Todd. From its earliest inception, this text has always been aimed at undergraduate students in their second or third year of undergraduate study. It has always presented itself as an introductory text, thus accounting for its being shorter than a number of other texts which are available. Alongside this, the text has always stressed that it is able to state the law briefly and concisely but without sacrificing clarity, whilst at the same time presenting high quality analysis. It has also always explained that trusts is a subject requiring a great deal of time, patience, and critical engagement on the part of its students. This edition is very much in this vein and continues with the spirit of focusing on principle more than detail (and particularly factual detail). It also continues to prioritize areas commonly taught on undergraduate courses, rather than attempting to encompass everything about trusts and equity. Thus, it continues to give little attention to those aspects which could in principle be included, but are in practice covered elsewhere in undergraduate programmes in law—such as land law, the law of contract, commercial law, and the English legal system. But in dispensing with what the book is not seeking to cover, there is plenty to say about what is in this particular edition of the text and its companion resources. There is also a good deal to say about how the book seeks to impart understanding about trusts and trusts law.

As already stressed, it has always been a feature of this text to provide clarity in coverage of key areas of trusts law, which reflects the size of the text. Alongside this, its distinctive approach focusing on principle rather than detail has also enabled it to punch above its weight as far as critical engagement and analysis are concerned. This particular edition continues in this more long-standing vein, and also in a more newly established one.

The 2011 edition made very significant stylistic changes to the materials and their presentation. This was to ensure that, as well as being an up-to-date and analytical and critically engaging account of trusts and trusts law, the text would focus as much on meeting current needs in and approaches to learning. This newer approach has been some time in conception, informed by my own activities as a teacher of trusts, by discussions with colleagues who share my passion for the subject, and also by my interest in promoting excellence in learning. The changing writing style for this book has been very strongly influenced by my experiences as a teacher of trusts in a number of institutions and across a number of years at the frontline of learning. This has made me acutely aware of how changing patterns of study in university education must have an impact on how textbooks prepared as resources supporting the LLB curriculum are written. There is of course the very notable influence brought to bear by modulariza-tion. Alongside this, there is also an increasing emphasis on learning as a dialogical process within which you are active participants rather than passive subjects. From these influences there have also been some presentational changes to the text in the more recent editions, as ever-greater use is made of shorter and more concise paragraphs to make information more manageable as you approach your learning. This has been assisted by taking every opportunity to provide inter-text 'headings' and different for-matting, which helps the text appear less daunting, and helps concentrate attention on how different things relate to one another or are different from one another.

Changes made in the 2011 edition received excellent feedback, and the newer stylistic approaches—both in actual writing and in modes of presentation—have been applied more extensively across additional chapters. Here, there is a great deal of emphasis in engaging with you as you build understanding, and using this approach to integrate forward and backward linkages between different topic areas. The re-ordering of the first chapters introducing the fundamentals of an express trust that was undertaken in 2011 has clearly worked very well, and so this format has been retained in this edition. And this new edition continues to work on encouraging reiteration of earlier learning experiences as we work through the text—and also ensures that 'iterative' attention is paid for materials still to come—through the continuing emphasis on chapter beginnings as well as the 'work-through' materials themselves.

This approach reflects that much of learning about trusts and trusts law is about iteration and reiteration and requires understanding the subject as a 'coherent whole', and much of this depends on appreciating the existence of linkages within it at an early stage, even if fuller understanding of them can only follow in time. For those of you who look at a particular chapter in isolation, this approach will help you to understand how a particular aspect of trusts law fits in with everything else: here you will be able to see very quickly whether a topic is regarded as part of the 'heart' of the law relating to express trusts, or concerns the law relating to 'special' types of trusts known as implied trusts or charitable organizations.

The two years since 2011 have produced a huge volume of key developments in statutory provision and especially case law, with much of it having significant impact on the law. Thus, in this new edition, changes made to the style of the text as well as its content have been greatly assisted by the amount of re-writing necessary on account of changes in law. Perhaps most significantly, in terms of the sheer volume of materials within this text's coverage, the enactment of the Charities Act 2011 has resulted in all three chapters—10 through 12—on charity being very substantially revised and, in the case of Chapter 12, Cy-près, actually re-written. Equally, the Supreme Court decision in *Jones* v *Kernott* [2012] UKSC 53 has provided the impetus for the very significant reworking of Chapter 8 on beneficial interests in shared family homes. Elsewhere, the continuing significance of 'commercial dealings' for understanding the fundamentals of the trust has resulted in additions to Chapter 3's study of certainty rules. The materials now provide more extended coverage of the significance of *Pearson & Ors* v *Lehman Bros Finance SA & Ors* [2010] EWHC 2914 (Ch) and note the importance of the decision in *Crossco No 4 Unlimited* v *Jolan Limited* [2011] EWCA Civ 1619 for this, which is considered further in Chapter 18. Also within the sphere of requirements for a valid trust, more attention has been paid in this edition (in Chapter 5) to *Kaye* v *Zeital* [2010] EWCA Civ 159 than was possible in the previous one, with this case also being considered in the light of the decision in *Curtis* v *Pulbrook* [2011] EWHC 167.

The chapter on trusts in commercial dealings, which was new to the tenth edition, has been expanded to reflect the increasing significance of commercial dealings for understanding trusts law. There are a number of new cases here, including *Mundy* v *Brown* [2011] EWHC 377 (Ch), *Du Preez Ltd* v *Kaupthing Singer & Friedlander (Isle of Man) Ltd* [2011] WTLR 559, *Global Marine Drillships Ltd* v *Landmark Solicitors LLP* [2011] EWHC 2685, and *Bieber* v *Teathers Ltd (in liquidation)* [2012] EWHC 190 (Ch) in the discussion of *Quistclose* arrangements. Elsewhere, *Crossco No 4 Unlimited* v *Jolan Limited* [2011] EWCA Civ 1619 does build on the observations made in 2011 about the significance of *Pearson & Ors* v *Lehman Bros* for appreciating the nature of modern trusts law and how it might develop hitherto. And in strengthening coverage on the issues arising from utilizing trusts in the context of insolvency, the text has discussed extensively the judicial statement of Peter Smith J made by His Honour following the collapse of the litigation against Farepak executives brought by the Insolvency Service following the outcome of *Re Farepak* [2007] 2 BCLC 1. There is also new material seeking to draw a number of these themes together to consider *why* commercial parties are so attracted to equity and its doctrines—and, for the purposes of this text, centrally the trust—*at all*, and, in this vein, looking at just how long-standing this attraction appears to be and how this might forecast developments.

Chapter 14, which covers trustees' powers and duties, has been able to note that the Trusts (Capital and Income) Act 2013 received Royal Assent on 31 January 2013, but more detailed coverage of this within the text will have to be held over for the next edition. But elsewhere in relation to trusteeship, extensive alterations have been made to the text this time around. Here, materials on the fiduciary nature of trusteeship within Chapter 13's introduction to trusteeship have been significantly reworked on account of changes to the law which appeared to flow from the litigation in *Sinclair Investments (UK) Ltd* v *Versailles Trade Finance Ltd*. The decision at first instance ([2010] EWHC 1614 (Ch)) generated considerable criticism, and was widely believed at the time to be a 'rogue' decision which could not easily be reconciled with a number of fundamental aspects of trusteeship and particularly equity's governance of secret profit-making by fiduciaries. However, the Court of Appeal's ([2011] EWCA Civ 347) endorsement of personal liability (rather than that by way of constructive trust) for particular species of profit-making has led to significant rewriting of the materials in this edition. This is likely to continue into the next edition, where more coverage will have to be given to distinguishing between different types of unauthorized profit-making. This will be extremely challenging given the size of the text, and the focus on principle rather than detail that has emerged from it, but at this point the text has said as much about *Sinclair* and its implications as possible, and even predicting what might be required next time around is problematic amidst *Sinclair*'s continuing contention. Indeed, as recently as 29 January 2013, a judgment handed down by the Court of Appeal in *FHR European Ventures LLP & 6 Ors* v *Mankarious, Cedar Capital Partners LLC and Cedar Capital Partners Ltd.* [2013] EWCA Civ 17 suggested that if *Sinclair* represents the law then there is the need to provide an overhaul of the entire area of the law of constructive trusts 'in order to provide a coherent and logical legal framework' and made a strong entreaty to the Supreme Court to do so, in the light of the important issues of policy at stake.

Elsewhere, the study of beneficiary actions relating to missing property has slightly expanded coverage of dishonest assistance on account of several cases which appeared subsequently to the Court of Appeal decision in *Starglade* v *Nash* [2010] EWCA Civ 1314. Ones included in this edition are *Aerostar Maintenance International Ltd* v *Wilson* [2010] EWHC 2032 (Ch), relating to the meaning of dishonesty, and applications of *Starglade*'s standard-setting relating to 'ordinary standards of commercial behaviour' can be seen in *Halliwells LLP* v *Nes Solicitors* [2011] EWHC 947 (QB) and *Secretary of State for Justice* v *Topland Group plc* [2011] EWHC 983 (QB).

Both these latter chapters, as well as those covering charity and shared family homes, which have been much more extensively revised, reveal the way in which the text is constantly under threat from the pressure to include new materials whilst at the same time avoiding increases in its overall size. There are sound pedagogic reasons for maintaining the current size of the text, as well as economic ones, but unfortunately it is also the case that even if 'the subject' of trusts law isn't actually increasing in size (with a central thesis of Chapter 18 being that this is happening), the materials required for understanding it are definitely increasing in volume. Here, charity, trustee-ship, family homes, and beneficiary actions, as well as all being stalwarts of Trusts and Equity English law syllabi that exemplify areas where there is rapid and extensive development in the law, also actually show that understanding the nature and significance of this requires understanding of existing/traditional approaches. This is because new developments are actually being built on these existing/traditional approaches, which in turn makes it very difficult to cut existing coverage to make way for new materials. This accounts for some lengthy chapters in this text, with those listed above providing illustrations of where this arises.

It is in this setting that the companion ORC for this text has acquired such a strong significance for it. It was always likely that the ORC was, in any case, going to be very important for areas experiencing rapid and extensive development, by providing a mechanism for very quick communication of key developments in law or policy movements which occur between editions. And the previous edition acknowledged that given the increasing pressure on 'text space', it was likely that the ORC would also have to be used as a location for areas which remain important for understanding trusts in the overall, but where tough choices need to be made on what remains actually within the text and what, although important to it, will have to be located elsewhere. For this edition, the chapter traditionally looking at 'Equitable Fraud' has been relocated to the ORC. Given the significance of a number of its key themes for understanding how equity works, where it is currently most active and why, this is undoubtedly a loss for the main text. It may be possible to relocate it within the text in subsequent editions—but this current decision could also be looked at differently. It could be regarded as a bold step which marks the ORC genuinely as an extension of the main text, rather than a location beyond it for a number of 'wider perspectives' or 'further reflections' on a particular matter. The latter is of course a very important function of the ORC for achieving a study of trusts and trusts law which is rounded and closely integrated with the scholarship which has grown up around it. But actually, in the context of the popularization of electronic learning resources alongside traditional paper-based ones, there is every reason to regard the ORC as an extension of the main text rather than as a supplement for it.

When commencing your study of trusts it is worth appreciating that concepts in trusts law are very difficult: this is not helped by the way in which many appear to be 'abstract' rather than tangible, and the way in which the accompanying terminology can on occasion be very confusing. And to assist this, as a matter of presentation, the text makes reference only to the words 'he' and 'his', used interchangeably for both genders. In recognition of this, every effort has been made to make the materials as accessible as possible, while trying to explain the concepts as fully as possible. And it is also worth remembering that although you will find things difficult at times, trusts is a really fascinating subject which is *definitely* worth the effort which it will take trying to get to grips with.

This was my impression as a student, and it certainly remains so now that I am a teacher myself. It is also the case that my own experiences both as a student and as a teacher strongly suggest that the best law students are not necessarily those who do the most work, but rather those who think hardest about the subject. I encourage my own students to email me, and each other, since this is a good way of discussing things. It also gives insight into areas of difficulty, and often encourages me to consider things I might have missed.

In terms of those to whom thanks are owed as a new edition of this text is published, as always I would like to thank my friend and colleague from the University of Leeds, Michael Cardwell, for our continuing and inspiring reflections on trusts. Special thanks are also due to Margot Brazier for her continuing support even after my departure from the University of Manchester. Thanks too to Jamie Murray for many inspiring shared perspectives on trusts, to TT Arvind for the support and encouragement I receive across a number of shared interests, and also to my York colleagues Stefan Enchelmaier and Jenny Steele. As always, very special thanks are due to my husband and colleague Gary Wilson for all the support he provides, both all the time and in this particular context, especially for his thoughtful and extremely valuable insights into trusts law.

And lastly (but certainly not least), I would also like to thank the editorial and production staff at OUP for all their hard work in helping to prepare this edition, and for their support and expertise, from which I continue to benefit considerably as an author.

It remains only for me to encourage you to enjoy your study of trusts.

Sarah Wilson

NEW TO THIS EDITION

- Chapter 12 has been entirely rewritten.

- Chapters 3, 8, 10, 11, 13, and 18 include substantial additions and rewriting.

- New coverage of the Charities Act 2011 and the Equality 2010.

- New material reflecting developments in all key areas, including family homes, trusteeship and beneficiary actions.

- Revision Boxes, which include exercises designed to reinforce learning, have been introduced at the end of each chapter.

OUTLINE CONTENTS

DETAILED CONTENTS

---

1 Law and equity and an introduction to the trust   1

---

2 The nature of the trust: its operation and applications in society and the economy   26

3 The three certainties and the significance of the 'beneficiary principle' 54

4 Formality and the creation of valid trusts 91

5 The constitution requirement for a valid trust 116

13   Introduction to trusteeship and an overview of the 'office of trustee'   302

14   Powers, discretions, and duties of trustees   337

15   Variation of trusts   355

TABLE OF CASES

TABLE OF STATUTES

TABLE OF STATUTORY INSTRUMENTS

1

Law and equity and an
introduction to the trust

The term 'trust' is used a great deal in everyday conversations and this book is all about what we mean by the term 'trust' when it is used in conversations about law, and specifically English law.

This chapter is designed to introduce the 'trust' arrangement that is found in English law, explaining its basic nature and also its jurisdictional basis within equity. It also seeks to give an initial overview of how and why trusts arise, and indeed where they can be found 'at work' within society and the economy. This is the starting point for the remainder of this text, which is concerned with explaining the framework governing the successful creation of trusts and also that which underpins how they operate once they have been created.

1.1 An introduction to trusts and the law

At the heart of everything that we learn about the trust is that it is a device found within English law where there are two types of 'ownership' of property that exist for the same property at the same time—so-called 'simultaneous existence of different types of title to property'. We will come to this shortly, but first we are going to learn a little more about the trust as it is understood as a legal device, from looking at two dictionary definitions of 'a trust'.

The *Cambridge Advanced Learner's Dictionary* explains a trust as 'a legal arrangement in which a person or organisation controls property … for the benefit of another person or organisation'.

The *Compact Oxford English Dictionary* explains that, in law, a trust is 'an arrangement whereby a person (a trustee) is made the nominal owner of property to be held or used for the benefit of one or more others'.

These two basic dictionary definitions introduce the way in which a trust is a legal device or arrangement that is brought into being *to provide benefits* for another person, which relate to some kind of property. By emphasizing the importance of *control over* property and *nominal ownership* of property in the pursuit of providing benefits for another or others, these basic definitions are an important introduction to the way in which the trust achieves this purpose through the *simultaneous existence of two types of ownership of property*, as indicated above. This paves the way for explaining that, in the trust arrangement, ownership of property is *divided into two types of ownership* in, or title to, property. These two titles to property are title 'at law' or 'legal title', and title 'in equity' or 'equitable title'. And, as suggested above, these distinctive titles will exist in the same property at the same time: this is their so-called simultaneous existence.

This introduction to the trust will consider how it is possible for two different titles to the same property to exist at the same time—the so-called 'jurisdictional basis' of the trust within English law. Here, we will learn that this is because equity was prepared to develop *equitable title to property*, and understanding why equity might have been prepared to do this will help us to understand how the trust instrument evolved. At that point, it will become clear how both equity's origins and also its modern significance within English law make the trust such a useful, flexible, and adaptable legal device in the twenty-first century.

The way in which this text discusses equity and equitable jurisdiction will focus on understanding the trust, given that this text is all about trusts and trusts law. This makes this text different from both examinations of equity occurring within texts on the 'English legal system', and also from other 'equity and trusts' texts on trusts, which are consciously about equity more generally. So we do need to appreciate the nature of equity to start our study of trusts, but what we learn about it here is all about helping to understand trusts.

At this point, we need to say more about the distinctive nature of the trust and to emphasize that the trust is able to confer benefits of property quite differently from other ways of doing this with which we are more familiar. Some of the detail of this is held over for discussion in Chapter 2, but we do also need to be aware at this stage that, in developing the trust, equity developed a unique way of using property to provide benefit and enjoyment.

This immediate discussion concerns the simultaneous existence of two types of title to (the same) property that characterizes the trust. It requires us to consider the significance of property in English law, and particularly the significance of ownership of property. Once again, in the same vein as it approaches its treatment of equity, this discussion of property and 'English property law' reflects that this text is one on trusts, rather than one that considers the nature of property within English law more directly: in this latter regard, 'land law' texts fulfil this function for the law of real property and works on commercial law provide extensive considerations of personal property. So what do we need to know about property and its recognition within English law in order to achieve an introductory understanding of trusts and trusts law?

In many respects, appreciating the importance of property within English law is key to understanding why equity has evolved the trust, and what uses and purposes it serves, or to which it could at some future point be applied. In being more specific about what we need to understand about property within English law, the trust is best understood from having some appreciation of the rights relating to property that can be found within private law.

In English law, a distinction is drawn between rights and entitlements that subsist at law and those that subsist in equity, whilst also being *capable* of having simultaneous existence across a number of 'interests', which are recognized by private law. As a number of texts on the English legal system make clear, the defining character of private law is that the law provides a series of rights and obligations that apply universally to everyone, which are supported by remedies for 'breaches' of these that have arisen, but then leaves decisions on using (that is, enforcing) these to individuals who have rights that have been breached.

Within property law itself, this can be seen reflected in a number of rights and entitlements to property, where rights and entitlements to property in law and equity are not only capable of having simultaneous existence, but also do commonly actually coexist. This includes the ultimate property right, which is, of course, ownership of property. We will discover that ownership of property at law and ownership of property in equity enjoy some shared similarities, and also that they are quite different. And the first step for appreciating this is to remember that, in a trust arrangement, ownership of property at law and in equity exist at the same time for the same property.

This book is all about the consequences of the simultaneous occurrence of these two types of ownership of property. And whilst this is not a text on property as such, we do need to appreciate that the implications of simultaneous ownership stem from the significance of ownership of property within English law.

1.1.1 The significance of ownership of property in English law

In the course of everyday dealings with property, it will be very clear that property is owned by a given individual, and much of the property that is encountered in everyday life will be identifiable with 'an owner'. There is an important point to be made in relation to ownership of land shortly, but this is the usual scenario relating to ownership, and within this all of the rights and interests relating to that property are those of the owner of property. Ownership of property is commonly theorized as a 'bundle of rights' relating to property, which form the basis of the way in which an owner of property is considered able to deal with property belonging to him in any way he pleases—including his ability to create entitlements to it for others. And as any encounter with English property law—however fleeting—will reveal, this is reflected in the owner holding legal title to the property. Here, title to property at law is the formal embodiment of a person's rights relating to property, which flow from his ownership of it. All that owning property entitles one to, and any responsibilities attaching to ownership, flow from holding legal title to the property concerned.

Ownership, legal title, and rights that are 'good against the world'
In expanding these key ideas slightly, in English law, legal title represents rights of the owner that are 'good against the world', which we will discover stems from the nature and intention of the English common law. This means that law recognizes the person who owns the property as the only person entitled to deal freely with that property, and this is how holding legal title to property provides the basis for free dealings with property. Ordinarily, this entitles a holder of legal title to property to sell it (where legal title will be transferred to a new owner in exchange for consideration), or to use the property to raise security. Both of these benefits of holding legal title indicate that this is capable of having considerable value, and thus title to property facilitates free dealings and dealings with confidence, because ascertaining that someone has legal title to property is crucial to knowing that it is his to sell or to use to raise security.

Notwithstanding that title to property is the basis for these transactions and that legal title is extremely valuable, one of the rights that an owner of property enjoys by virtue of being its owner is entitlement to give it to another. In this latter situation, when a gift is made, legal title to the property is transferred to the recipient because this is what its original owner wishes to happen. In this situation, the owner is not wishing to gain anything in return. Making gifts is something that happens so commonly that few will give any thought to how this happens and to what this amounts. We look at this more closely in Chapters 2 and 4, but for now you need only to appreciate that legal title (and thus ownership of) property will be transferred to another because the donor wishes that he should lose legal title to the property and that the recipient should acquire it.

The limits of legal title—and the limits of ownership:
an early insight into the trust
In the previous paragraph, it was noted that, *ordinarily*, legal title embodies rights and entitlements to enjoy property or to deal with it that are those exclusively of the owner,

and that this is formally represented by holding legal title to the property. This is the case because ownership of property is the ultimate property right, and in the materials in Chapter 4 we learn how law seeks to ensure that only an owner can properly deal with his property and that attempts by anyone else to purport to do so will not result in a rightful owner losing his property. These so-called 'formality requirements' for dealing with property seek to support the legal maxim *nemo dat quod non habet* ('none but the true owner can pass good title to property'). Ownership of property is a universal right at law, which means that it is good against (or enforceable against) any other person. However, it is also the case that, in some situations, holders of legal title are not in the position of universal entitlement regarding their property as ordinarily applies to owners. First, an owner of property can actually lose legal title to it, because ownership can lawfully be passed to another by someone other than him. This can happen through operation of exceptions that have developed to the *nemo dat* rule. This does have some peripheral significance for our study of trusts (as we will see in Chapter 17), but this is generally a consideration for studies of commercial law.

The other, very significant, reason why holding legal title does not always carry with it the bundle of rights ordinarily embodied in ownership is because this ordinary position arises only where ownership is not separated, and the only title to property in existence is legal title. Just because legal and equitable titles to property are capable of coexisting does not mean they will necessarily do so, and with most property that is identifiable with an owner, they will not. Ordinarily, only title at law will subsist, and the existence of equitable title to property is the signature feature that tells us that property is not owned outright by an owner and that it is instead subject to a trust. This means that ownership of property is actually separated into two distinctive titles to it. And, as we discover, where a trust is present, holding legal title to property acquires an altogether different significance.

1.2 Understanding the trust: appreciating the nature of equitable and legal title—*Westdeutsche Landesbank Girozentrale* v *Islington London Borough Council*

Unlike in the case of absolute ownership, in the simplest variety of trust, there will be two people simultaneously owning the property in question. However, the relationship that each person will have to the property will be quite different from that of the other. In this situation, where property is held on trust, there is a legal owner, who is called a 'trustee'. He has essentially a management role, and is subject to duties in respect of the property and the administration of the trust. The property will also have an owner in equity, who is called a *cestui que trust*, or 'beneficiary'. It is the beneficiary who is entitled to enjoy the property and whose position is therefore closest to being what a layman might consider to be an owner. So, in a trust situation, it is the beneficiary's equitable ownership of property that signals entitlement to enjoy the property in ways that we would associate with holding legal title to property where ownership is not separated. It is in respect of the beneficiary that the trustee's duties are owed and he can enforce them against the trustee.

There are a number of variations of the basic idea of the trust, and this most simple type identified above will arise where someone who owns property outright (at law) wishes another to benefit from this, but wishes to achieve this without making an outright transfer of ownership of the property to them. This makes a trust like a gift in some respects, but also different from it in others. More will be said about how effective gifts of property are achieved in Chapter 2, because understanding what is involved in making gifts of property can help us to understand what is involved in declaring a trust of property in terms of what is required and also what implications flow from this. At that point, we will discover just how differently a trust achieves providing benefits from property from other ways of achieving this. This is on account of the special 'signature' feature of the trust, which is the separation of ownership into two distinctive titles to property that occurs when property is settled on trust by its owner. At this point, the person(s) intended to benefit from the property acquires equitable title to it, while the person(s) responsible for ensuring that this happens is vested with legal title. What we need to understand at this stage is how ownership will become separated in this way and what will cause it to do so. The starting point for this is the illustration of a trust's creation in Figure 1.1.

	Before	After
Legal title—burdensome (managerial in nature)	Settlor	Trustee
Equitable title (beneficial: provides enjoyment)	None	Beneficiary or cestui que trust Note: either trustee or beneficiary may also be settlor

Figure 1.1 The creation of a trust.

As this figure suggests, this separation of ownership into equitable and legal titles (or 'estates', which is the terminology often used) in property is fundamental to the law of trusts. This provides the very foundation for the remainder of this book on the law of trusts, which is all about the creation of equitable ownership of property and the implications of its creation. The very premise of the book should suggest to you that equitable ownership of property is very important, and it will become clear just how valuable equitable ownership of property is. This is both in terms of the benefits that equitable ownership confers upon those who are so entitled, but also in terms of the ways in which it defines concomitant responsibilities and duties for those who are trustees of the property.

There is a lot of interesting discussion following from Figure 1.1 illustrating the creation of a trust, and a great deal of this is central for understanding how ownership will become separated and what will cause it to do so. This will also provide a lead in to understanding how a trust's jurisdictional basis in equity makes this possible.

Why will ownership become separated—and how will it become so?

An understanding of what will cause ownership to become separated is necessary before any substantive analysis of equitable ownership can be made. Understanding this is key to understanding how law knows when such an arrangement has come into being. The first thing that we need to appreciate is why Figure 1.1 tells us that, before a trust of property is created, the only type of title to property that exists is legal title—title at law. This is explained for us by the seminal House of Lords case *Westdeutsche Landesbank Girozentrale* v *Islington London Borough Council* [1996] AC 669. This is particularly so with the now very famous passage from the judgment of Lord Browne-Wilkinson, which insists (probably as part of the *ratio* of the case) that the owner of any property is vested with legal title alone. From this, it is apparent that only when separation of title is sought will distinct equitable ownership arise. Indeed, it is clear in light of *Westdeutsche* that distinct equitable title is not recognized as being capable of having an independent existence unless and until title to property becomes separated into these distinct components. According to Lord Browne-Wilkinson at 706:

> A person solely entitled to the full beneficial ownership of money or property, both at law and in equity, does not enjoy an equitable interest in that property. The legal title carries with it all rights. Unless and until there is a separation of the legal and equitable estates, there is no separate equitable title.

1.2.1 Title to property: legal and equitable interests

This analysis suggests that, in absence of a trust, equitable ownership of property does not exist, and thus that it has no intrinsic value. This does require some thought given that, even at this early stage of introducing trusts, equitable title is being associated with 'value' through its associations with entitlement, benefit, and enjoyment. We also know that, in a trust setting, legal title more readily connotes responsibility and burden, and that, as we will discover in Chapter 2 and especially Chapter 5, what is referenced as 'bare' legal title is usually regarded as having no value. However, it is also the case that, in absence of a trust, people who are legal owners of property believe, entirely correctly, that their ownership gives them extremely valuable rights. An explanation for this apparent paradox would be to suggest that, in absence of a trust, owners at law hold equitable title as well, and that it is the equitable interest in the property rather than the legal title to it that carries with it the valuable rights of ownership. And, in this context, while the duties of legal ownership are not any different in character, they cease to be burdensome—or even that obvious—when owed by one person to himself rather than to another.

Indeed, earlier editions of this book followed this latter analysis and earlier versions of Figure 1.1 showed the settlor, as the original owner, as being vested with legal title and also equitable title 'before' a trust came into existence. However, in the light of *Westdeutsche*, we must now regard the position as set out by Lord Browne-Wilkinson, that, in the absence of a trust, it is legal title to property that is valuable and all rights pertaining to ownership (the 'bundle of rights' proposition) of the property are embodied in legal title to it. We shall discover (in Chapters 6 and 17 in particular) that Lord Browne-Wilkinson's approach does, however, significantly affect how we analyse respectively resulting trusts and also tracing in equity, because we have to abandon ideas that settlors might simply be able to keep the equitable title to property that they have always had, having parted (only) with legal title to it. But, for present purposes, it does not matter a great deal, and the differences in the 'before and after' diagrams of today and yesteryear are semantic.

1.2.2 Separation of title into distinct ownership: the trust and the requirement of 'something more'

We are already aware that there are actually different types of trust about which we need to learn, and the best starting point for this is to take the simplest type of trust and to explain that the most common scenario for a trust to arise is that in which the legal owner of property makes a declaration—or statement—that the property is to be held on trust for the benefit of a person, or persons. This will most commonly involve transferring legal title of the property to the person(s) intended to act as trustees under the arrangement. Where this happens, the trust is said to be 'constituted', and this establishes that it has been successfully created. However, this is not tantamount to saying that a trust will automatically arise where ownership becomes separated into distinctive legal and equitable title, where the former comes into the hands of the trustee. Although the orthodox view is that a trust will arise whenever ownership is separated, there are factors that are fundamental to the existence of any trust. Centrally, a trust will arise only where the original owner of the trust *intends* for the property to become subject to a trust, and thus intends for a trust to arise.

The significance of an *intention to create* a trust will remain central throughout this study of trusts, in which it will be extremely prominent when we consider the requirements that must be met for creating a valid trust of property, and also (although much less directly so) when we assess the implications of a valid trust in terms of the entitlements of a beneficiary and the responsibilities of trusteeship. When we work through the materials of Chapter 2 and especially Chapter 3, it will become clear that, for a trust to arise, an owner of property must not only intend that another should benefit from the property, but also he must actually intend for this benefit to be delivered by way of a trust and not in any other way that it is also possible to provide enjoyment from property. So intention to create a trust is a central ingredient in what causes ownership of property to separate (in order to create an arrangement that is quite different from other ways of delivering benefits from property).

Operating closely alongside the need for an owner of property to intend to create a trust is a further key ingredient required for bringing a valid trust into existence. In *Westdeutsche*, Lord Browne-Wilkinson stated that the basis for all trusts is *conscience*. This suggests that, while distinctive equitable title will not exist unless and until ownership becomes separated, it is important to understand that the conscience element is central to creating a trust. This is considered in more depth in due course (especially in Chapter 6), but for now we need to understand what the conscience element actually means and why it is such an integral part of being able to tell that a valid trust of property exists.

Again, explanation is offered by Lord Browne-Wilkinson, at 705: 'Equity operates on the conscience of the owner of the legal interest. In … a trust, the conscience of the legal owner requires him to carry out the purposes for which the property was vested in him.'

Anyone who is familiar with equity's operations and its origins will already know that conscience, and indeed 'good conscience', provide its mainstay, and some reminder of this will be given shortly when we consider why equity invented the trust and how it was able to do so. In terms of how and why conscience is the basis for all trusts, very simply this is because, where there is an intention to create a trust of property, this is said to affect the conscience of the person who holds legal title to the property in this arrangement. Equity's 'operation' on, or imposition upon, the conscience of the holder of legal title means that equity requires him to hold property as owner at law on behalf of the owner of the property in equity. This is usually a person who has been selected to act as trustee for this very purpose, but it can also be the original legal owner of property who decides to settle it on trust and also to undertake trusteeship. We can now see that, whoever is acting as trustee, this type of legal ownership held by trustees is quite different from that which is unencumbered by obligations to another and which normally entitles the holder to deal freely with the property. This can be seen by looking back to earlier materials suggesting that, in a trust arrangement, what we normally associate with 'legal ownership' becomes transformed into something else, and this is further reinforced by looking back to the dictionary definitions. which reflect this position in language of 'control' of property and 'nominal ownership' of property.

So, when legal title to property is transferred to another in the presence of an intention to create a trust, this reasoning proposes that a trust actually arises by virtue of the fact that, and precisely because, the conscience of the legal owner is affected. This requires him to hold property as owner at law on behalf of the owner of the property in equity. Usually, the conscience of the legal owner is 'affected' in this way from his undertaking of trusteeship (and its attendant duties), which is voluntary in nature (as explained in Chapter 13, although, as Chapter 5 reveals, there can be some difficulty with this in circumstances in which the settlor is found to have declared himself trustee). However, it is also the case that actual imposition upon the conscience of an individual can arise where legal title, and thus (initially in absence of a trust) ownership of property, has been acquired through inequitable conduct on his part. Greater explanation is given of this latter type of situation in Chapters 6, 8, and 17, where it will become clear that the unconscionable conduct in these situations will actually bring a trust into existence—with the type of trust created a different type from the simplest one for providing benefit at which we are looking here.

1.2.3 The parties who can be identified in a trust arrangement

Some of this description is now getting very technical, because parties who arise in a trust arrangement are starting to be identified, and so the next step is to explain this properly. In turn, this will be followed by explaining *why* an owner of property would choose to make it subject to a trust in order to provide a benefit of it for another, and then some consideration of *how* this is actually possible on account of equity and equitable jurisdiction. But, to explain 'who's who', the owner of property who decides to settle it on trust, rather than to provide its benefits in other ways, becomes a *settlor* of trust property when he does this in order to confer some kind of enjoyment for another.

The person who is the recipient of this generosity is the *beneficiary*, who is the person entitled to the benefit of trust property. When a trust arises and ownership is divided into distinct titles, the beneficiary will own the property *in equity*. Crucially, it is only the beneficiary under a private trust who has *locus standi* to enforce it, to ensure that he can accrue the benefits intended by the settlor. The key to the beneficiary's enjoyment of the trust property is that the *trustee* has responsibility for it. When a trust arises, 'ownership' of the property leaves the settlor and becomes separated into two components: one is equitable title; the other is legal title. Legal title is title at law, which the trustee holds. But this is a different type of holding title from that normally arising from ownership, because in this arrangement a trustee holds this for the benefit of the beneficiary, and incurs a number of responsibilities and duties in respect of this.

In summary, the settlor is the original owner of property (who holds legal title to the property—according to *Westdeutsche*, there is no distinct equitable title to property at this stage) and creates a trust by conveying legal title to it to one or more trustees, manifesting an intention that it is to be held on trust for one or more beneficiaries. Upon this, and in the presence of intention and conscience (*Westdeutsche*), title becomes separated and a trust will arise. The trustees of property become its owners at common law and are given control of the property, but also responsibility for it. Thus trustees hold legal title in furtherance of the entitlements that the beneficiaries are due under the arrangement (the *conscience* element from *Westdeutsche*) and become subject to a number of duties reflecting this.

We shall see that, on account of this, the trustee becomes subject to a number of duties relating to expectations in his conduct in carrying out the trust. On top of this, the relationship between trustee and beneficiary is regulated by its recognition as a fiduciary relationship, which means that there are special rules by which trustees must abide, as well as expectations that they must meet in carrying out the trust. Much more will be said about this in both Chapters 13 and 14, but for now it is sufficient to clarify that legal ownership arising in the context of the trust can be particularly onerous. There are a few further basic points that accompany this simple outline of creating a trust and the terminology attached to the different parties who can be found within the trust arrangement. Making these points also signposts a number of detailed studies in this text and where they occur within it.

Settlors, trustees, and beneficiaries are not necessarily different people. Indeed, in a resulting trust scenario (referenced briefly in Chapter 3, and then considered more extensively in Chapters 6, 7, and also 8), the original owner of property will always become a beneficiary when his property becomes trust property. In other words, settlor and beneficiary are the same person in this situation.

A settlor can validly constitute a trust by declaring himself trustee of his own property on behalf of one or more beneficiaries. It is more usual for him to nominate others specifically for the purpose of being trustees, but, as we will discover in Chapter 5, not only can this happen as a matter of law, but also it does happen.

A trustee may be the sole beneficiary or one of a number of beneficiaries. Indeed, settlors can even be trustees and beneficiaries, and this is normal in the case of trusts arising from the family home, which are considered in Chapter 8.

Once a trust is constituted, the settlor ceases to be part of the arrangement. The law underpinning the successful constitution of a trust is considered in Chapter 3, and the practical effect of it is that the settlor will fall from 'the picture'. Once the trust is constituted, trustees become subject to a number of duties that arise in relation to the trust property and it is only the beneficiary who has the standing to enforce a trust. An original owner may, in practice, remain within the arrangement, but this is where he becomes a trustee or beneficiary, and thus he acquires capacity as a different trust actor.

1.2.4 The reasons for creating a trust: the trust as an alternative to making an outright gift

Earlier materials have suggested that the trust has much in common with the gift mechanism, in as much as both have at heart a benefit for someone whom the owner of property wishes to have such benefit from it. We will learn more about how to make an effective gift in Chapter 2, but we do already know that a gift involves an outright transfer of ownership (through transfer of legal title) from one person to another, and essentially a gift is an outright transfer of ownership of property that is gratuitous (without consideration). Ahead of finding out more about making gifts, we do already know that making gifts can be very straightforward, because it is an activity with which we are all very familiar—as donors and as recipients. At this stage, having only an awareness of this means that we can find out more about the trust and its nature.

Given that the most straightforward types of trust are created to enable the beneficiary to enjoy the property, and we know that trustees hold legal title to the property for this very purpose and become subject to a number of duties in order to ensure this, then why go to all of the trouble of making a trust arrangement? Why not simply give your property to the intended recipient?

As we will find out in Chapter 2, transferring property to another by way of a gift is actually very easy, especially as far as personal chattels are concerned (more requirements attach to making gifts of land and personal intangible property). With this in mind, it will quickly become apparent that there are reasons that are both settlor-oriented and beneficiary-oriented that suggest in favour of creating a trust rather than making a gift.

From the perspective of an *original owner of property*, declaring a trust (and thus becoming a settlor rather than simply a donor) is a useful device for being able to have a say in how your property is used and applied. This is not the case in an out-and-out gift of property to another, and the trust mechanism will thus allow a settlor to exercise some control over what happens to property that is intended to benefit another. The settlor will provide instructions to this effect in a trust arrangement, and this may well be underpinned by seeking to protect a recipient from his own financial fecklessness or it may well be motivated by a desire to ensure wealth remains within a family over successive generations rather than is 'lost'. We will discover in Chapter 2 that this type of arrangement is called a 'family settlement trust', and within this we can see two further advantages in creating a trust rather than making a gift as far as the settlor is concerned: first, the creation of trusts allows the same property to be used to provide benefits for several persons at the same time as making it hard to deal with freely; and second, as we see in Chapter 2, very wealthy people can actually save money through avoiding taxation by giving their property to others, and so there are tax-saving incentives for creating trusts.

From the perspective of a *recipient of property*, creating a trust is a useful device where it is the intention of its owner that someone should be able to benefit from property, but that the beneficiary should remain free of the responsibility that attaches to it. This can be seen both in relation to real property (because houses have to be maintained and any financial liabilities incurred on them have to be satisfied, etc.) and in relation to personal property, which might, for example, take the form of investments that must be looked after.

In addition to giving the intended recipient of property the benefits of property ownership without its responsibilities, the trust arrangement *creates enforceable rights* in relation to the property for the *beneficiary* under a trust. This is very important in terms of the way in which it contrasts with a contractual arrangement. A beneficiary under a trust is not a party to the trust arrangement; this is brought into being where the owner of property transfers title to it to a trustee, or declares himself trustee of the property. This is very significant because, under a contractual arrangement, the doctrine of privity will usually prevent anyone other than one of the contracting parties from enforcing the arrangement. Whilst the Contract (Rights of Third Parties) Act 1999 has mitigated this position in some respects, the creation of a trust has always given third-party enforcement rights to a beneficiary; indeed, it is only a beneficiary who can enforce a trust. The way in which innovation of the trust has traditionally had significance in overcoming the limitations of the doctrine of privity is considered further in Chapter 2.

Much more is said about how the trust 'shapes up' alongside other ways of providing benefits of property for others in Chapter 2. This is where we consider what the trust does and how it works alongside gifts of property, loans of property, and contractual agreements to provide a benefit for third parties. What follows now is some explanation of why equity invented the trust, and how doing so was possible for equity.

1.3 What does the trust owe to equitable jurisdiction and *what is* equitable jurisdiction?

We have suggested that legal title to property is good against the world and that it forms the basis of free dealings with property. In this respect, legal title is a highly visible indicator of property 'belonging' to another. Equitable interests are more complicated: their existence suggests that a holder of legal title does not enjoy all of the rights of ownership, and this is the key to understanding both the reasons for the existence of equitable title and also the difficulties to which holding equitable title to property can lead. Essentially, equitable title to property emerged as a response to the complexities of owning property and the injustices that can be caused by recognizing legal title alone. This, in turn, was possible on account of the historical emergence of equitable jurisdiction from medieval times onwards. Over time, this would give rise to the Court of Chancery, which has historically been administered entirely separately from the courts of common law; these jurisdictions were actually fused only in the late nineteenth century (in the Judicature Acts of 1873–75).

What follows is a brief account of equity's emergence and its historical development, and the emergence of the Court of Chancery. And, for this purpose, regarding legal title to property as good against the world is a sensible starting point because it is as good an illustration as any of the nature and operation of the common law, which equity developed alongside. Today, we can appreciate that equity had an important role as a complementary jurisdiction that was concerned with supporting the subsistence and enforcement of legal rights. This can be seen in the equitable maxim that 'equity follows the law', which has recently been applied by the House of Lords in *Stack* v *Dowden* [2007] UKHL 17, a case that we will encounter in Chapter 8 in relation to trusts and family homes. Anyone who has studied contract or tort law will know that equity is better known for being a more flexible jurisdiction than the common law for those whose legal rights would give them access to certain, but also inflexible, remedies. And equity is perhaps known best for being a jurisdiction focused on mitigating the harshness that can be caused for those who have no rights that law will recognize, and who—without equity's interventions—would be left without a remedy.

But how did all of this happen?

Equity's origins explained and the significance of the Norman Conquest

Because this is a text on trusts, rather than one focused more generally on equity, much of what follows is oriented towards explaining why equity invented the trust and how it achieved what many believe is its ultimate innovation. But, in starting at the beginning, equity's origins can be traced to the system of law that was put in place in England following the Norman Conquest.

The Conquest led to an entirely new system of law being introduced, which evolved into a series of rights and entitlements, and also obligations and responsibilities, which were 'universal'. This was very significant, because law had previously been much more 'localized', and had been formulated from the customs and practices of different tribes. These different groupings were often at war with one another and were 'governed' by quite different customs from one another. This new system put in place following the Norman Conquest was intended to apply to everyone, and was designed to sweep away local custom-based law and to become a universal law 'of the Kingdom'. This would take some considerable time to emerge, but because it was meant to apply to everyone, it became known as the 'common law'—and this is how the term 'common law' originated for 'English law'.

The common law was administered by the Common Law Court within the Royal Court. This reflected the common law as that of the kingdom and that which ultimately stemmed from the king. The Common Law Court heard matters concerning this universal set of rights and entitlements, and obligations and responsibilities, which were brought before the king, and this was all that the Court would 'hear'. The common law recognized only these universal rights 'at [common] law' as ones that governed relations between persons, and also as between individuals and the Crown, and so the only disputes that the Court would hear were those attaching to this emerging universal code.

This universal set of rights and entitlements, and obligations and responsibilities, which sought to put in place a 'certain' position that would apply to everyone, would be embodied in rights and entitlements, and obligations and responsibilities, across a number of spheres of 'interest'. And it sought to govern different 'interactions' both between individuals, and between an individual and the Crown.

From the earliest days of the common law, it became clear that, just because the common law applied *to* everyone, this did not mean that it would be respected *by* everyone—hence the function of the King's Court to hear disputes arising as a result. And so a set of responses or remedies grew up around these rights and entitlements, obligations and responsibilities, as they themselves emerged. These were for situations in which the King's Court was satisfied that one party had acted in breach of what the common law said he must or must not do by way of another's common law position. As a reflection of the nature of the common law, it made sense that the remedies administered for these matters brought before the Court produced universal and certain outcomes to accompany universal and certain rights and obligations.

As a result of these remedies being certain—by virtue of being universal—they were also rigid and inflexible. For example, any student of law will know that an award of damages is the usual remedy for a breach of contract, or the commission of a tort against a person or his property. Here, the damages award assumes that what the claimant has suffered as a result of his rights being breached by another can be compensated by means of a monetary payment being made by that other and, as any student of law also knows, while this will be the case in a number of situations, it will not always be what the aggrieved party actually wants.

But, even in the early days of the common law, it was recognized that remedies at common law had limitations, as well as advantages, flowing from being applicable to everyone. So there emerged the right to petition the king directly when a decision of the Common Law Court was considered unfair or unjust. Thus the office of King's Chancellor was created, in order to hear petitions presented to the king in this way. And it was from the powerful nature of this office that a system of 'discretion', which was distinct from the operation of the common law, was able to evolve.

1.3.1 The powers of the Chancellor and his exercise of discretion: how equity appeared

Essentially, the Chancellor became prepared to act in such a way notwithstanding that the common law was, of course, intended to apply to everyone. This was because, as a result of hearing petitions to the king, it came to be recognized that the strict application of (the universally applicable) common law could be inflexible and could cause significant hardship to some who became caught up in the common law's universal reach—and also its universal limitations. It was in these circumstances that the Chancellor came to use the powers and discretions attaching to his office to impose on the conscience of an individual. The Chancellor was able to be extremely powerful on account of the fact that—through hearing petitions made to the king—this office carried a number of powers and discretions, which were those of the Royal Court and which could be used against subjects as such. These were associated with issuing royal writs, acting against individuals, and even enforcing orders against them with imprisonment. Today, we can see this in the way in which contempt of court is underpinned with the power of imprisonment.

This would require that individual to act in ways that would produce a 'just outcome', which the particular circumstances called for. Originally, the office of Chancellor was an ecclesiastical post, which does explain the early emphasis of 'good conscience' for responses to the common law's certain, but inflexible, determinations. Over time, it became a role occupied by lawyers, and this discretionary use of power developed into a special court to deal with these special petitions; by the fifteenth century, the Court of Chancery was born.

It should be becoming clear that, surrounding the emergence of the common law as a set of cogent rules, equity's role appeared to be concerned with remedying failures of process. Chancellors would see themselves as perfecting the human defects of process that could arise at common law, by focusing on a person's conscience to achieve an outcome that was just. Here, equity's focus on the conscience of an individual ensured that there was no need for the formalism and technicality characteristic of the common law (which was itself still actively developing). It was also responsive to individual circumstances and, moreover, a Chancery decree would bind only parties to the suit—hence references to equity as a 'personal' jurisdiction.

This provided the foundations of equity on the basis that the Chancellor became prepared to use his powers and discretions to prevent injustice from arising in encounters between persons, across the spheres of 'interest' governed by the common law. This was made so by his mandating that someone who committed a 'wrong' must act in a particular way towards another affected by the wrong. The Chancellor achieved this through what is known as 'imposing on the conscience' of such a person.

1.3.2 From exercise of discretion 'ad hoc' towards a more formalized 'system' of equity

This recognition of the limitations of remedies at law led to equity developing its own remedies, which were not available at common law, and also a number of distinctive principles and doctrines that would inform how these different approaches should operate alongside the common law. However, these 'alternatives' were intended to be applied only in individual circumstances and would always be discretionary outcomes—that is, there was no entitlement to equity's interventions. This was because this alternative jurisdiction was supposed to reflect individual circumstances without affecting the universal position at law that applied to everyone.

To reflect this, equity's jurisdiction started off being ad hoc in nature—precisely because it was focused on providing an alternative where this was called for in individual circumstances without changing the universal position. Indeed, in many ways, it remains a 'personal' jurisdiction—that is, exercised against individuals in particular circumstances, where doing so is called for—which means that it also continues to be characterized by discretion. Indeed, the two jurisdictions continued to be administered separately until the late nineteenth century. Equity did gradually become more formalized, but the principles for granting 'relief' in equity remain largely unaltered even though the two jurisdictions of law and equity are now actually fused, and were so by the Judicature Acts of 1873–75.

But, in the early days of the Court of Chancery, although the Chancellor's power could in principle be exercised without altering the substance of the common law in question, the practical result of his jurisdiction was that the exercise of common law rights was affected significantly. Indeed, in the light of the Chancellor's ability to refuse to issue a writ to a claimant at common law, or to compel conveyance of property by its owner to someone else, scope for conflict between the two systems became manifest. But this would not emerge until much later; in equity's early days, the common law was itself not very clearly defined.

In the modern law, one of the reasons why equity remains very faithful to its historical origins in terms of operation, as well as purpose, is because retaining these early features has been necessary for it to avoid actual conflict with law. It is not difficult to see why equity would want to try to achieve justice for those who have no rights that 'the law' will recognize, and thus no access to actions or remedies at law. It is also easy to see why equity might try to provide flexibility for those who *do* have legal rights. But equity has also had to evolve in the context in which the common law originated in seeking to provide universal legal rights and obligations that were fundamental to the law of the kingdom. There was a significant debate during the nineteenth century, when law and equity fought for supremacy, and today modern equity does 'follow the law'. The twelve key 'maxims' of equity, and a number of principles that have emerged from them, reflect both equity's more formalized—and less ad hoc—operations and also the way in which it interfaces with law. They are central to the nature of equitable jurisdiction today, and for understanding *how* this is exercised and *to whom*, and *what* equity can actually do in the face of a wrong, which does in itself provide important insight into how equity governs its relationship with law—and they are as follows.

(1) Equity will not suffer a wrong without a remedy.

(2) Equity follows the law.

(3) Where there is equal equity, the law shall prevail.

(4) Where the equities are equal, the first in time shall prevail.

(5) He who seeks equity must do equity.

(6) He who comes to equity must come with clean hands.

(7) Delay defeats equity.

(8) Equality is equity.

(9) Equity looks to the intent rather than the form.

(10) Equity looks on that as done which ought to be done.

(11) Equity imputes an intention to fulfil an obligation.

(12) Equity acts *in personam*.

Although only these twelve are usually regarded as the definitive equitable maxims, equity has developed additional principles, which may be treated to all intents and purposes as if they numbered among the maxims. The following may not be an exhaustive list, but all of these principles will appear again in the book (bearing in mind that the language of these maxims and principles appears to vary slightly between different authorities).

(i) The principle that 'equity will not assist a volunteer' is fundamental to the discussion in Chapter 5, which relates to the constitution of trusts and the effecting of gifts.

(ii) Also at the heart of Chapter 5 is the mantra that 'equity will not perfect an imperfect gift'.

(iii)   The way in which 'equity will not construe a valid power out of an invalid trust' has very strong references to materials in Chapters 2 and 3, which reveal the nature of the trust, and also the conditions that must be satisfied in order for a valid trust to exist.

(iv)   That 'equity will not permit the provisions of a statute intended to prevent fraud to be used as an instrument for fraud' will be explained in materials relating to formality requirements for trusts, in Chapters 4 and 6, and this accommodates the need for a trust to operate in certain situations in which this might be difficult to achieve, as illustrated in Chapters 8 and 9.

(v)   The way in which 'equity will not permit a trust to fail for want of a trustee' is a theme that runs throughout this text in some form or another, and particularly in Chapters 3 and 13.

1.4 A brief reference to equitable remedies today—leading into equity's development of the trust

Although this is a text on trusts, it is useful to get a more general sense of equity's remedies and how different they are from those subsisting at common law. We will discover that many are personal ones, which can be applied against a specific individual in response to specific circumstances. As equity developed its own remedies, their first signature feature was not being available at common law, and equity would not administer common law remedies. However, the Common Law Procedure Act 1854 gave the common law courts some jurisdiction to give equitable remedies, and the Chancery Amendment Act 1858 would enable the Court of Chancery to award the common-law-derived remedy of damages, but only in addition to, or in substitution for, an equitable remedy. The courts would become fused in the latter part of the nineteenth century, but the principles governing equitable remedies were not affected by this and remain largely unchanged.

The equitable remedies with which we are most likely to be familiar are the *injunction* and also *specific performance*. For those that apply more specifically in breaches occurring in the context of trusteeship, there is discussion of breach of fiduciary duty and the *remedy of account* (in Chapters 13 and 16), and sometimes equity imposes a *constructive trust* (see Chapters 6, 8, 9, and 17). This text is more focused on those remedies available for breaches of obligations arising in equity for trustees and for those whom equity deems to treat as if they were trustees (such as those considered in Chapters 13, 16, and 17), including injunctions (in Chapter 13, for example, we see the use of injunctions to prevent the misuse of confidential information). But, for now, we do need to be aware of the significance of encountering, for example, specific performance in contract law, and also injunctions across a number of torts, especially in so-called 'continuing torts' such as nuisance and trespass.

Materials on the Online Resource Centre explain how special types of injunction can be involved in the protection of property and also in recovery of property from those who should not have it.

The discretionary nature of equitable remedies
The damages award for breach of contract or commission of a tort illustrates that the major difference between the two systems is that whereas common law remedies are available as of right, equitable remedies retain the discretionary nature of early equitable

jurisdiction. Although the creation of wholly new equitable rights and principles has been curtailed over the last two centuries on account of equity becoming more of a defined system, and one increasingly defined by precedent, its remedies remain discretionary, notwithstanding that discretion is exercised according to fairly clear and even rigid principles. The discretionary nature of the remedies can lead to dire consequences, because if an equitable estate or interest depends on the award of an equitable remedy, a refusal to grant the remedy effectively destroys the interest.

A common ground for refusal of a remedy is the behaviour of the party claiming the equitable remedy, because 'he who comes into equity must come with clean hands'. This can be seen in *Coatsworth* v *Johnson* (1886) 54 LT 520, CA, in which the claimant was in possession of land under a contract for a lease, where no lease that would be recognized at common law had been executed. The landlord in fact turned the claimant out, and the claimant sued for trespass. He would have won the action had he been regarded as a lessee, either at common law or in equity. Indeed, according to *Walsh* v *Lonsdale*, equity would normally regard the claimant as being an equitable lessee, but this particular tenant was already in breach of various covenants under the agreement. Thus the Court of Appeal refused to grant the equitable remedy and the claimant actually *lost his interest*. This then forced him to pursue the common law, which, because he had no lease at common law, meant that he lost altogether. This case thus illustrates the discretionary nature of equity's jurisdiction and remedies, while emphasizing the need to treat common law and equitable rights and remedies separately. It also shows that an entire interest can be lost where an equitable remedy is refused.

Much more is said about the general nature of equitable remedies in the materials relating to specific performance and injunctions that can be found on the Online Resource Centre.

1.4.1 Beyond *in personam*: how equity evolved beyond its origins and early rationale

That equity remains, at heart, a personal jurisdiction is embodied as one of the maxims, but this is not exclusively so. And, in focusing on the trust, much of this text's commentary on the trust and 'trusts law' reflects the particular nature of equity's development in relation to property. Over time, equity appreciated that some 'injustices' arising from recognizing only legal rights to property would be appropriately remedied by a specific mandate for a given individual in response to the particular circumstances, but that others would not be so.

This is how the trust evolved from equity's roots in good conscience and justice to give rights in equity that are more like common law rights in terms of who is bound by them. Understanding this requires understanding how the changes to English law brought about by the Norman Conquest applied to land—which is where we see the first trusts being developed.

Following the Conquest, William's attempts to assert supremacy over England's landowners met with resistance, and so he responded by confiscating all land in the wake of his victory. He then allowed land to be held by others in exchange for money or services. It remains today that *all* land is technically owned by the Crown, which remains supreme landlord, and thus those who 'own' land actually, strictly, own an interest in 'their' land. Under this new 'feudal' system, land could be held through a complex tenancy hierarchy whereby dues would be collected for the Crown, and this was achieved through a network of lords and 'overlords'. Overlords (sometimes called 'mesne lords') were able to hold land directly from the king, and rights at law to the land cascaded down to ordinary tenants.

Glossing over a great deal of the detail of the feudal dues, which comprised money and services for which holding land was exchanged, the early forerunner of the trust called 'the Use' emerged from the very strict dealings with land that characterized this system. For example, whenever land was succeeded by an heir, a payment fell due on this event, and where a tenant died without an heir, the land would revert to the lord, and a lord would have certain rights and entitlements where land was held by a minor. As long as any feudal dues remained valuable, the lords desired to protect them, and rules about title to land at common law were developed to aid this process. Many entitlements to property for the lords (particularly dues) that arose on the death of a tenant—especially in situations in which there was no heir or the heir was a minor—could be avoided by conveying the land to younger adult members of the family, or leaving the land by will. For this reason, taxes were imposed on conveyances, and until 1540 freehold estates could not be left by will, and rights and entitlements to land could, by law, pass only from a holder to his eldest son. The consequences of this protectionism were that it was virtually impossible to make provision for children, other than an eldest son, and even for a widow. And given that land could not be left by will initially, when flexibility was developed, it was so left through the 'conveyance route', which made it possible (although very costly) for a holder of rights in land to make a disposition (from the word 'disposal') of them whilst he was still alive.

We will come to understand that this is referenced in legal language as an '*inter vivos* transfer', and that what started to happen in the light of common law rules surrounding succession and inheritance was that tenants could provide for others whom they had in mind by conveying entitlements to altogether different persons, who became holders or owners 'by conveyance', and the original tenant would lose his legal entitlements to the land. Because of their status in communities and their positions of trust, it was common for clerics or religious orders to become owners by conveyance, and later this role also became occupied by attorneys. This is because these others would hold the property, which would then be 'to the Use' of the person(s) for whom the tenant wished to provide. Commonly, the person 'to Use' the property would initially be the tenant himself (who would still need to 'use' the property even though he no longer had legal entitlement to it); then use of the property would fall to his widow; and following her death it could come to the use of all of his children. This was possible on account of rules of survivorship attaching to joint tenancies in land, and many accounts of the emergence of the Use explain that an important catalyst for it was that many men fighting in the Crusades wished for their land to he held safely whilst they were away for years at a time.

Many Crusaders would not return at all, of course, and a transfer of title by conveyance would help to protect the position of his family in these circumstances; many decisions to do this will have been made from a generalized appreciation of short life expectancy. Because what was being done as far as legal title was concerned was permissible by common law rules, the common law position relating to transfers of rights in property was theoretically unaffected by this. At the same time, equity recognized this arrangement and would enforce it by, if necessary, imposing on the conscience of those to whom the property had been conveyed. This would be able to force the use of the land to be given to those whom the tenant wished to have it. These persons became known as *cestui que use*.

There are also a number of accounts of the way in which transfers of title by conveyance became a way of avoiding dues—or taxes—that would automatically fall on a holder's death and transfer of his entitlements to his eldest son. This regime was underpinned by common law rules that were very focused on retaining value attaching to land for the Crown (through this system of payment of dues and services for privi-leges), and was being undermined by the conveyance transfer. This is why Henry VIII famously banned the Use in the Statute of Uses passed in 1535, mindful to bolster transfer dues to fund his ever-hungry 'War Chest'. The Statute of Uses achieved this by looking only at an original holder and at the person who was to have the Use of the property, and ignoring those to whom the conveyance was being made to achieve this. The practical result of this was that it became impossible to transfer property to someone for the purpose of benefiting someone different. In other words, it became impossible to transfer title to land with the obligation to use it in a particular way for someone different.

From 'the Use of' to held 'on trust': the appearance of the modern trust

It was from these origins that the modern trust would start to emerge from around 1700, as equity became determined to produce a mechanism whereby a holder of legal title to property could be compelled to use it for others intended to benefit. This person, known as the *cestui que use*, became known as the *cestui qui trust* to reflect and accom-pany the way in which property became held 'in trust' for rather than for 'use of' the property. In turn, the holder of legal title became known as the 'trustee' to reflect this, and the *cestui que trust* became recognized as the owner of this property in equity—or its equitable owner. The basic rationale remains the same: to separate out enjoyment of property from its ownership, and to ensure that this happens by imposing duties upon the owner of legal title to the property.

The Use shows us that, from an early stage in equity's development, it became possible to impose on the conscience of a legal owner of property to ensure that those without entitlements to this property at law, and whose claims to the property law would not recognize, would not be disadvantaged. It was also recognized that the efficacy of this arrangement would depend upon those who would understand that its intention was to benefit others who might otherwise be victims of injustices arising from the common law recognizing only legal rights. This is why legal title was transferred to persons such as clerics and lawyers, on account of their standing and integrity. These two key ideas—of an arrangement that could benefit otherwise vulnerable persons, and that this could be achieved only where those who hold legal title recognize the position of others—would over time form the core tenets of trusts law that accompanied the development of the 'trust arrangement' into its modern formulation. Appreciating this becomes very important in due course, but for now we need to think about just what equity's willing-ness to impose on consciences of individuals who held property for the use of others actually enabled equity to do for these persons. This is, of course, that equity was able to create a special type of ownership of property for them: the type of title to property that arises when ownership of it becomes separated.

1.4.2 A beneficiary's ownership of trust property

A beneficiary's equitable ownership of trust property is not, of course, the only enti-tlement to or interest in property that can exist alongside others' legal ownership of property or legal entitlements to or interests in it. And today we see a range of interven-tions from equity, which tell us, on occasion, that equity will regard a purely personal response as that which achieves the just outcome in the circumstances. For example, there are 'equities' or 'mere equities', which we will discover are entitlements to prop-erty that are quite different from a beneficiary's equitable interest. This can be seen, for example, in the 'deserted wife's equity' (as in *National Provincial Bank Ltd* v *Ainsworth*

[1965] AC 1175), and the right to have a transaction set aside on grounds of fraud or undue influence (such as in *Barclays Bank* v *O'Brien* [1994] 1 AC 80 and *Royal Bank of Scotland* v *Etridge* (2001) 4 All ER 449). Although these are entitlements to property, they are not true interests in property itself. This can be contrasted with the way in which equity has also evolved interests in property that are intended to be universal in their reach in a way that has more in common with the essence of the common law than equity's *in personam* origins and operations.

We know that, under a trust arrangement, a beneficiary holds equitable title to the 'trust property' and is thus regarded as the equitable owner of this property. To achieve this, equity has had to adopt features of the common law in terms of rights and entitlements that are ones at law. In turn, this required equity to evolve beyond its personal operations to an extent that is considerable, and this has also meant equity evolving beyond its traditional character as a discretionary jurisdiction. These lengths reflected a spectrum of perceived seriousness of injustice capable of arising in relation to property; in some cases, it has required equipping claimants with a more certain position of their entitlement, and one that subsisted against more than one person.

From the days of the Use, which arose from discretions exercised by the Chancellor in the King's Court during medieval times, the modern trust embodies equity's protection against injustices arising from the ownership of property by separating out the benefit of property from its ownership. We now consider how equity ensures that legal owners of property do not use property in ways that will disadvantage those who do not have rights to it that the law will recognize.

In terms of understanding how a beneficiary under a trust came to be regarded as an owner of property in equity, we can see this through appreciating how equity originally sought to separate out the enjoyment of property from its formal ownership. From the very beginning, this was through *imposing on the conscience* of those who hold legal title to property in circumstances in which they needed to be mindful of others in how that property was used. Over time, impositions upon conscience have become hardened into duties to which owners of property become subject where a trust subsists, and also into rights that someone other than him can acquire. Most interestingly for us, the trust illustrates how equity's formulation of these entitlements of a beneficiary means that they not only apply to the original owner of property, but also to others who might acquire legal title where property is passed from one person to another. We can reason such entitlements as being different from ones that are *personal* against a particular defendant, and being instead rights and entitlements to the *property* itself.

Understanding the significance of equity's creation of the trust: the scope of equitable interests in property

This requires us to look at what are known as 'rights *in rem*'—that is, real rights and not ones that are simply a discretionary response against a particular individual—and at how equity has created these. Rights *in rem* are actually capable of interfering with legal rights and they are capable of affecting a number of persons. The equitable ownership of property under a trust is one such example of this: it *is* the 'paradigm' example in any case, but because this is primarily a text on trusts, it is the one on which we focus.

Equity's recognition of a beneficiary's ownership of trust property as a right *in rem* means that equitable ownership of property under a trust is potentially 'good against'—or enforceable against—persons other than an original legal owner of property. It is a world away from equity's personal jurisdictional activity, and allows a beneficiary to enjoy rights relating to property that are more like the universal rights conferred by law. We have talked briefly about why equity did this—recognizing that this was central for responding to some injustices—and now we need to think about how equity was *able* to do this, and also think about how we know that this is the case. This is important given what we have also said about legal title being at the heart of rights to property and the value of property, and also equity's own governance of its relationship with law. Thus we need to look more closely at the implications of equity creating entitlements that create real property rights for a claimant in property belonging to another.

1.5 Equity's development of real rights in property for those without legal title

In a way that is too abstract to appreciate now, but which will be a central theme as we discover more about trusts and trusts law, equity will not lightly come to the view that someone who owns property at law must share rights to it with someone who does not—and perhaps especially rights of ownership. Most of the time, equity will act on this only where this *should* happen because it is extremely clear that a holder of legal title has it only for the purposes of controlling and managing property for another. In short, equity will do this only where it is very clear that a trust is intended and that the conscience of a holder of legal title is affected as a result. This is the simplest type of trust that we have referenced up to now, and we will also find out (in Chapter 6, with hints in earlier chapters) that trusts can arise without their creation being intended—but, again, we will see that there are limits to when equity will deem it appropriate for a trust to be 'imposed'. Again, English law is very strongly focused on framing this by having due regard to the position of ownership within English law, which (ordinarily) regards title at law as the king of property rights.

In discussions that follow about when equity will deem it appropriate for someone other than a legal owner to 'own' property, we will consider the normative issues concerning whether equity makes too much deference to ownership at law. But we need to bear in mind that as equity evolved, and developed its own governance and remedies, it had to be careful not to conflict with law, which as we know became more tricky as the common law itself developed beyond infancy into maturity. In relation to property, this meant seeking to prevent and respond to injustices, whilst having due regard to the 'bundle of rights' embodied in ownership at law, rather than undermining these universal entitlements.

Authority that equity can create rights to property for a claimant that are property rights in the true sense (and thus equitable rights as rights *in rem*) is found in the key House of Lords decision in *Foskett* v *McKeown* [2000] 3 All ER 97. According to Lord Browne-Wilkinson at 109, in relation to equitable title to property under a trust:

> It is a fundamental error to think that, because certain property rights are equitable rather than legal, such rights are in some way discretionary. This case does not depend on whether it is fair, just and reasonable to give the purchasers an interest as a result of which the court in its discretion provides a remedy. It is a case of hard-nosed property rights.

As a result of this, he held that 'equitable interests are also enforceable against whoever for the time being holds those assets'.

1.5.1 **Are equitable rights *in rem* as good as 'legal rights'?**

However, *Foskett* also tells us that all equitable rights, even 'hard-nosed' ones that do not arise as a matter of discretion, 'are enforceable against whoever for the time being *holds those assets other than someone who is a bona fide purchaser for value of the legal interest without notice* or a person who claims through such a purchaser'.

The 'bona fide purchaser': how the rule explains the significance of notice for all equitable entitlements to property

What this means is that the holder of an interest in property in equity is more vulnerable than one who holds a legal interest in property because his rights can only ever bind everyone 'except the bona fide purchaser [of the legal interest] for value [provides consideration] and without notice [of the equitable interests]'. So equitable interests in property can be extinguished or defeated where legal title to the property is transferred to someone who provided value for this, and who did not know of the existence of these other interests. All equitable interests in property are subject to the rule, even those that are 'hard-nosed' and whose existence does not depend on being 'fair, just, and reasonable'. However, there are conditions that must be satisfied for this to happen. This means that there are conditions to be met before a holder of an equitable interest in property will lose this interest on account of a purchaser of legal title being one who is protected by the rule. It is worth stressing that we shall see this rule as it applies to the purchase of legal title to property, but in principle it applies to providing value for any legal interest in property and not simply legal title: for example, this would apply to a lender's interest in trust property that has been wrongfully pledged by a trustee as security for a personal loan to him on which he then defaults. Equally, it is not only a beneficiary's entitlements to property under a trust arrangement that fall subject to this rule, and in relation to property that is land an *equitable* lease or easement, or a restrictive covenant, is something that can, in principle, be defeated by a bona fide purchaser.

In terms of what must be satisfied before a purchaser can be deemed to be protected by the rule, one of the conditions rests on what he must provide in the way of value for the legal title that he is purchasing, which is considered shortly. We will now consider what must be fulfilled so that a purchaser can establish that he is one 'without notice' of the equitable interests that also subsist in the property. These are considerations of how these equitable interests of others can be 'known' about, and how knowledge or 'notice' of them can be acquired by another.

Although all equitable interests in or entitlements to property are, in principle, subject to the bona fide purchase rule, in practice this is now far less important than it once was. This rule provided the basis for the so-called 'doctrine of notice', which governed dealings with property and which, for transactions relating to land, has largely been superseded with requirements of registration. And, in relation to dealings with other types of property, *BCCI* v *Akindele* [2000] 3 WLR 1423 is authority that there is little place for the notice doctrine in dealings with personal property in commercial dealings. But in terms of understanding the essence of the bona fide purchaser rule, which is still very significant for a beneficiary's ownership of trust property (and its extension of this to others by way of concurrent jurisdiction, as explained in Chapter 17), essentially, to take property free from equitable interests, the purchaser must have not had:

- actual notice of the equitable rights subsisting;
- constructive notice of the equitable rights—that which would be gleaned if all usual enquiries and investigations appropriate to purchases of property of a particular nature had been carried out; and

- notice that is imputed to the purchaser—any actual notice or that which is constructive of a person working for the purchaser (such as his solicitor).

1.5.2 Explaining the significance of notice requirements

We will explore the bona fide purchaser rule more as it applies to trusts in Chapter 17, bearing in mind that much of the detail of it belongs to the law of real property. But by way of illustrating both its history and also its significance for studying the law of trusts, reference is now made to a very old case called *Cave* v *Cave* (1880) 15 ChD 639. *Cave* also illustrates for us why, at a very early stage, the modern law of trusts had to evolve in ways that are mindful of dishonest trustees. In this context, this is to help us to foster an appreciation that although equitable interests in property can be very strong, they are ultimately less so than legal interests, and that we will need to ask ourselves why this is the case.

In *Cave* v *Cave*, Charles Cave, as sole trustee and family solicitor, stole trust money and purchased a house with it. As a result of this transaction, the moneys in the trust fund were converted into land, so that the beneficiaries of the fund became beneficiaries of the land. The fraudulent trustee/solicitor then raised money by way of legal mortgage at a time when a legal mortgage took effect by way of a conveyance of the entire freehold estate to the mortgagee, with a covenant to reconvey the property to the mortgagor if the money loaned, plus interest and administration charges, were repaid to the mortgagee on a fixed date. When these conditions were met, equity enforced this covenant and also allowed the mortgagor to demand a later reconveyance, subject to repayment of the capital loaned, plus interest and administration charges. Here, the mortgagee obtained legal title, and he also provided value, in the form of the money advanced. Accordingly, Fry J held that he had no notice of the beneficiaries' interest. There was no suggestion that the mortgagee was acting in bad faith, and he was therefore a bona fide purchaser of the legal estate for value without notice of the beneficiaries' equitable interests, so legal title passed to the mortgagee free of encumbrance. This is because Charles Cave acted as solicitor for both the mortgagor and the mortgagee, and obviously he knew the truth, but Fry J held that his notice would not be imputed to the mortgagee since he was party to a fraud.

1.5.3 Conditions attached to the doctrine of notice: equity and the 'purchaser for value'

For a third party to take free of an equitable interest in property, the purchase must be one for 'value'. Value includes not only consideration recognized at common law, but also equitable consideration. Thus, for example, as well as value in terms of money or money's worth (recognized as consideration by both systems), equity also recognizes a future marriage as consideration (which is explained in Online Resource Centre materials for Chapter 5) and so it constitutes value for the purposes of the bona fide purchaser rule. On the other hand, the common law allows contracts under seal to be enforced even in the absence of consideration; equity does not take the same view, and such contracts do not provide value for the purposes of this rule (nor incidentally can such contracts be enforced using equitable remedies). Where the value is money, the purchaser must pay all of the money before receiving notice of the equitable interest.

1.5.4 The bona fide purchaser rule: why develop real rights subject to such a (really big) limitation?

Legal rights are universal and 'bind the world', and so legal title to property is the 'ultimate' property right, and operation of the so-called 'bona fide purchaser rule' means that those who hold equitable rights will not have entitlements to property that are as strong. This means that, on occasion, the interests of legal ownership will trump those who equity has deemed deserving of real rights, because the circumstances are such that the rights of the legal owner will prevail. Determining this is not easy, and we will touch on normative considerations arising from competing interests in property at points in this text. As far as this rule is concerned, it reflects that, by their nature, equitable interests in property are not as 'visible' as legal ones, which are created formally in ways that law prescribes and will recognize. As we know, in most situations it will be clear who owns property, but, as you will discover, it will not always be clear that someone is a beneficiary under a trust of that property. This means that it will not always be clear to a purchaser that legal title being held is *bare legal title* held by a trustee rather than outright 'ownership', given that those who hold legal title to property are ordinarily those who are vested with all rights of ownership. In these circumstances, those who are seeking to pass property to others have every interest in representing that they hold all rights of ownership, which is what a purchaser is giving value for. Sometimes, this will not be the case, and although the person who is seeking to do this knows it is not the case, the purchaser will not. Beyond the medieval period and into early modern times, the economy started to transform, and because of this property, including land, became a commodity to be bought and sold, and not simply something passed between generations.

In these circumstances, equity does, of course, wish to protect those who might be disadvantaged because they hold no legal rights in property that was intended to be used for their benefit—but given that equity is concerned with good conscience and justice, those who purchase property in good faith need to be sure that they are buying what they think they are buying. Thus equitable property rights, including 'hard-nosed' rights *in rem*, all developed subject to this significant limitation. This is because holding legal title to property provides the basis of free dealings with property, and thus represents the key to the value of property in capitalist societies. As you will discover later (especially in Chapter 17), equity has also developed responses for those whose equitable interests in property are actually lost; for now, referencing this underscores that they *can be* lost—and a beneficiary's equitable ownership of property will be lost if legal title to it comes into the hands of a 'bona fide purchaser'.

1.5.5 Rights in law, equity, and illegality: *Tinsley* v *Milligan* and *Rowan* v *Dann*

If all of this suggests that the doctrine of notice is a significant limitation of the strength of equitable rights that are rights *in rem*, then the case of *Tinsley* v *Milligan* [1994] 1 AC 340 gives us a different perspective. This case shows us that the 'hard-nosed property rights', as termed by the House of Lords in *Foskett* v *McKeown* [2001] 1 AC 102, subsist for those who hold them not simply regardless of what might be fair, just, and reasonable, but actually in circumstances in which their holder has behaved in ways that are contrary to equity's operating principles.

In this case, Stella Tinsley and Kathleen Milligan jointly purchased a home, which was registered in Tinsley's name alone. On the principles set out in Chapter 6 (and also discussed in Chapter 8), the beneficial interest would have been shared between Tinsley and Milligan in equal shares—but, to both Tinsley's and Milligan's knowledge, the home was registered in Tinsley's name alone to enable Milligan to make false claims to the Department of Social Security for benefits. After a quarrel, Tinsley moved out and claimed possession from Milligan. Milligan counterclaimed, seeking a declaration that the house was held by Tinsley on trust for both of them in equal shares. Tinsley argued that Milligan's claim was barred by the common law doctrine *ex turpi causa non oritur actio* and by the principle that 'he who comes to equity must come with clean hands'.

The House of Lords held (Lord Keith and Lord Goff dissenting) that, because the presumption of resulting trust applied (see Chapter 6), Milligan could establish her equitable interest without relying on the illegal transaction and was therefore entitled to succeed. The case supports the analysis, which was subsequently made in *Foskett* v *McKeown*, that Milligan's resulting trust interest was a property interest in its own right, which had an existence that was independent of the precise arrangement between the couple. In the context of this discussion of equity's innovation and modern recognition of rights to property that are rights *in rem*, had Milligan held no more than a collection of personal rights against Tinsley, then her claim would surely have failed. This is because, in these circumstances, she would have been unable to assert those rights without disclosing her fraud. Indeed, Lord Browne-Wilkinson went so far as to say, at 371:

> More than 100 years have elapsed since the fusion of the administration of law and equity. The reality of the matter is that, in 1993, English law has one single law of property made up of legal and equitable interests. Although for historical reasons legal estates and equitable estates have differing incidents, the person owning either type of estate has a right of property, a right *in rem* not merely a right *in personam*. If the law is that a party is entitled to enforce a property right acquired under an illegal transaction, in my judgment the same rule ought to apply to any property right so acquired, whether such right is legal or equitable.

The suggestions made in this statement that equitable property rights are strong even in the face of illegality does have scope to bring the law of property into conflict with criminal law, and also equity into conflict with law, notwithstanding Lord Browne-Wilkinson's view to the contrary. But, in this context, *Tinsley* and the decision of the Court of Appeal in *Rowan* v *Dann* (1992) P & CR 202 did provide for us, some time before *Foskett* v *McKeown*, an important statement that some equitable rights do also have the characteristics of rights *in rem*.

1.6 The emergence of the modern trust and the emergence of 'trusts law': an introduction to Chapter 2

The beneficiary's equitable ownership of trust property is the paradigm illustration of how equitable rights to property are capable of being rights *in rem*, and attention will now be focused on understanding more about the trust, and the significance and scope of 'trusts law'. This commences in Chapter 2, which introduces how and where trusts can be found in society and the economy in the twenty-first century, and will explain for us how understanding the 'timeline' for the appearance of the modern trust can help us to understand the modern trusts law that is the subject of study in this text.

Revision Box

1. Ensure that you can answer the following questions.
   (a) How did distinctive 'equitable jurisdiction' develop within English law?
   (b) What was the impetus for equity's development?
   (c) What was the special court administering equity called and when did equitable juris-diction cease to be administered separately from the common law courts?
   (d) From your reading so far, what kind of things does equitable jurisdiction appear to do?
   (e) In what ways is the operation of modern equity both similar to and also different from its early origins?
   (f) What is the significance of the so-called 'maxims' of equity?

2. From this, consider the following scenarios referenced in this chapter.
   (a) The doctrine of proprietary estoppel, which seeks to prevent a person going back on a representation made to another in relation to property on which the other person has been relied
   (b) The doctrine of promissory estoppel, which seeks to prevent a contracting party from reneging on his promise not to enforce his legal rights (such as seeking full payment due under the contract) upon which the other party has relied
   (c) The doctrine of undue influence, which seeks to prevent a party from exerting im-proper pressure on another in the formulation of legal agreements
   (d) The 'deserted wife's equity', under which a wife's a right to occupy a family home arises from particular circumstances
   (e) The personal remedy of specific performance, when one contracting party is un-willing to perform his contractual obligations
   (f) The use of an injunction to prevent 'wrongdoing' on the part of an individual

In relation to each one:

- identify the 'injustices' and/or inflexibility that recognizing only legal rights and/or accessing only remedies at law may present;
- think about the difficulties that might arise from equity intervening in these circum-stances to provide a more just/flexible outcome; and
- think about the particular problems that might arise where third parties—those other than the individual defendant and the claimant seeking equity—are potentially affected.

FURTHER READING

Hayton (2001) 'Developing the obligation characteristic of the trust' 117 Law Quarterly Review 96.

Parkinson (2002) 'Reconceptualising the express trust' 61 Cambridge Law Journal 657.

Todd (1981) 'Estoppel licences and third party rights' Conveyancer 347.

 online resource centre

For summaries of a selection of these articles, please visit <http://www.oxfordtextbooks.co.uk/orc/wilson_trusts11e/>

2

The nature of the trust: its operation and applications in society and the economy

It will become apparent shortly that the trust is put to a variety of uses in English law, and also that this is possible because of its special feature of dividing ownership of property into distinct legal and equitable title. To reiterate the key point made in Chapter 1, a trust involves a division of the ownership of property, and a trust is created where the settlor—the original owner of the property—confers legal title to it to one or more trustees, manifesting an intention that it is to be held on trust for one or more beneficiaries. The trustees of property become its owners at common law, and are not only given control of the property, but also responsibility for it.

What will become clear shortly is that this is what happens in the simplest type of trust arrangement that we encounter, which is known as an 'express trust'. It is so-called because it is a trust that has been expressly created by an owner of property, who settles it on trust for the purpose of benefiting someone else. It is important that we understand this at this stage because we will also encounter other types of trust in this text. Indeed, as early as Chapter 3 we will get a sense that other types of trust arise, and then we will consider trusts that are implied rather than express in Chapter 6 through to Chapter 9. When we study implied trusts, we learn that a distinctive body of 'trusts law' governs their creation and operation, and in Chapters 10, 11, and 12 we consider a body of law that has grown up around types of trust arrangement that are regarded as anomalous alongside the rest of trusts law. So a very important aim of this chapter is to explain that those trusts known as express trusts are the mainstay of trusts law, and indeed that the law relating to express trusts is regarded as synonymous with the general use of the term 'trusts law'.

So, much of this chapter will be concerned with introducing the 'express trust', which you will learn is actually correctly termed the 'express private trust'.

2.1 An introduction to the basic nature of the trust and some key features

The language of the express trust tells us that at the heart of this arrangement is a property owner's wish to create a trust of the property; the importance of his intention to do so was flagged up in Chapter 1 and will continue as a dominant theme throughout this text. Here, you will learn that the intention to create a trust is the linchpin in meeting the requirements in place for actually creating one, and also for the implications—the practical results—of having created one. It is also very helpful to appreciate early on that no trust will be created unless those who are intended to be trustees actually have legal title to the property. How this happens and the practical significance of this is considered in Chapter 5, where it becomes clear that even if an intention to create a trust is very clear, one will not arise unless trustees have legal title to the property. This is known as legal title 'vesting in' trustees, and this is achieved by a process called 'constituting' the trust. It is by this means that trustees come under equitable obligations that are enforceable by the beneficiaries.

Much of this chapter is concerned with understanding the express trust and appreciating how understanding what it is can tell us more about the special nature of the trust—and the significance of its very signature feature of separating ownership. This means that the materials will explain that the trust is very different from other ways in which those who own property can deal with it to benefit others. For this to happen, we need to consider key ways in which other means of using property to benefit others can be found in English law. This discussion gravitates around ownership of property, because ownership of property is the key to determining that property should be used to benefit others. In this discussion, we consider ways of using property to benefit others that do not affect its ownership at all, and others that involve outright transfer of ownership from one person to another. Both of these scenarios contrast with the trust: in the trust situation, ownership is affected by seeking to provide benefit, but not because it is transferred outright from one person to another. This allows us to see just how different the trust's separation of ownership is from all other ways of using property to benefit others.

For now, a little more is said about the trust, mindful that this chapter is all about introducing the trust as a special instrument and explaining what is special about it. In the next chapter, attention becomes firmly fixed on the express trust, which provides our guide for understanding the nature of English trusts law. Ahead of this, and taking us a step closer to understanding what is special about the trust, we need to do two things: first, we need to get an overview of just how important trusts are by considering where they are found to be created, why they are so created, and by whom; second, we need to get a sense of what is meant by the express trust arrangement by taking an overview of what other types of trust we will encounter in this text.

2.2 The trust in the economy and society in the twenty-first century

Taking the former first, we can regard this text as a celebration of the trust and all that it can achieve. We will see that trusts are ubiquitous across our economy and society, and we will also come to appreciate their diversity and ability to adapt to new uses in conferring benefits of property. Notwithstanding that the principles that will apply to each variety of trust are similar rather than identical, we will see that it is truly remarkable just how many applications have arisen from the same basic concept.

Remembering that Chapter 1 explained that the trust emerged from 'the Use' by the eighteenth century, the obvious starting point for us here is to consider what were the first modern trusts of property: family settlement trusts. These arrangements reflect that the rationale for many modern express trusts—that is, those that are deliberately created for the purpose of providing benefit from property—is retention of wealth by those who are wealthy. This is what will be seen to underpin many of the trusts that we encounter in this text and which arise today, and it was ever thus. The modern trust, and the entitlements of beneficiaries and duties of trustees arising from it, have grown up around arrangements that have sought over centuries to tie up wealth within a family. These arrangements sought to achieve this in two distinct ways: by being drafted to allow for limited free disposal of the property by individual family members; and also to minimize exposure to taxation (remembering that one of the key consequences of the Use was to avoid the duties that accompanied holding land). Trusts can be created by virtue of wills (as we will see shortly), but actually the law of taxation means that, in many cases, it is more advantageous that trusts come into effect *inter vivos*—that is, in the lifetime of the owner, or settlor.

2.2.1 Traditional uses made of trusts: trusts relating to family arrangements, and trusts associated with death and succession

Arrangements known as 'family settlements' are still found today, but they were immensely significant historically, in a much more socially polarized society in which there was a much larger aristocracy class. In providing a short explanation of why it is that trusts today owe so much to such arrangements for their origins, this text is not seeking to make normative judgements on their social desirability. It is only the legal dimensions of these arrangements on which the text is seeking to comment, whilst making the point that their very appearance in this book is a social commentary of sorts, albeit one that simply duly notes the social and economic inequalities that allowed them to flourish.

Under such arrangements, trustees are likely to be members of the family, and this has always been the case; they can also be the 'family solicitor', who is familiar with the family, its history, and its assets. However, the courts are not keen on these trustee arrangements because of the likelihood of conflict of interest arising from a trustee who is too close to, or too closely involved with, the beneficiaries. For these reasons, this type of arrangement was central in how the law relating to trusts actually developed. This will be proposed more explicitly shortly, but for now it is sufficient to suggest that it is likely that the very stringent nature of trustees' duties (considered in this text in Chapters 13, 14, and 16) in the modern law owes much to these arrangements.

2.2.1.1 How have family settlements influenced modern trusts law?

Family trusts are also now commonly administered by the trustee and executor departments of banks and the other professional specialist trusts service providers that are increasingly a characteristic of the legal management of trusts. The involvement of such service providers in these arrangements makes a more general point that proper professional administration is very important for maximizing tax benefits, but it is also the case that the professional trustee is a more recent phenomenon, and traditionally those who become trustees have been selected to undertake the task because of their general standing within particular social settings (and wider community) rather than because of their expertise in trusts or even in dealings with property. The rise of the professional trustee, and the impact that this has had on trusts law originally conceived around 'lay trustees', is considered in Chapters 14 and 16, but at this early stage it is worth noting that professional trustees will charge heavy fees for this expertise.

In due course, such charging for services will need to be explained in the light of the fiduciary nature of trusteeship considered in Chapter 13, but, returning to settlements more specifically, their defining feature is that they will create successions of interests in property. This is explained much more in Chapter 14, but essentially the same property is used to create benefits for different people over different time frames, as can be seen from the very simplest arrangement in which a settlor will settle property 'for B for life, and thereafter for C'. We can see how this creates different, and indeed successive, interests in the same property, through the terminology that is used to identify the different parties who will be involved in this arrangement. The settlor is the same as any other settlor that we have encountered—that is, someone who settles property on trust for one or more beneficiaries—and, as we already know, we will see those who are also family members or their agents acting as trustees, and it is how beneficiaries are termed that gives us most insight into the term 'settlement'. Chapter 14 will explain how this language has arisen, and its direct connection with the family settlement arrangement, but for now, in this scenario, B is known as the 'life tenant', is usually entitled to the immediate income from the property, and is often referred to as an 'income beneficiary'. After B comes C, who is the beneficiary entitled to capital, and is said to be entitled 'in remainder'. In citations of cases, 'ST' indicates a settlement trust and 'WT' a will trust.

This reference to 'WT' shows us that a number of trusts will be created by wills, and this provides a starting point for appreciating the significance of trusts for providing benefits of property following the death of its owner. As in the case of family settlements, trusts arising in the context of death have a long operating tradition in determinations of ownership of property following the death of its owner. We do find trusts at work here, but there is only limited significance for them for this text. So the main purpose of discussing them briefly is to explain that there is a tradition for trusts arising in relation to death and to explain the terms that are associated with this, which are actually significant at various points throughout the book.

When a person dies, the legal and beneficial entitlement to all of his property passes to his 'personal representatives'. If he made a will in which he appointed specific persons to be his personal representatives, these persons will be known as his 'executors', and their first task is to obtain probate of the will, which is to have the will registered by the registrar. After this, these personal representatives are responsible for ensuring that all debts and funeral expenses are paid from the deceased's property, and then they must distribute the rest in accordance with the instructions given in the will.

When a person dies intestate—that is, without making a will—a statutory scheme provided by the Administration of Estates Act 1925 will come into play for ensuring that his property is dealt with. These rules attempt to give effect to what most people are assumed to have intended to happen to their property after their death, by providing first for any widow or widower, then for children, and so on. This ensures that those who are most closely related to the deceased will benefit as a reflection of what the deceased would probably have wanted. The scheme extends outwards for situations in which the deceased has no close relatives, and in these circumstances his more distant relations will benefit. If he has no relations at all, the property passes to the Crown.

In circumstances in which there is no will, a deceased person's representatives will be 'administrators' rather than executors, and such persons acquire this capacity by being granted entitlement to administer the estate. Such persons will usually be those who are entitled to the property and so, in the first instance, a widow or widower will be looked for to be granted the right to administer the estate; where there is no widow or widower, this right passes to the children, and so on. The distinction between *executors* and *administrators* is not very significant for this text, but its importance can be seen in *Re Gonin* [1979] Ch 16.

Trustees, executors, and personal representatives
Whether the personal representatives are executors of a will or administrators on intestacy, their duties are the same, and many of the rules that apply to trustees (see

Chapters 13, 14, and 16) apply also to them. They hold their office for life, but their active duties will usually be completed within one or two years. As has already been indicated, during this time they must locate and acquire all of the deceased's assets, pay all debts owed by the deceased and expenses arising from his death, and then distribute the property either in accordance with the terms of the will or the statutory scheme, as the case may be.

Gifts, property, and the 'residuary legatee'

Wills commonly provide for specific gifts to relatives or friends. A gift of land is called a 'devise' and its recipient, a 'devisee'; a gift of personal property, including money, is a 'legacy' and its recipient, a 'legatee'. Property that is not specifically disposed of by will is called 'the residue' and the entitled person(s), the 'residuary legatee(s)'. If a specific bequest fails for any reason (possible reasons appear in Chapters 3 and 6), it is added to the residue. In practice, this often comprises a significant proportion of the property, because it is usual to provide small specific gifts to selected friends and relatives, and simply to leave the rest to the person whom one most desires to benefit.

Trusts arising on death

Trusts may arise on a death either because the will specifies that some property is to be held on trust, or because the intended recipient is under the age of 18, so that the legal title must be held for him until he reaches that age. Where trusts are deliberately created, it is usual to name the persons who are to act as trustees, and when the executors have completed their administration, they must transfer that property to the trustees. Often, the same persons will be named as both executors and trustees, and will continue to hold the legal title in their new capacity.

Death, the administration of property, and the role of executors

It is important to appreciate that the legatees, devisees, and beneficiaries under any trust created by the will have no beneficial interest in that property until such time as the executors appropriate (that is, earmark) property to meet the gifts or trusts created by the will. What they have is merely a right to demand the proper administration of the estate by the executors. Similarly, persons entitled under intestacy have no beneficial interest in the property until the administrators have paid off all of the liabilities affecting the deceased's property and prepared their accounts, showing what is available for those persons. For the sake of convenience, the persons entitled under intestacy are referred to as the 'next of kin' rather than as legatees, etc. It is possible for a partial intestacy to occur, for example where the deceased failed to specify his residuary legatee in his will, or where the residuary gift fails. In such a case, the property will pass to the next of kin, as provided by the statutory scheme.

2.2.2 Beyond family settlements and trusts arising from death: finding trusts elsewhere in society

As all of the foregoing has suggested, today we can find trusts across a number of spheres in society and performing a wide variety of functions. It has also been noted that although there will be variation in how trust principles operate in these different spheres, it is the basic nature of the trust that makes this possible—that is, the provision of benefits from property through separation of ownership into distinctive legal and equitable titles, or 'estates'. The following will give a flavour of this, giving emphasis to the different applications of trusts that can be found in this text.

2.2.2.1 Modern trusts of real property: trusts arising from cohabitation

Earlier, we learned that the first modern trusts of property emerged around land, and became synonymous with the family settlements that sought to preserve intact family wealth through limited free dealings with property and dispositions of property designed to minimize tax liability incurred on valuable property. As we know, such arrangements do still exist, but only in very limited social milieu. We do still find trusts playing a very important role in relation to ownership of family property in a much more 'everyday' sense, and in ways that are less overtly concerned with wealth, notwithstanding that, for most ordinary people, their 'home' is the most important asset that they will own over the course of a lifetime. The trusts that we find here are ones that arise from homes which are shared by families, and in situations in which formal ownership of this property at law may or may not include both partners in a traditional marriage or cohabitation arrangement. Here, the existence of a trust will be central in determining who will 'own' the valuable part of a home—the so-called 'equity'.

This is also known as 'beneficial interest' in the home, and effectively entitlement to the equity in a shared home arises from being a beneficiary under a trust that exists in relation to that home. This means that the person(s) who holds legal title to the home will do so not as owner, but as trustee for those entitled to its equity. As we will see in Chapter 8, who owns a family home in equity will normally become an issue upon the occurrence of a signature event. Normally, this will be upon breakdown of the relationship between the parties, but it can also happen where the parties remain a couple, but a third party is seeking to claim the home as its own. In this latter situation, the third party is typically a financial lender that has provided a loan secured by the property, on which the borrower (one of the parties) then defaults.

Chapter 8 will explain that, traditionally, there has been a typical scenario in which trusts have been used in order to determine ownership of a shared property, and this is the situation in which legal title to the property is held by one of the partners alone, which means that any claim for a proprietary interest by the other party must be one in equity. In these circumstances, equity must decide *whether* the claimant should have a beneficial share in the home. We will also see that trusts have become very significant for resolving disputed ownership where both parties are owners of their property 'at law', and what equity must decide here is not whether the claimant has a beneficial share of the property, but *what size* this should be. In understanding how trusts are so significant in these determinations, we will discover that, although we do find express trusts in this context, more commonly we actually find differently created and differently operating resulting and constructive trusts. Very simply, these trusts will arise in circumstances in which a claimant provides money for the purchase of the home, or in situations in which the legal owner has (effectively) told the claimant that the home belongs to both of them.

Ahead of this, Chapter 6 will explain what we mean by 'resulting' and 'constructive' trusts, and later on in this chapter we will learn that these are known as *implied* trusts. Chapter 8 will also explain that although proprietary estoppel has been very significant in disputes relating to shared homes over much of the last decade, this has changed recently. Here, we will learn that the House of Lords has restated not only the importance of the trust, but also that the trust is the most appropriate way of determining ownership of shared homes.

2.2.2.2 Trusts arising in personal asset maintenance and management

Up to now, the uses that we find being made of trusts are joined by a common thread: the ownership of property within what are 'private' familial arrangements. There are also a number of other ways in which trusts are associated with personal asset creation and also *maintenance*, but which signal their application outside the context of family wealth—where, historically, emphasis was very much on wealth preservation.

Creating trusts and avoiding tax

In linking these two themes, many trusts today are created as 'tax planning' devices, which is the accepted euphemism for minimizing tax liability through legal avoidance, rather than through illegal evasion. In Chapter 1, the introduction to the way in which the trust emerged from the Use explained that at the same time as seeking to protect those who might otherwise be disadvantaged from ownership of property, this device also appeared to reduce liability to 'dues' payable when ownership of property passed from one person to another. In the modern law of trusts, the avoidance of taxation through using the trust has become a dominant reason for creating trusts. Today, trusts are recognized as being central in tax avoidance schemes, which are perfectly lawful.

A full understanding of how trusts are central to tax avoidance requires an extensive discussion of the 'tax system' in the United Kingdom as it relates to private individuals (as distinct from corporations and charitable organizations, for example), currently comprising income tax, capital gains tax, and inheritance tax. This is too complex for this study and also too peripheral to its core purpose, so it is suggested very simply that much of the thinking behind trusts today can be illustrated with reference to capital gains tax and inheritance tax (but with income tax also being very important). Capital gains tax is the tax that is payable upon a *disposal* of an asset, including where a 'capital sum' has been accrued from the asset, and where there are some 'exemptions' (which apply to gains made on trust assets). Inheritance tax is payable upon transfers of property following a *death* and it makes 'chargeable' transfers of property at death, and upon transfers made by gift from the deceased within seven years before his death.

Essentially, trusts are used because all personal taxation works by 'charging' on accumulations of property—so the more property you have, the more you get taxed, and at higher rates. For wealthy people, this means that sharing property out between others is actually often the best way of preserving 'their' wealth. In this regard, because a beneficial owner can incur tax liability, passing beneficial interests to someone who has much less by way of taxable assets is going to result in less being lost from private wealth to the public purse. This is achieved by an owner passing beneficial interests to his children (particularly infants and young adults), or to a company that is controlled by the owner-cum-settlor. This advantage of minimizing loss outside familial interests is combined with the way in which, on principles considered in Chapter 1, the owner-cum-settlor will retain control over how this is done and how the property can be used, and there are also available various exemptions and 'reliefs' and transfers that are potentially exempt from tax in the context of a trust for owners and recipients alike. Other devices that allow an owner-cum-settlor to benefit more directly include so-called 'offshore' schemes, which are schemes located in jurisdictions known for their favourable tax regimes, which also help to establish that the arrangement is not liable under the UK regime at all.

When we consider trusts that are fixed and those that are discretionary, we will note that historically there were potentially considerable gains to be made from 'playing' changing tax regimes through arrangements whereby none of the beneficiaries has any right to the property at all unless and until the discretion is exercised in their favour. It will be suggested at that point that these arrangements have been hard hit by tax legislation, and this makes an important general point for understanding the relationship between taxation and trusts. In a number of cases, we will see that one of the parties to the litigation is the UK tax authority, and that this reflects the way in which there have been concerted efforts to limit tax avoidance given that what cannot be collected from taxation is then not available for the public purse. There is thus a tension between allowing trusts to be used as a device for wealth preservation and the ability to generate money for public utility, through ownership of property and dealings with it.

So, generally, many trusts are used strategically for avoiding tax, but there are other ways in which trusts can be used for asset management by individuals.

Trusts arising from pensions provision

As we will discover in Chapter 7, trusts have become very important in the context of pensions provision on account of the current spotlight on making financial provision for retirement, and the relative roles and responsibilities for state provision and private funding models. The increasing prominence of privately funded retirement provision is attributable to an ageing population in the light of a declining birth rate, and also because of current levels of 'expectations' in terms of living standards. This has meant that much political attention has become focused on legal questions arising from creating a workable framework for pension assets to be collected and safeguarded over extended periods of time, which, for most people, will be a period of forty years or more. Pension provision is one of the biggest socio-economic issues of current times, and the attractiveness of the trust arrangement in delivering investment benefits in the light of the challenges of safeguarding assets over such a long period into the future was crucially recognized by the *Report of the Pension Law Review Committee* (1993, Cmnd 2342), chaired by Sir Roy Goode. The Committee's recommendations resulted in the passage of the Pensions Act 1995. The 1995 Act sought to reflect the importance of rigorous regulation and supervision of pension schemes, and one of its principal tenets was its accommodation of the reality that the beneficiaries under a pension scheme differed from those under the normal trust arrangement; indeed, the entitlement of beneficiaries under a pension scheme could be seen to arise from contractual origins (provided by their contracts of employment).

In this respect, while the trust's traditional associations are strongly with wealth and its preservation, it is nevertheless significant that it is these age-old principles that are envisioned as the blueprint for this personal asset management into the twenty-first century. This is a testament to the trust's versatility and adaptability, and also to its endurance. This is so notwithstanding that demonstrating how pension funds are modelled on the trust instrument will reveal some crucial departures from 'ordinary' trust principles, as will become clear in Chapter 7.

Trusts arising in personal bankruptcy

Returning again to trusts involving people rather than purposes, the language used here has been quite deliberately so, and does actually mark out two key elements of considering how trusts arise in 'personal bankruptcy'. First, the language signals that this discussion of the importance of trusts is continuing a broad theme of narrating the lives of individuals, which has looked so far at preserving familial wealth, shared home ownership, retirement provision, and death. It also helps to separate this out from a more dedicated consideration of trusts arising in business and commercial dealings, which shifts focus from individuals to commercial arrangements and the business structures within which these operate. So, in continuing the narrative of individuals, bankruptcy or personal insolvency denotes legal recognition that an individual is unable to pay his debts. This brings into being a formal legal process whereby the person who is bankrupt loses control of his property, which becomes vested in a person known as his 'trustee in bankruptcy' for the purpose of being used to try to satisfy the claims of the bankrupt's creditors. The rationale for the bankruptcy process is clear: the bankrupt has incurred liabilities and those who are owed money by him are entitled to be paid; a long-standing aim of bankruptcy law is that as many of a bankrupt's creditors should be paid as possible, by as much as possible, given the amount of property that is available for this. This also recognizes that, once a person has become bankrupt, there is likely to be a shortfall between what is owed and what the bankrupt actually has.

Notwithstanding this aim, we see a special kind of trust that can be used to protect the bankrupt's property in certain ways from the full force of the bankruptcy process. The history of the so-called 'protective trust' dates back to the nineteenth century, when family settlements were more common than they are today. The protective trust would be based on a life interest in property (a type of interest in property that is as it sounds), which would be made determinable (or contingent) upon the bankruptcy of the owner, and would be combined with a discretionary trust in favour of the former life tenant, his spouse and children (if any), and ultimately his next of kin who would inherit in the event of his death.

The obvious advantages are that, upon bankruptcy, the debtor's interest in what is now trust property simply ceases to exist and cannot be claimed by creditors or the trustees in bankruptcy. The property itself remains in the hands of the trustees, who can distribute the income as they see fit in the circumstances. If the reason for the determination is the actual indebtedness of the former life tenant, it would clearly be pointless to make payments to him, because the creditors could then seize the money. But in these circumstances the lifestyle of the family can be maintained by paying the income instead to the spouse, or directly to those who supply the debtor's needs, since they can apply it for the 'use and benefit' of the former life tenant without placing money directly into his hands. It is not even necessary to set out in express terms the nature of the trusts, since s. 33 of the Trustee Act 1925 provides a model form that can be invoked simply by directing that the property shall be held on 'protective trust' for the benefit of the person who is to be the life tenant (called the 'principal beneficiary' in the section).

There are two main limitations on the operation of a protective trust, the first being that it is not possible to settle property upon oneself via such trusts; protective trusts are usually created by the parent of the principal beneficiary on his behalf. The second is that the life interest must be made *determinable* upon the relevant event. Beyond simply stating this, the law is complex, and involves making some very difficult distinctions between what is permissible and what will be considered void as being a device for defeating creditors.

The protective trust has most significance on account of the fact that, upon bankruptcy, a trustee in bankruptcy is likely to want to seek the sale of the family home in order to satisfy the claims of creditors. In this light, traditionally, it was the position that if a trustee in bankruptcy wishes to pursue this, it is only in exceptional circumstances (see, for example, *Re Solomon* [1967] Ch 573 and *Re Lowrie* [1981] 3 All ER 353) that he will not be able to do so. It is, of course, possible to analyse this contentious position of the family home as a reflection of deeply entrenched retributionist ideas that have, since Victorian times, associated bankruptcy with misconduct, or at the very least irresponsibility and improvidence, rather than *misfortune*. It might instead be seen more simply as part of the 'economic reality' of a creditor's entitlement to be paid for the money that he has advanced to the debtor.

In some respects, the Insolvency Act 1986—in which the law relating to personal insolvency is largely located, alongside that relating to corporate insolvency—entrenched further associations of indebtedness with irresponsibility, on the basis that it contends that, for some, bankruptcy might represent 'an easy solution for those who can bear with equanimity the stigma of their own failure' (Sir Kenneth Cork, at para. 191 of the *Report of the Review Committee on Insolvency Law and Practice*, 1982, Cmnd 8558). However, the provisions of s. 335A state that where an application for sale of a home is made, the court shall make an order that it considers just and reasonable, having regard to a number of factors relating to the family home's 'own claim to protection', as alluded to in the judgment of Megarry V-C in *Re Bailey* [1977] 1 WLR 278.

Predictably, the provisions focus on the interests of the bankrupt's creditors, who are identified in s. 335A(a). In addition, where the proposed sale includes a dwelling house that 'is or has been the home of the bankrupt or the bankrupt's spouse or former spouse', the provisions of s. 335A(b) determine that the court's calculus of 'just and reasonable' involves it having regard to a number of factors. These factors, located in s. 335A(b), relate to:

(i)   the *conduct* of the spouse, civil partner, former spouse or former civil partner, so far as contributing to the bankruptcy,

(ii)   the *needs and financial resources* of the spouse, civil partner, former spouse or former civil partner, and

(iii)   the *needs of any children* ... [Emphasis added]

In these circumstances, the court will also have regard to 'all the circumstances of the case *other than the needs of the bankrupt*' (s. 335A(c), emphasis added).

This is hardly a protection charter, though, because where an application for sale is made one year after the vesting of a bankrupt's property in the trustee in bankruptcy, the assumption will be made that the interests of creditors do outweigh all other 'competing' considerations, apart from those that reflect 'exceptional circumstances' (which itself appears to reflect the position prior to the 1986 Act). Thus this is a mechanism for *delay* rather than *protection* in many respects, but greater *delay* (and arguably also even *protection*) of a bankrupt's property does appear to flow from the Enterprise Act 2002. In spirit and intention, this enactment signalled a strongly changed emphasis across bankruptcy law, by seeking to align the consequences of bankruptcy (essentially, disqualification as a bankrupt and attendant impotencies) and prospects for rehabilitation to degrees to which a bankrupt could be deemed to have contributed to his bankruptcy. In relation to a bankrupt's family home, the Enterprise Act (which amends the Insolvency Act 1986) provides that where the trustee in bankruptcy has not sold the property or applied for an order of possession within three years of the date of the bankruptcy, the property reverts to the bankrupt, and thus is not part of the estate that can be applied to creditors' claims.

2.2.3 The significance *of* trusts relating to share holdings *for* understanding trusts law

Just before moving away from trusts arising in the course of personal dealings toward trusts arising from dealings between 'commercial parties', very brief mention must be given to trusts and shares. This is because shares are an enormously popular type of trust property, which will become apparent from the large number of cases that we will encounter in this text which involve shares as trust property, even though we will not focus on trusts and shares explicitly. We will encounter several cases involving creating trusts of shareholdings, which are accepted illustrations of the core elements of trusts law. For example, a number of cases involving attempts to make gifts of, and to create trusts of, shares will be central to our discussion of formality requirements and the role that equity can play where an attempt to constitute a trust has not been carried out sufficiently in order to be successful. This is because a very large number of all of the cases at which we will look concern attempts to create trusts of shares. In turn, this tells us that trusts of shareholdings are actually very common. Here, instead of being owned outright by a shareholder, they will be held on trust by so-called 'nominees', so that the returns made on the shareholding can benefit another. Most commonly, this happens where the holding is in what is known as a public, rather than a private, company (with the legal distinction drawn between whether or not shares are available for public purchase on the open share market); in this scenario, a nominee is likely to be a bank or a specialist trust service provider (often referred to as a 'trustee company'). In such a situation, legal title to the shares will be held by the nominee in trust for a shareholder. Shares generally will provide a standard 'investment' direction for trustees, whose duty it is to safeguard assets comprising a trust, to maximize opportunities for generating returns on 'equities'. From a different, but related, perspective, those who want others to benefit from their shareholdings will choose to create trusts of them rather than to make gifts of them, because managing shares by watching what is going on in the markets, and knowing when to buy and sell, is a skilled and time-consuming undertaking. Moreover, there will be a so-called 'portfolio' of shares where holdings are actually in not one, but several, different companies, and it does take time and expertise to make sure that the right kind of investments and disposals of shares are made at the right time. This is what we can see in what is known as a 'unit trust', thereby linking what has been said about pensions provision with the popularity of shares as 'trust property'.

2.2.3.1 Trusts arising in business and commerce

Chapter 18 comprises a dedicated consideration of how trusts found in the context of business and commerce actually operate; our purpose here is therefore only to introduce this, and also the significance of trusts that are found in this setting for our study of trusts more generally. This is particularly important because there is evidence suggesting that it is actually the trusts that are found in commercial and business contexts that are currently having most influence on how trusts law generally is adapting to reflect how trusts are being used in the twenty-first century. As we know, it was trusts arising in the preservation of familial wealth through 'family settlement' that helped to carve out the parameters of earliest modern trusts law, and also much of its detail. This is no longer the case in the twenty-first century. It is not even the use of trusts in relation to family homes that is having the most influence on how trusts law is developing in the twenty-first century, notwithstanding the increasingly ubiquitous opportunities for home ownership and also that a home is the most important asset that many individuals will own across their lifetimes.

The dedicated study of trusts and commercial dealings will provide an account of the way in which the strongest influences that are being brought to bear on the nature of trusts law in the twenty-first century are coming from outside private individual, or even family, circumstances, and are instead deriving from the increasing prominence of trusts and associated 'equitable obligations' in business and commerce.

In the dedicated study of trusts arising in business and commerce, we will learn that trusts can be found underpinning commercial loan arrangements because of their comparative advantages over ordinary contractual principles. It will become clear at this point how loans of property, which would ordinarily be governed by contract law, can arise using what are known as 'express trusts', which are the simplest type of trust, and also how different 'implied trusts' can be used to achieve this where no express trust has been created. There will be discussion of how trusts might arise in cases of insolvency, and how this might be both similar to and also different from how they arise in instances of personal bankruptcy. The material will also provide an opportunity to understand and reflect on just how significant business and commercial dealings, rather than 'private trust arrangements', have become as authorities for meeting validity requirements to create trusts, and also for the entitlements and responsibilities that arise from this. Very significantly, we will explain the ways in which business and commerce have sought to develop fiduciary obligations into their operating frameworks—that is, the fiduciary obligations that equity originally developed to protect beneficiaries under a trust. And in this vein we will look at how business and commerce has tried to claim for 'business dealings' actions relating to missing property that equity developed for beneficiaries under a trust for situations in which trust property goes missing, and which allow a claimant to recover the property or its substitute, and any increases in value that have occurred while it has been wrongfully taken. These latter reference points will involve us reflecting on how equity developed the trust, and the significance of extending equity's actions beyond those for whom these actions were developed (which is also considered extensively in Chapter 17).

2.2.3.2 Trusts for purposes rather than people

Up to now, everything that has been said about trusts has strongly associated their creation with providing benefits of property. However, before too long it will become apparent that sometimes people try to create trusts not so that others can benefit from the property, but rather to achieve particular purposes. When we learn about attempts to create trusts for the care of animals, for example, we can still see strong associations between using property and providing benefits, but this is less clear when we see attempts to create trusts to fulfil the building of monuments or the maintenance of monuments that have already been built. These are known as 'trusts for purposes' and, in Chapter 3, we will learn that legal issues associated with trusts designed for the upkeep of animals have more in common with ones seeking to build or maintain buildings or monuments than ones created to benefit people. But these arrangements 'for purposes' are not uncommon—particularly those concerning the upkeep of animals, given how strongly the British are identified as a nation of animal lovers.

2.2.3.3 Trusts arising in the context of organizations

Trusts can also be used to enable property to be held for the benefit of people who, for some reason, cannot hold it themselves. Interestingly, some of the earliest uses made of the trust instrument were for Franciscan friars for this very purpose. Incorporated bodies, such as companies, which are incorporated under the Companies Acts, and universities, which are incorporated by charter, have legal personality, and can therefore hold property themselves. So there is no need for treasurers or directors, among others, to hold the property on their behalf as trustees, and normally they do not do so. It will become apparent that they may owe fiduciary duties that are akin to those of trustees. This will also apply to certain charities that can be incorporated, and in which case are able to hold property in their own right. However, unincorporated charities, in common with other bodies lacking legal personality, are not able to hold property themselves. And, in the case of unincorporated charities, the property is held by trustees, who are often individuals, for the purposes of the charity, and donations to charity therefore commonly give rise to trusts. While it is possible for trusts to be used to hold property for unincorporated bodies such as members' clubs, we will discover in Chapter 7 that this is not the mechanism used. Here, we will discover that, in such un-incorporated associations, funds will be held by the present membership, and subject to contractual rights and duties; where property is held by club officers, such persons are usually regarded as agents rather than trustees. An exception to this general pos-ition is that of trade unions, which are in the unique position of being regarded as un-incorporated for most purposes, whilst at the same time sharing a number of features of corporate bodies.

2.2.3.4 Trusts and public organizations: the context of charity

In relation to charity specifically, when we study charity it will become clear that trusts and trusts law provide the basis for a special type of trusts law, which is called 'charity law'. Charity law reflects the governance of organizations that have historic-ally developed through recognition by equity as trusts that are quite unlike the other trusts that we will encounter. This is because charity law reflects the fact that charit-able organizations are actually charitable trusts that are publicly enforceable by the Attorney-General, and which do not need a beneficiary to enforce them. Indeed, what will become apparent is that charities are effectively trusts for purposes, rather than trusts for persons, and that, because of this, many of the 'requirements of a valid trust' arising in the context of a normal private trust for a beneficiary do not apply to them. In this context, there are trustees even though there are no beneficiaries as such, and these trustees have responsibility for the governance and administration of the charity. What this amounts to is that the law relating to charities is a body of trusts law that is quite different from the general law of trusts, and is actually regarded as anomalous on account of just how different organizations that are governed by charity law are not simply from the express private trusts, but also from all private trusts—including those arising in commercial dealings, as well as familial ones, whether these arise by way of an express trust or a trust that is regarded as implied.

2.3   Introducing different types of trust: express, implied, resulting, and constructive trusts explained

There have now been a few references to the way in which many of the trusts that are encountered in this text will be express trusts. This type of trust is the simplest type that we find, and it is one that arises from the expressed wishes of a settlor to settle property on trust. It is the easiest model or type of trust to understand, and it is used as a starting point to explain and illustrate the creation and operation of trusts more generally.

In Chapter 1, we encouraged you to associate the creation of trusts with providing the benefits of property, when we suggested that settling property on trust was one of the options available to an owner of property who was seeking to do this for another. At that point, we looked at reasons why an owner of property might seek to create a trust rather than utilize other ways of conferring benefits from property. What we can add to this now is that such a conscious creation of a trust for one or more of those reasons gives rise to a so-called 'express trust'. This is because the trust that arises in such situ-ations does so because the settlor has expressed an intention to set up a trust, and one will arise on account of his *express* intentions that it should.

2.3.1 Introducing the significance of the express private trust

So what is known as an *express trust* arises where an owner of property sets out to create a trust of property, and the one that arises from him doing so reflects his express intentions. As we will discover, it is the express trust that provides the basis for what we understand as the general law of trusts. It is, in many regards, a paradigm trust in as much as it embodies much of what is generally understood by the term 'trust', as well as provides the basis for the general law of trusts. This gives the first indication that there are other types of trust and, in discovering what these are, we need first to understand that the full name given to the express trust is actually the 'express private trust'. To explain this, we already know that, when we encounter charitable trusts in this text, we find trusts that are not private at all. The signature feature of a private trust is that it is enforceable by a beneficiary, and only by a beneficiary. What we now need to appreciate is that there are different types of private trust, with the express trust being the classic model trust.

We will find that doing so is central for understanding the vast number of different uses to which the trust is being put in current times, and to which it could also be potentially applied, because this does require appreciation of trusts that are resulting and constructive. These 'other types' of trust start to appear in Chapter 3, and by Chapter 4 it starts to become apparent that they are governed by trusts law that is different from that which is integral to the express trust. This is considered further in due course, and especially in Chapter 6 through to Chapter 9, but it is important to understand at this stage that this book on trusts law will consider different types of trust. At this stage, this involves noting that a trust can be created expressly by a settlor and also in other ways. And this requires us to grapple with an even more fundamental qualitative distinction between private and non-private trusts.

The distinction between private trusts and public trusts can be dealt with briefly at this stage because much of this has already been dealt with by the introduction to charity. The distinction is essentially one of enforcement and entitlement: whilst a beneficiary both is entitled to the trust property and is the only one who can enforce a private trust, when a trust is charitable property and is given to 'purposes' rather than persons, such an arrangement is enforceable by the Attorney-General.

2.3.2 Introducing private trusts that are not express trusts

From this, we need to appreciate that private trusts can be express trusts or implied trusts. The term 'implied' trust is used commonly to explain the arrangement that arises when a trust will not arise from a settlor's expressed wishes, and might not even arise from his wishes at all. Where an implied trust is based on a settlor's intention, this is intention that is not expressed, but is reasoned as being what he would have wished for in the circumstances. Opinion is divided on whether this is a particularly helpful classification for non-express trusts because, although it might be convenient, we will find that a settlor does not have to use the term 'trust' in order for an express trust to arise, nor does he even have to say anything at all, because an express trust can arise by way of conduct. Because of this, it is also important to qualify whether an implied trust is one that is resulting or constructive, which is considered extensively in the part of the text commencing in Chapter 6.

Ahead of this and for this introduction to the trust, an implied trust that is a 'constructive trust' will arise in a number of different factual situations, which will often appear to be diverse. However, all constructive trusts have in common the fact that they will arise where a trust is imposed by the courts irrespective of the intention of the owner (of what becomes the trust property), and will be so on account of some unconscionable conduct or situation. In this respect, they can be said to arise from the operation of law. An arrangement known as a 'resulting trust' can also be found in a diverse variety of factual situations, but these trusts are more difficult to pin down than constructive trusts, which are essentially (with limited exceptions) impositions of trusteeship in unconscionable situations. In seeking to understand resulting trusts, it is helpful to remember that all resulting trusts do have one element in common: although legal title is vested in a trustee, the settlor and the beneficiary are actually the same person. In understanding how this transpires, we need to grasp that it will do so for two reasons, and for present purposes we will explain this very simply, in anticipation of fuller consideration given in Chapters 6, 7, and 8. Broadly (and with emphasis on *simplicity* at this introductory stage), this will occur because the settlor has tried to create a trust in favour of a third-party beneficiary and because, although legal title has been transferred from him, he has failed to divest himself of equitable interest in the property. Here, equitable title never leaves him. Alternatively, a resulting trust will arise where property has been divested from the settlor, but it is for some reason later returned back to him.

This is a very simplistic introduction to resulting and constructive trusts, and one that is designed to signpost at this early stage that this text on trusts law is concerned with different types of trust. Once the text has considered the general law of trusts as it applies to the express private trust arrangement, Chapter 6 offers a comprehensive introduction to constructive and resulting trusts by way of introducing these less 'formal' (in terms of creation) trusts, and thereafter their essential characteristics and operational features. In Chapter 6 through to Chapter 9, the workings of resulting and constructive trusts will be explored by means of discussions of: the ways in which associations without legal personality can hold property, and also pension funds; trusts arising from cohabitation; secret trusts; and equitable fraud. Thereafter, Chapters 14, 16, and 17 include discussions of the application of constructive trusts to liabilities that arise, both for fiduciaries and also for those known as 'strangers to a trust', for unauthorized profits that are made from trust property, or the receipt of trust property that has been applied in breach of trust.

The other reason for such a short and simplistic introduction to resulting and constructive trusts at this early stage is to ensure that you are familiar with the terminology that you will encounter. In continuing this theme, there are other key terms that are commonly used in classifying and identifying different types of trust, and which it will be helpful for you to be aware of.

2.3.3 Explaining references made to express trusts that are 'fixed' and 'discretionary'

We will discover shortly (when looking at creating powers to provide benefits from property), and further in Chapter 3, that a trust is a 'mandatory' arrangement, which means that, once it has come into being, trustees *must* carry it out in accordance with a settlor's instructions. In furtherance of this, the classification of express trusts as ones that are fixed or discretionary will become very significant for meeting so-called 'certainty requirements' for validity. For now, we need to understand that where there is more than one beneficiary who is intended to benefit from the settlor's generosity, there arises what is termed a 'class' (the term used to mean a group) of beneficiaries, or 'objects' of a trust, and where this is the case it becomes very important to consider whether the trust being created is a 'fixed' trust or a 'discretionary' trust.

A trust is said to be *fixed* if, in creating a trust, a settlor sets out what property is settled amongst a class of beneficiaries, making it clear what share each of them is to have. The clearest example of this would be a trust that is created for four named beneficiaries, each of whom is to have equal share of the property. The shares in a fixed trust may or may not be equal, and what distinguishes a fixed trust is that this share or proportion of the trust property for each beneficiary is determined by the settlor at the time that the property is settled. Given that Chapter 1 identified amongst the reasons for creating trusts an owner's control over how property is intended to benefit others, would it not always be the case that, in creating a trust, a settlor will always make decisions about who is to receive what?

Actually, something different happens when a settlor creates what is known as a *discretionary* trust. In this arrangement, the settlor will leave it to trustees to determine who is to benefit from the trust property rather than decide this himself. Here, trustees will have discretion as to who will receive the trust property and how much they will receive. What happens is that the settlor will specify a particular class of beneficiary intended to benefit from the property, and then leave it to the trustee to determine who within this class should actually receive this and how much they should have. In this type of arrangement, those who are within the settlor's 'chosen class' are considered potential beneficiaries as far as the trust property is concerned, and will not have any interest in the trust property unless and until the trustee exercises discretion in their favour. The position is different in regards to enforcing a trust: we know that a beneficiary under a trust is the only person who can enforce it, and all those within a settlor's chosen class will have the *locus standi* to enforce a trust (and thus to force the trustee to carry it out in accordance with the settlor's wishes) even if this does not ultimately occur in their favour.

In Chapter 1, it was suggested that 'owner control' was one of the reasons why an owner of property might seek to create a trust of it rather than make a gift of it. If this is the case, then how can we explain the creation of trusts under which an owner gives discretion to others even as to who will benefit under the arrangement? We can do so by looking at some of the other reasons for creating trusts that we also encountered in Chapter 1. Here, we learned that trusts are very important for preserving wealth and that, closely related to this, they are also very significant in tax avoidance. Bringing those two ideas together, once again we find that family settlement trusts are very significant. It is the case that these were the first modern trusts of land, but they have a much more general significance for understanding the creation of trusts in English legal culture, and also the nature of the trusts law that has developed around this. These types of trust, which as we know sought to create successive interests in the same property, were trusts arising from ideas of 'owner control', but they were also a model for wealth preservation. Not only were they able to limit free disposal of property by individuals, but the family settlement is also how creating trusts for tax reasons became popular; in this context, this also popularized giving discretion to trustees. There were a number of advantages in giving discretion to the trustees, one of which was to enable trustees to alter beneficial interests in property to take advantage of changing tax circumstances. Another was that, in some circumstances, tax liability arises only where rights in property have been created, and so this suggested that advantages could be gleaned from circumstances in which none of the beneficiaries has any right to the property at all unless and until the discretion is exercised in their favour. Interestingly, discretionary trusts have been hard hit by tax legislation, however, and are probably less common today because of this.

So references to trusts that are fixed and those that are discretionary will be very important for our study of trusts. There are also some terms that are useful to be aware of even though they are of very little significance for this text.

References made to express trusts as being 'executed' or 'executory'

Following on from the way in which, much as it sounds, an express trust arises where a settlor expressly settles property on trust for a beneficiary or beneficiaries, in some cases and academic commentaries, reference will be made to trusts that are 'executed' and those that are 'executory'. You will notice in due course that very little significance is attached to these terms within this text, beyond simply noting them and explaining them as part of its introduction. As the heading suggests, both of these terms arise in the creation of express trusts, and the difference between them is that while, in an *executed* trust, the settlor has made clear the interests that are to be taken by the beneficiaries, in an *executory* trust scenario, defining the beneficial interests under the trust does not become clear until a further document is executed. In this latter situation, a valid trust is created, but it remains executory until the further 'instructions' are executed. This distinction does not really impact on this text's analysis at all, and it remains only to note that stricter rules of construction apply to executed trusts than to those that are executor. This is because, in the latter case, the courts are concerned with more 'open' questions relating to ascertaining a settlor's true intentions, in the absence of specific directions on the application of property to beneficiaries.

References made to trusts that are 'bare trusts'

Although they are not a feature of this text as such, it is useful for you to understand what is meant by the term 'bare trust'. A 'bare', or 'simple', trust is said to arise when property is held by a trustee in trust for an adult beneficiary, who has an interest in property that is described as 'absolute'. This pertains to situations in which, essentially, the beneficiary may at any time request that legal title is conveyed to him and, upon receiving this request, the trustee must comply. In circumstances in which a trustee must convey legal title to the beneficiary upon his request, it is perhaps not surprising that the trustee of a bare trust is not subjected to the duties relating to trusteeship that pertain to other 'special' trusts. A common illustration of this scenario is where a solicitor acts on behalf of a client. In certain transactions—most commonly, the purchase of a domestic dwelling house—a solicitor will hold money on behalf of a client in anticipation of completion; upon completion, the client will instruct the solicitor to pay over moneys falling due and the solicitor must do so. In this scenario, a bare trust arises *ab initio* on account of the fact that property is given to a trustee to hold on behalf of its original owner. It can also arise when, at some time after its creation, a trust *becomes* a bare one. This can be illustrated by a trust that confers a life interest in property to A that, upon A's death, passes to B absolutely: upon A's death, B becomes entitled to the property *absolutely* and the trustee must convey legal title to B upon his request.

Following the introduction to trusts and trusts law provided by this chapter, along with Chapter 1, the first part of this text focuses entirely on the express private trust, and specifically what is required to bring an express private trust into being. Given that much of what will be said in these early chapters is actually a reflection of the special nature of the trust and the distinctive way in which trusts deliver the benefits of property for others—especially those that have been deliberately created to do this—the material that follows now is designed to draw out just what is distinctive and special about the trust. We propose that much can be learned about what is special about the trust from looking at other ways of providing benefits from property.

As the introduction suggested, this will focus on key ways in which benefits from property for others can be achieved through outright transfers of ownership of property from one person to another. This is what happens first, and then there is also reference to using contract to benefit a third party. Here, we will glean just what is special about the trust not only in terms of its signature feature of separating ownership, but also the implications of this in terms of what rights equity grants to those who hold beneficial ownership of property in a trust arrangement.

2.4 Trusts distinguished from ways of providing benefits of property at common law

In Chapter 1, we learned that, in the trust arrangement, we find two types of ownership of property that exist simultaneously. This was presented then as something that is special, and distinctive, to the trust, made possible by equitable jurisdiction within English law. So we do have an impression that the trust works differently from what is found in law, but this is a long way from being able to point to exactly what a trust is and indeed what it does. Something else that we do know is that a trust will give a non-legal owner enforceable rights in respect of the trust property. However, while the function of the trust, and some of the implications of separating ownership into distinctive legal and equitable titles to property, might be clear and even straightforward to understand, what a trust *is* is not terribly easy to define. Part of the reason for this is that the trust is an extremely flexible instrument, as we shall see in this text.

This is, of course, connected directly to the attention that has already been drawn to the use that is made of trusts across widely differing social and economic situations, of which all of the foregoing examples are *illustrative*, but by no means exhaustive. It is, of course, the case that understanding *what* a trust *is* is in many ways a prelude to understanding *how* it is used, and in many respects it would be appropriate to have considered this more fully before looking at common uses made of the trust. However, it is also the case that appreciating how trusts are used might help us to understand more about what, fundamentally, a trust *is*. The trust is not easy to 'pin down' in many respects, and this is complicated further by the way in which other wholly different legal devices are applied to situations similar to those in which trusts are to be found. For example, it has already been suggested that members' clubs are normally based on contract, not trust, but that the property of charities that are unincorporated is held by trustees. It is also the case that while banks may be trustees if they are specifically constituted as such, ordinary accounts create only a debtor–creditor relationship, which is contractual. In the commercial–corporate sphere, company directors are not usually trustees, but it will become apparent (in Chapter 13) that they share many trustees' duties.

In light of these difficulties, this book has traditionally looked at concepts found within the common law to try to explain what a trust *is* by looking at what it *is not*. Indeed, by looking at what is special about a trust (and what is not a characteristic of a number of common law concepts), this approach can help to foster appreciation of *what* a trust is and *why* it is able to do the things it can. Over time, this text has developed an approach whereby the legal devices to which it draws attention in trying to explain the nature of the trust all have in common the function most usually associated with trusts—that is, providing the benefits of property for another. We already know from Chapter 1 that the trust achieves this in a way that is special and unique to it, and so, to draw out the significance of delivering benefits through the separation of ownership, we will now consider how an owner of property might more normally provide benefits for others using his property.

This approach of identifying more usual approaches emphasizes mechanisms that deliver benefits of property through outright transfers of ownership by an owner to the intended recipient. Here, we consider how benefits of property can be provided through the sale of property by its owner, and also its owner making a loan of it. It will discuss these mechanisms as a prelude for suggesting that, in many respects, the creation of a trust has most in common with making a gift of property. This will help us to draw out the significance of the trust's *modus operandi* of delivering benefit through separation of ownership. And finally, the nature of the beneficiary's entitlement under a trust is explained by looking at how an ordinary contract can be used to create benefits for third parties.

2.4.1 Using property to provide benefit: transfers of property 'for value'

A transfer of ownership of property for consideration, or value, is technically a way of providing benefit of property, because it is a way in which someone who really wants 'something' is able to acquire it. This can be seen in dealings with everyday things, such as food and clothing, or more 'one-off', but also very common, transactions such as the purchase of a home or acquiring property such as shares. In turn, all of these examples illustrate the same principle: they provide benefits from property through an outright transfer of ownership. And, as suggested, this is something that, when explained, can take us further in understanding what a trust is and how it works.

Without going into the technicalities of specialist sale-of-goods law and focusing on the proprietary nature of these transactions, ownership in property will leave a vendor and become vested in a purchaser all of the time in the everyday dealings that we make in 'contracts for consideration' with vending machines, with online interfaces, and the good old-fashioned way in shops. Here, someone who wants property is able to benefit from it by acquiring it from someone else who has it, and this will be a transfer of ownership that is permanent. However, what is significant about the transfer for consideration is that the person who wants to benefit from the property (namely, by owning it) has to provide something in exchange in order to be able to do so. In other words, the transfer will be permanent, but it is not gratuitous, and what amounts to consideration must satisfy common law rules relating to this.

2.4.2 Using property to provide benefit: loans of property from one person to another

Much like the way in which explaining a transfer of property for consideration could easily slip into a discussion of sale-of-goods law, it is difficult to say very much at all about loans of property without stepping into specialist considerations of banking and the law relating to security. However, from the perspective of dealings with property generally and understanding the nature of the trust more specifically, we can regard making a loan of property as another means for providing the benefits of property. This is because someone who wants or needs something is able to borrow it from someone who has it and who is prepared to lend it. But here the property is not intended to be 'kept' indefinitely by the borrower, and so it is advanced to the borrower subject to terms putting in place requirements for its return to the lender. There are lots of loans that will not involve transfers of legal title to a borrower. These will include everything from the commercial hiring of heavy plant and equipment to lending your car or a handbag to a friend or family member. This is because this type of property requires more than its receipt by another to pass title to another, given that there is not going to be an 'exchange', as in the case of a sale; so instead the former will be achieved through complex commercial borrowing arrangements, while the latter will not be considered as having intention to create legal relations.

But there *are* loans that will involve transfers of ownership of property from one person to another, and these are arrangements that can help to uncover more about the trust. Where money is loaned from one person to another, because of the nature of money in English law, there will be a transfer of ownership of it from lender to borrower. This applies to cash itself, and also with bank accounts, in which the relationship between a bank and customer is a (contractual) debtor–creditor relationship. So there is a transfer of ownership from its owner to a recipient, albeit that this is subject to agreed terms concerning its return—that is, its repayment—such as the time frame for this and the rate of interest falling due on repayment. Normally, this arises as a result of a lending or borrowing agreement being contractual, and it is important to take this on board now, because we will discover in Chapters 3 and 6, and especially Chapter 19, that loans of money can also arise from an agreement that actually amounts to creating a trust. But, in many respects, the 'trust loan' is significant precisely because it contrasts with the norm—that is, a 'contractual loan'. So, for now, we need to understand that, technically, a loan can provide benefits of property through a transfer of ownership, because there is someone who wants the property and there is someone else prepared to loan it to him. And, in appreciating this, we also need to understand that the nature of this benefit is intended to be temporary and will commonly be subject to incurring interest. This means that the benefit is also non-gratuitous on the part of the original owner, as well as not permanent, and this is significant for helping us to construct an understanding of what a trust might actually be.

2.4.3 Using property to provide benefit: creating a power to give property to another

Where lawyers talk about 'creating a power', this essentially describes the creation of a discretion or authorization to act in a particular way. The type of power with which we are most likely to be familiar is the power of attorney, which many will have heard about even without understanding precisely what it might involve. However, even without knowing much about a power of attorney, most people will have a sense that it provides authorization to act in the affairs of others to take account of particular situations or events. And, in relation to a power of attorney, this can be created for very specific situations or events, such as a person being temporarily legally incapacitated by virtue of being abroad or temporarily ill; it can also be a more long-term strategy for those who become old and who fear losing their faculties on account of degenerative disease. We do not encounter power of attorney in this study of trusts, but using it as an example can tell us much about the general nature of a power, and helps us to gain some appreciation of the power to give property, which we will come across. The general nature of a power is about ensuring that there is a course of action to follow should certain events arise, but that this will not be exercised unless they do. The language used in relation to a power is that it is the *donor* of a power who confers the power and the *donee* who holds the power to act.

Given that this is a discussion of the ways in which owners of property can use property to benefit others, the type of power that we encounter here is the so-called 'power of appointment'. Its full title is 'power for the appointment of property' and arises from using the term 'appointing' as a synonym for 'giving' property to another.

It will become clear in Chapter 3 that it can sometimes be difficult to tell whether a donor wishes his property to be settled on trust, or is providing authorization for it to be appointed to others, but also the discretion for it not to be given to them. Sometimes, it will be clear that what is being created is a power of appointment, because along with the instructions given will be a default provision—an alternative course of action for the property should this particular power to give it to another or others not be followed. From *Re Gestetner's ST* [1953] Ch 672, we know that the technical term for such a default provision is a 'gift over in default of appointment' (known for short as a 'gift over'), and very simply it is an 'alternative' provision for what happens to the property if the power is not carried out. We will also see that all powers can be classified as mere (or *personal*) powers and *fiduciary* ones, depending on the nature of the relationship between the donor of the power and the donee. In the context of property, the donor will be the owner of property, but why has such a device for providing the benefits of property actually emerged?

In many respects, a power of appointment (of property) is a 'hangover' from earlier times, when awareness of different ways of dealing with property to allow others to benefit from it was first developing. When an owner of property wished to make a gift of it (rather than to create a trust), empowering someone with discretion over whether to appoint property in favour of another could give flexibility to reflect changing circumstances and unforeseeable events. This could be especially significant in circumstances in which an owner was no longer alive to act accordingly himself.

As with discretionary trusts, the objects of the power have no definable interest in the property unless that power is exercised in their favour, but once it is, they will acquire ownership of it in a way that is gratuitous and permanent.

2.4.4 Using contract to provide benefits for third parties

In Chapter 1, we learned that one of the reasons for creating trusts was that trusts create enforceable rights for a beneficiary. So what we now know is called the express trust will give enforceable rights to the person intended to benefit from the property, and we also know that an express trust will arise where it is an owner of property's express intention that it should do so. And whilst we do not know very much about the actual mechanics of it at this stage, we *do* already have a sense that an owner actions his intentions in this way by appointing a trustee to carry out the trust, or by taking on the task of trusteeship himself. Once this happens, the owner-cum-settlor will lose all interest in the property and all control over the arrangement (unless he acquires a different capacity as beneficiary in the new arrangement, which does happen); it is only the beneficiary who can enforce the trust, and it is very unusual for beneficiaries to provide consideration. This is because, effectively, the beneficiary is the recipient of a gift of the property, albeit that this is a gift without an outright transfer of ownership and one that creates obligations for another—the trustee. In the trust arrangement, it is only the third-party beneficiary who can actually enforce the arrangement, as can be seen in Figure 2.1.

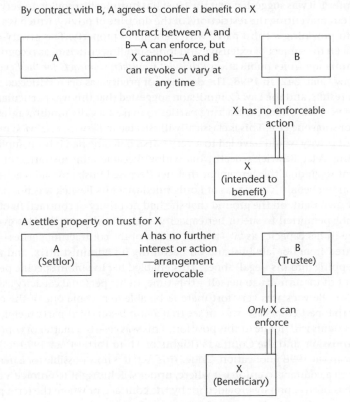

By contract with B, A agrees to confer a benefit on X

Contract between A and B—A can enforce, but X cannot—A and B can revoke or vary at any time

A

B

X has no enforceable action

X (intended to benefit)

A settles property on trust for X

A has no further interest or action —arrangement irrevocable

A (Settlor)

B (Trustee)

Only X can enforce

X (Beneficiary)

Figure 2.1 Trust and contract.

When this was suggested in Chapter 1, it was noted that, by giving a beneficiary enforceable rights, the trust contrasts with the position of the contract, in that traditionally this latter legally binding agreement is enforceable only by the parties to it on account of the doctrine of privity. This introduces the way in which, in principle, contract can be used by an owner of property to agree with another to provide benefits for a third party. Explaining how this could work will, in turn, expose the limitations of using contract and help to draw out the manifest strengths of the trust for achieving this purpose.

Taking the former first, we can see how contract can be regarded as one of the ways in which the benefits of property can be delivered to another, using the famous contract case of *Beswick* v *Beswick* [1968] AC 58. It is also the case that *Beswick* shows us that contracts to provide third-party benefits can also involve transfers of ownership of property—albeit to someone other than the person intended to benefit from the property. So, we can already see similarity between the contract and the trust, because a recipient will not acquire legal title to the property in either of these arrangements. *Beswick* v *Beswick* also shows us how contract *can* be used to provide benefits that are intended to be permanent and also gratuitous, and, much like a trust, in circumstances in which the intended recipient is not intended to have legal title to the property. This case involved Peter Beswick, an elderly coal merchant, who transferred his business to his nephew, who in return agreed (amongst other things) to pay £5 a week to Peter's widow following the former's death.

In Chapter 1, it was suggested that the trust has historically provided a very important means of circumventing the restrictions of the doctrine of privity, which is a significant obstacle to providing a third party with benefits of property. The privity-of-contract rule has been the subject of extensive and long-standing criticism, as recognized by the Law Commission in its publication *Privity of Contract: Contracts for the Benefit of Third Parties* (Law Com. 242) in 1998. The doctrine of privity has been criticized for producing harsh results, and the Law Commission suggested that this was particularly the case where the very reason for contracting parties to make a legally binding agreement is to provide for someone else. This is classically illustrated in *Beswick* v *Beswick*, in which the doctrine of privity would have led to a very harsh outcome had it been applied.

Following Peter Beswick's death, his widow became administratrix of his estate, and sought to enforce the agreement that her deceased husband had reached with his nephew on her behalf. The House of Lords ruled that Mrs Bewick was not permitted to sue in her own right, on the ground that she had no privity of contract. In other words, she was not permitted to sue in her capacity as the third party 'X'. However, she was able to sue in her capacity as 'A'—that is, as one of the contracting parties—which she had acquired from her late husband on becoming his administratrix, and was by this means stepping into his (legal) shoes. This enabled her to obtain specific performance of payment of the annuity to herself—this time, in her personal capacity as 'X'.

While Mrs Beswick was very fortunate to be able to become one of the contracting parties in that particular case, we can see that a number of third-party recipients of contractual benefits will not be in this position. This was clearly a matter of concern for the Law Commission, and the Contracts (Rights of Third Parties) Act 1999 followed very quickly from the 1998 publication. Under this Act, it is now possible for a person who is not party to a contract to enforce it where, under s. 1, his right to enforce a term of the contract has been expressly provided for by the contract, or where the term purports to confer a benefit for him. However, this may not be a 'third-party charter' because of s. 1(2), which provides that s. 1 will not apply to the former provision where, on proper construction of the contract, it appears that the parties did not intend the term to be enforceable by the third party. And even where the term purports to provide a benefit for a third party, the position here is more precarious than the rights conferred by the creation of a trust, on account of a further cardinal principle of contract law.

At the heart of English contract law has always been the right of the parties to agree to vary, or even cancel, their agreement. So, even in situations in which the contracting parties agree initially to provide a benefit for a third party, they can, at some future point, revoke this. This enables the contracting parties not simply to 'contract out' of giving the third-party enforcement rights, but actually to agree subsequently to revoke the benefit altogether. Here, the Law Commission's recommendation that the contracting parties may expressly reserve the right to vary or cancel the third party's reliance or acceptance is provided for by s. 2.

In its main focus on the trust, this chapter—and the text overall—is seeking to show just how much can be understood about the trust by looking at its features and operations alongside those of the contract. Studying the doctrine of privity and its 'reform' by the 1999 Act reveals that contract is an altogether more precarious deliverer of third-party rights. It may well be that those who make agreements for third-party benefits will honour them and will not seek to revoke them, and thereby give rights of enforcement that are rights in a meaningful sense. However, this is in stark contrast with the rights that arise on the creation of a trust. For one thing, the creation of a valid trust is an arrangement that is permanent and cannot be revoked, and so this establishes the position for the third-party benefits that are provided by it. This means that, once created, there is no opportunity for a settlor to revoke the terms of a trust arrangement unless he has expressly reserved for himself what is known as a 'right of revocation'. This is because, once constituted, altering the arrangement to X's detriment would be akin to making a gift to him and then taking it back again. Because of this, the rights of enforcement attaching to an express trust are recognized by equity as arising 'as of right', just as the rights of a party to a contract to enforce it are recognized by law as arising as of right. This flows from the 'hard-nosed property rights' that *Foskett* v *McKeown* [2000] 2 WLR 1299 tells us characterize a beneficiary's interest in trust property (see Chapter 1).

Thus, although the 1999 Act has forced us to re-evaluate the crucial distinction that has traditionally subsisted between the trust and the contract, it is also the case that the legislation is not a third-party charter and that the trust is altogether a less precarious way of creating third-party rights.

Further consideration of the historic interactions of the trust and the doctrine of privity can be found on the Online Resource Centre. For present purposes, we are keen to reinforce the core characteristic of the trust as providing benefits of property that are both permanent and gratuitous, and also that a beneficiary's rights of enforcement reflect that, under a trust, he enjoys a type of ownership of property. This is what makes the trust very much like a gift, which is what now remains to be considered.

2.4.5 Using property to provide benefit: creating a gift for another

Chapter 1 introduced the way in which fuller understanding of the trust, what it is and what it does, can be achieved from comparing creating trusts of property with making gifts of it. We are now going to look at the gift, so that we can understand more about what we now know is called an express trust—that is, the type of trust that arises because an owner of property is seeking to provide benefits for another using that property. Looking at the gift will provide the basis for understanding how different the gift and the trust actually are, and especially of the reasons why this is the case.

The gift has been held over as the last of these different mechanisms found in law that enable an owner of property to use it to benefit another. This is because, in getting closer to learning more about the trust, it is in the gift that we can see the greatest number of features in common, notwithstanding that all of these (other) arrangements work differently from the trust, with its very special operating feature of separated ownership. Whilst the loan and the transfer for consideration both provide benefits of property for those who want it from those who have it, the recipient must pay for this: the benefit is not gratuitous as it is with a trust, and nor is it even permanent, in the case of a loan. In the case of a contract for benefiting a third party, the benefit is gratuitous, but it might or might not be permanent, because it can be revoked. In a gift situation, the benefits provided are always gratuitous, and they are also always permanent and irrevocable once an effective gift is made. An effective gift is one that the law will recognize has given the recipient ownership of the property *at law* even though he has provided nothing in return.

We can see that these characteristics make the gift very like the trust in many respects, whilst we already have a sense of how differently these two mechanisms work. We know that the signature feature of the trust is that it delivers the benefits of property through separating ownership of property into distinctive titles to that property, and now we need to appreciate how a gift of property might be achieved, so that we can make these comparisons. The way in which the gift, like the trust, seeks to create benefits of property that are both permanent and irrevocable, and also entirely gratuitous, can be seen from the key authority *Milroy* v *Lord* (1862) 4 De GF & J 264. This is a highly significant case for studying the creation of express trusts, which we will encounter in Chapters 3, 4, and 5 (and also Chapter 18). At this point, *Milroy* explains, at 274, that an owner of property who wishes to provide such benefits can do so as follows:

> [I]n order to render a voluntary settlement valid and effectual, the settlor ... may of course do this by actually transferring the property to the persons for whom he intends to provide, and the provision will then be effectual, and it will be equally effectual if he transfers the property to a trustee for the purposes of the settlement, or declares that he himself holds it on trust for those purposes.

To clarify the language used here, as we will find out in Chapters 4 and 5, use of the term 'effective', or 'effectual', is a synonym for something being 'valid'. This is a term that most would recognize, and it becomes very significant when considering transfers of property that are 'invalid' or 'ineffective'. What is likely to be less familiar at this stage is the use of the term 'voluntary'. We did actually encounter this embodied in one of equity's maxims—that 'equity will not assist a volunteer'—and once again this will become more significant in Chapters 4 and 5. What we need to understand here is that the term 'voluntary settlement', or 'voluntary transfer', refers to one that is made by an owner of property in favour of another that is gratuitous on his part, and will not involve consideration. In this type of arrangement, a recipient is known as a 'volunteer'.

In this famous passage from Turner LJ's judgment in *Milroy*, we can see the similarities between the mechanisms of trust and gift, and also in their intended effects. Here, both will involve an owner of property losing ownership of the property because this person wants another to have the benefits of owning property permanently and also gratuitously. The simplest way of defining a gift, which also explains how technically this will be achieved, is as a gratuitous transfer of ownership of property from one person to another. The parties in a gift arrangement are known respectively as 'donor' and 'recipient', and what will happen upon making a gift is that the donor will lose the bundle of rights to the property embodied in its ownership, and these will be acquired by the intended recipient of the property. We know from Chapter 1 that outright ownership is itself represented by holding legal title to the property, and so, when making a gift, ownership of property is passed from one person to another through making a transfer of legal title to the property.

At some levels, making a gift is simple: a gift of property will arise because this is what the owner of property wants to happen. We are familiar with this through the custom of making gifts for birthdays and family occasions, and also to mark religious and cultural occasions, but because making gifts is so deeply entrenched in our psyches, many of us will never give any thought to the legal mechanics that are involved. What we are doing when we make a gift on such occasions is passing ownership of property that we own to another person because we want that other person to have it. What we will not be familiar with is how the way in which we do this actually reflects legal rules developed around making gifts that are effective and valid—and which, once they have been made, cannot be revoked.

Legal rules for making valid gifts have developed because this is a transfer of ownership in property, and it is also—unlike a transfer for consideration—one that occurs gratuitously and without an exchange. So there will be fewer visible indices of transfer of ownership that can make it clear that this is what the owner of property actually wants. It is very important that this is capable of being ascertained and established, because the owner will lose that ownership of the property to another. Because of this, law has developed rules that govern how any transfers of ownership from one person to another must be conducted for law to be prepared to accept that this has happened and to regard it as 'effective'. As we will discover in Chapter 4, so-called 'transfer formality requirements' are designed to prevent secret dealings with property, and to ensure that only an owner of property can pass good title to it and that a new owner of property will properly be recognized where this has happened.

Much more is said about formality generally in Chapter 5, but, in this discussion concerning gifts, we can see that formality requirements surrounding gratuitous transfers are concerned with two things: first, with what the law requires is present in any transfer of ownership of property from one person to another; and second, with ensuring that this is what the owner of property wants, because it is clear that he does. In a sale of property, the latter function will be served by the 'exchange' involving consideration, whilst in a gift situation it requires an owner of property to show his intention to lose ownership of property gratuitously in favour of another. In relation to actual requirements of transfer, what the law requires will depend on the nature of property rather than its value.

When these two elements are taken together, we can see that what is required to make an effective gift of property has resulted in different approaches being adopted, according to how property is classified in English law. What is required will depend on whether the property is, first, *real* property or *personal* property, and then, in relation to personal property, whether the property is *tangible* or *intangible*.

How does an owner of property make a gift that is effective?

To be a gift that is effective and one that will confer upon a new owner the bundle of rights that law recognizes as ownership, all gifts require an owner's *intention* that this should happen. This can be clear from a written deed of gift, or from an owner delivering that property to the recipient, making it clear that it is to become the property of the recipient (and that he is not simply making a loan of it, nor offering it for sale, etc.). For personal property that is a chattel—or a chose in possession—this is all that is required, which reflects the fact that dealings with chattels are commonplace in everyday life. Indeed, the common law has even developed the more flexible approach of 'symbolic' delivery, where actual physical delivery is difficult on account of the size of the property or, on occasions, its value, as illustrated by *Jaffa* v *Taylor Gallery Ltd*, The Times, 21 March 1990.

Even without the detailed discussion of formality requirements that is still to come, we already have a sense that prescriptions regarding how property is passed from one person to another are seeking to protect ownership by preventing unintended dealings with property. In this light, it is not surprising that law has developed additional requirements for types of property that are dealt with less in the course of everyday dealings than chattels. And in respect of dealings with land and intangible personal property (choses in action), establishing intention through a deed of gift or through delivery to the intended recipient is only the starting point for achieving an effective transfer.

Taking land first, no transfer of title to property that is land will be effective unless this is made by way of a written conveyance. This is according to s. 52 of the Law of Property Act 1925, and means that an owner can tell another of his wish to give that other his house, but unless there is a proper deed for the conveyance, then no title to the property will pass from its owner to the intended recipient. In respect of intangible personal property, what is actually required will depend on the actual species of chose in action itself, but clusters around requirements of writing and endorsement (that is, signing), and sometimes registration. This reflects a general appreciation that intangible property is itself less visible than a chose in action, and thus there is scope for dealings with it to be less visible and a concomitant need to make ownership of it more visible in these circumstances. So, in this regard and in relation to some common types of intangible property:

- *cheques* must be endorsed for title to pass by virtue of the Bills of Exchange Act 1882;
- *copyrights*, etc., must be in writing to pass title on account of s. 90(3) of the Copyrights, Designs and Patents Act 1988; and
- *shares* must be transferred by the completion of the appropriate form, plus registration of the transfer, by virtue of requirements currently set out in the Companies Act 2006 (and a long-standing requirement of 'companies legislation').

Gifts that are considered ineffective at law

Where these requirements have not been met, this attempted transfer of ownership is not one that law will recognize, and it will fail. Such a failed transfer is known technically as an 'incomplete transfer', or one that is an 'ineffective transfer'. In a number of cases, reference is also made to incomplete or ineffective transfers as ones that are 'imperfect' because they are flawed, and as such are incapable of transferring ownership effectively.

The normal outcome in this situation is that the original owner will retain ownership, because the intended recipient cannot acquire ownership at law. The reference to 'normal outcome' is to the way in which, as far as the law is concerned, the transfer has failed, and the attempted gift is not an effective one. This can be seen in Turner LJ's judgment in *Milroy* (see the start of section 2.4.5). However, because equity is concerned with achieving just outcomes, there are occasions on which equity is prepared to be more flexible than law, and so is prepared to recognize a valid transfer of ownership in circumstances in which law would not be prepared to do so.

We shall find out more about equity's role in incomplete property transfers when we study formality requirements. For present purposes, it is enough to explain that making a gift involves an outright transfer of ownership, and also to reinforce that, to make a gift, there is an outright transfer of ownership required, and this is quite different from the trust, which *separates* ownership.

2.5   From introducing the trust to the substantive law of trusts and the initial link provided by 'ownership'

Following on from the introduction made to the trust in this chapter and the last, Chapter 3 marks the beginning of our study of the substantive law of trusts. This will take a detailed look at what is required to create a valid express trust, and will be a chapter-by-chapter study of the main requirements of a valid trust. Chapter 3 begins this with a consideration of so-called 'certainty requirements', which is then followed by discussion in Chapter 4 of formality requirements, with a meeting point for a number of these considerations being the focus in Chapter 5 on how a trust is constituted. In this regard, Chapters 3, 4, and 5 can be seen as a corpus of chapters concerned with the creation of trusts by focusing on what is required to create a valid trust.

Much of this core material applies to trusts that are expressly created by a settlor for the very purpose of providing benefits of property—whether this is directly to provide benefits for (a) specific person(s), or less directly by seeking to avoid full exposure to taxation. This reflects a proposition that will be referenced at several points throughout this text: that the general law of trusts has evolved and developed to reflect these deliberate attempts to create trusts of property in mind. This will be borne out when we consider implied trusts in the next part of the text, where it will become clear that even though these are also what we can regard as 'private trusts', the law governing their creation and operation can be quite different from arrangements that law recognizes as deliberate attempts to settle property on trust.

By way of an introduction to the general law of trusts, which at this point reflects how an express trust is validly created, we also need to understand that property can be settled on trust only by a person who owns it at law. This is one of the requirements of a valid trust, but is one that can be dealt with briefly here before moving to the main requirements that flow from this basic premise. It is known as the 'capacity requirement', and in this regard we can see a legal owner's right to settle property on trust for another as part of his entitlement to deal freely with property. This is, of course, part of his 'bundle of rights' embodied in ownership of property, which is represented formally by his holding legal title to it.

 Revision Box

1. For very fundamental issues, explain the following.
   (a) What is meant by the term 'express trust'?
   (b) What 'roles' or 'actors' can be identified in an express trust arrangement?
   (c) If ownership is separated into distinct components in a trust, who holds each type of title and what happens to the original owner of the property?
   (d) Why create a trust rather than make a gift of property from the perspective of each of the actors encountered in an express trust arrangement?
2. In focusing on express trusts directly, explain what is meant by the following.
   (a) An express trust that is 'fixed'
   (b) An express trust that is discretionary'
   (c) A 'power', and how 'powers' are encountered in the study of trusts.

FURTHER READING

Conaglen (2005) 'The nature and function of fiduciary loyalty' 121 Law Quarterly Review 452.

Emery (1982) 'The most hallowed principle: certainty of beneficiaries of trusts and powers of appointment' 98 Law Quarterly Review 551.

Harris (1971) 'Trust, power and duty' 87 Law Quarterly Review 31.

Hopkins (1971) 'Certain uncertainties of trusts and powers' 29 Cambridge Law Journal 68.

Millett (1985) 'The *Quistclose* trust: who can enforce it?' 101 Law Quarterly Review 269.

Thompson (2002) 'Criminal law and property law: an unhappy combination' 66 Conveyancer 387.

 online resource centre For summaries of a selection of these articles, please visit <http://www.oxfordtextbooks.co.uk/orc/wilson_trusts11e/>

3

The three certainties and the significance of the 'beneficiary principle'

This chapter marks the beginning of our study of the substantive law of trusts, by focusing on certainty requirements. It also marks the beginning of a core of chapters concerned with the creation of trusts, which focus on what is required to create a valid trust of property. Unlike some of the other requirements that we will find here in this first part of the text, certainty requirements apply across all private trusts. Having made that point, it is also the case that these requirements are at their most direct and explicit when we are referring to deliberate settlement of property on trust through creation of an express trust—and perhaps especially so when we consider what is known as 'certainty of intention'. The same is the case for this chapter's other, but closely related, focal point: the beneficiary principle. This is regarded as a cardinal principle of trusts law, and applies in some manifestation to all trusts except for charitable ones— although, once again, it is in the express private trust that its application is clearest and most obvious.

Traditionally, this chapter has commenced with passages explaining why the certainty requirement exists for creating a valid trust and why no trust can be valid without it. In this edition, a different approach has been chosen, and the rationale for this requirement will be used to close the passages on certainty. This is for two reasons: one reflects the substantive materials on certainty; the other reflects the structure of the chapter. In relation to the latter, this chapter is subdivided into two distinct parts, albeit that these parts are closely related. We will find that looking at the beneficiary principle follows on naturally from considering the certainty-of-objects requirement, but also that a quite distinct set of issues will be discussed within it. In relation to the former, you will find the material on certainty lengthy and at times complicated. This is perhaps especially so given that, when we look at certainty-of-objects requirements for trusts, we will also have to touch on how these requirements operate in what are known as 'powers', which were introduced in Chapter 2. So it is hoped that being able to wrap up by reflecting on what meeting these requirements is all about will be a helpful way of starting to clarify your understanding.

Part I Certainty and the creation of a valid trust

3.1 Certainty requirements: a general overview

The starting point that is almost always used for studying certainty requirements is the famous passage in Lord Langdale's judgment in *Knight* v *Knight* (1840) 3 Beav 148. The classification of certainty requirements that has been distilled from this judgment can be criticized, and it has indeed been the subject of criticism, but it is the classification that has traditionally been adopted by the courts and it remains at the heart of judicial approaches to certainty requirements. It is from this that what have become known as the 'three certainties' have emerged—but, ahead of revealing what these actually are, it is probably helpful to have a sense of what is meant when the term 'certainty' is used.

In this context, when we are considering what is necessary to bring into being a valid trust, whenever reference is made to 'certainty requirements', this is reference to making it *clear* that creating a trust of property is being attempted. So *what* has to be clear or certain is, according to Lord Langdale:

> As a general rule, it has been laid down that when property is given absolutely to any person and the same person is ... to dispose of that property in favour of another ... it will be considered a trust ... First, if the words so used, that upon the whole they ought to be considered as imperative, secondly, if the subject (of the arrangement) be certain, and thirdly, if the objects or persons intended to have the benefit of the recommendation or wish also be certain.

So, to summarize *what* must be clear or certain on the basis of Lord Langdale's adopted classification, we can glean that, to create a valid trust (with these rules being clearest in application for an express trust):

- it must be certain that the settlor *intends* to create a trust of property;
- it must also be certain *what* is intended to be trust property; and
- it must be clear *who* is intended to benefit from the settlement of property on trust.

In turn, requiring that it is clear that a trust is intended has become known as 'certainty of intention', whilst 'certainty of subject matter' is the term given to requiring the property that is being settled to be made clear. And the requirement that it is clear who is intended to benefit from this arrangement is known as the 'certainty of objects' requirement.

Satisfying certainty, and the absence of certainty?
Everything up to now has suggested that this is one of the core validity requirements for private trusts and, generally, when we speak of 'validity requirements', the position is that if any of these is not met or complied with, then the attempt to create a trust will not succeed and no trust can arise. However, with certainty requirements, the practical consequences of such a failed attempt to create a trust for others will depend on the circumstances. This will become clearer as we look through the requirements themselves and explain at each stage how absence of a particular certainty requirement will affect attempts to create trusts. But at the outset it is probably worth noting that the consequences of there being no certainty of *intention* to create a trust will produce different results from when it is clear—or certain—that creating a trust is what was intended, but this cannot happen because it is not clear *what* is being settled on trust or for *whom*. It would be helpful to try to understand this general position at this stage, but it will, of course, be explained at the relevant junctures in the text, when it will be easier to see what happens in its proper context.

What follows now is a detailed examination of all three components that embody the certainty requirements which must be satisfied for a trust to arise. As we work through the material, we must remember that, for a valid trust to be created, all three must be satisfied, even though the precise consequences of failing to meet the individual requirements will differ. The net result is that the trust which the owner of property appears to be trying to create cannot and will not come into being.

3.2 Certainty of intention

The certainty-of-intention requirement is what we can distil from Lord Langdale's requirement that 'words so used' must be clear or certain so as to indicate that a trust is intended. This is sometimes misleadingly termed the requirement of 'certainty of words'. This is not unreasonable given that this is actually what Lord Langdale says, but it is one of the reasons why his classification has been criticized. This is more appropriately termed the 'requirement that it must be clear that a settlor intends to create a trust' for a number of reasons. Essentially, these are as follows.

The practicalities surrounding the creation of trusts
Although we learned in Chapter 2 that, in practice, a large number of express trusts are documented in writing, this is because they are being used strategically in tax planning and not because there is any requirement that they are so. Indeed, as signposted in Chapter 2, Chapter 4 explains that, ordinarily, trusts can be declared orally and have no requirement to be in writing.

That the courts have taken an approach according significance to words used, but not regarding them as conclusive
We see evidence that the courts have taken an approach that accords significance to words used, but does not regard them as conclusive, in this chapter's discussion of precatory words, and also in the approach in *Harrison* v *Gibson* [2006] 1 All ER 858, which is authority that, where words are used, the courts will interpret them in their individual context rather than take a literal objective reading of them. And because equity looks at intention rather than form, this means that creation of a trust can be inferred from even very simple and untechnical language, and without ever using the term 'trust'. So this points to certainty of intention being something different from, or certainly something that cannot be collapsed into, certainty of words. This becomes even more apparent when we consider the way in which the courts have adopted the spirit, rather than the letter, of Lord Langdale's approach by accepting that, on occasions, a settlor's conduct (in the actual absence of words) can be evidence of his intention to create a trust.

The approach taken in *Harrison* v *Gibson* [2006] 1 All ER 858 reflects the way in which many trusts will be created in writing, either because they arise under a will (and are thus testamentary trusts, denoted by the 'WT' suffix) or because they are used for tax planning purposes. In the latter situation, making a written declaration of trust provides documentary evidence of when a trust was created, which is at the heart of tax planning. In this setting, a modern trust 'precedent' will be carefully documented to meet an individual settlor's tax planning needs, and will be highly intricate and designed to provide for almost all conceivable contingencies, with *Harrison* suggesting that even identical wording used can have quite different meanings when used by different people in different contexts.

3.3 **The modern law relating to certainty of intention**

Here, we learn more about how an owner of property makes it clear (or 'certain') that he wants to create a trust of his property rather than do something different with it. In *Knight* v *Knight*, Lord Langdale spoke about conveying an 'imperative', which will become clearer shortly. For now, it should not be too surprising to learn that an owner of property can make it certain, or clear, that he intends to create a trust by saying that the property is to be 'given to B, on trust for C'. This would make things very clear, but successfully settling property on trusts commonly arises without making things *this* clear.

The title for this section is deliberate because it is, of course, important for a text of this nature to give most emphasis to the law as it is. Again, the starting point is Lord Langdale's famous passage in *Knight* v *Knight*, showing how the courts have adopted this and refined it for current conditions. In this regard, it will become clear that this modern development of *Knight* reflects that trusts arising from commercial dealings are as important, if not more important, than the traditional trusts, which were concerned very much with family arrangements. But we also need to look at historical readings of Lord Langdale's judgment to explain what the courts will not regard as acceptable in the modern law, as well as what they will—whether this is in the context of traditional trusts, or in the way in which trusts are increasingly being found in commercial dealings.

For these reasons, there will often be a written document that evidences intention to create a trust, which will then be interpreted according to *Harrison* v *Gibson*. But we also now know that a trust can arise without this, and even without settlors making their intention clear through use of the term 'trust'. Here, examining the key case of *Paul* v *Constance* [1977] 1 All ER 195 and also a line of cases descending from *Re Kayford* [1975] 1 All ER 604, we can see how flexible the courts are on finding intention even where this is not expressed as such, or even at all. Here, we find cases that are authority that less will suffice, and that words, or even conduct, can provide evidence of intention and give rise to a valid trust.

Paul v *Constance* involved a cohabiting couple, Mr Constance and Mrs Paul, and the fate after Constance's death of money that she had placed in a bank account. The claim against the money was brought by Constance's wife, to whom he remained legally married whilst he had set up home with Mrs Paul. Originally, £950, which was compensation obtained by Constance following an accident at work, was placed in a bank account that was held in Constance's name alone. There was evidence suggesting that it was always Constance's intention that the money was held for both him and Mrs Paul, notwithstanding that the bank account in Constance's name gave him ownership of the money at law. Indeed, there was evidence that the couple had been advised against opening a joint account by the bank manager, so as not to cause embarrassment to Mrs Paul. Following this initial deposit, there were a number of movements of money in and out of this account. One withdrawal of £150 was made, which was divided equally between them, and several deposits were made of winnings at bingo, which was regarded as a joint venture by the couple. When Constance died, the issue was raised whether Mrs Paul could claim any share of the fund. If the money in the account had belonged solely to Constance, then his wife, Mrs Constance, would be entitled to it on his death.

The Court of Appeal held that the money was not owned absolutely by Constance, and that Constance instead held the money on trust for himself and Mrs Paul, which gave Mrs Paul an equal share of the money. This was so notwithstanding that no words of trust were used; instead, Constance's certainty of intention was inferred from a combination of what he did say to Mrs Paul, his conduct surrounding the arrangement, and the nature of his relationship with Mrs Paul. Indeed, showing intention to create a trust in this way was an entirely appropriate reflection of Constance's unsophisticated character and demeanour, as Scarman LJ noted at 531:

> When one looks at the detailed evidence to see whether it goes as far as that—and I think that the evidence does go as far as that—one finds that from the time that the deceased received his damages right up to his death he was saying, on occasions, that the money was as much the plaintiff's as his. When they discussed the damages, how to invest them or what to do with them and when they discussed the bank account, he would say to her: 'The money is as much yours as mine'.

Scarman LJ also suggested that this was a borderline decision, the reasons for which will be considered shortly, but in giving considerable scope to what is permissible for amounting to showing certainty of intention to create a trust, Scarman LJ also insisted that, however it is shown, there is a definite factor that has to be present in the utterings and doings of all—sophisticated or otherwise—for the courts to find that a trust is intended: '[T]here must be clear evidence from what is said or done of an intention to create a trust ... an intention to dispose of property or a fund so that somebody else to the exclusion of the disponent acquires a beneficial interest in it.'

Paul v Constance *and the significance of 'the circumstances' for finding certainty of intention*

Paul v *Constance* was applied in *Rowe* v *Prance* [1999] 2 FLR 787, showing that the courts continue to make rulings on certainty of intention in the context of family relationships. In addition, there is a line of cases dating from the same time as *Paul* v *Constance* showing us that, increasingly, the courts are having to make these deliberations outside family dealings, and actually in commercial and business dealings. Here, a line of commercial cases dating from *Re Kayford Ltd* [1975] 1 WLR 279 reveal more about what must be shown by words or conduct in order for a trust to be intended.

Like others that have followed it, the *Re Kayford* litigation arose from a company experiencing financial difficulty, and is one of a number of cases in which these organizations have been held to have declared trusts of money that has been received by them, which has been contributed by their customers or others with whom they deal. We will come back to these cases again, as we will *Paul* v *Constance* and others that we will encounter shortly in this chapter (notably, *Jones* v *Lock* and *Richards* v *Delbridge*) when we look at how trusts are validly constituted in Chapter 5. But, for now, *Re Kayford* and subsequent cases illustrate for us that the courts will allow certainty of intention to be established from conduct alone, and that, for this to happen, there are requirements regarding what must be shown.

In *Re Kayford*, a mail order company that was in financial difficulties and the directors of which feared insolvency sought to protect customers who placed orders with it. To do this, the company sought to set up a separate bank account, which was to be called the 'Customers' Trust Deposit Account', to hold the customers' deposits and payments until their goods were delivered. The intention behind this was that the customers' money should be kept separate from the company's general funds, but the company's bank advised it that instead of opening a new account, it should instead use an existing, but dormant, account already in existence and held in its name, which contained a small credit balance. When the company was wound up, it was held that the money in the account (minus the small credit balance) was held by the company on trust for the customers. This meant that instead of being ordinary creditors of the company who would have to stand in line with other creditors for assets that could be available for repayment, those customers who had not received their ordered goods were actually beneficial owners of the money, which would not fall to be distributed by ordinary rules of winding up.

As Megarry J explained, at 282, 'it is well settled that a trust can be created without using the words "trust" or "confidence" or the like: the question is whether a sufficient intention to create a trust has been manifested'. In this regard, Megarry J insisted that it did not matter that the money had not been placed in a separate account as had originally been intended. This involved an extended discussion around the way in which ordinary debtor–creditor relations could be transformed by finding intention to create a trust: in these circumstances, 'the obligations in respect of the money are transformed from contract to property, from debt to trust'. This is so albeit that Megarry J reasoned this with reference to the decision in *Re Nanwa Gold Mines Ltd* [1955] 1 WLR 1080. Strictly speaking, *Nanwa Gold Mines* was actually a *Quistclose* arrangement (so-called after *Barclays Bank Ltd* v *Quistclose Investments Ltd* [1970] AC 567, which is discussed briefly in this chapter, before being considered extensively in Chapter 18), whereby a trust arises in what would normally be a straightforward contractual debtor–creditor relationship, because this is what the creditor (rather than the debtor in a *Kayford* situation) intends. *Kayford* does now appear dated in the light of modern consumer protection legislation, and Megarry J's judgment on the requirements of declarations of trust must, on one level, be read in light of this.

Nevertheless, reading *Kayford* as a commentary about the circumstances that can give rise to declarations of trust is still of utmost importance for trusts lawyers, who must be able to appreciate and understand a number of fundamental values, and how they have developed. There will always be a need to consider how these 'trusts values' might be applied in novel situations, as the more recent cases show. It is also the case that only the context for *Kayford* is dated, and that its principles can actually be seen in operation in a number of cases that have followed it. What the customers in *Kayford* needed to show in order to recover the money in the account was a proprietary interest in the money, to which they could assert a claim, and which would operate to privilege their claims over others that may have been made against the fund. This required identifying the fund containing the contributions as trust property. This was possible on the basis that the money never dropped below the amount of the initial deposit amount (so that the excess amounts were clearly the contributions), and this situation arose from the company's intentions for the money in that account. Setting out the entire passage from Megarry J's judgment, at 282, will make understanding what has been said so far easier and will also aid developing these ideas further:

> [T]he money was sent on the faith of a promise to keep it in a separate account, but there is nothing in that case or in any other authority that I know of to suggest that this is essential. I feel no doubt that here a trust was created. From the outset the advice (which was accepted) was to establish a trust account at the bank. The whole purpose of what was done was to ensure that the moneys remained in the beneficial ownership of those who sent them, and a trust is the obvious means of achieving this. No doubt the general rule is that if you send money to a company for goods which are not yet delivered, you are merely a creditor of the company unless a trust is created. The sender may create a trust by using appropriate words when he sends the money (though I wonder how many

> do this, even if they are equity lawyers), or the company may do it by taking suitable steps on or before receiving the money. If either is done, the obligations in respect of the money are transformed from contract to property, from debt to trust. Payment into a separate bank account is a useful (though by no means conclusive) indication of an intention to create a trust, but of course there is nothing to prevent the company from binding itself by a trust even if there are no effective banking arrangements.

So what were the company's intentions as far as the money was concerned in *Kayford*? We know that this account contained only customers' money, and was intended to be kept separate from the company's other assets, and we get a better sense of what its intentions actually had to be for a trust to arise from the way in which *Re Kayford* was applied by the Court of Appeal in *Re Chelsea Cloisters Ltd* [1980] 41 P & CR 98. This case concerned a 'tenants' deposit account', which was set up to hold deposits against damage and breakages. Notwithstanding the absence of expressions of trust, it was found that there was intention to create a trust because the act of setting up the account was an irrevocable step that would deprive the company of all beneficial interest in the money. This is what also lay at the heart of *Kayford*, in that the company understood that the fund containing the customers' money was not a fund on which it could draw. And in his discussion of *Nanwa Gold Mines* in *Kayford*, Megarry J spoke of the use of a separate bank account as useful, but not conclusive, evidence of intention to create a trust. This is very significant, given the decision in *Re Multi Guarantee Co. Ltd* [1987] BCLC 257, in which the Court of Appeal distinguished the two previous cases, because, although there was a separate account, no final decision on what to do with the money in it had been taken and so an irrevocable intention was not established.

Very recently, and in the context of the aftermath of the Icelandic banking crisis, a *Kayford* argument failed in *Du Preez Ltd* v *Kaupthing Singer & Friedlander (Isle of Man) Ltd* [2011] WTLR 559. This was so on the grounds that 'mere acceptance by a bank of instructions from its customer could not be analysed as a declaration of trust by the bank', and it was found that the facts before the court were 'far removed from that line of authorities'. In similar vein, and very controversially, *Re Farepak* [2006] EWHC 3272 (Ch) produced a result that is widely regarded as out of line with the application of *Kayford* in *Chelsea Cloisters* and the distinction drawn in *Re Multi Guarantee*. It has even been analysed by some as a harbinger of different times in which the courts will be less open to finding certainty of intention to create a trust in certain situations, with a strong suggestion that this is particularly the case in situations of financial distress that result in insolvency.

This case arose from a Christmas savings scheme, operated by Farepak, which allowed customers to spread the costs of festive season purchases over the year. The scheme operated through a system of agents who would collect customers' money and pass this onto Farepak. On 11 October 2006, Farepak's directors decided to cease trading and Farepak went into administration on 13 October. The moneys paid to Farepak by the customers had largely gone, but in the final three days leading up to the administration the directors sought to ring-fence moneys received by customers in that period, so that they could be returned to them if necessary. A deed of trust was executed, but this contained a mistake as to the bank account identified in it. It was argued by the administrator that moneys received in the administration period, and the period from 11 October to 16 October, were held on trust for the customers. Reasonings included *Quistclose* principles (making it an implied resulting trust), the expressly executed declaration of trust, an implied declaration arising out of the related facts, and even a rather bizarrely reasoned constructive trust.

The existence of a trust was rejected in *Farepak* even though the mistake in the trust deed could be rectified, because this trust deed was said not to alter the character of the relationship between *Farepak* and its customers from one that was contractual to one giving rise to obligations arising from existence of a trust and concomitant proprietary entitlements. There was insufficient evidence that a trust was intended, and the trust deed instead pointed to a mere declaration of intent to use the funds in a particular way. This could look consistent with *Multi Guarantee*, in which there was a separate bank account, but no definite and irrevocable course of conduct for its content. However, the Farepak directors had drawn up the trust deed because they did intend for customer money to be ring-fenced so that it could be returned to them if necessary. Although this sounds like a textbook re-run of *Kayford*, there was actually no reference in *Farepak* to *Kayford* or to its Court of Appeal approval in *Chelsea Cloisters*.

If the courts are becoming less willing to recognize trusts in these situations, then we need to try to understand why this might be the case. The line of thinking that is critical of both *Kayford* and especially *Quistclose* principles suggests that trusts are being used instrumentally in order to avoid the ordinary consequences of insolvency law. This is especially an issue with *Quistclose* trusts (considered in Chapter 18), which can very easily be seen as a creditor's intended avoidance of the ordinary consequences of insolvency law. This is not a study of insolvency law, but these criticisms flow from the position that, once it is clear that a business cannot be saved, the policy of insolvency law is to ensure that as many of its creditors can be paid from the assets that are still available for this purpose. There is a statutory list for prioritizing payment amongst creditors in which customers and ordinary creditors (who have taken no security for their loans) rank below a number of other creditors, and are unlikely to be paid, given that the very reason the business has become insolvent is because its financial liabilities outstrip its assets.

Critics of *Kayford* and *Quistclose* arrangements suggest that those who are owed money by failing businesses are effectively able to become secured creditors by showing that their loan was made on trust principles rather than ordinary contractual ones, and this means that what is deemed 'trust property' never becomes part of the general pool for distribution amongst creditors. This is explained more fully in Chapter 17, but essentially it is possible on the basis that a beneficiary's equitable ownership of trust property confers a proprietary entitlement, which is protected in the event of the insolvency of the party who holds legal title to the property.

Here, *Farepak* is viewed by some as evidence of changing judicial attitudes to finding trusts, given how much business failure current economic conditions have already produced and are forecast to continue to produce. This proposed influence of policy on judicial willingness to 'find' the existence of a trust—by casting doubt on intention to create one—implied in *Farepak* is more openly discussed in *Pearson* v *Lehman Bros Finance SA* [2010] EWHC 2914 (Ch). Although he was prepared to acknowledge the importance of policy only 'at the margins', Briggs J did insist that any ruling that property that would otherwise be available for distribution amongst unsecured creditors—in accordance with insolvency law—is subject to a trust should not be made 'lightly'. Certainty-of-intention rules do generally seek to ensure that no trust is created lightly. But restating this basic rule in this context makes explicit that 'finding' a trust where there is an insolvency can too easily compromise legal mechanisms to ensure fairness in these circumstances (see the discussion in Chapter 18).

Farepak has been criticized for not applying *Kayford* principles where, on the facts of the case, certainty of intention could have been found. The use of *Quistclose* reasoning was criticized in any case, but *Kayford* arrangements are based on the same premise, whilst also working differently by reflecting a debtor's intention rather than a creditor's. It is possible that this marks the beginning of a conscious policy against finding a debtor's declaration of trust. But in arriving at the conclusion that there was no trust for the customer depositors, it is suggested that the application of *Quistclose* principles in *Farepak* was wrong in those particular circumstances, because the attempt to create the trust was made by the debtor in what appeared to be a textbook application of *Kayford*.

Quistclose *principles and a creditor's certainty of intention*

However, *Quistclose* principles and decisions made on them are highly significant for this discussion of certainty of intention. *Quistclose* arrangements are so called after *Barclays Bank Ltd* v *Quistclose Investments Ltd* [1970] AC 567, the key House of Lords case that gave recognition to them. As Chapter 6 explains and Chapter 18 develops, these arrangements are trusts arising from loans made by creditors to debtors, which are non-express and are recognized as being a type of resulting trust. They are important here because they illustrate how circumstances that are distinct from *Kayford* arrangements can give rise to certainty of intention to create a trust. For our purposes here, *Quistclose* arrangements are non-express trusts that arise where, although no words of trust are used, money is lent to a debtor for a specific purpose, and carrying out this purpose subsequently becomes impossible. At this point, the creditor is entitled to the return of what is his property, which—because it is subject to a trust—is regarded as being separate from the debtor's other property, even if it has not been kept physically separated from it. Like *Kayford* arrangements, *Quistclose* trusts are very strongly associated with financial distress and business failure, but key to their operation is that although any creditor will lose legal title to money lent (whether this is on contractual principles or trust principles), because of his intention that it must be used only for a specific purpose, title becomes separated and he will retain equitable title to it. This is what enables him to claim as his property that which is held by a debtor who becomes insolvent.

Again, like *Kayford*, a trust will not automatically follow from circumstances of financial distress, and a loan will be treated as an ordinary contractual arrangement unless intention to create a trust can be found. For *Quistclose* arrangements, the key requirements are that money is advanced for a specific purpose, and although the existence of a separate bank account is not conclusive evidence of this, it is regarded as being very strong evidence in favour of a trust. When we discuss *Quistclose* arrangements in Chapter 18, it will become apparent that a core requirement for being able to enforce this arrangement is that the purpose for which the money was advanced cannot be carried out, and the way in which the courts have interpreted this has attracted a great deal of criticism.

For a *Quistclose* trust to arise, as far as certainty of intention is concerned, the most important cases are *Twinsectra* v *Yardley* [2002] 2 WLR 802 and *Du Preez Ltd* v *Kaupthing Singer & Friedlander (Isle of Man) Ltd* [2011] WTLR 559. Both cases point to (*Quistclose*) trusts arising from the intention of the *parties*, with this being ascertained from their dealings and the circumstances of the case. Given that it is conventionally understood that trusts arise from a *settlor's* intention, this suggests that different considerations may apply to satisfying certainty of intention in commercial dealings, in which contractual relations are the norm and the parties are bargaining 'at arm's length'.

This proposition is discussed at length in Chapter 18, but we can see it specifically noted in *Kayford*, in which Megarry J believed that he was not seeking to develop principles to be applied to commercial or 'trade creditors', and was instead concerned with the position of members of the public and especially those who could ill afford to lose out financially on account of the circumstances. Much more recently, and well beyond the somewhat dated context of *Kayford*, such sentiments can be found expressed by the Law Commission. The remarks were made in the context of the Law Commission's work on trustee exemption clauses—its Consultation Paper, *Trustee Exemption Clauses* (CP 171), was published in 2003 and its report of the same title (Law Com No. 301) in 2006—but in making it clear that it was acutely aware of the growing use of trusts in the sphere of commercial dealings, the Law Commission also suggested that some features of trusts arising in this context distinguished them from trusts arising elsewhere. Indeed, as the Law Commission noted in 2006, the parties found within such arrangements are likely to be market participants of equal strength, and thus well versed in the needs of business and the nature of business risks, and better placed to find out about the technical operation of trusts than an ordinary individual. In turn, this would mean that parties who become settlors in these arrangements would have much more familiarity with what is done and what needs to be done than those within a more traditional type of trust.

On the other hand, the Law Commission has also identified the precarious and actually genuinely ambiguous position of very small enterprises, termed 'micro businesses'. Couched within its work on reforming insurance contract law (see, for example, its paper *Reforming Insurance Contract Law: A Summary of Responses to Consultation*, published in 2009), the Law Commission's emphasis of the similarities between micro businesses and 'ordinary consumers' means that we need to be cautious in concluding that businesses are better able to bear losses than ordinary consumers. This is notwithstanding that, as *Farepak* shows, many participants in 'saving schemes' are from the very poorest groupings in society, with this reflecting the 'mail order' shopping patterns at the heart of *Kayford*.

Whatever *Farepak* actually stands as authority for, and putting aside for one moment criticism that these arrangements privilege some creditors at the expense of others and so thwart the intentions of insolvency law, these cases illustrate a very important point: they show that determinations on certainty of intention are being influenced increasingly by commercial dealings, rather than by private familial ones. And in this context *Farepak* is part of a lineage of cases showing us that certainty of intention to create a trust can arise within business dealings, which are ordinarily governed by contractual principles, without the term 'trust' ever being used.

3.4 A core requirement for satisfying certainty of intention

Beyond the business context, these cases are also part of a larger body of trusts jurisprudence that demonstrates that making your intention to create a trust clear or certain does not actually require you to say anything, and also that this is capable of being read into an extensive range of conduct. However, it also becomes clear, from looking at a different body of decisions, that the courts are very inflexible about one key criterion in determining whether or not the certainty of intention requirement has been satisfied. This is the case law that descends from *Milroy v Lord* (1862) 4 De GF & J 264.

You will remember that we looked at *Milroy v Lord* in Chapter 2, when learning about the different ways in which an owner of property can deal with it to provide benefits from it for others. One of the things that we could draw from *Milroy* at that point is that it set out two ways in which an owner of property can provide benefits for another that are both gratuitous and permanent. These are, of course, making a gift and declaring a trust, and two cases from the lineage of *Milroy* tell us that satisfying certainty-of-intention requirements mean that an owner of property must not simply intend for another to benefit from the property, but that he must also intend that the benefits be delivered by way of a trust.

In the modern law, this means that whatever an owner of property actually says or does in relation to his wishes for his property, for him to satisfy the certainty-of-intention requirement, he must make it clear that he is declaring a trust of his property rather than making a gift of it. This requirement can be seen illustrated in the key cases of *Jones* v *Lock* (1865) LR 1 Ch App 25 and *Richards* v *Delbridge* (1874) LR Eq 11. We will encounter both cases again in subsequent discussions of formality requirements and constituting trusts, but for now they are authority that the certainty-of-intention requirement will be satisfied only where it is clear or certain that an owner of property is seeking to create a trust. When we speak of 'declaring a trust', as Chapter 1 suggested, this is some kind of a statement on the part of the owner of property that property belonging to him is to be used to benefit others; in this context, this is key to satisfying the certainty of intention (to create a trust) requirement.

In *Jones* v *Lock*, a father handed a cheque to his 9-month-old son, uttering words that made it clear that he meant the child to have the sum represented by the cheque. He then removed the cheque for safe keeping, but died before he could endorse it in his son's favour. As will be explained in Chapter 4, endorsing the cheque was required to pass title to the child—that is, to make a valid gift of it—and so the only way in which the child could still receive the property was as beneficial owner under a trust. However, the court refused to construe the father's actions and statement that 'I give this to you, baby' as evidence that he was seeking to create a trust of the property, under which he (as holder of legal title) would be trustee. This is because Lord Cranworth LC ruled that the father's actions had not manifested an irrevocable intention to create a trust: essentially, there was no certainty of intention to create a trust.

A similar result arose in *Richards* v *Delbridge*, whereby Delbridge wished to give Richards—his infant grandson—the lease that he had on his place of business as a bone-and-manure merchant. He endorsed the lease with the wording 'This deed and all thereto belonging I give to Edward Benetto Richards from this time forth, with all the stock-in-trade', but this was not sufficient to make an effective legal assignment of the property, and the grandfather's death meant that this could not be done properly. The court once again refused to construe the grandfather's actions as manifesting intention to create a trust. Instead, like the father in *Jones* v *Lock*, the grandfather was deemed to have intended to make a gift of the property, which had failed because what was required to make an effective gift had not been carried out.

In his judgment, Sir George Jessel MR in *Richards* v *Delbridge* took care to emphasize that intending to make gifts and intending to create trusts were very different, and would be treated as being very different by the courts. A theme that runs through all of these cases is that, in looking for certainty of intention, the courts are looking for a point at which property ceases to be entirely at the disposal of its owner and becomes that in which he retains no interest, and this is intended to be a permanent arrangement. Once we have grasped the idea of a permanent and irrevocable cession of an owner's interest in his property, we need to be able to link this benchmark for identifying intention to create a trust with the significance attached by Lord Langdale to 'imperative' in *Knight*.

We know that the signature feature of the trust is that ownership is separated, and we also know that this is what makes it fundamentally different from a gift. So, in trying to clarify how intention to create a trust might be different from intention to make a gift, we need to think about why ownership becomes separated in the trust arrangement. Ownership becomes separated in the trust arrangement so that a beneficiary can enjoy the property whilst another has responsibility for the property and must use it only for this enjoyment of another. This is where we can start to understand the significance of 'imperative', as stressed by Lord Langdale. The idea of imperative is central to creating a trust, because those who hold legal title to property in this arrangement are not the owners of the property; instead, they are custodians of it, who are obliged to use it for the beneficiary's enjoyment.

Understanding this is very important because the material that now follows shows us that whatever words or conduct are used, they must be of a particular character. Here, Lord Langdale's insistence upon (words and/or conduct) conveying imperative translates into words and/or conduct that convey obligation or duty to use the property in a particular way—namely, to provide benefit for another. This is very important, because several cases tell us that words denoting anything different are not capable of evidencing intention to create a trust.

Words of a particular character: the history of precatory words
The intention that must be found must seek to impose on the holder of legal title the obligation to act in a particular way in relation to another, rather than to appeal to him to use the property in a particular way. This can be shown by judicial responses to donors of property who use words that express hope, wish, or desire. These are known as 'precatory words', and judicial approaches to them can be understood by means of an appreciation of the complex history between precatory words and certainty-of-intention requirements.

In the modern law, it is clear that the general position on precatory words is that they will not be regarded as capable of manifesting intention to create a trust. Authority for this is commonly regarded as coming from *Re Adams and the Kensington Vestry* (1884) 27 ChD 394, in which it was established that recipients of property were no longer to be made trustees unless this was the testator's clear intention, and a gift to the widow 'in full confidence that she would do what was right as to the disposal thereof between my children, either in her lifetime or by will after her decease' was treated as giving the widow an absolute interest unfettered by any trust in favour of the children. Cotton LJ felt that it was necessary to establish such a position, with other cases from this vintage, such as *Lambe* v *Eames* (1870–71) LR 6 Ch App 597, testifying to this.

From looking at *Adams* alone, it is not altogether apparent why the courts would need to make this clear, given that Lord Langdale's insistence on imperative pre-dates these decisions by a number of decades—and by half a century, in the case of *Adams*. However, there is a reason for this, because precatory words actually do share a complex history with satisfying certainty-of-intention requirements. At the heart of this is the law relating to executors of wills and the significance of the Executors Act 1830.

It is, of course, the case that, where someone has left instructions for disposal of their property by way of a will, this is actually the only way for ascertaining intention and there is no scope for asking for further direction. It is also the case that the history of precatory words, as far as intention to create trusts is concerned, exposes a further complication that, at one time, attached to ensuring that property would be dealt with according to what a deceased person apparently intended. Up until the middle of the nineteenth century, the courts were actually very predisposed to have regard to almost any expression of desire that an owner of property was seeking to create a binding trust of that property. This is because, historically, administration of estates lay with the ecclesiastical courts, which permitted an executor to keep for himself any undisposed-of residue of property after the specific bequests had been satisfied. When this jurisdiction was taken over by the Court of Chancery, it preferred to treat the executor as trustee of such residue for the testator's family, and almost any expression of desire or hope would be seized upon to effect this policy. Even this solution was not entirely satisfactory. Widows and eldest sons of gentry were often provided for in any event by a marriage settlement, or entail of the estate, and the courts were suspicious of their ability to manage the family property in prudent fashion (that is, to keep it in the family). This meant that a similar approach, which was developed for executors, began to be applied also to actual legatees under a will. To effect this, precatory words such as 'wish', 'hope', or even 'in confidence' that the legatee would use the gift to benefit others would be taken to create binding trusts.

3.5 The modern law on precatory words and the significance of intention

This lenient view taken of precatory words largely disappeared with the Executors Act 1830, which specifically required executors to hold property in an appropriate manner. Since 1830, therefore, the courts have felt able to tighten up their attitude, and cases such as *Adams* and *Lambe* provide authority for this. However, because a settlor's intention is all-important, cases such as *Paul* v *Constance* show us that the courts will have regard to language that is not ordinarily associated with creating trusts, with *Re Kayford* and subsequent cases showing us that this can even be inferred from conduct. What also becomes clear is that, when ruling on whether the certainty of intention requirement has or has not been satisfied, it is still possible for a trust to be created by precatory words if it appears, from looking at the entirety of a document and the settlor's conduct, that a trust was in fact what he intended.

We already know that looking at the entirety of circumstances is very significant generally, and this means that just because precatory words may be capable of signalling intention to create a trust in some circumstances, those same wordings will not always have the same effect. This can be seen in *Re Hamilton* [1895] 2 Ch 370, in which Lindley LJ said, at 373 (of a testamentary gift):

> You must take the will which you have to construe and see what it means, and if you come to the conclusion that no trust was intended, you say so, although previous judges have said the contrary on some wills more or less similar to the one you have to construe.

Similarly, in *Cominsky* v *Bowring-Hanbury* [1905] AC 84, the House of Lords found a trust on the basis of words very similar to those employed in *Re Adams and the Kensington Vestry*—that is, 'absolutely in full confidence that she [the widow] will make such use of [the property] as I would have made myself and that at her death she will devise it to such one or more of my nieces as she may think fit'.

The exception to this general position is the situation in which a testator reproduces the exact language of an earlier will that has previously been held to create a trust. In these circumstances, it may be possible to infer that he intended to use the earlier will as a precedent. In this situation, there is authority that the court, in construing the later case, should follow the earlier decision, at least unless that decision was clearly wrong: *Re Steele's WT* [1948] Ch 603. Although this case attaches great significance to the actual precatory words used, it is not really an exception to the foregoing flexible approach, because all of the circumstances do indeed point to an intention to create a trust. It follows that draftsmen should make clear beyond doubt that precatory words are intended to indicate desire alone, unless, of course, a trust is indeed intended.

3.6 Criticism of the modern law on certainty of intention

Where it is held that there is no certainty of intention, there can be no trust. This means that any transfer of title to property (provided that this satisfies formality requirements) from its owner to another will be treated as an outright gift in his favour. This means that the recipient takes the property as its owner and free from any obligation to use it in ways that consider the interests of others.

The function of the certainty-of-intention requirement is to ensure that, where an owner of property is seeking to deal with it in ways that involve him losing his rights to it as owner, what he is trying to achieve from this is actually what will happen. So where there is evidence that an owner of property is seeking to make a gift of it, this is what should happen to the property. Here, the courts are insistent that a trust should arise only where there is the clearest intention that creating a trust is what the owner of property wanted. Here, *Milroy* v *Lord*, and particularly its application in *Jones* v *Lock* and *Richards* v *Delbridge*, is authority that the courts will more readily conclude that an owner of property is trying to give it away outright than to create a trust of it. This is because although an outright gift will involve an owner of property losing all entitlement to property, creating a trust will not only involve his loss of interest in the property, but also has far-reaching consequences for others. It will create enforceable rights for a beneficiary, of course, but the corollary of this is that it will create extensive and burdensome duties and obligations for another. The function of the certainty-of-intention requirement is to ensure that doing this is what an owner of property actually wants to achieve, and that this will not happen unless this is so.

We will look again at *Paul* v *Constance* as a key authority for constituting trusts, but for present purposes it signals a very accommodating approach to finding certainty of intention to create a trust. This follows from what was said about the case by Scarman LJ in his judgment. Scarman LJ considered this a 'borderline' case, and one in which it was difficult to pinpoint a specific moment at which the money in the bank account ceased to be owned outright by Constance (who had legal title) to become held by him in order to benefit them both. It was difficult to point to a moment before which Constance could do as he pleased with the money and after which he would have to use it in ways that reflected Paul's beneficial ownership of it. If it had not been possible to do this, then arguably no trust should have arisen, because trusts are, in principle, irrevocable and there must be a moment at which this irrevocable commitment is made.

In this regard, *Pearson* v *Lehman Bros Finance SA* [2010] EWHC 2914 (Ch) provides a salutary reminder that the courts will look carefully at the circumstances when determining whether certainty of intention to create a trust has been demonstrated. Briggs J insisted that express reference to 'ownership', 'belonging', and 'title', and actually to the word 'trust' itself, will be regarded as persuasive rather than conclusive evidence of a trust's existence, and that a different conclusion might be found on an objective reading of the agreement or relationship. This is probably more directed towards trusts arising in commercial arrangements than more traditional ones, with this core idea being developed further in *Crossco No 4 Unlimited* v *Jolan Limited* [2011] EWCA Civ 1619 (about which more is said in Chapter 18). But this reminds us that even the clearest words are not conclusive, and that equity focuses on the substance of what is intended rather than the form of its expression in determining the existence of a trust.

Paul v *Constance* is authority that words and/or conduct of a simple and unsophisticated nature will, in appropriate circumstances, be regarded as evidence that a trust is intended, at the heart of which is supposed to be the objective of distinguishing attempts to provide gratuitous benefits of property by way of a gift from ones that will involve heavy responsibilities for some. This is supposed to explain the results reached in *Jones* v *Lock* and *Richards* v *Delbridge* on the ground that no trust could arise in either case because there was no evidence of an intention to create one from what was said and done. This is what makes *Choithram (T) International SA* v *Pagarani* [2001] 1 WLR 1 such an interesting case. Not only does it illustrate how accommodating the courts are capable of being in finding certainty of intention from what is said and done, but it also shows willingness to find certainty of intention to create a trust on the part of an owner of property from his use of the word *gift*! We will look at *Choithram* more closely in Chapter 5, but for present purposes we need to understand that apparently, although the wording used by the settlor was what might be expected in the case of a gift, it provided evidence that a trust was intended. This was because 'Although the words used by [the donor] are those normally appropriate to an outright gift', the term 'I give to X' was nevertheless capable of demonstrating intention to create a trust because 'their only possible meaning in this context' was to effect the creation of a trust, and here the donor's actual use of these words were 'essentially words of making a gift on trust'.

This case does show the kind of contextual interpretation of words used emphasized in *Harrison* v *Gibson* [2006] 1 All ER 858, but it does raise issues of whether the courts are being mindful enough of the function of certainty of intention, or whether they are too accommodating of finding trusts. Perhaps this is justifiable in what are non-commercial arrangements, in which some reverse logic—if not actual reverse engineering—is necessary because an owner of property has died and is no longer capable of explaining his intentions. But this can lead to uncertainty in dealings with property, which is contrary to policy that emphasizes the essence of certainty when it comes to dealings with property. The long-standing view of *Paul* v *Constance* is that it is a borderline case, which is very fact-specific, and it does not obviously provide a general authoritative position. There are reasons why this should also be the analysis of *Choithram*, given the scope for difficulties arising from such positive use of language that ordinarily runs contrary to creating trusts.

As the courts become mindful of the greater scope for creating trusts in the commercial context, there should be considerable caution in any possible importing of *Paul* v *Constance* and *Choithram* ideas into business dealings, given their scope for creating uncertainty in dealings with property. Perhaps this is unlikely because, in the commercial context, the relationships between the parties are contractual and conducted at 'arm's length'. However, given the scope for confusion in dealings with property that might arise from *Paul* v *Constance* and *Choithram*, one wonders whether any recourse should be had to them in making any determination that a trust of property was intended and thus (subject to satisfying all other requirements) that one should arise.

3.7 Certainty of subject matter

Whilst certainty-of-intention rules tell us that no trust can arise unless the owner of property intends this to happen, the fact that there are actually 'three certainties' tells us that more is still required. In this regard, we can analyse certainty of intention as necessary, but not sufficient; once certainty of intention is established, then there is still more that an owner of property must make clear (or certain) in relation to the trust property and those who are intended to benefit from the trust that he is trying to create. Taking the former first, satisfying certainty of subject matter means meeting key requirements that attach to the property itself that is being settled. This involves two elements whereby it must be clear (or certain) that the property *itself* can be identified *as trust property*, and what *amount or size of* this property is to be received by a given beneficiary.

This requirement sets out that if property to be the subject of the trust is not specified in a way that makes it clear that it is intended to be 'trust property', then no trust is created. In these circumstances, it is not regarded as 'sufficiently certain' that property is actually 'trust property', and so the intended trust cannot be valid. What follows now is an examination of each of the limbs in turn, which gives an analysis of the key cases and also is an attempt to present a rounded account of the issues arising in the application of it. There is also woven through this an examination of the way in which the courts take quite different approaches when applying the different elements of the 'certainty of subject matter' rule.

3.7.1 The first limb of certainty of subject matter: property must be identifiable as 'trust property'

This is the requirement that property being given to another *can* actually be identifiable *as* trust property. To satisfy the test, it appears to be necessary that the trust property be defined in objective, rather than subjective, terms, and so cannot be expressed in ways in relation to which opinions are capable of differing. This can be illustrated by the key case of *Palmer* v *Simmonds* (1854) 2 Drew 221, which is where we do get a clear statement on what is required and what will not suffice. In this case, a testatrix left on trust 'the bulk' of her residuary estate and, after consulting a dictionary, Kindersley V-C found, at 226, that the term 'bulk' was inadequate to specify any portion of the property as trust property:

> What is the meaning then of bulk? The appropriate meaning, according to its derivation, is something which bulges out … Its popular meaning we all know. When a person is said to have given the bulk of his property, what is meant is not the whole but the greater part, and that is in fact consistent with its classical meaning. When, therefore, the testatrix uses that term, can I say that she has used a term expressing a definite, clear, certain part of her estate, or the whole of her estate? I am bound to say that she has not designated the subject as to which she expresses her confidence; and I am therefore of opinion that there is no trust created.

Since it was not possible to carve out from the residue that portion which was to be held on trust, the trust failed, and the residuary legatee took the whole amount of the property absolutely and thus free from any trust. This same approach can be seen in *Curtis* v *Rippon* (1820) 5 Madd 434, and also *Sprange* v *Barnard* (1789) 2 Bro CC 585, in which the testatrix instructed that 'whatever was left' of property originally bequeathed to her husband was to be given to others upon his death. From these cases, and as stated in *Palmer* itself, for it to be sufficiently clear or certain that property can be identified as trust property, the requirement is that 'a term … expressing a clear and certain part of the property, or the whole of the property' is used. If this is present, then it is said to be sufficiently certain that particular property is property that an owner wishes to settle on trust for the benefit of others.

On looking at these old cases, the purpose of *Palmer* does seem to be clear, as is the mischief that it is seeking to avoid: the use of virtually meaningless terms in the creation of arrangements relating to property that we now know are permanent and irrevocable, and which create rights in that property for some and concomitant duties in respect of it for others. However, we see how strictly the courts apply this even in situations in which this mischief is not necessarily present. This can be seen in the decision in *Re Kolb's WT* [1962] Ch 531 to disallow the term 'blue chip' as one that distinguished what was to be trust property from what was not. This term is commonly used in investment rhetoric in respect of shares in large public companies, which are considered an entirely safe investment, but it was found to be a term without technical or objective meaning. Thus Cross J ruled that its meaning, in the context of the will, must depend on the standard applied by the testator, which could not be determined with sufficient certainty to enable the clause to be upheld.

These cases tell us that the courts are incredibly strict in deeming that language used by a settlor has not made clear enough what is or is not intended to be trust property, and the consequence of this is that no trust can arise, because it is not clear enough what is or is not intended to be trust property. Shortly, it will be suggested how this very strict approach might contrast unfavourably with that which is taken in the second limb of the certainty-of-subject matter requirement; before this, brief mention is made of a case that does actually appear to be at odds with the cases under this first limb: the decision in *Re In the Estate of Last* [1958] 1 All ER 316.

Last shows a very unusual outcome for an 'anything which is left. . . ', which, on the basis of the foregoing discussion, should result in a disposal of property in favour of another being an absolute gift to him, and one free from any subsequent obligations to deal with the property for others (namely, free from any trust). A number of texts do not deal with it, because it does seem at odds with the *Palmer* case law, in as much as a trust was found to attach to 'anything which is left' following the death of the original recipient of the property. However, it would seem that there was a clear objective for reaching this result, and this suggests that *Last* is not really an authority and was instead a decision confined to its facts.

3.7.2 The second limb of certainty of subject matter: ascertaining the size of beneficial shares of 'trust property'

Once it is sufficiently certain that property is trust property rather than property not subject to a trust (and has thus satisfied the *Palmer* v *Simmonds* requirement), then there is the question of how much of it an individual beneficiary is to receive. Issues about this will arise in situations in which, in making clear what is or is not trust property, a settlor has left the issue of how much unclear. This is a question of quantifying the size of a beneficiary's interest or share in the trust property, and a number of decisions point to the courts taking a much more relaxed approach than they do to determinations of whether property is or is not trust property. A key case here—and one that does show very clearly how generous the courts are here, as compared to a very similar situation, which arose in *Re Kolb*—is *Re Golay's WT* [1965] 1 WLR 969.

In *Golay*, the testator had directed his trustees to allow a named recipient to 'enjoy one of my flats during her lifetime and to receive a reasonable income from my other properties'. Ungoed-Thomas J felt able to uphold the gift because the trustees could select a suitable property, and a 'reasonable income' could be quantified objectively by the court. In taking this view, the judgment suggests that if the entitlement were to what the testator or another specified person considered to be reasonable, then the trust would fail, because the test would then be subjective. Indeed, courts are 'constantly involved in making such objective assessments of what is reasonable'.

The judgment in *Golay* is very short, and the case appears to be out of line with the others considered. The test cannot simply be whether the income could be objectively quantified by the court, since a court could equally well quantify 'the bulk' or 'blue-chip securities'. Can it really be supposed that a court, faced with a statutory provision that applied to 'blue-chip securities', would be unable to apply the provision, and that it should be unable to do so even armed with the commonness of that term in accepted and standard investment parlance? Because Ungoed-Thomas J is clearly correct in stating that courts are constantly making such objective assessments, is it—dare one say—*reasonable* for them to be so easily defeated by a commonly used term such as 'blue-chip securities'.

Golay has been criticized extensively, and it appears that Ungoed-Thomas J has not really taken on board the function of the certainty requirement. Much more will be said about this at the close of this part of the chapter, but it is not too much of a spoiler to suggest that certainty requirements are very strongly concerned with making it possible for trusts to be carried out. In the context of property, objectivity is important for enabling trustees to determine whether property is trust property, and to differentiate it from that which is not. And in this regard the only justification for upholding the courts' powers to make determinations of reasonableness is to say that trustees should forever be coming to court to obtain directions. Another view of this differential approach between the two limbs of certainty of subject matter is that, as a matter of general policy, the courts should strive to uphold trusts rather than to strike them out, and if this requires some judicial application of reasonableness, then this is something in which the courts are well rehearsed to engage. If this is the case, then current approaches do reflect the way in which it is justified for a very strict view to be taken on the 'is it or is it not trust property?' question, and that, once this is satisfied, a trust should not actually fail for absence of certainty of subject matter.

There are problems, however, in taking a lenient approach to determining beneficial shares in property, which can be seen in *Hunter* v *Moss* [1994] 1 WLR 452, which was followed by *Re Lewis's of Leicester Ltd* [1995] 1 BCLC 428. *Hunter* involved an oral declaration of trusteeship of 50 shares of a company's issued share capital of 1,000 shares, which succeeded, even though the particular shares were not ascertained or identified. However, the company was precisely identified, all of the shares in that company were identical, and the quantification (50 shares) was obviously precise. Moreover, as long as the trustee retained all 1,000 shares, there would be no point in identifying which 50 shares were subject to the trust. On its facts, therefore, the decision in *Hunter* might seem uncomplicated. However, difficulties can arise where the facts are not so neatly configured, such as if the same trustee of the same property had subsequently split up the fund, sold the shares, and reinvested the proceeds in a number of funds, some of which performed well and others less so. On the assumption that this case is correct, this latter situation would raise issues that are considered in Chapter 17, and a beneficiary's entitlement to the substitute property would depend on the principles established by *Re Hallett's Estate* (1880) 13 ChD 696 or *Re Diplock* [1948] Ch 465.

3.7.3 Possible difficulties with *Hunter* and the significance of *Re Goldcorp*

However, this hypothetical situation does show that *Hunter* could give rise to some problematic circumstances, and it has been subjected to fairly heavy academic criticism as a consequence (see, for example, Hayton [1994] 110 LQR 335). It is regarded as being inconsistent with the Privy Council decision in *Re Goldcorp Exchange* [1995] 1 AC 74 (see also Chapters 13 and 17), in which an argument was unsuccessfully advanced that a seller of gold bullion (who had gone into liquidation having taken money from the purchasers) had become a trustee of an undivided share in his stocks. Peter Birks [1995] RLR 83, 87, even went so far as to argue that, from the reasoning of the Privy Council in *Re Goldcorp Exchange Ltd*, 'One inference is that the Court of Appeal's decision in *Hunter v Moss* [1994] 1 WLR 452 must be wrong'. In fact, neither case mentions the other—possibly because they were decided at virtually the same time—and there are quite significant differences between the two cases.

In *Goldcorp*, there was no declaration of trusteeship by the vendor, so there is a certainty-of-intention problem; the trust property was not constant, since the vendor's gold stocks were being traded all of the time. There is also much authority pointing to the courts' reluctance to import notions of equitable property into commercial sales of goods, primarily for reasons connected with certainty, with this being evident in decisions as early as *Re Wait* [1927] 1 Ch 606, which was followed in *Re London Wine Co. (Shippers) Ltd* [1986] PCC 121 and *The Aliakmon* [1986] AC 785. These seem perfectly convincing grounds for distinguishing *Hunter* and *Goldcorp*—assuming, that is, that both cases are correct. A different distinction was, however, drawn by Neuberger J in *Re Harvard Securities* [1997] 2 BCLC 369. Here, the view was taken that, if forced to make a choice between *Hunter* and *Goldcorp*, the Court of Appeal should be followed in preference to the Privy Council, but in any case Neuberger J also took the view that, at any rate, for dealings in shares, *Hunter* was a correct statement of the law.

The distinction between shares and other property seems difficult to justify in principle. Notwithstanding its critics, *Hunter v Moss* does not seem to be a problematic decision, but it is also one that is different from *Goldcorp*. Reiteration of *Hunter* as a correct statement of law can be found in *Pearson v Lehman Bros Finance SA* [2010] EWHC 2914 (Ch). This arose as a result of assessing whether *Hunter*'s position—that unsegregated, interchangeable property can satisfy certainty-of-subject-matter requirements—could be applied to 'the constantly fluctuating mass of security interests [mainly bonds and equities] in [several deposit] accounts' held by Lehman Bros. Briggs J found that a trust of property, the individual units of which are capable of mutual substitution, will satisfy certainty-of-subject-matter requirements provided that the property itself is sufficiently identified (thereby satisfying the requirements of *Palmer v Simmonds* (1854) 2 Drew 221) and provided also that the beneficiary's proportionate share of it is itself not uncertain. This is at one with *Hunter v Moss* and, in stating this, *Lehman Bros* might bolster critics of the approach taken in *Golay* to ascertaining certainty of share or proportion. Beyond this, it will be interesting to see how a further finding of Briggs J might be developed in the future—that is, his suggestion that a trust does not fail for want of certainty merely because its subject matter is, at present, uncertain if the terms of the trust are sufficient to identify its subject matter in the future.

Certainty of subject matter: a summary of what needs to be understood
These cases do involve an understanding of not only property, but also commercial law, to get any kind of grasp of them. Here, cases like *Re London Wine Co* and *Re Goldcorp* show us that even where the property in question is certain as trust property, the dimensions of commercial law and practice, which are also involved, make determining, in practice, how much of it is owned beneficially by a particular beneficiary very complicated. These cases also show us something else—namely, that sometimes in these commercial dealings it is not even that clear when something is or is not trust property, and thus whether even the first limb of the certainty of subject matter has been satisfied.

A number of these commercial-type cases arise from disputed ownership of property, and you will get a sense of this from your reading. You will also get a good sense that there is plenty going on that requires understanding of specialist 'commercial law'. What is most important at this point in time in this text is that you understand what is meant by satisfying certainty-of-subject-matter requirements, how this is achieved, and what the consequences of failing to do so will be. For these first aspects, you will need to be sure that you understand that the courts take a very strict approach to determining whether something is or is not trust property, and why this might be the case, as illustrated in *Re Kolb* and some of the commercial cases. You will then need to appreciate what arguments might be made both in favour of and against a different and more lenient approach being applied to secondary questions of 'what' or 'how much' a beneficiary is to receive, being aware of the difficulties that this might create.

What happens if it is not 'sufficiently certain' that property is trust property?

Where it is not deemed to be 'sufficiently certain' that property is trust property, no *express* trust is created. This has the overall result that the original owner of the property who was trying to settle the property on trust retains the property. This is ordinarily on a resulting trust mechanism, which will arise where legal title to the property has already been transferred to a trustee with every intention of bringing the express trust into being. Here, ownership is separated, but it is not possible to create the express trust that was intended, and the settlor retains a beneficial interest in the property. Most commentaries do not distinguish this situation from what happens when the owner of property is intending to act as trustee under the trust that he intends to create. Most analyses consider that, technically, the intended trust is now constituted (as long as certainty of intention is present, for reasons that become clearer in Chapter 5), and beneficial ownership remains with the settlor on a resulting trust, but there is also the view that the settlor simply retains this absolutely. It can also transpire that passing legal title to another to act as trustee has been attempted, but failed (for formality reasons, usually, as well as trust property not being certain). In this case, technically, ownership never leaves the settlor and no trust is brought into existence, suggesting the settlor retains the property absolutely. This general position of a resulting trust for the settlor (or residuary legatees, in the case of an attempt to establish a trust by will) is subject to one exception, which applies by virtue of *Hancock* v *Watson* [1902] AC 14. This rule applies where there is an absolute gift of property in the first instance and trusts are subsequently imposed on that property: if the trusts fail for any reason, the property is not held on a resulting trust for the settlor or his estate, but will vest absolutely in the person to whom the property was given.

3.8 The certainty-of-objects requirement

The material will now introduce the remaining 'certainty' requirement for a valid express trust, and will do so by providing a complete picture of the three certainties. The certainty-of-objects requirement for creating a valid trust is the lengthiest and most complex of the certainty requirements, but it is also what will draw this first part of the chapter to a close. At this end point, there will also be an opportunity to reflect on why there is the certainty requirement, and why, if any one of the three elements is missing, this will invalidate a settlor's attempt to create a trust.

Focusing for now on the certainty-of-objects requirement, if we look back to Lord Langdale's speech in *Knight*, we see that 'the objects or persons intended to have the benefit ... [must] also be certain'. So immediately we see that 'objects' is a word for people, and thus 'beneficiaries' in the trust scenario. We will think more generally about the policy of this particular aspect of certainty rules shortly, but at this stage we need some overview of why Lord Langdale identified this as a requirement. This involves us thinking through something of which you will already be aware and also introducing you to something with which you will not yet be familiar.

We do already know that it is only a beneficiary who can enforce a private trust, even if it will become clear only in the second part of this chapter that this is what underpins the so-called 'beneficiary principle'. The beneficiary principle requires that, for a trust to be valid, 'there must be somebody, in whose favour the court can decree performance'. As we will find out, this requirement comes from a very famous case—*Morice* v *Bishop of Durham* (1805) 10 Ves 522—and makes identifying a beneficiary under a trust very important generally; as we will discover, this has particular significance where a trustee refuses to carry out a trust or does so improperly.

In developing this latter idea, we also now have to be aware that a trust is what is known as a 'mandatory' arrangement that relates to property. This means that any trust that is valid (because it has satisfied all validity requirements) is one that *must* be carried out, and the obligations that arise under it for a trustee are thus said to be 'imperative'. The mandatory nature of a trust is reflected in one of equity's principles, which comes into play where a trustee who has been appointed under the arrangement is not able to, or refuses to, carry out the trust. In these circumstances, the court will carry out the trust if no one else can be found to do so, because 'equity will not permit a trust to fail for want of a trustee'. If this happens, it becomes especially important to be able to identify those who are intended to benefit. But generally, because a valid trust must be carried out, when considering whether a settlor's wishes should create a valid arrangement, regard must be given to whether a trust is actually capable of being administered. This may well be impossible when the 'class of objects' or beneficiaries of the trust is too vaguely described or too large, but determining this means that it must be possible to identify, or to *ascertain*, beneficiaries in the first instance.

Ascertaining certainty of objects: identifying approaches taken by the courts

This means that we must now study how beneficiaries under a trust are identified and how this is reflected in ensuring that the certainty-of-objects requirement is satisfied. At this point, we are going to see how these central ideas of enforcement of the trust, and also its workability and administration, can be seen in two key tests adopted by the courts to establish whether any given trust does satisfy certainty-of-objects requirements. These are approaches that are used to determine whether who is intended to benefit under the arrangement is sufficiently clear or certain, and they can be summarized as follows.

- The *individual ascertainability test* asks whether it is possible to tell, with certainty, whether any individual coming to the court to enforce the trust has sufficient interest to do so. It is necessary to establish whether or not he is part of the class of objects, and essentially it is an 'is or is not' test.
- The *class ascertainability test* requires that a list of all of the objects within a class can actually be drawn up. This is a 'class list' test, and it will be satisfied only if a 'complete list' of all objects within a class *can* be drawn up.

It will become clear that the class test is a far more stringent one, but before looking at where the tests can be seen applied to arrangements concerning property that are trusts, we need to understand that there are other types of arrangement relating to property in relation to which there are also certainty-of-objects requirements. We are focusing only on those relating to trusts, but before we can do this and for reasons that will shortly become apparent we need to understand that there are different types of arrangement for the disposal of property by one person in favour of another (often called 'dispositions' of property) that are subject to certainty-of-objects requirements.

These arrangements include, of course, the *trust*, on which we are focusing in this material, and a disposition of property will create a trust where there is a duty to distribute specified property amongst a class of objects, or beneficiaries. At points, trusts can look like powers (which are identified and explained next), and the distinguishing characteristic of a trust is that a trust is mandatory: in this arrangement, a settlor instructs and a trustee must act accordingly. We will find out shortly that trusts are further classified as 'fixed trusts' and 'discretionary trusts'. A disposition of property will create a *power* if there is specified property and a class of persons intended to benefit, but there is no duty to distribute property in the way that there is in the trust situation. As Chapter 2 explained, powers of appointment of property are in many ways a hangover from the past, and sometimes a power will clearly identify itself with the presence of what is known as a 'gift over in default' (or simply 'gift over')—that is, the provision of an alternative for what happens to the property if the power provided is not exercised.

There is also what is known as a gift, or series of gifts, subject to a 'condition precedent'. This is also subject to certainty-of-objects requirements, but ones that are not as stringent as those for trusts or even powers. What this is can be illustrated best by the key case, which is *Re Barlow's WT* [1979] 1 WLR 278, in which the executor of a testatrix was directed by her to allow any of her friends to make purchases from her art collection at below market value. So here the condition for being able to claim the right to make the discounted purchases was to have been a friend of the testatrix; to be a valid gift subject to a condition precedent, the term 'friends' had to satisfy certainty-of-objects requirements, which it did. But, as we will find out, there will be a different outcome where this term is applied to trusts, on account of the stricter test that is applied to them.

Why are powers ever a consideration when looking at certainty of objects in trusts?

We will discover that even looking only at trusts involves making some references to powers, and so you need to be aware of the way in which powers, as well as trusts, are classified. Generally, and also when relating specifically to entitlement to property, powers will be *fiduciary* if the relationship between the donor and holder donee is a fiduciary relationship (that is, a relationship of utmost loyalty, as we will discover in Chapter 13), while a *personal* or 'mere' power arises from a purely personal relationship between the parties. Fiduciary powers are particularly important for us as we look at trusts and their administration by trustees, given that, as we will discover, the office of trustee is a fiduciary one, but unfortunately the way in which fiduciary powers are sometimes termed 'trust powers' does create scope for confusion. But why do we have to think about powers at all in looking at certainty-of-objects requirements?

We have already learned that, like trusts, powers of appointment are subject to certainty-of-objects requirements that must be satisfied if they are to be valid, but it has also been suggested that powers of appointment of property are, in many respects, a hangover from the past. So why is it that we need to consider powers at all when we look at what is required for a trust in terms of satisfying certainty-of-objects requirements? Things will become much clearer shortly, but, very briefly, there was a period between 1955 and 1971 during which powers were used almost as a standard alongside discretionary trusts, because it was widely believed that all trusts were subject to very stringent requirements on the identification of beneficiaries. However, since 1971, powers have fallen into disuse again, because liberalized certainty-of-objects requirements mean that it is much easier to create valid discretionary trusts.

The significance of these dates and the nature of their developments will become clear shortly, but what follows now is a brief overview of the key case law relating to certainty of objects for powers.

The nature of powers and the tests for certainty, and the significance of distinguishing trusts and powers

Given the nature of a power, a donee is perfectly within his right not to exercise it, and so the need to establish certainty of objects may not be quite as obvious as (it will become clear) is the case for a trust. But it will still be necessary to be able to establish whether any given individual is or is not an object of the power, since only objects of the power will have *locus standi* to enforce it, even if the extent of this is preventing a donee from acting otherwise than in accordance with it. It is also necessary because, as Sir Robert Megarry V-C made clear in *Re Hay's ST* [1982] 1 WLR 1202, donees are required to get a feel for the width of the class. In *Re Gestetner's Settlement* [1953] 1 Ch 672, Harman J had to consider the validity of a power given to trustees to distribute among a very wide class, including directors and employees, or former employees, of a large number of companies, with a gift over in default. Since membership of the class constantly fluctuated, it was impossible to draw up a list of the entire class at any one time. He held that it was not necessary to know all of the objects in order to appoint, and that it was not fatal that the entire class could not be ascertained.

In *Re Gulbenkian's Settlements* [1970] AC 508, trustees were given a power to apply income from the trust fund to maintain, among others, 'any person in whose house or in whose company or in whose care Gulbenkian may from time to time be residing', and there was a gift over in default of appointment. In upholding the power, the House of Lords held that the individual ascertainability test applied to powers, meaning that a power would be valid if it could be said with certainty who was *or was not* a member of the class. Like in *Gestetner*, the power would not fail because it was impossible to ascertain every member of the class; also like *Gestetner*, the provision in *Gulbenkian* had to be a power because there was a gift over in default of appointment. This would not arise in a discretionary trust because trustees are mandated to appoint property in accordance with a settlor's instructions.

Given that this heading signposts not only the *Gulbenkien* test, but also its significance, first, the emphasized words *'or was not'* are important for when we consider how this test is relevant for trusts. Second, the House of Lords expressly rejected Lord Denning MR's test in the Court of Appeal in *Gulbenkian* [1968] Ch 126, suggesting that validity should depend on being able to identify only one beneficiary as being clearly within the class. This was because this approach took no account of the trustees' duty to carry out the power in a fiduciary manner. The Denning test would really be appropriate only of the donees were at liberty to distribute to the first person who came to hand, and it has been shown that this is not the case.

3.8.1 Introducing certainty of objects in trusts: types of trust and types of certainty

When we look at what is required for it to be sufficiently clear or certain who is intended to benefit from the trust, it will become clear that what is required depends on the distinction between different types of express trust identified in Chapter 2—that is, whether a disposition is a fixed trust or a discretionary trust. We now need to understand that there are differences in what is required as between different types of trust, and also to be aware of how validity can be affected by two key types of certainty.

- 'Linguistic' or 'semantic' certainty relates to whether the language used to describe the class of beneficiaries or objects is conceptually certain, and asks us to think about, for example, what is different about 'men who are 7 ft tall' from reference to 'tall men'?
- 'Evidential' certainty arises in questions of whether it can be shown of a particular person whether he is actually a member of a particular class. In the example above, this would ask whether it can be established whether a person is a 'male who is 7 ft tall'.

3.8.2 Approaches to certainty of objects in fixed trusts

The test for certainty of objects in fixed trusts is set out in *IRC* v *Broadway Cottages* [1955] Ch 20. This demands that, to satisfy this requirement, it must be possible to draw up a complete list of the members of the class, and this requires both linguistic and evidential certainty. If this cannot be done for any arrangement that is seeking to create a fixed trust, then the arrangement cannot be a valid trust and will fail to be so, on grounds that it is not sufficiently clear or certain who is to benefit from the settlement of property on trust. The rationale for the class list approach is made by Jenkins LJ in this case in his insistence that 'There can be no division in equal shares amongst a class of persons unless all the members of the class are known'.

Although the class test is a very stringent one, even here there is some flexibility for helping to ensure that 'conceptual certainty' requirements do not cause the trust to fail. *Re Tuck* [1978] 2 WLR 411 is authority that a settlor can provide for a third party to give meaning to a term that would otherwise be conceptually uncertain. It is clear that this can be trustees themselves or an expert whose opinion is sought specifically for the issue in hand. In *Tuck* itself, this related to a requirement that a beneficiary was 'of the Jewish faith' and 'married to an "approved" wife', giving the Chief Rabbi authority to determine this. However, *Tuck* is also subject to limitations and, reading it alongside *Re Jones* [1953] Ch 125 and *Re Wynn* [1952] Ch 271, it is clear the court is the final arbiter of what is acceptable in determining a trust's validity and what is not.

Although a fixed trust cannot be valid without it being possible to draw up a complete list of all beneficiaries, which is the only way in which to ensure that such an arrangement can be carried out according to a settlor's instructions, it does not follow from this that there are no issues arising from the application of the class test to fixed trusts. For trustees to be able to carry out a trust, they must not only be able to ascertain beneficiaries, but they must also be able to locate them. In this regard, the class or group of beneficiaries does not have to be large for it to be extremely difficult to find one of its members, and it may even be the case that, although a class is conceptually certain, someone within it is not actually known to exist by the trustees. So what can a trustee do in these circumstances, given that the essence of a fixed trust is that the settlor instructs and the trustee acts accordingly?

These two situations raise the same practical difficulty of whether to distribute a trust or to delay this on account of unknowns, but they are treated differently as far as the law is concerned. In relation to the beneficiary about whom trustees do not actually know, trustees are permitted under s. 27 of the Trustee Act 1925 to distribute a fund without having regard to a beneficiary of whom they have no notice, with trustees who have advertised the trust in the *London Gazette* and in any locality in which any land subject to the trust is located being deemed to have no notice of such a claimant. In relation to the latter—the missing beneficiary—a so-called *'Benjamin* order' (deriving authority from *Re Benjamin* [1902] 1 Ch 723) allows trustees to distribute the trust. This does not vary or destroy a beneficiary's interest, and so if one who is missing subsequently returns, then he is still entitled to his share. Thus, in granting a *Benjamin* order, the court will require those who are receiving the fund to make an undertaking to return to the missing beneficiary that to which he is entitled should he reappear.

3.8.3 Approaches to certainty of objects in discretionary trusts

The test for certainty of objects in discretionary trusts is set out in *McPhail* v *Doulton* [1971] AC 424 as substantially the same as that laid down in *Re Gulbenkian* for fiduciary powers—namely, the individual ascertainability test.

This is, of course, how the *Gulbenkian* test becomes significant for discussion of discretionary trusts, and now is the time to explain more of the background to this. Earlier, the significant dates were identified as 1955 and 1971, and in taking the former first, in the aftermath of *IRC* v *Broadway Cottages Trust* [1955] Ch 20, the class ascertainability test became applied to discretionary trusts as well as to fixed ones. This was reasoned by Jenkins LJ as being justified on grounds of 'ultimate enforcement'. This reasoning proposes that, because a trust is a mandatory arrangement, it is one that must be carried out; if no willing trustees can be found, then it will fall to the court to carry out the trust, because 'equity will not allow a trust to fail for want of a trustee'. In these circumstances, it would not be appropriate for the court to exercise discretion as between objects, and the only course of action available to it in these circumstances would be to distribute the property equally amongst all of the beneficiaries within the class: 'equity is equality'. To do this, it would need to be possible to draw up a complete list of all of the beneficiaries within this class.

This reasoning was dismissed for discretionary trusts in the House of Lords' ruling in *McPhail* v *Doulton*. This was the first phase of the infamous and long-lasting litigation concerning a disposition in one Bertram Baden's will 'to or for the benefit of any of the officers and employees or ex-officers or ex-employees of the company or to any relatives or dependants of such persons'.

It was the decision in *Broadway Cottages* that caused the resurgence of powers between 1955 and 1971, when it became virtually impossible to create valid discretionary trusts. This led to the appearance of creating a 'power and trust over in default' because the certainty-of-object test for powers was thought to be less stringent than that for discretionary trusts. In other words, an instrument that was valid as a power might be invalid as a discretionary trust if there were a wide range of objects. It therefore became common practice to draft powers with a wide range of objects, which were valid, while confining the trust over to a narrow range of objects. Such an instrument could be valid, whereas if drafted as a trust alone, it would fall foul of the certainty-of-object requirements.

However, in *McPhail* v *Doulton*, the House of Lords decisively rejected the principle of equality of distribution in situations in which equal distribution would have made a nonsense of the settlor's intention, and ruled that the court could, in the final scenario, apply discretion as amongst objects. Thus the reasoning in *Broadway Cottages* was inapplicable (and indeed *Broadway Cottages* was overruled), and what was required instead was that it was possible to tell whether any individual coming to court to enforce a trust or power had sufficient interest to do so. In other words, the question was whether or not this particular individual was within the class of objects.

The key points in Lord Wilberforce's judgment can be summarized as, first and foremost, that the appropriate test should reflect that, in most cases, equality of distribution was probably entirely at odds with the settlor's intention, precisely because he had elected to create a trust in which some within the class of objects would not actually benefit at all. Thus, at 456:

> the test for the validity ... *ought to be similar to* that accepted by this House in *re Gulbenkian's Settlement* ... namely that the trust is valid if it can be said with certainty that *any given individual is or is not* a member of the class. [Emphasis added]

It is important that we emphasize that, for Lord Wilberforce, this did not represent complete assimilation between trusts and powers, and that, overall, a stricter standard applied to trustees than to donees of a power. However, even if all of these requirements were satisfied, there may be circumstances that make the trust administratively unworkable, and thus which ought to invalidate a trust that has actually satisfied the certainty-of-objects requirement.

Considerations of McPhail v Doulton, *ahead of introducing* Baden's Deed Trusts (No. 2)

There is a lot of force in Lord Wilberforce's observations on why there should be a departure from a *Broadway Cottages* approach to discretionary trusts, but aspects of this decision do need some thought. Although Lord Wilberforce *was* careful to stress that this did not amount to complete assimilation of trusts with powers, his judgment does raise issues about the fundamental nature of trusts and powers, and differences subsisting between them. This is particularly so in relation to how these fundamental differences manifest in questions of effective administration in a trust, and that trustees are fiduciaries who are duty-bound to carry out the trust. Further consideration of this is available in material written for the Online Resource Centre that accompanies this book.

The next phase of the Baden litigation: *introducing* Re Baden's Deed Trust (No. 2)

The litigation returned to the Court of Appeal as *Re Baden's Deed Trusts (No. 2)* [1973] Ch 9 to consider application of the *McPhail* test to the words 'relatives' and 'dependants' used in Bertram Baden's will. It was found that there were no certainty issues with 'dependants' (for reasons about which you will read shortly), but 'relatives' did lead to differences in opinion, largely thanks to a very clever argument made by counsel for Baden's estate, John Vinelott QC. At this stage, twelve years had passed since Baden's death, and the litigation had both paralysed the legacy and consumed a considerable amount of it in funding the litigation; it was therefore, as Sachs LJ observed, a situation that 'lacks attraction'.

Vinelott QC argued that it could not be shown that any person definitely was or *was not* within the class, as required by the *Gulbenkian* test. Had this argument succeeded, it would have had enormous implications for the *McPhail* ruling on approaches to certainty of objects in discretionary trusts. Indeed, as Megaw LJ observed, it would have meant a virtual return to the rejected class ascertainability test. The Court of Appeal did reject the argument, but the individual judgments did so on the basis of quite different considerations. Also, as evident in the judgment itself, it was made very clear to Baden's next of kin that they should not pursue the litigation any further, which meant that this case did not go to the House of Lords. This means that which approach *would* be adopted in subsequent litigation remained unclear and that a clear statement in this area is not possible to make. In absence of this authority, what we can do is make a reasoned assessment of which one of these three approaches *should be* adopted in the light of the issues that are raised when difficulties arise in ascertaining whether someone is or is not in the settlor's chosen class of beneficiary.

The judgment of Sachs LJ avoided the difficulty by emphasizing that the court was concerned only with conceptual certainty, so that it should not be fatal that there might be *evidential* difficulties in drawing up John Vinelott QC's list. This effectively destroyed the Vinelott argument, which was addressed primarily towards *evidential* difficulties in drawing up the class. Sachs LJ also took the view that the courts would place the burden of proof, in effect, on someone claiming to be within the class. This seems acceptable if ultimate enforcement is the issue and the test is of the *locus standi* of the claimant, but it does not help the administration of the trust.

Megaw LJ adopted a different solution requiring that, as regards a substantial number of objects, it can be shown with certainty that they fall within the class. This is rather a vague test: clearly, it is not enough to be able to show that *one* person is certainly within the class, because this test was rejected in *Gulbenkian* (see 'The nature of powers and the tests for certainty, and the significance of distinguishing trusts and powers' earlier in this chapter). Presumably, the test requires evidential, as well as conceptual, certainty. Perhaps Megaw LJ adopted it simply because he could find no other way of rejecting Vinelott's argument without returning either to the rejected *Broadway* test or to the Denning test, which had been rejected in *Gulbenkian*. Indeed, none of the judges in the Court of Appeal was able to find a satisfactory solution to this difficulty. The test may have the merit, however, of ensuring that the trustees will be able to get a feel for the width of the class, which they need to be able to do to exercise their discretion.

Stamp LJ's test is probably the strictest of the three, and he seemed to be quite impressed by the Vinelott argument. He emphasized that it must be possible for the trustees to make a comprehensive survey of the range of objects, but he did not think it would be fatal if, at the end of the survey, it were impossible to draw up a list of every single beneficiary. He would have taken the view that the trust failed had he not felt compelled to follow an early House of Lords authority, which had held that a discretionary trust for 'relations' was valid—'relations' being defined narrowly as 'next of kin'.

Of the three tests, that of Sachs LJ will usually be the easiest to satisfy, but it relies heavily on an additional administrative unworkability test, the extent and application of which, as will become clear in the next section, are quite unclear. At this point, and by way of a summary, the following is also suggested.

- The distinction drawn by Sachs LJ between conceptual and evidential uncertainty has its origin in Lord Wilberforce's speech in *McPhail* v *Doulton*, and indeed there are traces of a similar distinction in *Gulbenkian*. The justification is that evidential distinctions can always be resolved by the courts, but, as was explained earlier, the courts can also resolve conceptual uncertainties. But surely, once the *Broadway* equality of distribution principle has been abandoned, the justification for certainty rules is not to assist the courts, but rather to assist the trustees in administering the trust? And trustees will be defeated just as easily by evidential as by conceptual difficulties.

- If a class is conceptually certain, then the only reason why a list of the entire class cannot be drawn up is evidential. The class test, if it was ever meaningful at all, must have been an evidential test: if the test were simply conceptual, then there would be no difference between the individual and class ascertainability tests.

- This suggests that no good basis can be found for the distinction drawn between conceptual and evidential uncertainty. Supporters of Sachs LJ's view would view the administrative workability test (see section 3.9) as sufficient to ensure that the trust is workable, but in that case why is any test other than this one needed? In any case, evidential issues would now need to be dealt with by the administrative workability test, and it is not obvious that that is an improvement over dealing with them as part of the individual ascertainability test itself.

- Megaw LJ's test is evidential and addresses the problem of making the trust workable for trustees. It is therefore suggested that this is preferable to Sachs LJ's test.
- Stamp LJ's test is also evidential (indeed, entirely so, since 'next of kin' is not itself conceptually certain), but once the *Broadway* equality-of-distribution principle has been rejected, it is difficult to justify a test as strict as that of Stamp LJ, since his test amounts virtually to a return to the class ascertainability test.
- This, then, is an argument for preferring Megaw LJ's test, or at any rate a test similar to it.

The consequences of a discretionary trust being void for uncertainty of objects

Looking no further than at who was pushing the *Baden* litigation tells us exactly what happens when a discretionary trust fails for not satisfying certainty-of-objects requirements: it was executors for Baden's estate, acting on behalf of his next of kin pursuing the litigation. This is because where a disposition that is a trust fails for lack of certainty of objects, there will be a resulting trust for the settlor or, in the case of a testator, his next of kin.

3.9 Beyond satisfying certainty-of-objects requirements: the significance of 'administrative unworkability' for the validity of discretionary trusts

In *McPhail*, Lord Wilberforce suggested that even dispositions that *do* satisfy certainty-of-objects requirements could *still fail* (to be valid) on grounds that the class specified by the settlor rendered the trust administratively unworkable. The context for this is, of course, that a trust *must* be carried out and that, because of this, it must actually *be capable* of being carried out.

So what did Lord Wilberforce actually mean when suggesting that a trust could be capable of being 'administratively unworkable'? This is not actually very clear from the judgment, in which Lord Wilberforce's actual words were: '[T]he meaning of the words used is clear, but the definition of beneficiaries is so hopelessly wide so that the trust is administratively unworkable … perhaps "all the residents of Greater London" will serve [as an example].' This actually raises more questions than it provides answers. Is it the size or width of the class that makes a trust administratively unworkable, as suggested in *McPhail*? There was suggestion in *Re Manisty* (1974) Ch 17 that this arises where the terms of the trust 'negate any sensible intention on the part of the settlor' and thus amount to being capricious; *Re Hay's ST* (1982) 1 WLR 202 intimated that it arises because the terms make it impossible for a trustee 'to survey the field of objects and make a rational decision' as to whom to apply property to (and who not to exercise discretion in favour of).

Although both cases concerned the validity of powers, once again powers act as a benchmark for discussing what should happen in the case of a discretionary trust. This is because powers (and especially fiduciary powers) have a number of similarities with these trusts, and they are also fundamentally different because there is a duty to carry out a trust. Mindful of this, the judgments of both *Hay* and *Manisty* allude to the challenges arising for trustees in the mandatory distribution of property amongst a class of beneficiaries when how to do this (and indeed to whom) is within their discretion.

The enormity of the trustee's task was recognized in *Re Hay's ST* by Megarry V-C, who contrasted the trust with the position of the holder of a power, who can exercise this 'in favour of such of the objects who happen to be at hand or claim his attention'. Although 'not required to make an exact calculation' as between deserving claimants, a trustee under a discretionary trust *must*, said Megarry V-C at 210:

> first consider what persons or classes of persons are the objects ... there is no need to compile a complete list ... or even make an accurate assessment of the number of them: what is needed is an appreciation of the width of the field [of objects] and thus whether a selection is to be made merely from a dozen or, instead from thousands or millions ... Only when the trustee has applied his mind to the 'size of the problem' should he then consider in individual cases whether, in relation to other possible claimants, a particular grant [or exercise of discretion] is appropriate.

'Administrative unworkability' applied to discretionary trusts

The leading case here is *R* v *District Auditor, ex parte West Yorkshire Metropolitan County Council* (1986) RVR 24. The case arose when this local authority, acting under statutory powers, set about creating a trust 'for the benefit of any or all or some of all or some of the inhabitants of the county of West Yorkshire'. The class of objects was deemed sufficiently certain (that is, it satisfied the *McPhail* individual ascertainability test applicable to discretionary trusts), with the term 'inhabitant' accepted as satisfying conceptual and evidential requirements. However, because the class of potential beneficiaries numbered some 2.5 million 'inhabitants', it was deemed administratively unworkable because the class was far too large. This decision is authority that size of class is definitely a key consideration of administrative (un)workability, and appears to point to the way in which a large class combined with little or no guidance for the trustees is likely to invalidate the trust. But this also suggests that the acceptable width of the class presumably depends on the exact nature of the trustees' duties, and whether they must actually survey the entire field—which is what Lord Wilberforce appeared to appreciate, even if he did not develop his explanation of it as far as he could have done. Relevant here is a very interesting article by Harpum (1986) CLJ 391.

3.10 Drawing conclusions: understanding certainty requirements for a valid trust

We now know what fulfilling certainty requirements means and actually involves, and now we can use what we have learned to try to understand why they exist and why any attempt to create an express trust will fail unless they are satisfied. We can also use this as an opportunity to appreciate the interrelationships between certainty requirements and formality and constitution requirements for validity.

- *We can see certainty of intention as a mechanism for ensuring that, by his words or conduct, an owner of property really wants to create a trust.* Because doing this has such considerable implications for entitlements to property that are quite distinct from making a gift of or loaning property to another, no trust should be created unless it is very clear—or certain—that this is what an owner of property is seeking to achieve. Here, the courts will play very safe and are very unwilling to infer the creation of a trust in absence of clear evidence this was intended. This was also evident in the constitution cases relating to self-declarations of trusteeship, in which the courts are effectively looking first at whether certainty of intention to create a trust is present.

* *Where it is clear that property is intended to be settled on trust, it is important for trustees to know how to administer a trust.* In order to do this, trustees will need to be able to ascertain who is to benefit from it, the nature of the property, and how it must be distributed. Here, certainty requirements provide a source of instructions for the trustees. Where property is not to be given to another absolutely, but is instead subject to a settlor's instructions, trustees must know how to carry these out. Knowing what is or is not trust property is prerequisite for trustees to acquire legal title to it (through the process of constitution, which requires compliance with formality requirements), which in turn is essential for trustees to be able to deal with it to secure its benefits for a beneficiary. In terms of what trustees must do with trust property in carrying out the trust (which is a mandatory arrangement), they need workable instructions, and not ones incapable of being carried out because it is not clear what property is being settled or to whom it is to be applied. This is particularly the case where a settlor is now deceased, so that there is no scope for him to provide guidance beyond what he has actually made clear.

There is also a further justification for making it clear that property *is* subject to a trust, what this property actually is, and who is intended to benefit: fear of the 'fraudulent trustee', which, as a number of cases that we will encounter suggest, is a well-founded concern. We have not encountered this yet, but we will do so in due course. It is a justification that operates in close conjunction with the requirement that there be identifiable beneficiaries and reflects that it is only a beneficiary who has *locus standi* to enforce a trust (including to pursue a fraudulent trustee), and so the courts are very strict when it comes to being able to point to someone who can enforce a trust as a test for its validity.

Part II   The beneficiary principle

Introducing the beneficiary principle is very important in drawing this chapter to a close, in as much as this provides a logical 'end point' for the material on certainty, as we continue on to examine validity requirements for express private trusts. In addition, these requirements also provide a very effective forecast for the study of charity once we have looked at the creation of private trusts. We already know from Chapter 2 that charity law is a special body of trusts law that is considered anomalous with the rest of trusts law, and what will become clear is that charitable organizations are actually publicly enforceable 'trusts for *purposes*' rather than 'trusts for *individuals*'.

This last point is very significant because studying certainty has shown that the trust is a mandatory arrangement that must be carried out. It also became apparent, when we looked at certainty of objects, that a trust will be valid only if there is someone who has the standing to enforce the arrangement, and this reinforced earlier material suggesting that a key feature of the trust is that only the beneficiary can enforce it. All of these ideas converge in the seminal statement from Sir William Grant MR in *Morice* v *Bishop of Durham* (1805) 10 Ves 522, as authority that 'there must be somebody, in whose favour the court can decree performance'. This is what has become known as the 'beneficiary principle'.

So, as a general rule, for a private trust to be valid, there must be someone who can be identified as having sufficient *locus standi* to enforce it. This is why certainty-of-objects rules have emerged, and this is why trusts will be 'void for lack of certainty' if the relevant test for certainty is not satisfied (that is, either the class ascertainability test set out in *IRC* v *Broadway Cottages* [1955] Ch 20 for fixed trusts or the individual ascertainability test from *McPhail* v *Doulton* [1971] AC 424 for discretionary trusts). Thus the reason for having stringent certainty-of-objects requirements is to ensure that there is always someone in a position to enforce the trust.

Where a trust is one for human beneficiaries, the position is straightforward, subject to satisfying the relevant test. The difficulties that not having a human beneficiary in whose favour the 'court can decree performance [of the trust]' can create can be seen in attempts that are made from time to time to create private trusts (that is, those that are not publicly enforceable) *for purposes* instead of for individuals.

When we look at charity law, it becomes clear that the beneficiary principle does not apply to charitable organizations, because the Attorney-General is under a duty to enforce them should this need arise. However, attempts to create *private trusts* that are trusts for *purposes* rather than for persons are fraught with difficulties, and this is most often because there is no one who is obviously in a position to enforce them. This is now explained, along with why these dispositions are ever valid when they contravene the beneficiary principle.

Introducing private 'purpose trusts' and their links with charity law

Before looking at the attempts made to create express private-purpose trusts, and the difficulties caused by doing so, the significance of the beneficiary principle for private trusts is proposed through some signposting of what is to come when we look at charity law. The link between the application of the beneficiary principle to private trusts and charitable organizations, which do not need beneficiaries, can be seen in *Bowman* v *Secular Society Ltd* [1917] AC 406, in which, in echoing *Morice* sentiments, Lord Parker decreed that 'A trust to be valid must be for the benefit of individuals ... or must be in that class of gifts for the benefit of the public which the courts in this country recognise as charitable'.

Thus the beneficiary principle (and the rules for certainty of objects that are built on this) should mean that, where a trust is a private (non-charitable) trust, but has no human beneficiaries, it will be void on the ground that it infringes the beneficiary principle. This is the general position, but we do need to consider the few anomalous exceptions to this rule and the problems that are associated with them. Here, most attention is paid to how these arrangements create difficulties because they infringe the beneficiary principle, but, as we will discover, there are a number of potential difficulties arising from decreeing that any private trust can be valid without human beneficiaries.

Why create trusts for purposes rather than for individuals?

Before looking at the validity of trusts that have no human beneficiaries, it might be a good idea for us to try to understand why attempts are ever made to do such a thing. Indeed, everything up to now has suggested that trusts (and certainly 'express trusts') are created because an owner of property wishes for another to benefit from it, and so we need to find out why trusts would ever be consciously created in which property is not intended to benefit beneficiaries.

Much of this becomes easier to understand once the cases start to tell the stories, and these cases are typically a reflection of the desire of an owner of property to use it to 'provide for' some*thing*, rather than for someone. We will see that this is often a favourite pet (an 'animal beneficiary') or, in the case of *Re Thompson*, a favourite pastime. They also arise where someone wishes to erect or maintain a grave, or to create a monument to another—or even to *himself*! Typical illustration of this kind of desire can be seen in *Pettingall* v *Pettingall* (1842) 11 LJ Ch 176, which concerned an annuity of £50 for the testator's 'favourite black mare', and which was designed to ensure that she could live out her life in green and lush surroundings, free from the burden of being ridden, etc. This kind of action is regarded neutrally by many as being eccentric, and indeed very 'English', and has also been less kindly referenced as 'weakness in human sentiment' in a key case.

3.11   The validity of private trusts that are trusts for purposes

It is clear from a number of cases that the courts *have* accepted the validity of a limited number of non-charitable purpose trusts, and ones that are even recognizable as limited categories of arrangement. This can be seen in a number of key cases, which are valid notwithstanding that they do infringe the beneficiary principle. As suggested, this can be seen in a cluster of what might be termed 'pets and graves' cases. We have already encountered the provision in *Pettingall* v *Pettingall* for a favourite mare; others seeking to take care of animals include *Re Dean* (1889) 41 ChD 552 and *Re Kelly* [1935] IR 255. *Mussett* v *Bingle* [1876] WN 170, *Re Hooper* [1932] 1 Ch 38, and *Pirbright* v *Salwey* [1896] WN 86 are all cases involving building and maintaining monuments, and particularly memorials. *Bourne* v *Keane* [1919] AC 815 concerned private Catholic mass, while *Re Thompson* [1934] Ch 342 is the 'pastime' case involved in upholding a trust for the promotion of fox hunting. As we will discover, a number of these cases point to the multiplicity of difficulties that can befall attempts to create such arrangements and, in illustrating this, we shall discover shortly that *Mussett* is a particularly interesting 'graves' case.

However, the validity of these cases must be read alongside *Re Astor's ST* [1952] Ch 534, which is said to be authority for the general position that non-charitable purpose trusts that violate the beneficiary principle are void. *Re Astor* itself concerned a trust that instructed trustees to hold a fund upon various purposes, including 'the maintenance of good relations between nations [and] … the preservation of the independence of newspapers'. This was struck out as being void because there were no human beneficiaries capable of enforcing it. Thus *Astor* provided restatement of the principle established in *Morice* v *Bishop of Durham*, dating from the early nineteenth century—that, in order to be valid, a private trust must be one for human beneficiaries. This was an important restatement on account of the fact that, notwithstanding *Morice*, it marked recognition of one of the cardinal principles of trusts law; the nineteenth and early twentieth centuries had actually produced a number of trusts that were valid despite contravening the beneficiary principle.

The way in which these contravening trusts were explained in *Re Astor* is the reason why it was such a significant case and is considered to be authority for the modern law. In *Re Astor*, Roxburgh J ruled that these arrangements were 'exceptions' and did not negate the general principle, which is that, in order to be valid, there must be 'someone in whose favour the court can decree performance'. There was also some discussion of the way in which their validity could be explained by virtue of being enforceable by the 'residuary beneficiary' (as explained in Chapter 2, one who receives property that has not been specifically bequeathed in the case of a will, or one who is the intended object of such an attempt, but the gift has failed for some reason). There is extensive discussion to be found in Sheridan (1953) 17 LQR 46, and it is the case that the residuary beneficiary point will work for a number of these arrangements, but it will not obviously explain all of them. A different view of the anomalous exceptions in *Astor* is that there is nothing wrong with these arrangements being valid if they are construed as trusts of imperfect obligation—that is, they are valid, but not enforceable (see Brown (2007) 71 Conv 148). A further view is that it would have been more satisfactory for *Astor* actually to have declared these exceptional cases as ones that are incorrect. However, it is also the case that this was a first-instance decision, and so Roxburgh J may well have felt that he lacked the authority to so declare. Thus it might be unfair to suggest that Roxburgh J missed an opportunity in the same way as might be said of the Court of Appeal in *Re Endacott* [1960] Ch 232.

A missed opportunity? Re Endacott

Re Astor was upheld in *Re Shaw* [1957] 1 WLR 729, also at first instance, which concerned George Bernard Shaw's famous, but ill-fated forty-letter alphabet. Then, in *Re Endacott* [1960] Ch 232, the Court of Appeal had the opportunity to consider the *Re Astor* approach. In *Endacott*, a bequest 'to North Tawton Devon Parish Council for the purpose of providing some useful memorial to myself' was held void, and at one level this *did* provide important Court of Appeal authority for *Re Astor*. In this spirit, there was insistence that a number of the valid purpose trusts (including those that we have just considered) were to be regarded as 'anomalous and not to be extended', and were not even to be *followed*. It was even suggested that such arrangements reflected 'weakness in human sentiment'. One cannot help but wonder if this was on the strength of the appellate court's views; it is a pity that this was not considered an opportunity either to overrule the earlier cases or to clarify the basis on which the trusts were to be enforced. This is because it is difficult to know exactly what they stand for, or even on what principles they actually operate. This would have required some consideration of Roxburgh J's residuary beneficiary suggestion, or critical appraisal of analysing private purpose trusts as ones of imperfect obligation.

3.12 **Other problems with creating valid non-charitable purpose trusts**

The view that *Re Endacott* was a missed opportunity in relation to these 'anomalous' valid trusts, which both *Astor* and *Endacott* clearly considered troublesome, becomes even more powerful given that the validity of these arrangements does not only offend the beneficiary principle; such arrangements that are upheld as valid trusts are also troublesome in a number of other ways. Indeed, even if a non-charitable purpose trust falls within these limited categories and is not invalid for offending the beneficiary principle, there are other 'pitfalls' that it is also likely—if not certain—to encounter. That *Re Endacott* is also authority that such an arrangement will be valid only if the purpose is defined with sufficient certainty (that is, is sufficiently clear) in order to be valid suggests that these purposes can lack certainty. But the cases suggest that the most significant difficulty beyond infringing the beneficiary principle is that they will often infringe what are known as 'perpetuity' rules. Perpetuity requirements are now covered substantively by this text only in the Online Resource Centre, reflecting the declining interest in them within undergraduate study and recent reform of the law.

Generally and in brief, in order to be valid, a private trust must not infringe either of the two perpetuity rules. The policy behind having such rules is to ensure that there is a time limit for how long property can be tied up on trust. The basis for this is that if trusts were able to exist indefinitely, then this would very seriously affect free dealings with property *across* generations. This can be seen in the words of Deech (1981) 97 LQR 593, at 594, describing the rule against perpetuities as:

> necessary … to strike a balance between on the one hand the freedom of the present generation and, on the other, that of future generations to deal as they wish with the property in which they have interests. If a settlor had total liberty to dispose of his property among future beneficiaries, the recipients, being fettered by his wishes, would never enjoy that same freedom in turn.

This policy against 'dead hand rule'—that is, preventing the dead from dictating what it is possible for current and future generations to achieve—has traditionally been manifested in two key rules, which comprised a complex mixture of common law and statutory provisions, and which, if violated, would render the trust void. The first is the rule against remoteness in vesting, which requires that a beneficiary's interest in trust property must 'vest' in him within the perpetuity period. The second is the rule against perpetual duration, which requires that, in any valid trust, there must be no possibility that property will be tied up in the trust for a duration that is longer than the perpetuity period. This puts limits on how long a trust can 'last', and a trust will be valid only if it provides that it will come to an end within a time frame that is lawful, and this is what has raised issues for private purpose trusts.

As the materials available on the Online Resource Centre explain, perpetuity law has recently been reformed courtesy of the Perpetuities Act 2009. However, this legislation has left untouched the position of private purpose trusts, which (expressly by s. 18 of the 2009 Act) remain governed by common law limits on duration. The common law period is a 'life in being' plus twenty-one years. In plain English, this means the lifetime of a human being who is alive at the date on which the trust is created. The life in being that is chosen by settlors is often the monarch or a member of the royal family, and historically the use of a so-called 'royal life [in being]' clause reflected associations made between royalty and longevity. So the perpetuity period would be for the lifetime of this person plus twenty-one years. This is much easier to see in relation to *Re Hooper* [1932] 1 Ch 38 and *Re Kelly* [1935] IR 255, than in the abstract. Further, you should be aware that some of these 'purpose trust' dispositions have been upheld on this basis, while others have failed because they infringe this rule. However, the cases also suggest that it is only human, as opposed to animal, lives that are to be considered for these purposes, even if the trust relates to an animal, with *Re Kelly* providing authority for this.

Re Hooper is authority that a gift for a non-charitable purpose to last 'for no more than twenty-one years', or 'so long as the law allows', is capable of being upheld for twenty-one years, but one that does not specify any time limit would infringe the rule and so be void. However, *Mussett* v *Bingle* [1876] WN 170 suggests that some latitude may be granted. This concerned a gift of £300 for the erection of a monument and one for

£200 to provide interest for its maintenance. The latter was indeed held void, because it infringed the perpetuity rule, but the former was held valid, on the assumed basis that the tomb would be erected within the perpetuity period.

3.13 Attempts to create private purpose trusts that avoid all of these 'pitfalls' for validity

There have been some attempts made to create valid trusts for purposes, rather than individuals, which are non-charitable (and thus subject to the law of private trusts), which will avoid the 'validity difficulties' that have become apparent up to now. The most pronounced one is infringement of the beneficiary principle, and the attempts to create arrangements that avoid this can be seen both in the conduct of those who wish to bring them into being and the courts that determine what should happen to them. The reason why these cases might appear to be different, certainly at first glance, is that, unlike *Re Astor* and *Re Shaw*, they do seem to be seeking to benefit actual people—either directly or less so. In this regard, cases such as *Re Astor* and *Re Shaw* can often be found referenced as 'pure' purpose trusts, in which the benefit is entirely abstract and there is no attempt to tie benefit to any individuals or group of individuals.

In this regard, the cases that we encounter now are focused on actual people—directly or indirectly. This notwithstanding, however, it will be suggested that even where an analysis of an arrangement given by the court claims that it avoids all of the pitfalls and that a valid purpose trust has been created, actually none of these cases contradicts the view expressed in *Re Astor* and *Re Endacott* that all private purpose trusts remain void, apart from the anomalous exceptions. This can be seen in three key cases, around which this discussion is clustered.

Re Abbott [1900] 2 Ch 326 concerned a trust for the maintenance of two old ladies, in which the property came from contributions made for this purpose from the community in which they lived. There was no question of the trust being invalid, even though the fund was clearly intended to be used for a purpose, rather than simply given to the two ladies. However, this case is probably best analysed as an ordinary trust for the two ladies, with a direction to the trustees to apply the fund only for their maintenance. This is possible without regarding this as a purpose trust at all, and instead as an ordinary 'beneficiary trust'.

Leahy v *Attorney-General for New South Wales* [1959] AC 457 concerned property to be held on trust for 'such order of nuns of the Catholic Church or the Christian brothers as my executors and trustees shall select'. The trust was not charitable, and it was held that it could not be valid as a private trust notwithstanding that individual 'objects' selected had sufficient interest to enforce the trust. The ruling was that this could not be a valid trust, because those objects, although having *locus standi* to enforce the trust (which is, of course, a key tenet of certainty of objects rules), were not actually being granted a full beneficial interest in the property under the trust's terms. The judge reiterated the conventional view that 'a trust may be created for the benefit of persons as *cestuis que trust*, but not for a purpose or object unless the purpose or object be charitable'.

However, what might appear to be a different type of decision can be seen in *Re Denley's Trust Deed* [1969] 1 Ch 373. This case concerned a gift of land for use as a sports ground 'primarily' for the benefit of the employees of the company concerned, and also for the benefit of 'such other persons as the trustees may allow to use the same', which was upheld because the class of individuals to benefit was ascertainable. The judgment of Goff J explained that *Astor/Endacott* principles operate to invalidate only those purpose trusts that are 'abstract or impersonal' purpose trusts, and that '[w]here [a] trust, though expressed as a purpose, is directly or indirectly for the benefit of an individual or individuals, it is in general outside the mischief of the beneficiary principle'. The intended effect of *Denley* is clearly supposed to be that some trusts which are purpose trusts are capable of being valid, and should not thus be subject to *Re Astor*, but what is not clear from the judgment is how this distinction works as a matter of legal principle.

Furthermore, notwithstanding the intended import of the *Denley* decision itself, the view taken of *Denley* in *Re Grant's WT* [1980] 1 WLR 360 is that it is not a purpose trust at all and is instead an ordinary trust for individuals. As Vinelott J explained at 370:

> That case [*Denley*] on a proper analysis, in my judgment, falls altogether outside … purpose trusts. I see no distinction in principle between a trust to permit a class defined by reference to employment to use and enjoy land in accordance with rules to be made at the discretion of trustees on the one hand, and, on the other hand, a trust to distribute income at the discretion of trustees amongst a class, defined by reference to, for example, relationship to the settlor. In both cases the benefit to be taken by any member of the class is at the discretion of the trustees, but any member of the class can apply to the court to compel the trustees to administer the trust in accordance with its terms.

Similar views can be found expressed by Peter Millett QC (1985) 101 LQR 269, 280–2, and whatever *Denley* decides, pure purpose trusts, such as *Re Astor's ST*, are unaffected by it and are still void. It is also clear that the individuals to whom direct or indirect benefit is given must be ascertainable within the certainty-of-object requirements: in *R v District Auditor, ex parte West Yorkshire Metropolitan County Council* [1986] RVR 24, an alternative argument that the disposition created a valid private purpose trust failed, since, whatever *Denley* decided and indeed even if there were objects with full beneficial interests, they were not ascertainable under the certainty-of-objects rules.

 Revision Box

1. What can we learn about the fundamental nature of the trust by looking at how certainty requirements relating to intention and to trust property can be satisfied, and what happens when they are not?

   Here, you will need to link your study of certainty back to the study of the essence of trusts in Chapter 2 and explain:

   – what is meant by the requirement of certainty;
   – the function of the certainty of intention requirement within certainty more broadly;
   – the key factors underpinning certainty-of-intention rules;
   – how trust property becomes significant in the light of what is meant by the requirement of certainty;
   – what the rules relating to satisfying certainty in relation to trust property actually are; and
   – what the consequences of failing to satisfy certainty in relation to trust property will be and why this is different from the outcome of failure to establish certainty of intention.

   →

> 2. What is the significance of *Re Baden's Deed Trusts (No. 2)* [1973] Ch 9 in the context of certainty of objects?
>   - Read the submission to the Court of Appeal by John Vinelott QC, counsel for Baden's estate, and summarize the main points of his arguments on why the disposition should fail on grounds of absence of certainty of objects.
>   - Ensure that you understand why, had Vinelott's core argument succeeded, the implications for the *McPhail* v *Doulton* [1971] AC 424 ruling would be considerable and indeed unacceptable. (NB *McPhail*'s treatment of *IRC* v *Broadway Cottages* [1955] Ch 20 is central here.)
> 3. Explain what is clear and what is less so about the significance of 'administrative unworkability' in determining the validity of express trusts.

FURTHER READING

Birks (1995) 'Establishing a proprietary base' Restitution Law Review 83.

Bond (2012) 'All in it together: the Supreme Court's verdict on the Lehman Brothers "client money" case' 27 Butterworths Journal of International Banking & Financial Law 267.

Brown (2007) 'What are we to do with testamentary trusts of imperfect obligation?' 71 Conveyancer 148.

Deech (1981) 'Lives in being revived' 97 Law Quarterly Review 593.

Dilnot and Harris (2012) 'Ownership of a fund' 27 Butterworths Journal of International Banking & Financial Law 272.

Eden (2000) 'Beneficial ownership of shares: the implications of Re Harvard Securities' Parts 1 and 2 16 Insolvency Law and Practice 174 and 137.

Gravells (1977) 'Public purpose trusts' 40 Modern Law Review 397.

Harpum (1986) 'Administrative unworkability and purpose trusts' 45(3) Cambridge Law Journal 391.

Hayton (1994) 'Uncertainty of subject matter of trusts' 110 Law Quarterly Review 335.

Martin (1996) 'Certainty of subject matter: a defence of Hunter v. Moss' 60 Conveyancer 223.

Martin and Hayton (1984) 'Certainty of objects: what is heresy?' Conveyancer 304.

Matthews (1984) 'A heresy and a half in certainty of objects' Conveyancer 22.

Millett (1985) 'The *Quistclose* trust: who can enforce it?' 101 Law Quarterly Review 269.

Pawlowski and Summers (2007) 'Private purpose trusts: a reform proposal' 71 Conveyancer 440.

Sheridan (1953) 'Lionel Astor: trusts for non-charitable purposes' 17 Law Quarterly Review 46.

 online resource centre

For summaries of a selection of these articles, please visit <http://www.oxfordtextbooks.co.uk/orc/wilson_trusts11e/>

4

....

Formality and the creation
of valid trusts

When we make a study of how trusts are constituted in Chapter 5, we will discover that very close relationships subsist between how a trust is successfully *constituted* and what is required by way of *formality* to achieve this. For now, we will try to separate out these two requirements by making a detailed study of the formality requirements found in the creation of a trust and those that, if not complied with, will prevent formation of a valid trust. In belonging squarely to the study of the creation of express trusts, the material here applies to express trusts, whilst it will become clear that formality requirements are differently configured or even absent when it comes to private trusts that are implied by virtue of being constructive or resulting. But, for clarity, these requirements also apply for express settlements of property that are made to charity.

By way of a reminder from Chapter 2, when any reference is made to 'formality' in connection with legal arrangements, we speak of ways in which law specifies that particular legal proceedings must be conducted. And by way of clarification, whilst law will not accept proceedings that do not comply with what is required, where what is prescribed has been complied with, then law will recognize this as being valid and will thus give effect to whatever the parties participating in the proceedings were seeking to achieve. This suggests that formality can be found in a number of proceedings in which individuals and other legal actors engage across a number of interests that are governed by law.

This particular text is, of course, concerned with formality requirements that arise where trusts of property are created by those who own property in order to provide its benefits for others, which suggests that we need to establish what law requires in two distinct respects.

It is, of course, the case that formality will be required for a number of legal proceedings and arrangements, but because trusts involve property and its ownership and enjoyment, we need to understand how formality governs dealings with property generally. From this, we need to appreciate what formalities might apply to the creation of trusts specifically.

In Chapter 2, we already became aware that what law prescribes in the way of required form in dealings with property will be strongly influenced by the type of property with which it is being dealt; we also became aware that special formality clusters requirements relating to writing, signing, and registration.

This is very important for appreciating what 'required form' applies in the creation of trusts. Or, more accurately, it applies to the creation of express trusts (whether this is a private one for a beneficiary, or for the benefit of a charitable organization), because a different body of law governs private trusts that are implied, in which case some formality requirements will be completely disapplied. So what formality requirements do we come across in the express creation of trusts of property?

Here, we encounter two types of formality, which give rise to distinct requirements. First, there is formality attaching to any type of dealing with property that involves transferring ownership of property from one person to another. What is required here will apply equally to recipients of outright ownership (legal title) following a sale of property or a gift of it, and to a trustee who takes charge of the property by receiving legal title to property where ownership is separated. Second, we encounter formality that will arise only in the creation of trusts. Here, we encounter prescribed ways of dealing with property that apply only in situations in which its owner is actually creating a trust of it, which are not found more generally in dealings with property.

The function of prescribed form: why is there formality in property transactions?

We will learn much more about these different types of formality and what they actually require to be fulfilled shortly, but at this stage we need to understand that all formality requirements have a key underlying rationale or purpose: the objective of protecting the parties involved in property transactions *by protecting the property itself* from unintended dealings by its owner, or even ones that are kept secret from him.

We touched on this in Chapter 2, and particularly when we discussed making gifts of property that law will regard as effective, but actually understanding the purpose of prescribed ways of dealing with property means that we have to look further back still to the materials of Chapter 1. This is where we learned that ownership of property embodies an owner's entitlement to deal freely with it, and that ordinarily an owner of property is able to deal with it pretty much as he chooses. Where property is owned outright, an owner's 'bundle of rights' is embodied in holding legal title to property, and this entitles him to sell the property or to give it away, as well as use it to raise security and also to settle it on trust.

This raises the question of *how* it is possible to tell that an owner of property is seeking to deal with it in such a way as will involve him creating rights for others in it, and also the closely related one of *why* it is so important for us to be able to establish that he is trying to do this. Taking the latter first, it is very important to be able to establish that an owner is trying to do this because any sale of property to a purchaser or gift made of it will result in the owner losing all rights of ownership of that property to another. Equally, if he creates a trust of that property, he is no longer able to deal with it freely as owner—even if he retains legal title to it by becoming a trustee. All of these situations will fundamentally change the relationship that an owner of property once had with it, and in all of them he will forgo the 'bundle of rights' embodied in ownership. It is for these reasons that the question of *how* we can tell that an owner of property is seeking to do this becomes crucial.

This is why legal requirements have evolved around particular dealings with property. These are designed to ensure that what is happening in respect of the property is what the parties are seeking to achieve by dealing with the property and that everyone involved is aware of this. This applies particularly for an owner of property because of the significance attached to ownership of property in English law, and the way in which ordinarily only an owner of property can pass title to it to another. Because of this, any attempt to deal with property in these ways that fails to comply with what law has prescribed for them will result in law not accepting that anything has happened, and the *status quo* of ownership will remain.

Prescribed formality: protecting the parties in dealings with property

It is not only an original owner who benefits from requiring things to be done in particular ways; for a new recipient of the property, too, being able to point to fulfilment of procedural requirements is evidence that ownership of that property now vests in him. Where dealings with property are ones for consideration, it is also the case that consideration will be important evidence of intention to deal with property in particular ways. Formality supports this by ensuring that all dealings with property are intended and also that they are visible. And so formality requirements might have an especially significant role in dealings with property that do not involve consideration. This is especially the case with a gift, but we shall see that it also applies to creating a trust. These dealings with property tend to be much less visible in any case, and it would be even less easy in these cases to see who has entitlements to property were it not for prescribing particular procedures for dealings with it.

In summary, for an owner of property, formality requirements help to prevent unintended transactions with property, and thus are central to reinforcing the position that the person who holds legal title to the property is the one entitled to deal freely with it, or retain it unencumbered. For a person acquiring property, formality requirements support the intention to pass ownership and all of the entitlements of ownership from one party to another. The formality surrounding the transfer helps to vindicate the legally binding agreement reached between the parties where there is a contract; it also concretizes the position of an intended recipient where there is a gift made or a trust created in his favour.

This gives us a general sense of why formality is so important, and that requirements of how things must be done in dealings with property will protect an owner of property's universal rights to it and also the position of any recipient of this, by making it clear to whom the property belongs. Once we understand this, we can apply it to the trust arrangement and the 'trust actors' we find within it.

In a trust arrangement, there are at least two parties involved and (because often, although he can do so, a settlor does not choose to act as a trustee) there will commonly be three actors who need to be considered in the light of justifying formality in dealings with property. The basic overriding objective is to protect *all* of the parties, and indeed the trust property, and formality requirements do so by preventing 'secret' transactions involving trust property. This therefore helps to ensure that all dealings with trust property are visible and ascertainable should query about them arise. From this basic premise, it is possible to see how all potential parties arising in the trust scenario can benefit from requirements that help to ensure 'open dealings' with trust property.

To understand this, think back to how the actors associated with the express trust arrangement were introduced in Chapters 1 and 2. Then remember how these basic ideas were developed in Chapter 3 in the course of identifying and explaining certainty rules. Here, we need to remember the 'settlor' perspectives that were embodied first in certainty of intention and then in the other two certainties. And we also need to remember how, at every stage, it was so important for settlor, trustee, and beneficiary to be clear about what is happening. At the heart of what is happening is property, which is, of course, 'trust property'.

The application of the general rational underpinning formality rules can be found in materials for this chapter available on the Online Resource Centre, but in essence the comparative invisibility and vulnerability of equitable ownership of property (alongside legal ownership) suggests that dealings with trust property must be readily apparent. Here, trust property can be protected by requiring dealings with it to be undertaken 'with formality'. The most obvious way to do this is to require writing, and the earliest modern embodiment of this is the Statute of Frauds 1677.

What is the tax angle of formality requirements found in the creation of trusts?

In this chapter, we shall see two things that remind us of what was said about the importance of tax in the creation of trusts initially in Chapter 1, which were then developed in Chapter 2. This provided a brief outline of how trusts are important for tax planning, with this being a term that is applied to minimizing exposure to tax liability.

The first is confirmation that trusts are used for tax planning purposes, evident from the way in which a large number of trusts are created formally without any formality being required by law for them to be valid arrangements concerning property and its ownership. This is because using trusts instrumentally in this way will mean that it is important to be able to establish who actually owns property and from when. Thus creating trusts in writing will make it absolutely clear who has beneficial ownership of the property (and significantly who does not) and also the exact date on which the arrangement was created. Both of these matters reflect how trusts are used as *avoidance* devices—that is, as a way of avoiding tax liability in a way that is lawful (and not to aid tax evasion, which is not lawful).

The significance of taxation for the creation of trusts can, second, be seen from how much of the litigation in this chapter involves the United Kingdom's tax authority, the nomenclature of which has changed over the years and which has most recently been renamed Her Majesty's Revenue and Customs (HMRC). Whatever the name under which it appears, its presence in litigation involving the creation of private trusts has been stalwart and dates back into the nineteenth century. This is because, mindful of the use of trusts as avoidance devices, it has been in the interest of the authority to take an interest in what is going on, with a view to maximizing what can be collected for the 'public purse', and to take steps to try to secure this by litigating any uncertain areas. We see a similar approach in our study of gifts made to charitable purposes in Chapters 10–13. But, for now, there are many examples of tax authority interest in the creation of private trusts, with much of this occurring around formality requirements and what formality can reveal about ownership of property, which is at the heart of tax liability. This is shown in this chapter, and also in Chapter 5 concerning the constitution of trusts, where—it has already been suggested—considerations of formality are much in evidence. Using trusts instrumentally for tax avoidance makes it very important to establish exact dates on which property is settled, given that, for taxation purposes, it is very important who owns what at particular points in time. So creating trusts in writing will provide an important 'evidence trail' for this, even where this is not strictly required by law for the arrangement to be valid, which we will find out is actually the case for most trusts.

Beyond this, a number of settlors will wish to provide written instructions on carrying out the trust to trustees, and will thus record declarations of trust in writing as part of this even if they are not required to make them in this way as a matter of law in order for the trust to be valid. What follows from this is that we now need to learn what law does require by way of formality for the creation of trusts.

4.1 What formality requirements relate to settling property on trust?

As suggested, we encounter, in the creation of trusts, formality prescriptions that relate to property dealings generally, and also ones that are found only in the creation of trusts. This actually gives us three types of formality at which to look closely. First, we find 'transfer formality' requirements, which attach to any dealings with property that result in its ownership leaving one person and becoming vested in someone else. In the second category—that is, those found only in the creation of trusts—we actually encounter two types. Here, we find formality attaching to making it clear that property is no longer owned outright and is now the subject of the trust, which is known as 'declaration formality'. We also find here what is known as 'disposition formality', which arises where there is a trust already in existence and a beneficiary's equitable interest (or part of it) in what is already trust property is being passed to someone else.

Having distinguished formality in this way, we are now going to discuss these requirements through a distinct structure. We look first at formality that arises initially in the creation of a trust from property that is owned outright, and thereafter at what is required for dealings with property that is already trust property. This means that we look first at *declaration* formality, then at *transfer* formality, and last at *disposition* formality. We look at the creation of a trust and initially at the first stage involved in creating any express trust of property: an owner's declaration or statement that the property is to become trust property. We then look at any transfer formality that is required as a result of this statement that property is now trust property.

At the outset, we need to understand that what is actually required by law in any given attempted creation of a trust will depend on the nature of the property being settled on trust. Thus what formality is prescribed by law will reflect legal distinctions drawn in English law between 'real' property and personalty, and then between personal property that is tangible or intangible. It is also worth pointing out that if what is required is not complied with, then as far as law is concerned what is intended and being attempted will not be recognized as having happened. We shall find out that there are some respects in which equity applies some flexibility, but generally where particular procedures required in the creation of a trust (or the assignment of an existing equitable interest under a disposition) are not complied with, then a trust cannot be valid and its attempted creation will fail.

4.2 Prescribed form for declaring property subject to a trust: declaration formality

Remembering that formality refers to prescribed procedures that must be complied with if law is to recognize the trust as valid, the formality requirements that we find operating in relation to declarations of trust are an example of prescriptions that we find arising *only* in the creation of trusts, and not in other dealings with property. As we know from Chapter 3, a declaration of trust is some kind of statement from a legal owner of property that property which has been held by him absolutely is now subject to a trust, and that it is being held on behalf of one or more beneficiary. We encountered declarations of trust when we considered what was meant by satisfying the requirement that it must be sufficiently clear or certain that an owner of property intends to create a trust of it.

When we looked at certainty of intention, it became clear that the courts were prepared to conclude that a trust is intended from what an owner of property says or from what he does, and for the most part this is sufficient. Providing intention to create a trust is manifested, and that it is clear from such words or conduct not simply that an owner of property intends another to benefit from it, but that these benefits must be delivered by way of a trust, then that is all that is required most of the time. This is because there are no declaration formality requirements for creating trusts of personal property. As far as declaring a trust is concerned, trusts of personalty can be declared orally and they will be valid if made this way.

Notwithstanding that written declarations of trust are not required for trusts of personal property to be valid, many will be so in practice because a large number of trusts are used in tax planning. The strict legal position is that declarations of trusts of personal property can be oral, but there are situations in which declarations of trust have to be made in writing. This arises where the property that is being settled as 'trust property' is land, which is subject to special rules relating to declarations of trust found in s. 53(1)(b) of the Law of Property Act 1925, which provides that 'a declaration of trust respecting land or any interest in land therein must be manifested and proved by some writing signed by the person who is able to declare such a trust or by his will'.

While a first-glance reading of this might suggest that the declaration must be made in writing, there is actually more subtlety than this and also in the effect of the absence of writing, with both suggesting that more must be said at this point.

In setting out a requirement of writing, it appears that the function of the requirement is to provide written evidence or documentation that the declaration has actually been made, rather than to require that the declaration itself is made in writing. This is the significance of the terms 'manifested and proved', but note that there is the requirement that this is signed by the person who is seeking to create the trust. And, in referencing the 'person who is able to declare such a trust', this takes us back to our initial thoughts—at the end of Chapter 2—on what confers capacity to settle property on trust. As the section itself clarifies, what is required is holding legal title to land, or holding any other legal interest in it that is being settled.

The effect of a declaration made without being evidenced in signed writing is that the declaration will be unenforceable, and it is very important to distinguish this from being actually void. Where something is considered in law to be *void*, it will have no legal effect whatsoever and is treated as if it never happened. Instead, the import of s. 53(1)(b) is that the declaration is valid, but unenforceable. Because of this, theoretically it is possible that such a declaration *could* become enforceable if written evidence of it were to be made or were to appear subsequently. There is no clear authority for this idea, and that which is cited at all is *Gardner* v *Rowe* (1828) 4 Russ 578, which is unfortunate, because *Gardner* itself appears to turn on another point.

What has been said up to now applies to what are known as *'inter vivos* trusts', which are ones that take effect while the settlor is still living. Where declarations of trusts are made by will and are thus regarded as trusts that are *testamentary*, regardless of the nature of the property, the will itself must satisfy the provisions of s. 9 of the Wills Act 1837, noting that this has itself been amended by s. 17 of the Administration of Justice Act 1982.

4.3 Formalities from general dealings with property arising in the creation of trusts: transfer formality

It is easy to see how we might encounter declaration formality when we are talking about creating trusts, but how we encounter other more general formality in the context of trusts specifically may not be so clear. This is where we need to explain how formality that arises in general dealings with property may become relevant for the creation of trusts specifically. This can be seen from the transfer formality requirements, which were explained in Chapter 2 as ones that arose from any dealings with property that involve transfers of title to it from one person to another. So, at that stage, we encountered transfer formality requirements in explaining the nature of transfers of property for value, and also gratuitous voluntary transfers, which are most commonly known as gifts. So how might transfer formality requirements arise in the creation of trusts?

How transfer formality requirements apply to the creation of trusts will become clearer still in Chapter 5, when we consider constituting a trust. At that point, we will learn how an owner of property can *become a trustee* of the property *himself* (thus explaining what we have already noted on a few occasions), as well as ask someone different to become a trustee, and thus hold the property and carry out the trust. More on the origins of this and its mechanics will be explained in Chapter 5, but for now we need to understand that transfer formality requirements will commonly arise because, in most express trust arrangements, a settlor will want to appoint specific trustees to carry out the trust. Wherever a settlor wishes for someone other than himself to act as trustee, then the legal title that he has to the property as its owner must be transferred *from* him *to* the person(s) who will act as trustee(s).

Where legal title to what becomes trust property is transferred to the trustee, then the trust is said to be constituted, but this will happen only where what is required *by law* to transfer title to that type of property is complied with. In these circumstances, it is clear that meeting equity's requirement that the trust is constituted requires satisfying law's requirements related to passing title to property by way of a gift. For this, we need to remember that a gift is a transfer of title to property that benefits an individual where that individual has *not* provided value for it—that is, when the individual is a 'volunteer'.

Ordinarily, this means satisfying law's requirements, but Chapter 2 suggested that equity can be more flexible about recognizing new owners of property, depending on the circumstances. But this mention was only fleeting, and there are still some bases to cover before revisiting law's requirements for making gifts of property and how, and indeed when, equity can add flexibility to this. This requires us to think about why a transfer of legal title to a trustee will be considered analogous with a gift for the purposes of satisfying transfer formality, and also to have an awareness of why it is so important for those who are trustees to have legal title to trust property.

The nature of property and the significance of intention

More will be said about the significance of intention in Chapter 5, but essentially a trustee must have legal title to the property because this is what gives him the authority and the capacity to deal with it so that it can be used to benefit the beneficiary. We will discover that an owner of property can become a settlor-trustee of it, but this is unusual in express trusts; ordinarily, others will be appointed, and where this is so they need to acquire legal title to the property. In these circumstances, ensuring that trustees have legal title to trust property has much in common with a gift, because it does involve a transfer of title that law will have to recognize for a trustee to be able to deal with trust property. And so it, like any other transfer of legal title from one person to another, must satisfy transfer formality requirements. There are *different* intentions behind transfers intended as a gift to a recipient and those intended to give legal title of trust property to a trustee: in the former instance, the owner of property wishes the recipient to become its owner; in the latter, the owner recognizes that a trustee must have responsibility for the property so that the beneficiary can benefit from it. But, as far as satisfying legal requirements, what is required for law to regard each transfer as effective is the same in both instances.

When legal title to property is transferred to an intended trustee in the creation of a trust, we know from Chapter 1 that his conscience is said to be 'affected' by receiving this property, understanding that he holds it for another's benefit. But if any 'transfer formality' requirements are not met, then an attempted transfer to a trustee will fail. This is clear from looking at *Milroy* v *Lord* (1862) 4 De GF & J 264, which was introduced in Chapter 2. *Milroy*'s actual reference is to 'imperfect gifts', but this principle applies equally to what Chapter 5 will tell us are known as 'incompletely constituted trusts'. What incomplete gifts and incompletely constituted trusts have in common is that attempts to transfer title to property in respect of them have failed to satisfy legal requirements that apply to them on account of the nature of the property concerned.

4.3.1 Equity and incomplete property transfers

In terms of what is required to satisfy law that property has a new legal owner, the material in Chapter 2 explained that this would depend on the type of property concerned, with simplest requirements attaching to ordinary chattels, and more onerous ones pertaining to intangible personal property and also to property that is land. As far as chattels are concerned, this is its delivery to the recipient with the intention that he should acquire ownership of it; for intangible personal property, this would require additional evidence of dealing drawn from endorsement, writing, or registration. Property that is land must be passed from one person to another by way of a written deed. The only thing that is different when making a gift of this property from transferring title of it to a trustee is the *type of intention* that the original owner of the property will have whilst making the transfer of legal title. In the case of the former, the owner must intend to pass ownership gratuitously to the recipient, while in the latter he must intend for the trustee to hold the property as custodian of it for another. Both involve transfers of legal title to property, but the nature of legal title transferred is very different: in one case, this is outright ownership; in the other, it is ownership stripped of all entitlements to the property.

So that is what law requires when property is transferred from one person to another, and law will not recognize any purported transfer of legal title where what is required has not been fulfilled, and will regard such as a transfer that is ineffective because it is 'incomplete'. The outcome of such an incomplete transfer is that ownership will remain where it originated. We now need to return to the suggestion made in Chapter 2 that, in some cases in which law would regard a transfer as incomplete, equity will recognize the transfer as one that is effective in equity. We need to understand the basic principles at work in achieving this before we can apply them to what happens in the creation of a trust.

Gifts that are incomplete at law are gifts that are not effective and will fail
This heading clarifies for us that the normal outcome in this situation will be that the original owner will retain ownership because the intended recipient cannot acquire ownership at law. The reference to 'normal outcome' is to the way in which, as far as law is concerned, the transfer has failed and the attempted gift is not an effective one. This can be seen in Turner LJ's judgment in *Milroy* v *Lord*, which we first encountered in Chapter 2, but at which we now look less selectively in order to understand that:

> in order to render a voluntary settlement valid and effectual, the settlor must have done everything which, according to the nature of the property comprised in the settlement, was necessary to be done in order to transfer the property and render the settlement binding upon him. He may of course do this by actually transferring the property to the persons for whom he intends to provide, and the provision will then be effectual.
>
> (*Milroy* v *Lord* (1862) 4 De GF & J 264, *per* Turner LJ at 274)

Authority that the normal application of *Milroy* v *Lord* to a gratuitous transfer of legal title to property will result in an incomplete transfer that fails, in which case ownership will remain with its original owner and not be transferred to a new one, can be seen in the outcomes of *Jones* v *Lock* (1865) LR 1 Ch App 25 and *Richards* v *Delbridge* (1874) LR Eq 11. We already encountered *Jones* v *Lock* in Chapter 3 on certainty of intention, and we did so at this point precisely because, in handing the cheque to his 9-month-old son, uttering 'I give this to you, baby' and removing it for safe keeping, the father had not done what law requires for this to have been an effective gift of the amount represented by the cheque. To achieve this, the father had to endorse the cheque in his son's favour, but he died before doing this.

Because more was required to be done by the father for law to recognize this gift to his son, it was regarded as a gift that failed on account that it was incomplete. In these circumstances, ownership remained with the father, which is exactly what happened in *Richards* v *Delbridge* when Delbridge wished to give Richards—his infant grandson—the lease that he had on his place of business as a bone-and-manure merchant. Delbridge endorsed the lease with the wording 'This deed and all thereto belonging I give to Edward Benetto Richards from this time forth, with all the stock-in-trade', but this was not sufficient to make an effective legal assignment of the property, and the grandfather's death meant that this could not be completed properly. If any of these requirements are not met, then an attempted transfer to another person will fail, because *Milroy* v *Lord* is authority for the application of the equitable principles that 'equity will not perfect an imperfect gift' and also that 'equity will not assist a volunteer'. Here, both *Jones* v *Lock* and *Richards* v *Delbridge* are authority for this position, and that such an attempted transfer to another person will fail.

Gifts that fail at law and equity's pursuit of 'just outcomes' ...
However, because equity is concerned with achieving just outcomes, there are occasions on which equity is prepared to be more flexible than law and is prepared to recognize a valid transfer of ownership in circumstances under which law would not be prepared to do so. In terms of understanding why this might be the case, equity's desire to be flexible is strongly connected with it wishing to give effect to instances in which, in substance, property has ceased to be owned by one person and belongs to someone different, even if law will not recognize this as yet. In taking this view, equity also recognizes that the ability of a new owner to become one recognized at law can be delayed temporarily from the way in which a number of formality requirements are tied into bureaucracies, which are associated with registration of a new title holder. We can see this in due course in relation to the registration of title to land with the Land Registry, and also registration requirements relating to shareholdings prescribed by companies legislation.

Property has a new owner in substance, if not, as yet, in form ...
This is so because equity is concerned with intent rather than form, and means that, in practice, equity will be prepared to be more flexible in two broad situations. The first situation in which equity deems it to be more flexible is where the recipient is not a volunteer at all, because he has provided value. In these circumstances, a recipient does have rights at common law to damages if the transfer is not completed in his favour. But equity can also effect the transfer because, in substance, the property has a new owner and equity is regarding as done that which ought to be done. For this, the consideration given needs to be recognized as value by equity, which, like the common law, will recognize money or money's worth. But unlike the common law, and because it is concerned with substance, it will not recognize agreements without consideration. Equity is also more flexible, however, and will accept what is known as 'love and affection'

consideration (which is considered in *Re Rose, Rose* v *IRC* [1952] Ch 499), and also that which is known as 'marriage consideration' (which can be found discussed on the Online Resource Centre within the materials relating to covenants to settle property on trust). And, in this regard, the strongest justification for recognizing that property has a new owner is where the property is unique, as is the case with land and shares in a private company, and a number of species of intangible personal property (for chattels, there is no additional formality to be tied into bureaucracy beyond delivery).

How does this apply to voluntary transfers?
Situations involving consideration are actually very unusual, and in its approach to incomplete property transfers, equity is much better known for its flexibility towards volunteer recipients of property—that is, those who are intended recipients of property by way of a gift. Thus, in some situations, equity will deem it unjust for a volunteer recipient not to be able to establish ownership of the property, and will seek a just outcome for him accordingly. For this type of transfer of ownership—that by way of a gift—which is entirely gratuitous at the behest of the owner, equity has historically focused on what an owner of property would need to do in order to achieve this. In this regard, the passage already quoted from Turner LJ's judgment in *Milroy* v *Lord* has been interpreted as having regard to whether an owner of property has done all that he can possibly do to ensure that he loses ownership of the property and that another will acquire it. In these circumstances, equity will be prepared to recognize that a transfer of ownership is effective 'in equity' until such a time as the legal formalities are completed, when it will also be effective *at law*. And, in taking this approach, *Milroy* distinguishes this situation from ones in which an owner of property has not done everything that is possible for him to do to effect the transfer, and that, because of this, a transfer failing to be effective at law should also remain unrecognized *by* equity *as* effective. This is what explains for us the outcomes of both *Jones* v *Lock* and *Richards* v *Delbridge*.

4.3.2 Applying *Milroy* v *Lord*'s 'last act' principles to the creation of an express trust

Where a transfer of legal title is made to a trustee, although consideration can be given, this is very unusual. So, in most cases, this will be a voluntary transfer like a gift; just like a gift, such attempts to make transfers of legal title to a trustee will be governed by the maxims that 'equity will not assist a volunteer' and 'equity will not perfect an imperfect gift'. Both are clear from the key passage from *Milroy* v *Lord*, and once again the only difference is that where an intended transfer to a trustee is incomplete *at law*, it is termed an 'incompletely constituted trust'. According to Turner LJ, at 274:

> in order to render a voluntary settlement valid and effectual, the settlor must have done everything which, according to the nature of the property comprised in the settlement, was necessary to be done in order to transfer the property and render the settlement binding upon him. He may [transfer outright] the property to the persons for whom he intends to provide ... and it will be equally effectual if he transfers the property to a trustee for the purposes of the settlement ... but, in order to render the settlement binding, one or other of these modes must ... be resorted to, for there is no equity in this Court to perfect an imperfect gift.

Milroy v *Lord* is also regarded as authority that, on occasions, 'equity will complete an imperfect gift' (which, for these purposes, includes a voluntary transfer of property to a trustee), even where this involves assisting a volunteer. This suggests that, on occasions, equity will regard recognizing a volunteer recipient under an incomplete transfer *as owner* as a just outcome, and the reason for this can be found in Turner LJ's judgment. This passage has been interpreted as the requirement that an owner of property must do all in his power to transfer the property, and not that he has actually succeeded. Indeed, if he had succeeded, title would have passed at law and there would be no need for equity's intervention. *Milroy* is authority that equity will recognize that property has a new owner where it is clear that no more can be done by an owner of property to effect the transfer. The theory behind this, in having regard to substance and intent, is that equity recognizes, *from* an owner of property doing all that he can to pass this to someone else, that there *will be* a new legal owner of the property once legal formality for its transfer *has* been complied with. This has become known as the 'last act' doctrine, and indeed as the 'rule in *Re Rose*' on account of the leading case for its application.

Discussion of the 'last act' doctrine now belongs squarely to that relating to constituting trusts, which will be considered in Chapter 5. What that discussion will show us is that any transfer of title to trust property to a trustee will be governed by the same transfer formality requirements as apply to any other transfer of title to property from one person to another. This is notwithstanding that the nature of legal title that is transferred to a trustee is different from that which is passed ordinarily in a gift or a transfer of value. This means that what is actually required by law will depend on the type of property, rather than the purpose of the transfer. We also know that, most commonly, a transfer of legal title to a trustee will be a voluntary transfer, and that this becomes very significant when legal formality is not complied with. In these circumstances, the only scope for a trustee (like a volunteer donee) to acquire title to the property is if equity is prepared to recognize the transfer as one that is effective.

If equity will do this, then the trust will be constituted, and the beneficiary will receive the benefits of the property as intended by the settlor. If equity will not recognize that the trust has been constituted by the settlor's 'last act', then the beneficiary will lose out, because no valid trust will arise.

Everything that has been said up to now in our substantive discussion of formality arising in trusts has concerned what is required in the creation of a valid express trust. As suggested earlier, ahead of looking at how what we have encountered here maps onto the requirement that the trust is constituted, there is still one formality type left to consider. So we now move to a different situation: instead of being concerned with the creation of an express trust, we now encounter formality that concerns dealings with property that is *already* subject to a trust.

4.4 Formality required for dispositions of equitable interests

Where a fully constituted trust already exists, then there is already a beneficiary who owns trust property in equity. In this setting, when we speak of 'dispositions of equitable interests', we are referring to situations in which a beneficiary under a trust chooses to give (or to assign) his equitable ownership of the trust property—or part of it—to another. The central issues here reflect that equitable interests already existing under a trust are being altered, and this will affect an existing beneficiary's entitlement under the trust. This final part of the chapter looks at formality governing these situations and the consequences of not complying with what is required at law.

4.4.1 The key legal provision: s. 53(1)(c) of the Law of Property Act 1925

The provisions of s. 53 (1)(c) of the Law of Property Act 1925 require that all such dispositions of equitable interests must be in writing to be valid. This is so regardless of the nature of the property concerned (in contrast with the position of declarations of trust), and covers both realty and personalty. Accordingly:

> a disposition of an equitable interest or trust subsisting at the time of the disposition must be in writing and signed by the person disposing of the same, or by his agent thereunto lawfully authorised by writing or by will.

It is clear from s. 53(1)(c) that any disposition *itself* must be in writing, and not merely evidenced by writing, and so immediately we can see a different position at work from that which applied to declarations of trust of land. What this means is that any purported disposition will be void (and not merely unenforceable) if the requirements of this section are not complied with. In terms of trying to identify a policy for this, we can see draw on the judgment of Lord Upjohn in *Vandervell v IRC* [1967] 2 AC 29. We shall see shortly that this is one of two key *Vandervell* cases that form the basis for this material on requirements for making valid dispositions of equitable interests.

According to Lord Upjohn, at 311:

> the object of the section [53], as was the object of the old Statute of Frauds, is to prevent hidden oral transactions in equitable interests in fraud of those truly entitled, and making it difficult, if not impossible, for the trustees to ascertain who are in truth his beneficiaries.

The strict nature of these provisions is designed to reflect the nature of beneficial interests. We have already encountered on a number of occasions suggestion that equitable interests in property are much less visible than legal ones, and are thus more vulnerable than them. So requiring that any movement of beneficial interests from one person to another is recorded in written documentation will help to ensure where these interests actually are, and who is holding them are clear.

Section 53(1)(c) of the Law of Property Act 1925, dispositions, and litigation

As we examine the key litigation—including two *Vandervell* cases—it becomes clear that much of this concerns the meaning of the term 'disposition' in the light of the s. 53(1)(c) requirement. From this, it becomes clear that the meaning of 'disposition' has attracted a considerable amount of attention, and has resulted in a large number of parties being prepared to engage in lengthy and costly litigation over it.

As the cases reveal, two types of taxation have had very considerable significance in the litigation, thereby pointing to their importance for the creation of trusts in the pursuit of tax advantages. Although most of the cases date from the 1970s or earlier, many of us will, of course, recognize references to 'stamp duty'. This is the duty that is payable on drafting certain legal documents, including those that transfer ownership of property from one person to another. This is most commonly associated with sales of real property—what is currently termed 'Stamp Duty and Land Tax', or SDLT). But as HMRC information relating to what is now called 'Stamp Duty Reserve Tax' (SDRT) explains, this tax is incurred on paperless transactions involving the purchase of shares or a number of interests or options relating to shares. References to 'stamp duty' in the older cases manifest in ones to fixed or nominal 'stamp' applicable to all documents under seal, regardless of value and also duty *ad valorem*, attached to the actual value of the property being transferred. These older cases also reference so-called 'surtax', a type of income tax directed at very high-earning people.

'Disposition of equitable interest': certainty in transactions involving relocations of beneficial interest and their status

Determining exactly what is and amounts to a disposition of an equitable interest does, of course, make a crucial difference in terms of requirements for validity. We already know that declarations of trust are treated differently as far as formality affects validity, and we also have some understanding from Lord Upjohn in *Vandervell* of why it is so important for understanding dispositions of existing equitable interests in property that they will actually be void if made in contravention of this and not simply unenforceable. What we need to think about now is what we actually mean by a 'disposition', and how we can see this meaning being determined by key litigation in this sphere.

In terms of ascertaining what exactly is treated as a disposition, which requires writing in order to be valid, we can get closer to understanding this by having some sense of what is *not* treated as a disposition by law. This can be illustrated by reference to key dealings involving equitable interests in trust property.

- *Vandervell No. 2 [1974] Ch 269 is authority that the extinguishment of a trust is not required to be in writing.* We shall consider *Vandervell No. 2* shortly, and in this situation s. 53(1)(c) has no application. By way of clarification, when we speak of 'extinguishment' of a trust, this refers to situations in which there is a trust in existence, and in which subsequent dealings will result in beneficial and legal interests becoming merged by coming into the hands of the same person.

- *Where there is a disclaim of a beneficial interest under a trust, s. 53(1)(c) has no application.* A refusal to accept any beneficial interest under a trust is said to result in this interest being disclaimed. In terms of how this is treated by law in the light of s. 53(1)(c), *Re Paradise Motor Co* [1968] 1 WLR 1125 is authority that disclaiming beneficial interest operates by way of avoidance and that, because the person concerned 'avoids' obtaining equitable interest in this way, he does not actually acquire anything he needs to dispose of. This means that s. 53(1)(c) has no application.

- *Release or surrender of beneficial interests* should *require application of s. 53(1) (c).* Surrender occurs when a beneficiary indicates that he no longer wishes to benefit under the trust, and thereby is said to 'surrender' his interest under it. Based on what has been said so far about s. 53(1)(c) and its policy, it *should* apply here because the beneficiary's beneficial interest is being relocated away from him, but there is actually no direct authority on this point. In contrast, the position of transactions that involve transfers or assignments of equitable interests *do* appear to be within the scope of disposition, and thus must be in writing in order to be valid. This can be seen from the litigation that has arisen in the light of establishing what is meant by a disposition.

4.5 Litigation arising from the meaning of 'disposition': *Grey* v *IRC*

Grey v *IRC* [1960] AC 1 considered whether 'disposition' should be interpreted in a broad or a narrow manner in order for the application (or otherwise) of s. 53(1)(c) to be ascertained. This involved construing the meaning of 'disposition' under s 53, in light of the reach of its predecessor, s. 9 of the Statute of Frauds 1677. The result of *Grey* is that the term 'disposition' was to be given its natural meaning, and thus would appear to cover any transaction in which a beneficiary's beneficial entitlement under a trust would be altered in any way.

The litigation in *Grey* arose from the way in which Grey initially transferred some shares owned by him into the names of two trustees on trust for himself. Sometime later, he orally declared that they should hold these on trust for grandchildren. The trustees then executed a confirmatory transfer of the shares into the settlement for the children. The transaction was an 'avoidance' device, which would succeed or fail as follows: if the transfer of the beneficial interest had actually occurred upon the written declaration, then *ad valorem* duty *was* payable; if the oral direction had transferred the equitable interest in the shares, then *ad valorem* duty was *not* payable and the transfer was merely confirmatory.

Grey is authority that a transfer of an equitable interest in property to another comes within the ambit of a disposition, and thus must be in writing in order to be valid. Hence the transfer of the equitable interests from Grey for the benefit of his grandchildren required writing to make an effective transfer of the beneficial interests. Thus his oral declaration was ineffective under s. 53(1)(c) and *ad valorem* duty was payable on the written transfer. Lord Radcliffe explained his view that s. 53 merely consolidated the earlier Statute of Frauds:

> if there is nothing more in this appeal than the short question whether the oral direction that Mr. Hunter gave to his trustees on February 18, 1955, amounted in any ordinary sense of the words to a 'disposition of an equitable interest or trust subsisting at the time of the disposition', I do not feel any doubt as to my answer ... Where opinions have differed is on the point whether his direction was a 'disposition' within the meaning of section 53 (1) (c) of the Law of Property Act 1925, the argument for giving it a more restricted meaning in that context being that is to be construed as no more than a consolidation of three sections of the Statute of Frauds, sections 3, 7 and 9. So treated, 'disposition', it is said, is merely the equivalent of the former words of section 9, 'grants and assignments' ... I am entirely in agreement, that a consolidating Act is not to be read as effecting changes in the existing law unless the words it employs are too clear in their effect to admit of any other construction ... But, in my opinion, it is impossible to regard section 53 of the Law of Property Act 1925 as a consolidating enactment in this sense.
>
> (*Grey* v *IRC* [1960] AC 1, *per* Lord Radcliffe at 16)

4.6 Formalities, dispositions, and taxation: the *Vandervell* litigation

As suggested, there are two *Vandervell* cases, part of a plethora of litigation arising from an elaborate avoidance scheme. Although this text quite consciously focuses on being a commentary on the law of trusts rather than a collection of stories of those who settle properly on trust, it is, of course, the case that some narrative background is often important for illustrating the legal significance of their settlements. The story of Guy Anthony ('Tony') Vandervell is told in more detail than is strictly necessary for this, on account of his very high profile and his larger-than-life persona. Significantly, the story of Tony Vandervell's settlements of property on trust can tell an important story of its own, which is very helpful for contextualizing our study of trusts. This relates to the length to which those who have accumulated wealth will go in order to preserve it in their dealings with property—and appreciating this comes from understanding just how important trusts are for tax avoidance schemes.

Tony Vandervell was a prominent English inventor, industrialist, and philanthropist, who was also a very famous motor racing financier and founder of the Vanwall Formula One (F1) racing team, which enjoyed a string of successes in the late 1950s and won the Constructors' Championship in 1958. This stemmed from a passion for racing cars and motorcycles in his youth; after World War II, he concentrated on developing racing cars using his industrial kudos and acumen, which arose from the way in which he made his personal fortune, in that his company—Vandervell Products—manufactured revolutionary closed-cage thin-walled bearings. His development of racing cars, altered by his mechanics using thin-walled bearing technology, started when he customized a Ferrari 125; this was then used as research by British Racing Motors (BRM), a British F1 racing team that raced from 1950 to 1977, and which won seventeen Grand Prix races during this period and in 1962 won the Constructors' Title. Vandervell even used this as an opportunity to provide Enzo Ferrari himself with a detailed critique of the Ferrari 125. After winning the Constructors' Championship in 1958 and after years of living life 'in the fast lane' in various ways, Vandervell retired to a more sedate lifestyle. His high-profile pursuits had made him a very wealthy man and this spawned a number of settlements of his property. Some of these settlements have become very high-profile in their own right—certainly amongst trusts lawyers! It is also significant for us that he died in 1967.

Like any ardent and prudent tax planner, Tony Vandervell made settlements in favour of family members, and shortly we will look at the legal significance of one settlement made in favour of his children. The first settlement that is significant for us is the gift of £150,000 that he wished to make to the Royal College of Surgeons (RCS) to endow a chair of pharmacology. Vandervell was equitable owner of a substantial number of shares in Vandervell Products Ltd, a private limited liability company that he controlled and which had produced the Vanwall racing car that won the Constructors' Championship in 1958. The legal interest in Vandervell's shares was held by a bank as nominee (as explained in the introduction in Chapter 2 to the significance of shares and shareholdings in the creation of trusts).

To endow the chair, Vandervell arranged with the bank, orally (in order to avoid paying stamp duty on any written document), for both legal and equitable interests in these shares to be transferred to the RCS. It was not Vandervell's intention that the College should receive the shares absolutely, with all of the implications that would have had for control of Vandervell Products Ltd; this was not, of course, what the RCS would have wanted either. Instead, the intention was that the RCS would receive dividends on the shares, which would be capable of generating the £150,000 for the chair, and because the RCS was a charity it would not be paying tax on the property (on which see further Chapters 10, 11, and 12).

Because it was the financial value of the shares that was being given to the RCS, rather than the corporate voice and control that was also embodied in the shares, Vandervell retained an option to repurchase the shares themselves for a nominal amount (£5,000). However, he did not retain this in his own name, because doing so would have left him liable to pay surtax on the dividends. Instead, he set up a trustee company, Vandervell Trustees Ltd, to which the option was granted. More is said about trustee companies in Chapter 14, but for now it is significant that the option was granted to the company rather than to Vandervell personally, and that this was an attempt by Vandervell himself to avoid incurring surtax liability.

The RCS actually received some £266,000 by means of this avoidance device, and so was clearly much benefited by it. However, things were more complicated for Vandervell: at this stage, the legal interest in the shares had been transferred to the RCS, while Vandervell Trustees Ltd had the legal interest in the option. If the equitable interest in either remained in Vandervell himself, however, he would be liable to surtax, on the basis of s. 415 of the Income Tax Act 1952. Clearly, to avoid this outcome, Vandervell had to show that he had divested himself of the entire benefit of the shares.

Although the particular income tax provision at issue in *Vandervell* has been long since replaced, the principle of using trusts—and in particular charities—as a means of avoiding taxation still survive. The principle is essentially that liability to income tax can be minimized by ensuring that the income is received by those whose taxation liability is least. The so-called 'granny trust', under which the income is paid to infant grandchildren, is a good example of this principle. Further examples of the use of the trust to avoid taxation are considered in Chapter 15.

In *Vandervell* itself, as a high earner, Mr Vandervell's personal liability to income tax was very high (note that surtax was being claimed at well over the marginal rates that would have been applicable for standard-rate taxpayers). As a charity, however, the RCS paid no income tax at all. It was important to show, therefore, that it was the charity and not Vandervell himself who was entitled to the income from the shares. The same principle applies today when trusts are being used as a device to save income tax: the settlor must ensure that he divests himself effectively of all interest in the trust property, since even the most tenuous connection with the trust may result in the income being deemed to be that of the settlor (see Figure 4.1).

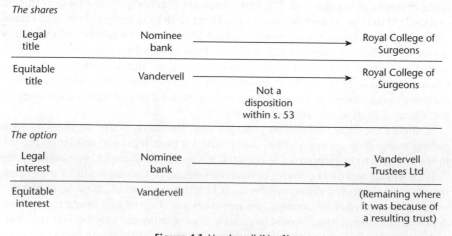

Figure 4.1 Vandervell (No. 1).

That was essentially the issue in *Vandervell* itself, as we shall see by considering Vandervell's position in relation to the shares and also the option in turn. There are also two phases of the *Vandervell* litigation in which we can see initial rulings on Vandervell's position in relation to the shares and the option, and also his subsequent position in relation to both of them considered by the Court of Appeal in the context of Vandervell potentially incurring further surtax liability.

In *Vandervell v IRC* [1967] 2 AC 29 ('*Vandervell No. 1*'), the meaning of 'disposition' arose in the context that, in order to avoid liability for surtax, Vandervell had to establish that he had divested himself of the entire equitable interest in both the shares and the option.

In respect of the shares, the Inland Revenue had argued that the oral instruction from Vandervell was ineffective because it was a disposition requiring writing, adjudicating that s. 53(1)(c) applied. The House of Lords ruled that the section had no application where a beneficial owner solely entitled instructs his nominee (who thus holds the legal title as bare trustee) with regard to the equitable and legal interests in the property. Thus Vandervell had successfully divested himself of equitable (and indeed all) interest in the shares, and therefore Vandervell would incur no liability for surtax. In respect of the option, the House of Lords ruled that Vandervell had not successfully divested himself of his equitable interest in the option. Whilst legal interest was held by the trustee company, equitable interest could not simply hang in the air, and so Vandervell held it on resulting trust and thus was liable to surtax. An interesting aside is that *Re Rose* [1952] Ch 449 (from which the 'rule in *Re Rose*' derives, as will be discussed in Chapter 5) was approved because the transfer was effective as soon as Vandervell had performed his last act.

The next chapter in the *Vandervell* litigation arose in *Re Vandervell's Trusts No. 2* [1974] Ch 269, which concerned surtax liability and the location of beneficial interests. This can be seen in Figure 4.2.

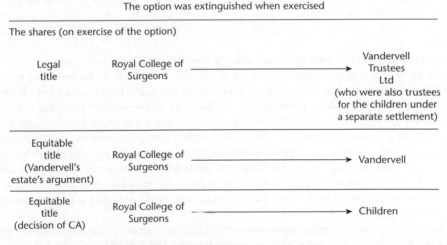

Figure 4.2 Vandervell (No. 2) (1961–1965).

Here, Vandervell's liability depended on the whereabouts of equitable interest in the shares when the option to repurchase had been exercised by the trustee company in 1961, using money from the children's trust. From 1961 to 1965, all of the dividends were applied by the trust company to the children's trust. It was argued by the Inland Revenue that equitable interest was still vested in Vandervell, while the legal interest had moved from the RCS to the trustee company. Vandervell argued that equitable interest in the shares lay not with him, but with his children. However, Vandervell then died and his estate sought to claim the dividends for the period 1961–65 on the same basis as the Revenue sought to assess Vandervell's liability in relation to surtax— namely, that Vandervell had not divested his beneficial interest, because there was no written transfer until 1965.

In the Court of Appeal, it was found that equitable interest in the option to repurchase the shares was held to have been destroyed when it was exercised, and that the *extinguishment* of Vandervell's interest was found not to be a disposition within the meaning of s. 53 and so did not require writing to be valid. In respect of equitable interest in the shares themselves, the children were found to be owners of the beneficial interest of the repurchased shares, under trusts that were precise and clearly defined. In terms of analysing the extinguishments of earlier trusts and the creation of new ones, the termination of a resulting trust did not amount to a disposition for the purposes of s. 53 and thus no writing was required, whilst the creation of a new trust in favour of the children was a trust of personalty (rather than land), which required no formality for its creation. As Lord Denning explained at 320:

> A resulting trust for the settlor is born and dies without writing at all. It comes into existence whenever there is a gap in the beneficial ownership. It ceases to exist whenever that gap is filled by someone becoming beneficially entitled. As soon as the gap is filled by the creation or declaration of a valid trust, the resulting trust comes to an end. In this case, before the option was exercised, there was a gap in the beneficial ownership. So, there was a resulting trust for Mr Vandervell. But, as soon as the option was exercised and the shares registered in the trustee's name, there was created a valid trust of the shares in favour of the children's settlement. Not being a trust of land, it could be created without any writing.

Lord Denning's ruling and the issues arising from this analysis

Lord Denning analysed the position as being a termination of the resulting trust of the option in favour of Vandervell and a fresh declaration of trust of the shares in favour of the children (presumably on the part of the trustee company). Lord Denning thought that, as to the first part, there was no writing requirement for terminating a resulting trust and, because the trust being declared in the children's favour did not relate to land, there was no writing requirement for this either. So, as far as the formality aspects of the *Vandervell* decisions are concerned, at no stage did s. 53 operate to defeat a transaction in either case, and because none of the transactions could have been kept secret from the trustees, this reasoning is in accordance with the policy of s. 53.

However, there are some difficulties with this analysis and a number of questions arising from it. For example, it is not clear where we can find the requisite intention to create the trust for children that is required for satisfying certainty of intention (as considered in Chapter 3), and it seems instead that the parties had assumed their interest in the property. We also need to consider whether it was really the case that Vandervell had no interest at all in the shares and that he had only an interest in the option. For Vandervell to be able to avoid the outcome in *Grey*, the declaration of the trusts in favour of the children had to have occurred before the option was exercised; otherwise, a resulting trust of the beneficial interest to Vandervell would occur.

4.7 *Oughtred* v *IRC*: disposition and specifically enforceable oral contracts for transferring subsisting equitable interests

Oughtred v *IRC* [1960] AC 206 is an important House of Lords decision that belongs to this discussion of s. 53, but it is also quite different from *Grey* and *Vandervell* in a number of respects. This is because it is almost entirely a pure taxation case, rather than one that illustrates any particular policy rationale for formality requirements.

The formalities interest from this case comes from the general position that contracts for the sale of personalty do not require writing and that, in cases in which the equitable remedy of specific performance is available, equity recognizes that the buyer has an interest as soon as the contract is made. Here, a possible route around s. 53 (and therefore stamp duty) might therefore be to have an oral contract for the sale of the property concerned, followed later by a formal transfer. The argument is that the oral contract, not the written transfer, conveys the equitable title. The logic of such an argument is that the subsequent formal transfer merely conveys the bare legal title, which is worth hardly anything for the purposes of *ad valorem* stamp duty.

This was the essence of the scheme in *Oughtred* v *IRC*, in which, once again, the property was shares. Mrs Oughtred owned 72,700 shares in William Jackson and Son Ltd absolutely. In a separate holding, 200,000 shares in the same company were held on trust for Mrs Oughtred for life, and then for her son Peter absolutely. The parties orally agreed to exchange their interests: Mrs Oughtred would obtain Peter's reversionary interest when he would obtain outright ownership of the shares (meaning that Mrs Oughtred would then have the 200,000 shares as outright owner); in exchange, Peter would obtain Mrs Oughtred's 72,700 shares, which would avoid his having to pay estate duty on them following her death. The contract was later performed, with the trustees of the 200,000 shares transferring legal title to them to Mrs Oughtred and Mrs Oughtred transferring her 72,000 shares to her son (actually to his nominees, which Chapter 2 explains is common in dealings with shares and why), with consideration of 10 shillings being provided for both transfers.

The Inland Revenue claimed stamp duty on the transfer of the reversionary interest in the 200,000 shares, the actual transfer of which involved writing, on the basis that it was a 'conveyance of sale'. Oughtred's argument was that the equitable interest was transferred on the oral contract for sale, and that the later writing transferred only the bare legal title, and so there was no value being transferred in this latter document and thus no stamp duty payable on it. The logic behind Oughtred's argument—and indeed behind the entire avoidance scheme—was that, until legal title could be passed in the respective transfers, both parties were bound by obligations of conscience to carry out the agreement. This brought into being a constructive trust, which is exempt from s. 53(1) requirements on account of s. 53(2), and thus the transfer would be valid without any written instrument that would incur *ad valorem* stamp duty.

The argument was rejected by the House of Lords, but it was a majority decision with Viscount Radcliffe and Lord Cohen dissenting. The essence of the majority view was that, although equity in appropriate circumstances can grant specific performance of a contract for the sale of shares (at any rate, in a private company, in which the shares are unique, but not in a public company, in which equivalent shares are freely available on the stock market) and although, in that case, a constructive trust arises immediately in favour of the purchaser (on principles that are explained in Chapter 6), the buyer does not have a full beneficial interest until the formal transfer. The situation was regarded by the House of Lords as being analogous to a sale of land, where the deed of conveyance is the effective instrument of transfer (and so liable to stamp duty).

The minority view, on the other hand, was that the purchaser obtained a full beneficial interest immediately. By way of clarification, conveyancing practice has always seen stamp duty fall payable on transfer, whilst beneficial interest passes on exchange of contract. Lord Jenkins' judgment explains the position of the majority and explains as follows in relation to shares in a private company:

> Under the contract, the purchaser is, no doubt, entitled in equity as between himself and the vendor to the beneficial interest in the shares, and (subject to due payment of the purchase consideration) to call for a transfer of them from the vendor as trustee ... But it is only on the execution of the actual transfer that he becomes entitled to be registered as a member, to attend and vote at meetings, to effect transfers on the register, or to receive dividends otherwise than through the vendor as his trustee.
>
> (*Oughtred* v *IRC* [1960] AC 206, *per* Lord Jenkins at 240)

The reasoning of the majority was followed by the Court of Appeal in *Neville* v *Wilson* [1997] Ch 144. On this reasoning, the purchaser will not have full beneficial interest until transfer has occurred, but the minority position is explained in Lord Radcliffe's dissenting judgment in *Oughtred*, at 228:

> There was no equity to the shares that could be asserted against her, and it was open to her, if she so wished, to let the matter rest without calling for a written assignment, from her son ... it follows that, in my view, this transfer cannot be treated as a conveyance of the son's equitable reversion at all.

Jerome v *Kelly* [2004] UKHL 25, which concerned liability for capital gains tax (CGT), can also be found in this discussion of the interplay of contract and beneficial ownership, clustering around contracts for land being specifically enforceable ahead of completion. Like many of these cases, *Jerome* had complicated facts, but in essence concerned CGT liability attaching to a contract for land with considerable development potential. Although the contract had a date for completion, but also scope for early completion and for the prospective purchaser to rescind in the event of particular planning permission complications, it was subsequently completed. Ordinarily, Jerome would have incurred substantial CGT at this point, but in the intervening period beneficial ownership of the land had changed, having been assigned from Jerome. The House of Lords found in favour of the taxpayer, with Lord Walker insisting that it would be 'wrong to treat an uncompleted contract for the sale of land as equivalent to an immediate, irrevocable declaration of trust (or assignment of beneficial interest) in the land. Neither the seller nor the buyer has unqualified beneficial ownership'.

4.7.1 **From *Oughtred* to some points of summary for formality requirements**

As stressed at the outset, *Oughtred* is a taxation case, albeit one that can enhance understanding of what formality is required for transfers that amount to dispositions of equitable interests. This closes our present discussion of formality focused on the formality requirements that we find in the creation of trusts and those arising where a trust is actually operational. Whilst doing this, we have learned about why formality is important in principle in dealings with property generally and how this can be applied more specifically to trusts—both to their creation and in dealings with equitable interests in trust property once a trust has been created. In respect of this latter point, we can now understand how important it is for the whereabouts of equitable interests in property to be clear, because generally these are less visible than legal ones, and we also know that ultimately they are less strong on account of being subject to the bona fide purchaser rule. This is why the writing requirement for dispositions of equitable interests has developed and is strictly enforced. And, on this latter matter, material located on the Online Resource Centre considers further the origins of writing requirements for trusts and assignments of benefits under existing trusts in light of the policy of preventing the perpetration of fraud. From looking at *Oughtred* following our discussion of *Grey* and *Vandervell*, we now have a better appreciation of the instrumental use of trusts in avoidance schemes—and also of the length to which those who have accumulated wealth will go in order to avoid paying tax. Indeed, in *Jerome*, Lord Hoffmann remarked that most tax legislation 'is concerned with economic reality and efficiency of collection'. There is not the scope for this text to consider the normative questions arising from tax avoidance, but quite clearly there are distributive justice issues arising from enabling the most wealthy in society to contribute a much smaller proportion of what they have to public funds than is expected from those who have accumulated much less.

But, returning once more to formality, in the discussion of constituting trusts that follows, it becomes clear that formality requirements continue to be very significant in the context of creating a valid trust.

4.8 Epilogue to formality: gifts that are made *donatio mortis causa* and the rule in *Strong* v *Bird*

There are now very brief accounts of two doctrines that have been much more important historically than they are today, and which do not obviously belong in a better place than this chapter on formality requirements, even though they do not obviously belong here either, because they concern making gifts rather than creating trusts. So they have been placed here because they are situations in which normal transfer formality requirements applicable to gifts do not apply, and in which instead equity will recognize that property has a new owner on account of the circumstances.

A gift made *donatio mortis causa* (broadly meaning 'gift by reason of death') is one that is literally made in contemplation of death, and is also conditional upon the owner of property actually dying for an intended recipient to be entitled to it. It is unlike an ordinary gift because the recipient's title to the property does not come into existence until the death of the donor and so, until that time, it can be revoked. Equally, it is not a testamentary gift taking effect under a properly attested will, and actually it can be made to a donee even in circumstances under which a formal will appears to contradict the *donatio mortis causa*. Serious illness is a common context in which such gifts arise: an owner of property will tell someone that he is to have some (or something) of the owner's property should he die. In these circumstances, the potential recipient will have custody of the property, but this will not become 'his' unless and until its owner dies. Upon death, equity regards the recipient's title to the property as perfected, notwithstanding that it is unlikely that formality will have been complied with. And this means that the perfected conditional gift made *donatio mortis causa* will override any alternative provision made for that property in a valid will.

Historically, *donationes mortis causa* (the plural) reflected an owner of property's desire to keep the existence of a mistress and any children born outside wedlock secret from his legitimate family, and his reluctance thus to make provision for her either *inter vivos* or under a will. However, the *donatio mortis causa* has more general application for situations in which the prospect of imminent death does not permit 'proper' arrangements concerning property to be made.

What needs to happen for equity to recognize a gift made donatio mortis causa?

Because gifts made *donatio mortis causa* are effectively gifts that are made without proper formality, stringent conditions have to be satisfied, given that the very purpose of formality is to protect property from unintended transactions. The necessary conditions for a *donatio mortis causa* to be upheld were set out by Farwell J in *Re Craven's Estate* [1937] Ch 423. And ahead of the three specific requirements, there must, of course, be an intention to give the property and not simply to secure it: there is no *donatio mortis causa* if there is a desire simply for another to 'look after' the property.

The three specific conditions that must be satisfied are as follows.

1. Property must be handed over in contemplation of a real possibility of death, and so in anticipation of a clear hazard to the owner's life. This is usually a serious illness, but it could also be a highly hazardous activity such as motor racing; it must be more than exposure to everyday risks such as air travel.

2. The gift must be conditional upon death occurring, and otherwise revocable, meaning that the donor must intend to keep the property if he survives.

3. The donor must have effectively parted with dominion (or autonomy, or control) over the property concerned. This is most obviously achieved through property actually being handed over, but it can also be so through transferring the means of access to the property, such as giving the recipient the key to the bank deposit box in which the property is lodged. The test is whether the donor has put it out of his power between the dates of gift and death to alter the subject matter of gift and substitute other property for it, as illustrated in *Re Lillingston* [1952] 2 All ER 184 and *Woodard v Woodard* [1995] 3 All ER 980 (in which the Court of Appeal inferred a *donatio mortis causa* of a car from the handing over of its keys, where the donor had also said: 'You can keep the keys—I won't be driving it any more').

The requirements of donatio mortis causa illustrated through key cases

It is also possible to transfer property that is not capable of physical delivery by handing over indicia of title, such as a a bank savings book or (presumably) a bill of lading covering a consignment of cargo aboard a ship, with the test being whether handing over the document 'amounted to a transfer' by virtue of this conveying to the recipient entitlement to the property.

Long after most students of the law of trusts must have thought that *donatio mortis causa* cases were ancient history, a *donatio mortis causa* was successfully argued before the Court of Appeal in *Sen v Headley* [1991] Ch 425. It had long been thought that it was impossible to have a *donatio mortis causa* of land, because the third of Farwell J's conditions cannot be satisfied, even by delivery of the title deeds. Here, an elderly man close to death gave the claimant the keys to a box containing the title deeds to his house, saying: 'The house is yours, Margaret. You have the keys. They are in your bag. The deeds are in the steel box.' Title to the house was unregistered and it appeared that the deceased had lived with the claimant as if married for around thirty years. Following his death, this

gift was challenged by his next of kin, and while there were no difficulties for the claimant with Farwell J's first two criteria, Mummery J held at first instance—*Sen* v *Headley*
[1990] Ch 728—that the deceased had not parted with dominion and it was not possible
to make a *donatio mortis causa* for land. There was no transfer of title deed executed within
the deceased's lifetime and any declaration of trust would require writing in order to be
enforceable, and Mummery J's view was that the doctrine of *donatio mortis causa* was
anomalous with the judicial caution that it should encourage, and its use should not be
permitted for, attempts to avoid the Wills Act formalities (on which, see Chapter 9) or the
perfection of an imperfect *inter vivos* gift. Mummery J's view was clearly the orthodox
one: that it was not possible to create a *donatio mortis causa* for land.

This finding was reversed in the Court of Appeal, by analogy with extensions of the
doctrine in previous cases. In *Snellgrove* v *Bailey* [1744] 3 Atk 213, the doctrine had been
applied to a gift of money secured by a bond, by delivery of the bond; in *Duffield* v *Elwes*
(1827) 1 Bli (NS) 497, the House of Lords had applied the doctrine to a gift of money
secured by a mortgage of land, by delivery of the mortgage deed. In each case, transfer of
indicia of title was all that was required, but one problem with this reasoning was that,
in *Duffield* v *Elwes*, Lord Eldon thought that the doctrine would not apply to a gift of land
by delivery of the title deeds. The Court of Appeal accepted that the doctrine was itself
anomalous, but stated that this did not justify creating anomalous exceptions to the
admittedly anomalous doctrine. The only reason why, with unregistered land, transfer
of the title deeds did not transfer title to the property was because of a formality statute.
All *donationes mortis causa* avoid formality provisions—usually ones pertaining to wills.
There was no reason why the formality provisions relating to land should be regarded
as presenting any greater obstacle than any other formality provisions, and no reason
why this case should be treated differently from other gifts made *donatio mortis causa*
that had been upheld.

It does not necessarily follow that this will necessarily work with all species of property. For example, there are difficulties with shares in private companies, which cannot
be physically transferred, and because registration of a new owner may be refused, as
we will find out in Chapter 5. So a situation involving shares would not be regarded as
directly analogous to land. However, where the subject matter is in principle capable of
being subject to such an arrangement, *Wilkes* v *Allington* [1931] 2 Ch 104 appears to be
authority that the gift is valid even if the donor dies sooner than expected and even if
from a different cause. The donor was suffering from an incurable disease and made the
gift knowing that he had not long to live; when he then died even earlier than expected
of pneumonia, the gift was held to be valid. Whether the same principle would apply
even if the death were completely different from the donor's expectation, for example
if he actually dies of food poisoning, is less clear.

4.9 The rule in *Strong* v *Bird*

The rule in *Strong* v *Bird* (1874) LR 18 Eq 315 is actually a very narrow doctrine that does
not concern us greatly, but which does provide a further exception (along with the 'last
act' doctrine and gifts made *donatio mortis causa*) to the principle that 'equity will not
assist a volunteer' (and it is also an example of the presumption that equitable title follows legal title when property is transferred from one person to another, which we will
consider in Chapter 6).

The rule in *Strong* v *Bird* can be invoked where a person (A) hands to another (B) his
property—say, share certificates—but fails to procure the transfer and registration of

(B) as the new owner, and then dies appointing this person (B) as his executor, but makes someone completely different (C) legatee of all of his personal property.

Equity will treat A's earlier gift to B as perfected, with A's property now vested in B as his executor, which will override C's claim to the property. The same principle operates if B owes A money, but A makes no effort to collect his debt and appoints B his executor: these were the facts of *Strong* v *Bird* itself. The appointment is, as it were, a conclusive release of the debt. But it must be clear that there was an intention to make the gift or to release the debt, and that this intention continued until death. In this case, the appointment of a debtor as executor for his creditor's estate has the effect of extinguishing the debt at common law because it is impossible for an executor to sue himself. In *Strong* v *Bird* itself, the debtor was the stepson of the deceased creditor and, after making some repayments to her as agreed, the deceased verbally released him from the remainder of his debt. This was not an effective release at law, though, and the litigation arose when her next of kin sought to enforce his repayment of that which remained outstanding. *Strong* v *Bird* is authority that, in such circumstances, equity will acquiesce with the common law position and accept that the debt should not be repaid, subject to the requirements relating to intention.

In *Strong* v *Bird*, the intention was to release the debt, but, as we saw at the outset, it can also apply to intention to make a gift. So, in *Re Stewart* [1908] 2 Ch 251, Neville J applied the same principle to perfect an imperfect *inter vivos* gift of bonds by appointment of the intended donee as executor. Equity will not interfere with the common law transfer of title, but it does require an attempt to make an immediate *inter vivos* gift of specific property, a continuing intent to make the gift until death, and the vesting of legal title in the donee. We can see the same idea at work given that the rule is also regarded as a mechanism for constituting a trust. There is also authority that *Strong* v *Bird* applies in situations in which a deceased person's death leads to the appointment of an administrator rather than an executor (on principles explained in Chapter 2). This was the view of Farwell J in *Re James* [1935] Ch 449, in which a housekeeper had herself appointed one of two administratrices of the testator's estate. But this was questioned in *Re Gonin* [1979] Ch 16, which arose when the claimant alleged that her parents had verbally agreed that the parental home and its contents should become hers upon their death, and this was in return for her returning home from being called away during World War II to look after them. In *Gonin*, the father had died intestate in 1957 and, following the death of her mother in 1968, the claimant took out letters of administration to her estate, and began an action to determine whether she was entitled, as administratrix, to vest the freehold in the property in herself. She claimed both land and contents (furniture) under the rule in *Strong* v *Bird*, on the basis that the claimant's mother intended to give the claimant the house on her death and the gift was perfected by the claimant taking out letters of administration. Walton J took the view that the appointment of an administrator was quite different from the appointment of an executor, since it is not a voluntary act of the deceased, but of the law. It was also often a matter of pure chance which of many persons entitled to a grant of letters of administration actually took them out:

> Why, then, should any special tenderness be shown to a person so selected by law and not the will of the testator, and often indifferently selected among many with an equal claim? It would seem an astonishing doctrine of equity that if the person who wishes to take the benefit of the rule in *Strong* v *Bird* manages to be the person to obtain a grant then he will be able to do so, but if a person equally entitled manages to obtain a prior grant, then he will not be able to do so.
>
> (*Re Gonin* [1979] Ch 16, *per* Walton J at 315)

Walton J did not actually need to decide whether the earlier authority was correct, because it was found that even if *Strong* v *Bird* applied to administrators, there was no evidence of a continuing intention on the part of the claimant's mother to give the house to the claimant. There is, however, academic support for *Re James* from Kodilinye [1982] Conv 14. Also, *Re James* was applied in *Re Ralli's WT* [1964] Ch 288, but the situation there was different because no intention at all was needed on the part of the transferor.

Revision Box

1. Using the chapter materials and further discussion on the Online Resource Centre, explain what is meant by 'transfer formality' and ensure that you:
   - understand why any transaction involving a transfer of title from one person to another will require transfer formality;
   - are able to provide examples of why and how transfer formality required will depend on the nature of the property;
   - understand how, in the context of trust creation, transfer formality can be linked to the 'less visible' nature of equitable interests in property;
   - understand when transfer formality will arise in express trust creation and when it will not; and
   - understand how requiring transfer formality in trust creation can be seen to protect the interests of each of the 'trust actors' identifiable in an express trust arrangement.
2. Explain what is meant by 'declaration formality' and, using cases and statutory materials as appropriate, where this is encountered in express trust creation.
3. Using cases and statutory materials as reference points, ensure that you understand the way in which the courts have approached 'dispositions' in the context of formality, and what this reveals about how and why express trusts are created.

FURTHER READING

Garton (2003) 'The role of the trust mechanism in the rule in *Re Rose*' 67 Conveyancer 364.

Halliwell (2003) 'Perfecting imperfect gifts and trusts: have we reached the end of the Chancellor's foot?' 67 Conveyancer 192.

Kodilinye (1982) 'A fresh look at the rule in *Strong* v *Bird*' 46 Conveyancer 14

Lowrie and Todd (1998) '*Re Rose* revisited' 57 Cambridge Law Journal 46.

Millett (1985) 'The *Quistclose* trust: who can enforce it?' 101 Law Quarterly Review 269.

Tham (2006) 'Careless share giving' 70 Conveyancer 411.

online resource centre For summaries of a selection of these articles, please visit <http://www.oxfordtextbooks. co.uk/orc/wilson_trusts11e/>

5

The constitution requirement
for a valid trust

As we progress through examining the requirements of a valid trust, the constitution requirement is that, for a private express trust to be valid, the person(s) intended to act as trustee(s) under the arrangement must acquire legal title to it. A trust cannot be valid without this happening, and thus if an attempt is made to ensure that trustees do acquire legal title to property and this fails, no trust can be created. But in terms of appreciating what is required to satisfy the constitution requirement, and why it might be a requirement at all, we need to return briefly to how Chapter 1, and then Chapter 2, started to explain the nature of the trust by looking at it alongside and against different ways in which an owner of property could use it to provide benefits for others. In Chapter 2, this became concentrated on the gift, because both devices deliver to others benefits of property that are gratuitous and also permanent. We can see this similarity in objective and purpose from the way in which *Milroy* v *Lord* (1862) 4 De GF & J 264 identifies the choice that an owner of property can make when seeking to use his property gratuitously to benefit others. But we can also see that they are different from the way in which they are explained as alternative ways for an owner of property to achieve benefits for others:

> He may of course do this by actually transferring the property to the persons for whom he intends to provide, and the provision will then be effectual, and it will be equally effectual if he transfers the property to a trustee for the purposes of the settlement, or declares that he himself holds it on trust for those purposes.
>
> (*Milroy* v *Lord* (1862) 4 De GF & J 264, *per* Turner LJ at 274)

Indeed, we do already have an understanding that there is a fundamental difference between the trust and the gift. We know from Chapter 1 that the gift is achieved by an outright transfer of ownership from the original owner to its intended recipient, and also that, when property is settled on trust, enjoyment for the latter is achieved through the simultaneous existence of two types of ownership of what becomes 'trust property'. This is the key to understanding the constitution requirement that attaches to valid trusts.

When we looked at certainty of intention, we understood that, when an owner of property is said to have 'certainty of intention' to create a trust, this means that he does not only intend to confer benefits of property, but also to achieve this through the separation of ownership of property into constituent equitable and legal titles. This will enable the beneficiary to enjoy the property without having any responsibility for making this happen, because the responsibility for making this happen is that of the trustee. This is the significance of the conscience requirement that underpins all trusts: that a person who is a trustee understands that he is responsible for the property, which he must use in furtherance of the beneficiary's interests under the trust.

The practical consequence of the conscience requirement is that equity will not permit a trustee to use trust property as his own, and we will learn more about this when we consider the duties to which those who are trustees fall subject, and how equity will react where trustees use trust property for personal gain (Chapter 13) and even where the result of an honest mistake by a trustee causes losses for a beneficiary (Chapters 16 and 17). What is significant here is the *raison d'être* of the constitution requirement. This is because, without the conscience requirement, it might be too easy for a trustee to use trust property as his own, which is precisely because he *does* hold legal title to the property, which means ostensibly that he is its owner. Appreciating why equity has developed the conscience requirement will in turn help us to understand the constitution requirement, because in many ways it is a reaction to it.

The constitution requirement demands that, for a trust to be a valid one, those who are to act as trustees must have legal title to the property. Given what has been said up to now about how equity must be able to prevent those who are trustees treating trust property as their own, perhaps we need to understand why a trustee is ever in the position in which he can appear to be an owner of property that is actually trust property. Is this not a very risky position for trust property, and especially for equitable owners of personal property, where there is no formality requirement even to provide evidence that the trust was ever created? Generally, equitable ownership of property— even where this is land—is much less readily apparent than legal ownership of it. So why do trustees ever have legal title to trust property, let alone that they *do have* legal title has developed into a *requirement* without which a trust cannot be valid?

Background to the significance of constituting a trust

The rationale for the constitution requirement reflects that the elemental feature of a trust—the achievement of enjoyment of property without any responsibility—is actually indicative of its own inherent weakness: that the trust arrangement is entirely dependent upon the utmost integrity of those who do have responsibility for ensuring this enjoyment for someone different. The reason for this is that it is actually possible to separate the responsibility for property from its enjoyment only by vesting legal title to the property in those who are trustees.

Trustees are responsible for ensuring that property settled is able to benefit those who are entitled to it, and this means managing property and dealing with it in ways that will ensure that it can be used to best effect. This will mean investing trust property, and ensuring that it is in the right place to generate appropriate returns. For many trustees, this will mean investment in equities, which requires them to keep a close eye on the markets to ensure that investments remain wise ones and to move assets around if necessary to achieve this. This will also commonly involve selling existing trust property in order to purchase new investments for the trust, precisely so that a beneficiary can enjoy the kind of benefits intended by the settlor. In short, a trustee is a custodian of trust property because, whilst he will not benefit from it, his responsibility for it is key to the beneficiary's entitlements under a trust.

This is because the law will recognize only dealings with property that are conducted by those who own it 'at law', and we know from the previous chapter that this is because the law seeks to protect property from transactions that are not intended by its owner. So a trustee must be able to purchase and transact with property *as its owner* if he is to achieve the desired benefits for a beneficiary. And in terms of how the law seeks to protect all parties who deal with property, equally those to whom trustees sell (trust) property will want to be confident that they are dealing with persons who are entitled to sell it and from whom they can acquire good title to it. If this does not happen, then settling property on trust will never be able to achieve its desired benefits. Equity will ensure that a trustee has only nominal ownership of the trust property and is never able to treat the property as his, but this is couched within the reality that the only way in which to achieve optimum benefits for the trust is for such a person to have legal title to the property. This is reflected in the language of a trustee being entrusted with trust property because he must have legal title to it. That a trustee must have legal title to trust property is why constituting a trust is a requirement for a valid trust.

5.1 Achieving effective constitution of a trust

So what actually is meant by 'constituting' a trust, and how is it achieved? We had some introduction to this in Chapter 1, which briefly alluded to constituting a trust as vesting trustees with legal title to the property. Essentially, constituting a trust involves ensuring that those who are intended to be trustees under an owner's settlement of property on trust will have legal title to it, because this is what they need to have in order to be custodians of the trust property. Where those who are intended to have custody of trust property do have legal title to it, the trust will be valid from this perspective (it might still fail if other validity requirements are not met) by virtue of being what is known as a 'fully constituted trust'.

Ordinarily, this will mean that legal title to the property must be transferred from its owner to the intended trustee, but we will discover that this is not the only way of achieving an effective constitution. In this ordinary way, what will typically happen is that a person who settles property on trust will decide who is to act as trustee and will make arrangements for the property to be conveyed to that person. In this way, constituting an express trust will be as conscious as actually deciding to settle property on trust. It is also possible for a trustee to acquire title to property that he is intended to hold as trustee, but for this to happen in a way that was different from the way in which the settlor envisaged it would happen. In this latter situation, constitution is said to be 'accidental', but *Re Ralli's WT* [1964] Ch 288 is authority that such accidental constitution is equally effective constitution as would have been the case had the trustee actually acquired title to the property in the precise way in which the settlor envisaged he would. As an illustration, *Re Ralli* concerned a covenant to settle property on trust (see the Online Resource Centre for more on this case) and, in this context, the rule in *Strong v Bird* (1874) LR 18 Eq 315 (which was considered in Chapter 4) is believed to be authority that transfer of legal title to a deceased person's executor who was also intended by him to act as a trustee under a settlement of property will have the effect of constituting the latter arrangement.

Accidental constitution under *Re Ralli* and *Strong v Bird* is very unusual, and this book considers instead what is more usual in the creation of trusts. To get a sense of what is usual, we need to look once again at *Milroy v Lord*. We already know that *Milroy* explains how the benefits of property that are permanent and gratuitous can be achieved in one of two ways—namely, by making a gift, or by settling property on trust. Before we think about what *Milroy* stands as authority for in this regard, we can get a sense of how trusts are normally constituted from looking at the best-known application of *Milroy v Lord*: the Court of Appeal's decision in *Re Rose, Rose v IRC* [1952] Ch 499. We encountered *Re Rose* briefly in explaining formality requirements for making gifts of property in Chapter 4, where it was also noted that this is a central case for understanding the effective constitution of a trust. This is because the 'transfer formality' principles attaching to both can be the same; in helping to illustrate this, *Rose* actually conveniently concerned an attempt to make a valid gift and also to create an express trust.

Re Rose, *and drawing out the significance of the constitution requirement and how it is achieved*

The litigation in *Rose* arose from the way in which the deceased's estate was potentially liable for estate duty on account of two transfers of shares that the deceased wished to make, which were executed by him in March 1943. One transfer was intended to take effect as an outright gift to his wife; another sought to make her trustee of the shares for the benefit of the couple's children. Rose executed the transfer by completing the required paperwork in March 1943, but title to the shares at law could not pass from Rose until the directors of the company concerned registered the transferee as the shares' new legal owner. Under the company's constitution, its directors had a veto over any proposed transfer, but in the event the transfer was registered by them in June 1943. Rose died in 1948, and it was argued by the Inland Revenue that estate duty was payable because his death had occurred within five years of the transfer. The case turned on the way in which this would be the case if the transfer were regarded as having taken place in June 1943, when title to the shares passed at law from Rose to his wife.

We shall explore what actually happened in *Rose* shortly, but here it illustrates a number of introductory points. First, although making gifts and creating trusts are alternative ways of creating gratuitous and permanent benefits from property, they do arise together more commonly than this language of alternative might suggest. Second, *Rose* provides us with a reminder of how much litigation surrounding the creation of trusts is driven by taxation considerations—and indeed, by the awareness of HM Revenue and Customs (HMRC), known as the Inland Revenue in the case, of the lengths to which those who own property can be prepared to go in order to avoid paying tax. Third, and most significantly, it provides a way into understanding the significance of *Milroy* v *Lord* for what amounts to effective constitution, by pointing to the way in which constitution of a trust is most commonly attempted.

Where an owner of property seeks to settle property on an express trust, he will most commonly choose a trustee at this point. This is what actually happened in *Milroy* v *Lord*, which involved the settlor executing documentation for the purpose of transferring shares to a trustee to be held on trust for the claimants. In turn, *Milroy* v *Lord* tells us what is required to achieve this, but at the same time it also tells us that there are two ways in which a constitution that is effective can be achieved. By focusing on *Milroy* in this way, and on the trust as an alternative mechanism from an outright transfer of the property, and moving it away from voluntary dealings with property more generally, we can see that Turner LJ sets out the way in which a trust can be successfully constituted in one of two ways:

> ... if he transfers the property to a trustee for the purposes of the settlement, or declares that he himself holds it on trust for those purposes; ... but, in order to render the settlement binding, one or other of these modes must ... be resorted to ...
>
> (*Milroy* v *Lord* (1862) 4 De GF & J 264, *per* Turner LJ at 274)

From this, we can see that there are two ways in which legal title to property *can be* given to, or become vested in, a trustee. And if we join this with the rest of Turner LJ's famous passage, we can start to understand what *must be* done to achieve this.

The starting point for this is appreciating that the accepted ways of validly constituting a trust can be summarized as:

- the settlor must have *done all in his power* to transfer legal title to the person intended to act as trustee; or
- the settlor must have *declared himself to be trustee* of the property.

Whichever of these methods is used, the process of constituting the trust is what transforms legal title from the ultimate property right into 'nominal' legal title, which is characterized by duty and responsibility. As we look at each one in turn, we will see that determining whether *Milroy* has been satisfied raises a distinct set of legal issues. In looking at each one in this way, we also find that different normative considerations arise concerning whether the approach actually adopted is the one that should be. So what must actually be done is now explained by Turner LJ in *Milroy* at 274:

> [I]n order to render a voluntary settlement valid and effectual, the settlor must have done everything which, according to the nature of the property ... was necessary to be done in order to transfer the property and render the settlement binding upon him. He may, of course, do this by actually transferring the property to the persons for whom he intends to provide ... and it will be equally effectual if he transfers property to a trustee for the purposes of the settlement, or declares that he himself holds it on trust ... but in order to render the settlement binding, one or other of these modes must ... be resorted to, for there is no equity in this court to prefect an imperfect gift.

Although we will see that the two mechanisms, or modes, of valid constitution under *Milroy* raise distinct issues, there is also a common thread that runs through them. This flows from what was said at the very outset of Chapter 4 in anticipation of the material here. The beginning of Chapter 4 suggested that, when we came to Chapter 5 on constituting trusts, it would become clear that very close relationships subsist between how a trust is successfully *constituted* and what is required by way of *formality* to achieve this. The time has now come to explore this by understanding how each of the *Milroy* approaches for achieving effective constitution of a trust is grounded in formality requirements.

Part I **Transferring legal title to a trustee: satisfying *Milroy*'s first limb**

Transferring legal title to a trustee is the first 'mode' referenced in Turner LJ's judgment, and it is probably so because it is the normal occurrence in the creation of express trusts and is actually what was attempted in *Milroy* itself. Here, the settlor attempted to constitute a trust by appointing a specified trustee, Samuel Lord, to hold the property on behalf of the claimant, Milroy. The settlor did not actually succeed in doing this, but this is what he attempted to do—in common with most settlors of express trusts. The reason why the attempted transfer of legal title to a specified trustee did not succeed was that the voluntary deed attempting to achieve this, which had been executed by the settlor, was actually incapable of transferring legal title on account of the formality that was required to transfer legal title to the shares. As we know from looking at this earlier—in Chapter 2, briefly, and then more closely in Chapter 4—this requires registration of the name of the new owner in the books of the company or, in this case, a bank.

Because what was required to transfer legal title from settlor to trustee had not been complied with, it was held in the Court of Appeal that no trust had been constituted and thus Samuel Lord never became trustee of the shares. All constitutions are designed to ensure that those who are trustees hold legal title to trust property, and in this type of constitution this requires that legal title leaves the owner-cum-settlor and moves to someone else—namely, the person who is intended to carry out the trust. Because this will involve a transfer of legal title from one person to another, we can conclude from this that this type of constitution requires the satisfaction of transfer formality requirements.

Milroy's first mode of constitution: constitution governed by transfer formality requirements

We know from initial groundwork on transfer formality in Chapter 2 that what is required to pass legal title in property from one person to another depends on the nature of the property rather than the type of transaction. This was developed in Chapter 4, which suggested that transfer of legal title to a trustee was treated by law as any other transfer of title from one person to another in terms of what is required. Understanding this required taking on board that whilst the intention behind the transfer might be different where legal title is transferred to a trustee (as compared with ownership that is passed to the recipient of a gift), what was required for law to recognize the transfer has taken place at all was the same and governed by the type of property. So differences in intention behind the transfer will make the difference between what type of legal title is transferred, but the legal requirements for actually achieving this at all are governed by the nature of the property and not the type of transfer.

To recap on what is actually required, Chapter 2 and then Chapter 4 explained that title to an ordinary chattel is passed through requisite intention that ownership should pass being accompanied by its delivery to the intended recipient. The material also explained that additional requirements had been developed for transfers of ownership of intangible personal property, and also land, for different reasons: respectively, the much less 'visible' nature of intangible personalty and the intrinsic value of real property, and also its special nature within English law. And in terms of identifying 'themes' in these additional requirements, the additional protection being provided tends to be clustered around requirements of writing, endorsement, and registration.

So what is required at law for a third-party trustee to be recognized as the new legal owner of property that has been settled on trust will depend on the way in which the property is classified within English law. This mirrors everything that we have learned in respect of 'formality' for transfers of property. When we looked at transfer formality requirements, we also learned that whilst, as far as law was concerned, the transfer had failed because it was 'incomplete', equity was on occasion prepared to be more flexible. And what is meant by equity being 'more flexible' is that equity being prepared to recognize a transfer that law regarded as 'incomplete' as one that was effective in equity. We will now learn that equity adopts the same position for what, because formality required to effect successful constitution has not been complied with, law would regard as an 'incompletely constituted trust'.

When introduced to equity's flexible approach to incomplete transfers of property in Chapter 4, we learned that this would arise in situations in which recognizing a transfer in equity would be considered to have achieved a just outcome. It was explained that, in these circumstances, justice would be attached to recognizing that property does in substance have a new owner, and that this should not be denied on account of satisfying legal form, given that this can take time and is commonly tied into bureaucracy.

The most obvious justification for this arises where the recipient has provided value for the property. In this instance, as explained in Chapter 4, equity would look at intent rather than form and regard as done that which ought to be done, which means that the transfer is not really incomplete. We also learned that, on occasion, equity would also recognize a volunteer recipient as a new owner of property notwithstanding that 'equity will not assist a volunteer', in addition to its being unable to 'complete an incomplete gift'.

Explaining equity's just outcome for volunteer recipients of incomplete transfers of title

When we learned about equity's approach to a volunteer recipient, it was suggested that sometimes the circumstances are such that equity regards it as just to recognize an incomplete transfer, and that, in these circumstances, there will be a different outcome from the normal operation of equity not assisting volunteers and completing transfers, which can be seen in *Jones* v *Lock* (1865) LR 1 Ch App 25 and *Richards* v *Delbridge* (1874) LR Eq 11. At that point in Chapter 4, we considered that the 'last act' doctrine provided the benchmark for where equity would regard an incomplete transfer as effective, and when equity would leave it to fail for not satisfying legal requirements.

What we need to understand now is that equity's approach to volunteer recipients, in the case of a gift that would fail as far as law is concerned, also governs the position of what law will regard as an incompletely constituted trust for the same reason—namely, the absence of legal formality. This is because, whilst the intention is to transfer nominal legal title to a trustee, law's requirements are the same. Equity's response is the same because, characteristically, transfers of legal title to a trustee will be ones without consideration, which makes them, in the language of equity, 'voluntary transfers', and indeed a beneficiary under a trust is a volunteer on account of being a gratuitous recipient of a settlor's generosity. This means that equity will, on occasion, recognize an incompletely constituted trust as effective where this has arisen by a failed attempt to pass legal title to a trustee. This also means that the occasions on which equity will recognize this are governed by the 'last act' doctrine.

Authority for the 'last act' doctrine comes from the way in which Turner LJ's judgment in *Milroy* v *Lord* has been interpreted as requiring that an owner of property has done all in his power to transfer legal title to the recipient (this time a trustee), rather than that he has actually succeeded in so doing. And, as we now know, *Re Rose, Rose* v *IRC* [1952] Ch 499—the leading authority on the last act—involved an attempt to transfer legal title to a trustee and an attempt to make an outright gift. Now, it is time to understand how the 'last act' doctrine can be seen as an application of *Milroy*, how its results are reasoned as 'just outcomes', and how it actually works.

Initially, this requires reference to the judgment in *Re Rose, Rose* v *IRC* itself, and also to two earlier decisions that were cited in the judgment as authority for the particular approach and outcome in *Re Rose, Rose* v *IRC*: one is *Re Fry* [1946] Ch 312; the other, confusingly, is also called *Re Rose—Re Rose, Midland Bank Trustee Co* v *Rose* (1949) Ch 78. Then, as we consider other relevant case law in the area, we will encounter cases that arise from attempts—successful and otherwise—by owners of property to make outright gifts, and also ones arising from attempts—also successful and otherwise—by owners of property to transfer legal title to trustees. What we need to bear in mind is that, as we focus on the requirements of creating a valid trust, both types of case are authority for constituting a trust *in equity* through the last act of the settlor.

5.2 The rationale for the 'last act' and its application, illustrated in *Re Rose*

The facts of *Re Rose, Rose* v *IRC* have already been set out, and we know that the litigation concerned two purported transfers of shares, and also that liability for estate duty would fall due for both transfers based on the date on which legal title left the deceased and became vested in his wife, which was June 1943. The Court of Appeal ruled that the transfers were effective in equity in March 1943, when the deceased had executed the transfers in his wife's favour. In these circumstances, the intended outright transfer of the shares had taken effect in equity on this earlier date, and so had the intended transfer of legal title to her as trustee on account of the fact that Rose had done all that was possible to divest himself of ownership of these shares at that point. This meant that estate duty did not fall due on either transfer, because the gift was completed and the trust constituted by his 'last act', and what happened in June 1943 through the directors' consent to and registration of the transfers was merely law's formal approval of this. In coming to this view in the Court of Appeal, Evershed MR made clear at 511 that he adopted in full the words of Jenkins J in *Re Rose* [1949]:

> I was referred on that to the well known case of *Milroy* v *Lord*, and also to the recent case of *In re Fry* ... Those cases, as I understand them, turn on the fact that the deceased donor had not done all in his power, according to the nature of the property given, to vest the legal interest in the property in the donee. In such circumstances it is, of course, well settled that there is no equity to complete the imperfect gift. ... In *Milroy* v *Lord* the ... document was not the appropriate document to pass any interest in the property at all. In this case, as I understand it, the testator had done everything in his power to divest himself of the shares in question.

It was suggested earlier in the chapter that the 'last act' doctrine is a testament to equity's more flexible approach to entitlements to property, on this occasion manifested in taking decisions that, in substance, result in property having a new owner, even if law requires this to be 'rubber-stamped'. It is also the case that the just outcomes behind such a focus on substance are easy to relate to when the application of the 'last act' rule produces outcomes like that in *Re Rose*. In many ways, *Re Rose, Rose* v *IRC* is the textbook illustration of all of these matters, and it is hard not to think that *Rose* had the feel of a 'right result' in those particular circumstances. Working from this, we can see that what is possible under *Rose* might have even stronger rationale in cases like it where an owner of property actually dies before being able to carry out everything that must be done for law to recognize that property has a new owner: surely helping to fulfil a donor's wishes for his property is an appropriate direction for equity's pursuit of just outcomes? However, application of the 'last act' doctrine has also given rise to some difficulties, and these are ones that, on occasion, actually cast doubt on the inherent soundness of it as a doctrine. These can be seen to cluster determining *when*, and indeed *if*, the owner of property really has done *all* that he can and *has* performed the last act, which, as the cases show, will have crucial consequences.

5.3 The application of the 'last act' doctrine and the difficulties that it has exposed

Where a settlor is found to have performed the last act, a valid trust will come into being and, as we know, *Rose* is authority that the doctrine applies to donors in outright 'gift' transfers, as well as to trusts. If it is found that a settlor has not performed the last act, then the potential recipient (an intended beneficiary under a trust, or recipient of an intended gift) will lose out because equity does not complete incomplete gifts and neither will it complete incomplete trusts. So the consequences of being found on the right or wrong side of a settlor doing or not doing all in his power to effect a transfer of property are considerable. In this context, it is significant that the application of this principle can be seen in cases in which some very fine distinctions appear to have been drawn.

In contrast to the outcome in *Re Rose*, a 'last act' argument failed in *Re Fry* [1946] 1 Ch 312, because more could have been required from the testator for an effective transfer of title to the shares to be achieved. The reason in this case that the shares could not be registered was because consent had not been obtained from HM Treasury, as required by the Defence (Finance) Regulations 1939, under which shares could not be registered until Treasury consent was obtained. Although all of the requisite forms had been filled in by the donor, the required Treasury consent had not been obtained before he died. This appears at first sight to be similar to *Rose*, but it is clear from what was explained by Romer J that, in this case, the testator may not have done all that was required, so that the principles later elaborated in *Re Rose* could not apply:

> Now I should have thought it was difficult to say that the testator had done everything that was required to be done by him at the time of his death, for it was necessary for him to obtain permission from the Treasury for the assignment and he had not obtained it. Moreover, the Treasury might in any case have required further information of the kind referred to in the questionnaire submitted to him, or answers supplemental to those which he had given in reply to it; and, if so approached, he might have refused to concern himself with the matter further, in which case I do not know how anyone else could have compelled him to do so.
>
> (*Re Fry* [1946] 1 Ch 312, *per* Romer J at 317)

5.4 The 'rule in *Re Rose*' and the search for guiding principles

It is not entirely clear what mechanism is operating in *Re Rose*, and the case is not without its difficulties. Some of these issues were explored in Lowrie and Todd (1998) 57 CLJ 46. One possibility is that once the settlor has done all that he needs to do to constitute the trust (or to effect an out-and-out transfer), he is treated as if he has declared himself trustee of the property until legal title is actually transferred to the trustees (or, in the case of an out-and-out transfer, to the transferee). This is problematic, however, because it would appear to conflict with the requirements relating to *Milroy*'s second mode of constitution, which will be discussed shortly. At that point, we shall see that there is a long line of authorities showing that the courts are very reluctant to infer a self-declaration of trusteeship by the settlor in absence of clear intention on his part to become a trustee. Indeed, this is especially difficult given that one of the transfers in *Rose* intended to make a gift of the shares to the owner's wife, and where very clearly Rose did not intend to become trustee of them.

Another possibility is that equity imposes a constructive trust over the intervening period, which seems to be the view currently held by a number of academic commentators and also seemed to have judicial approval in the Court of Appeal decision in *Pennington* v *Waine* [2002] 1 WLR 2075. Much earlier than *Pennington*, judicial favour for a constructive trust reasoning can also be read into the Court of Appeal's decision in *Mascall* v *Mascall* [1984] 50 P & CR 119, on the ground that this concerned property that was land, and s. 53(1)(b) of the Law of Property Act 1925 imposes a writing requirement for evidencing declarations of trusts of land unless they are ones that can be categorized as implied, resulting, or constructive trusts (on which see Chapters 2, 4, 6, and 8).

In *Mascall*, the Court of Appeal applied *Re Rose* to registered land, but since the requisite writing to transfer title outright was present, there was no discussion of what type of trust would have arisen during the intervening period. The transferor had executed a transfer and sent it to HM Land Registry, and had also handed the land certificate to the transferee. At this stage, before the transfer and land certificate had been sent to the Land Registry for registration of the transferee as proprietor, the transferor changed his mind, after a quarrel with the transferee. The Court of Appeal held the transfer to be effective, since it was for the transferee to apply to the Land Registry for registration as proprietor, and the transferor had done everything that he had to do to complete the transfer.

Although *Mascall* v *Mascall* is silent on whether the trust in *Re Rose* is express or constructive, it is difficult to see what resemblance, in any way, the testator in *Rose* bears to those whose conduct is unconscionable (considered in Chapter 6 and also Chapter 17). Indeed, Lowrie and Todd (1998) 57 CLJ 46 suggested that, far from there being reasons why equity would wish to impose a constructive trust on Rose and people like him, there were sound reasons of policy why equity would wish to look kindly on those who wished to dispose of their property in favour of others. Moreover, the alternative solution—that the donor is taken to have declared himself trustee for the intervening period—also looks wrong in principle, given that he had intended a gift and equity will not normally infer a declaration of trusteeship from an incomplete gift (as we shall see in 'Part II The settlor must have declared himself to be trustee of the property: Milroy's second limb'). Furthermore, on closer examination, *Re Rose* is very difficult to distinguish from *Re Fry*, since the directors in *Rose* were not under any obligation to register the transfer (although they may well have routinely done so in practice), and so could presumably, had they felt so inclined, have refused to do so or have required further particulars from the donor. It is here that both cases (*Fry* and *Rose*) contrast with the position in *Mascall*, in which the Land Registry was under a statutory duty to register the title.

5.5 The 'last act' doctrine and more recent developments

While it is the case that *Re Rose* has the feel of a right result for the family in question in relation to liability for estate duty, any analysis that is based on trusteeship would also entail Rose being liable as trustee, and thus charged with the obligation of looking after the shares on the beneficiary's behalf and also open to attendant liability. Happily, this was for a short time only, and the directors (of whom the testator was one) were unlikely not to effect the transfer in favour of his wife (also a director). Nevertheless, it is not difficult to envisage that, on different facts, the outcome might not have been so positive. However, much as *Re Rose* might appear to be wrong in principle, it must be regarded as good authority not only because it was applied in *Mascall* v *Mascall* (notwithstanding express argument that *Rose* was wrong), but also because, as we know from Chapter 4, it was approved by the House of Lords in *Vandervell* v *IRC* [1967] 2 AC 691. In this regard, Lowrie and Todd (1998) 57 CLJ 46 suggest that there is an alternative analysis in the light of *Westdeutsche Landesbank Girozentrale* v *Islington LBC* [1996] AC 669, which is considered in Chapter 1 and also briefly in Chapter 6 in this context. This proposes that *Rose* can now be explained in such a way that it avoids the difficulties of articulating it around a trust analysis. We shall come back to this again shortly, after looking at some more recent developments.

It has been a long-standing view expressed in this text that continuing to use a trusts analysis for accounting for how the 'last act' doctrine actually works raises a number of difficulties, and that a more considered explanation within the case law would be extremely timely and welcome. When making these points, the Court of Appeal's decision in *Pennington* v *Waine* [2002] 1 WLR 2075 did not seem to be a development that could be regarded as either timely or welcome. This was because rather than taking up the invitation to forge some principled parameters within which the 'last act' doctrine could operate, *Pennington* seemed to cast aside the 'last act' doctrine altogether and sought to put in its place an approach that was even less principled. The Court of Appeal seemed to ignore completely the difficulties arising from applying the rule in *Re Rose*. And, in doing so, the Court of Appeal also ignored judicial concerns that it could operate in a more principled way, and even offerings on how this could be achieved from the Privy Council in *Pehrsson* v *von Greyerz* [1999] UKPC 26. We will come back to *Pehrsson* shortly, but for now we need to consider *Pennington* v *Waine*.

5.6 *Pennington* v *Waine*: an alternative approach to equity's recognition of new owners of property

When *Pennington* appeared, it suggested that the courts were taking a bolder approach to determining whether equity should or should not recognize that property has a new owner in circumstances in which law would not do so. This would not be governed by whether an owner of property had done all in his power to transfer the property; instead, the approach would be to ask whether it would be unconscionable for equity not to complete the transfer (whether this is in pursuit of a gift or a trust) in favour of the intended recipient. As with *Re Rose* and a number of these cases, the disputation concerned the gift of company shares, the formalities of transfer requiring the registration of the new owner on the company's register of shareholders under s. 182 of the Companies Act 1985 (with these provisions now being located in s. 770 of the Companies Act 2006). This ensures that the possession of share certificates provides evidence of share ownership, but does not effect it, and thus that mere delivery will not alone achieve transfer of ownership.

In 1998, the donor, Ada Crampton, executed a form for the transfer of 400 shares held in a family company in favour of her nephew, Harold Crampton. The transfer had been drawn up by the company's auditors, and in due course she signed it and returned it to the auditors, who placed it on the company's file. Ada's wish was also that her nephew should become a director of the company. Thus the auditors wrote to Harold, informing him of Ada's instructions in respect of the transfer of the shares, stating that, in respect of this, no action on Harold's part was required. However, Harold's consent to act as a director *was* required, and he was asked to complete a prescribed form for this purpose. The auditor took no further action to transfer the shares and Ada died in November of that year without the transfer having been sent to the company for Harold's registration as the shares' new owner. The Court of Appeal found that the gift of the shares to Harold was effective in equity, notwithstanding that Ada had not done everything in her power to effect the transfer. Clarke LJ regarded the execution of the share transfer form as constituting the transfer in equity of the shares. This in turn generated a bare trust upon Ada, under which she could have been compelled to procure the process of registration of the shares into Harold's name, thus completing the transfer at law.

The conscionability approach and perceived limitations of the 'last act' doctrine

What is particularly interesting about this judgment is the view of Arden and Schiemann LJJ of the role of conscionability in the determination of equitable assignment in circumstances in which the donor had not done everything in his power to *effect* the transfer. This approach suggests desire to replace the 'last act of the settlor' approach originating in *Milroy* v *Lord* with one based not on his actions, but on his hypothetical state of mind. This alternative test is constructed around the conscionability or otherwise of a donor's (often hypothetical) ability to revoke an incomplete gift in certain circumstances. *When* such an alternative test (of the donor's actions) would be invoked is not very clear, but the essence of the conscionability test was to be a matter for the courts to determine, having regard to all of the circumstances of the case. And although there could not be any comprehensive list of factors that define and constitute unconscionability, Arden LJ made reference to a number of relevant factors, including: that Ada had informed Harold of the gift; that she had signed the form and delivered it to Mr Pennington for him to secure registration; and also that Ada's agent had told Harold that he need take no action. Harold also agreed to become a director of the company, which he could not have done without shares being transferred to him. Arden LJ concluded that it should not have been possible for Ada to revoke the gift from the date on which Harold had formalized his consent to act as a director.

In considering *why* it might be that the Court's attention became focused on the donor's conscience rather than his actions in this case, Clarke LJ did have some sympathy with the argument advanced by counsel that the *Re Rose* test was fallacious because 'there is almost always something more which the donor could have done'. Because of this, equity could not be regarded as intervening only where the donor has done 'all that he can', because this would seldom be the case; hence it was held sufficient that the stock transfer form had been executed in circumstances in which there was no intention of revoking it in the future.

Whether this view is persuasive or not, it is the case that *Pennington* did address some of the concerns about *Re Rose*. This can be seen, for example, in the Court of Appeal's acknowledgement that, on occasions, donors might try to change their minds and that, in some circumstances, it should be permissible for them to do so, while in others it should not be so.

However, *Pennington* did generate a great deal of criticism, much of which focused on the vagueness of the conscionability test, and the scope that this had for undercutting equity's own mission statement as it is embodied in the maxims and equitable principles. The view taken in this text was that *Pennington* sought to give far too much accommodation to the position of would-be donees and would-be beneficiaries, who are actually volunteer recipients of another's generosity. It is difficult to see the very premise of a gift as not being inextricably connected with the intention of the donor, and the rules surrounding equity's strictness in not perfecting transfers that are made voluntarily, but imperfectly, must surely reflect an owner of property's rights to deal freely with his property.

Equity does follow the law, and from this a donor should remain free to revoke a gift (or a transfer seeking to create a benefit under a trust) before the point at which it is irrevocably made, albeit that equity will approach this by looking at substance rather than form. It appears from the facts of the case, and the convincing representation of them in Arden LJ's judgment, at [4] and [57], that the gift to Harold was intended. In this respect, *Pennington* v *Waine* appears directly analogous with *Rose* v *IRC*, in as much as both point to situations in which on their facts, each donor was extremely unlikely to have changed his mind. Although there is much to suggest that this *was* the intention both in *Rose* v *IRC* and *Pennington* v *Waine*, arguably equity should not be considering intervening at all where this type of intention is not present. And it is equally easy to envisage situations in which the issues surrounding intention are more equivocal and far less clear-cut.

A cavalier approach to gratuitous dealings with property

For the purposes of this text, *Pennington* showed the Court of Appeal adopting a highly cavalier attitude towards the principle of *Milroy* v *Lord*, which is founded upon the interests of certainty when ascertaining the wishes of the donor and is a cornerstone of the rules surrounding making gifts: a gift will be construed as such if a gift is intended. It appears to be putting in its place a test that subjects donors, their actions, and their intentions to a test of conscionability. *Milroy* v *Lord* and the case law that followed it (notably, *Jones* v *Lock* and *Richards* v *Delbridge*) might be seen to have produced some harsh results, and indeed the rule against imperfectly constituted gifts has led to harsh and seemingly paradoxical results. At one point, Arden LJ made clear her views that an alternative test based in conscionability provides a less paternalistic framework for the consideration of gifts and giving, and one that leads to a 'benevolent construction' of gifts, which gives effect to the clear wishes of the donor.

There is much that is intelligent and considered in this alternative construction of gifts, and it is the case, of course, that Arden LJ positioned paternalism alongside its ideological opposite—that is, autonomy and respect for individuals. Thus she framed her alternative test as a mechanism for ensuring that respect is given to the original intentions of the donor, asserting that approaches which (often hypothetically) permit donors to change their minds could be regarded as paternalistic. However, notwithstanding the strength of such views, there is also one central objective that *must* inform the courts' approach to the status of imperfect gifts and the position of the parties involved, which suggests that this should be cautious rather than cavalier. This was, in fact, clear from the very next sentence in Arden LJ's judgment, which spoke of the need 'to safeguard' the position of the donor. While the donor is central to any act of giving property, it seemed that *Pennington* created too much scope for working against the donor's interests (albeit mainly hypothetically), and could operate to privilege the position of the potential donee at the former's expense.

Gifts and the creation of trusts: Pennington v Waine, donors, and their wishes

It is the case that both *Rose* and, more recently, *Pennington* concerned transfers that were intended as outright gifts, as distinct from property intended to become subject to a trust. However, the difficulties raised by *Pennington* do have important application in situations in which the donor (at the outset at least) does intend to divest himself of all interest in the property, but this time in favour of a third party who is intended to hold the property on trust for an intended beneficiary, as was the case in one of the transfers in *Rose*. *Pennington* v *Waine* does suggest (despite Arden LJ's insistence to the contrary) that rather serious inroads might also be made into the closely related principle that equity will not infer a perfect trust from an imperfect gift. Trusts law is constructed around the essence of the trust as an arrangement that is irrevocable, as well as one that creates responsibility for property as well as entitlements to it, and quite rightly attaches considerable significance to the intention of the donor when determining whether a trust exists. While it is the case that, once the trust is in place, its enforcement is at the hands of the beneficiary, ordinarily to the exclusion of the donor (unless he is a party to the trust or becomes a beneficiary under it), this position arises once—and *only* once—the trust is fully constituted. Equally a gift, once given, is irrevocable—but again this happens only once a gift has been made and correct 'transfer' formalities have been complied with.

5.7 Concerns about new directions and the value of traditional approaches

In trying to get a measure of *Pennington*, *Choithram (T) International SA* v *Pagarani* [2001] 2 All ER 492 is a particularly interesting development. As part of the *Pennington* vintage, it suggests that an extremely low bar is set for determining whether it would be unconscionable for a recipient to be deprived of the benefit of the property. We also look at this case again shortly, slightly differently, but its facts concerned the deathbed creation of an *inter vivos* trust, which was intended to have nine trustees, of which the settlor intended to be one. The settlor stated that he *gave* all of his wealth to a foundation that he had established and of which he was one of the trustees, but he died before his assets were transferred and it was found, at first instance and on appeal, that there was no effective constitution under either limb of *Milroy* v *Lord*. This was reversed in the Privy Council, even though no transfer formality had been effected and notwithstanding that use of words of 'giving' to the foundation meant that there was not obviously the clearest evidence that a trust was intended. It was found that even saying 'I give to the foundation' would make it unconscionable for the trustees of the property not to be constituted as trustees, because 'although equity will not aid a volunteer, it will not strive officiously to defeat a gift'. On this criteria, it is difficult to imagine a situation in which it would be considered permissible (that is, conscionable) for a donor to resile from his 'gift'—which can actually be a trust, even if it is called a 'gift' on its face. One has to wonder from this whether the intention of the courts is that equity should recognize any incomplete transfer of property whatever the circumstances, and should actually adjust its maxims and principles 'governance statement' accordingly.

The traditional approach embodied in the last act is an outgrowth from the policy expressed in *Milroy* v *Lord* to seek to ensure that what happens to a person's property is what was intended, and that this complies with what the law requires. In turn, this reflects that, in these situations, valuable property rights are at stake: the rights and entitlements relating to the property, which pass to a recipient through making a gift or declaring a trust in his favour. It is thus suggested that, instead of focusing on the role of transfer formalities in outright transfers of property, and certainty of intention and the irrevocability of the trust arrangement, all of which are consistent with the nature of the gift and of the trust respectively, the doctrine of conscionability in conception might undermine the way in which making gifts and creating beneficiaries from recipients of trust property are, and *should be*, at the behest of the donor.

5.8 Judicial approaches post-*Pennington* v *Waine*

Whilst *Pennington* attracted a great deal of criticism from academic quarters, it was unclear how it would fare in the courts. This text's view has always been that, given that Clarke LJ was himself moved to remark in *Pennington* v *Waine* that hard cases make bad law, it is a great pity that the Court of Appeal seemed far less interested in the wishes of the donor than it should have been. Although this text has always stressed that promoting certainty in dealings with property through looking at what is actually said and done (even if this produces harsh results) is a preferable and sounder approach than taking a much vaguer, more nebulous, and even paternalistic one embodied in conscionability, it was mindful that the courts did appear to be favouring the latter.

This conclusion was drawn from the way in which *Pennington* appeared to be part of a 'pedigree' of a more liberal age for equity's system of governance, through the development of its principles and maxims in ways with which equity lawyers felt uncomfortable. Indeed, *Choithram (T) International SA* v *Pagarani* [2001] 2 All ER 492 seems to be reinventing equity's mission statement to account for the fact that while it would not aid a volunteer, equally it would 'not strive officiously to defeat a gift', even though it is not actually obvious from the case law that equity has ever striven to defeat gifts. This view of *Pennington*'s intentions also reflected the way in which it did not seem occupied with the concerns about the 'last act' doctrine that were evident in the earlier case of *Pehrsson* v *von Greyerz* [1999] UKPC 26. In this Privy Council case, Lord Hoffmann appeared to try to limit the situations in which the 'last act' doctrine should be applied to enable equity to recognize a transfer prior to ownership passing at law *only* 'when the donor has clothed the [recipient] with the power to obtain [ownership]'. Here, for Lord Hoffmann, *Re Rose* was authority that equity would regard the transfer as complete where 'no further act on the part of the donor is needed to vest the legal title in the beneficiary and the *donor has no power to prevent it*' (emphasis added).

5.9 A 'blueprint' for future development?

Given all of this, *Kaye* v *Zeital* [2010] EWCA Civ 159 (appearing under the name *Zeital* v *Kaye* in some reports) appears to be a very significant development. It concerned a probate case with extremely complicated facts, which required a ruling on ownership of an apartment held by the deceased through his beneficial interests in shares in a limited company. The deceased then died intestate, and there was a dispute about who owned the shares, which was further complicated by the way in which the company concerned had been liquidated (that is, its legal existence was being brought to a close), and it was the liquidator (the person actually effecting this) who sought the court's direction about where beneficial ownership lay. The deceased's widow had lived separately from him for more than twenty years; and the deceased's more recent partner insisted that he had given the shares to her informally. It was decided on appeal that the deceased's actions to pass the shares to his partner were not capable of transferring beneficial ownership of the shares to her. This is because he was not actually the registered owner of the shares (that is, owner of the shares at law), and so he could not execute a share transfer in her favour. Here, the company was in liquidation and no share certificate was handed over, and so it had to be concluded that the deceased had not done all that he could to transfer the shares to her.

If nothing else, *Zeital* stood as important recognition that the courts will actually deem some transfers as being *ineffective* in equity as well as at law. And, in doing so, it might have suggested the courts might be less results-focused than indicated by *Pennington* and even *Rose* itself. But it is not obvious that the judges in *Pennington* would have decided this differently, because *Pennington* is not authority that, in all cases in which there is a failed transfer (at law), equity will find it unconscionable for the recipient not to receive the benefit of the property. Instead, despite suggestions about its very low threshold, *Pennington* does indicate that, in some circumstances, equity will find it unconscionable for the recipient to be deprived of the benefit of the property, while sometimes it will not.

The implications of abandoning the conscionability approach and returning to the 'last act' doctrine

This text has a tradition of criticizing the courts for being too 'results-focused' rather than being 'principles-focused' when determining whether equity will recognize a transfer as effective. This was a criticism of the application of the 'last act' doctrine before *Pennington* appeared to sweep this away in favour of an approach that was very favourable to recipients rather than donors, even if it was not actually a 'recipient's charter'. What is interesting is that the language used in *Zeital* to explain why the gift had failed stated that this was because the deceased had 'not done all he could to transfer [the property]'. This *is* the language of the last act, and this decision may well be signalling current judicial favour for this—whether this is a restatement of orthodox approach, or a retreat from *Pennington*—notwithstanding that there was no overt criticism of *Pennington*.

Zeital must now also be considered in the light of *Curtis v Pulbrook* [2011] EWHC 167. Here, in a way that appears to bring together elements that are identifiable from *Rose*, *Pennington*, and *Zeital*, and attempts to present a cohesive approach, Briggs J appeared to endorse the view that there were three ways in which equity could recognize a transfer that is incomplete at law as effective:

> The first is where the donor has done everything necessary to enable the donee to enforce a beneficial claim without further assistance from the donor ... The second is where some detrimental reliance by the donee upon an apparent although ineffective gift may so bind the conscience of the donor to justify the imposition of a constructive trust ... The third is whereby a benevolent construction an effective gift or implied declaration of trust may be teased out of the words used.
>
> (*Curtis v Pulbrook* [2011] EWHC 167, *per* Briggs J at [43])

The first is attributed to the *Re Rose* principle and is strongly suggestive of continuing recourse to the position of a 'last act'. This embodies what this text would analyse as the *Pehrsson v von Greyerz* approach to the last act, thereby alluding to the need for consistency in application. The second recognizes that it may be appropriate for the courts to be 'pro-recipient' in circumstances under which the recipient is not a completely passive 'windfall donee', as illustrated by *Pennington* and indeed *Rose* itself. The third is more problematic and could embody the least attractive aspects of *Pennington*. But it remains to be seen how much significance is attached to Briggs J's thoughts on the triggers for equity's interventions, and how they might be applied. However, there is an inherent difficulty that will persist even in the emergence of a balanced and coherent approach to transfers of property, which will require at the very least revisiting the key cases to consider questions of consistency in application of the 'last act'.

This is because even a balanced and coherent approach to transfers of property requires us to confront the way in which any recognition of ownership *by* equity *of property ahead of* its recognition at law means that ownership of property will become separated. The separation of ownership is strongly associated with the existence of a trust, and for many property lawyers the separation of ownership can mean only that a trust of property subsists (albeit that a different analysis is offered in Lowrie and Todd (1998) 57 CLJ 46). On the conventional analysis, any separation of ownership gives rise to a trust: the temporary separation of title to property that arises when equity recognizes that it has a new owner will have the effect of transforming—albeit temporarily—property that is being given away by its owner into trust property.

This has the effect of transforming those who are giving their property away into trustees of it. On this reasoning, where an owner of property is trying to create an express trust, a different trust from that which he intended will come into being, although only temporarily. This will also have the effect of transforming into a trustee someone who has signalled in the strongest possible terms that he does not intend to be a trustee by attempting to appoint others to undertake the task. The reasons why it might not be appropriate to reason equity's role in incomplete property transfers by way of a constructive trust have been set out, but it is also the case that a number of academic commentators are comfortable with doing so, and this is also evident from the absence of critical appraisal for this from the courts. So while it is to be welcomed that the courts do seem keen to move away from *Pennington* v *Waine*, the appearance of *Zeital* can be seen to expose the need for future approaches to be developed in a much more considered way.

Part II **The settlor must have *declared himself to be trustee* of the property: *Milroy*'s second limb**

Whilst the first limb of *Milroy* v *Lord* may illustrate how most express trusts will be constituted, *Milroy* also allows this to happen by an owner of property declaring himself to be trustee of (what was) his own property on behalf of one or more beneficiaries. Here, there are no transfer formality requirements, because legal title is already being held by the person who becomes trustee; the person who becomes a settlor on account of his intention to do this will keep hold of legal title himself, but, because a trust has come into existence, equitable ownership also now subsists. This is held by the beneficiary and this means that the legal title now in existence is nominal legal title, which is held by a trustee in furtherance of obligations to the beneficiary. It *is* still being held by the same person, but it is a *different type* of legal title from that found in absolute ownership.

This type of constitution of a trust is most commonly called 'self-declaration of trusteeship', and although there are no transfer formality considerations here, we do know from Chapter 4 that, in the creation of express trusts, we also find so-called 'declaration formality'. For most trusts, this will not affect how a settlor makes his statement that the property is to be settled on trust. This is because although trusts of personal property are, in practice, created in written instruments, this is often because they are being used strategically in tax avoidance, or because a helpful settlor wishes to provide trustees with assistance from written instructions. For trusts of personal property, there is no requirement of law that a declaration of trust must be in writing in order to be effective. However, we also know from Chapter 4 that s. 53(1)(b) of the Law of Property Act 1925 requires declarations of trust relating to property that is land to be manifested and evidenced in writing, and signed by the settlor, in order to be enforceable.

Beyond this, there is a much less obviously close relationship between formality requirements and this type of constitution, but, as we will discover, there are still formality issues of which we need to be aware. Immediately, this suggests that, in satisfying this requirement, there are different issues arising here from those that we encountered in relation to transfer of property from owner-cum-settlor to a trustee. As we will find out, for declarations of trusteeship by the settlor, the courts are looking for evidence that an owner of property is seeking to undertake the obligations of trusteeship himself and not at whether he has tried to transfer legal title to another for these purposes. However, it is worth stressing that, while the courts might be looking for different things under the respective limbs of *Milroy* v *Lord*, the effect of the courts not finding that an owner of property has declared himself trustee is the same as the courts not finding a last act or (to the extent that *Pennington* remains good law) that it would be unconscionable to deprive the recipient of the benefit of the property: the trust is not constituted and any attempt to create an express trust will fail.

5.10 What the courts are looking for: satisfying *Milroy*, declarations of self as trustee, and 'failed gifts'

It will become apparent shortly that the courts will not conclude that an owner of property has decided to become a trustee on top of choosing to settle it on trust for another unless there is the clearest evidence that this is what he intended to do. In this regard, what the courts look for here is very closely related to satisfying certainty-of-intention requirements, and indeed we will find a number of certainty-of-intention cases discussed here. This becomes an issue where there is no attempt to transfer legal title to a trustee. In this instance, the courts must be sure that, in any pronouncement that an owner of property is to act as trustee, he did in fact seek to create a trust at all. In this regard, the courts insist that they will much more readily find that an owner of property is seeking to give his property away altogether than conclude that he is volunteering his services as a trustee. But given what we know already about satisfying certainty of intention, surely the question of whether an owner of property has declared himself a trustee is supplemental to establishing that he intended to create a trust rather than to provide benefits by some other means? In theory, this is a straightforward 'yes', but the case law that is found as authority for self-declarations of trusteeship suggests that the issues can be much more complex in reality.

The cases that we encounter in this section of the chapter suggest that questions about self-declarations of trusteeship have commonly arisen in relation to attempts to make outright voluntary transfers (gifts), which have failed for not satisfying law's requirements. We do already have a sense of this from Chapter 3, where we saw *Richards* v *Delbridge* (1874) LR Eq 11 as a certainty-of-intention case, and now we find out explicitly how it came to be the leading authority for what is required to be present for the court to find that an owner of property has declared himself to be trustee. Here, we will see that the law relating to self-declarations of trusteeship has historically been very influenced by 'failed gifts', and we will then consider how this has persisted in the modern law.

Self-declarations of trusteeship: background, context, and key issues
The starting point for understanding the modern law relating to self-declaration of trusteeship is that the courts will not lightly rule that this is what an owner of property intended for himself when deciding to settle the property on trust. Because a trust creates permanent rights for the beneficiary and makes onerous demands of trustees, we know already that certainty-of-intention rules operate to ensure that this happens only when it is intended. In situations in which these responsibilities will actually be those of the settlor, the courts have ruled that there will be a very high threshold for concluding that this is what an owner-cum-settlor wanted to achieve.

Whether enough attention is paid to the enormity of trusteeship in making these determinations is something that we will consider shortly, but, for getting a general sense of approach, we need to understand that the courts are very cautious in doing so. Here, we need to be aware that a number of cases clustered around the key *Milroy* v *Lord* authorities—*Jones* v *Lock* (1865) LR 1 Ch App 25 and *Richards* v *Delbridge* (1874) LR Eq 11—establish that:

- the courts will more readily find that an owner of property intends to make a gift of his property (that is, through an outright transfer) in favour of another than that he intended to declare a trust of the property;
- such 'outright transfers' often become embroiled in questions of self-declarations of trust because they fail for want of transfer formality, which is why their status and validity has come into question;
- these failed transfers are incapable of amounting to gifts, and so the only way in which they can be 'saved' (by satisfying *Milroy* v *Lord*) is by 'finding' an intention to create a trust; and
- in this case, *if* property is deemed to be held on trust, the theory is that absence of a transfer of title to a trustee can be 'explained' by finding that the owner of property is not only seeking to settle it on trust, but is also intending to act as trustee himself, in which case no transfer of legal title is required.

While the consequences of finding that there has or has not been a self-declaration of trusteeship by a settlor will be the same as a last act being found or being absent, the issues surrounding and actually determining validity are quite different. In the 'last act' cases, the context was the transfer of property; in the case of self-declarations of trusteeship by the settlor, the courts are looking for evidence that an owner of property is seeking to undertake the obligations of trusteeship himself and not at whether he has tried to transfer legal title to another for these purposes.

5.11 Satisfying *Milroy* v *Lord*: self-declarations as trustee, and 'failed gifts'

In Chapter 4, we learned that, in *Jones* v *Lock* (1865) LR 1 Ch App 25, an attempted gift of a cheque to a baby failed because his father did not endorse it before his death. What we can do now is explain properly why we had, by that time, already encountered this case in Chapter 3—that is, because an attempt was made to rescue this failed gift by establishing that the father's conduct had sought to create a trust of the cheque, to which he kept legal title on account of intending to act as trustee himself. Lord Cranworth refused to construe his actions as amounting to a self-declaration of trusteeship because no intention to create a trust of the property had been manifested. The intention was to make a gift, not irrevocably to settle it on trust, which is what would be required if a trust (and a self-declaration of trusteeship) were to be found. A similar argument was made, and with the same outcome, in *Richards* v *Delbridge* (1874) LR Eq 11, which we already know concerned a failed attempt to transfer the lease of a business from a grandfather to his grandson. It was found that there had been no transfer of the lease to Richards, nor a declaration of trust in his favour, and Sir George Jessel MR made clear his refusal to infer a declaration of trust from the failed gift.

We can see from both *Jones* v *Lock* and *Richards* v *Delbridge* that the courts will not respond favourably to attempts to save failed gifts through claims that donors' real intentions lay in creating trusts. This determination not to let gifts blur into trusts is clear from the courts' response to attempts that are made to do so, which have arisen from clever legal argument seeking to 'blur' them by exploiting their similarities. However, in rejecting such attempts as are made and on which the courts do have to make rulings, we are still left with case law that often seems to 'fudge' explanations of why gifts cannot be trusts rather than to clarify them. This becomes transposed into other judicial decisions, and means that legal commentaries are perhaps not as clear on these points as they might be. The quality of judicial reasoning is dependent, to a significant degree, on what is being argued by opposing parties in litigation, but the courts have perhaps unwittingly fuelled the ambiguity between making gifts and creating trusts in one significant respect: both *Jones* and *Richards* insist that dealings with property will more readily draw the inference of a gift rather than creation of a trust, because a trust creates an irrevocable arrangement characterized by responsibility.

The implication here is that there is a hierarchy of intention, which will make intention to create a trust the most difficult to satisfy. The problem with this is that, even to the most casual observer of a gift, this has the effect of depriving an owner of property of all interest in his property in a way that is permanent and irrevocable. We can see that, in the context of self-declaration of trusteeship, the courts are seeking to say that retaining a trustee's legal title has more lasting implications for an owner of property than giving it away, but what the courts do not stress nearly enough in making this point is that giving property away is actually very significant for its owner. It is fine to attach particular requirements to self-declaration of trusteeship, but the starting point for this should be that any dealing with property in which its owner will lose ownership should be treated very seriously by law.

So perhaps a more useful way of mapping intention to create a trust with making a gift is not to see them in a hierarchy, but actually horizontally—that is, as having equal significance, but being differently focused. Taking this approach would still reflect the outcomes of *Jones* and *Richards*, and their reasoning, but it would also require the courts to spell out that although establishing intention to make a gift of property is very important and will be regarded as so by the courts, this is wholly *different* from the way in which the courts will approach the creation of responsibilities for that property for someone other than its intended recipient. Taking this approach might actually lead to a more rounded approach to how the courts currently find a self-declaration of trusteeship on the part of an owner-cum-settlor.

5.12 *Richards* v *Delbridge*: what is required for satisfying *Milroy* v *Lord*?

Looking at the failed gifts cases, we now understand how *Richards* v *Delbridge* has become an authority for certainty of intention to create a trust (by virtue of the absence of this from the case itself), and this is key to understanding how it has become the leading authority for self-declarations of trust. Both *Jones* v *Lock* and *Richards* v *Delbridge* are cases in which, if intention to create a trust had been found, the resultant trust could be constituted only by a self-declaration of trust, on account of the transfer formality implications of appointing a third-party trustee. The prominence of failed gifts in explaining this mechanism of constitution helps to reinforce the earlier observation that most express trusts will be constituted by the appointment of a third-party trustee, and that self-declaration of trusteeship is more unusual. In fact, everything that we have learned up to now suggests that self-declaration of trusteeship really arises only where there are 'issues' about whether a trust was intended at all. This is not always the case, but traditionally this has been the more unusual mode of constitution of express trusts.

In the course of ruling that there had been no declaration of trust by Delbridge in favour of his infant grandson, and thus no self-declaration of trusteeship by him, Sir George Jessel set out what would be required for it to be found that an owner of property has declared himself a trustee of it, and what can be permitted in order that this can be found on the part of an owner of property who settles it on trust. This forms part of a very famous passage that points to the fundamental nature of a gift and a trust, and provides a reminder for us of their similarities and fundamental differences:

> A man may transfer his property ... in one of two ways: he may do such acts as amount in law to a conveyance or assignment of the property, and thus completely divest himself of the legal ownership, in which case the person who by those acts acquires the property takes it beneficially, or on trust, as the case may be; or the legal owner of the property may, by one or other of the modes recognised as amounting to a valid declaration of trust, constitute himself a trustee, and, without an actual transfer of the legal title, may so deal with the property as to deprive himself of its beneficial ownership, and declare that he will hold it from that time forward on trust for the other person. It is true that he need not use the words, 'I declare myself a trustee', but he must do something which is equivalent to it, and use expressions which have that meaning ... for a man to make himself trustee there must be an expression of intention to become a trustee, whereas words of present gift shew an intention to give over property to another, and not to retain it in the donor's own hands for any purpose, fiduciary or otherwise.
>
> (*Richards* v *Delbridge* (1874) LR Eq 11, *per* Sir George Jessel at 14)

5.13 Applying *Richards* v *Delbridge*: what is required, and what can be permitted, to satisfy *Milroy*?

The first point to make about this very famous passage relates to its emphasis on the fundamental difference between the trust and the gift. From this, it should come as no surprise that the courts will refuse to infer a declaration of trusteeship from a failed gift.

This is because a donor of a gift retains no interest after the property has been transferred, whereas a trustee's fiduciary obligations continue. In doing this, the judgment does not really give any attention to how losing all interest in property is actually no small thing either, thus fuelling this idea of a hierarchy of owner intentions in which giving property away is somehow less significant than creating a trust. But, putting this aside, we can glean plenty from the passage in terms of how it can be shown that an owner of property has intended not simply to create a trust, but actually to undertake the responsibilities of trusteeship.

In this regard, Sir George Jessel observed that showing this does not actually require the settlor to have used the words 'I declare myself trustee'. However, Jessel MR was insistent that, for a settlor to be taken to intend such, he must do something that is equivalent to saying 'I declare myself trustee'. In many respects, in taking this as the starting point, Jessel MR is suggesting that the most effective way of making it clear that these obligations are being undertaken *is* actually to say 'I declare myself trustee'. But not stipulating this as a requirement acknowledges that, in real life, declarations of trust will often arise in circumstances under which such an expression is not actually uttered.

In acknowledging this, Sir George Jessel did, however, insist that something must be done that is equivalent to saying 'I declare myself trustee'. And it is clear that cases applying *Richards* v *Delbridge* are effectively determinations of what *will* be regarded as equivalent to saying 'I declare myself trustee' and what *will not* be regarded as equivalent to it. This is very significant given that, in the latter scenario, no trust can come into being, because the trust cannot be said to have been constituted.

5.14 Applying *Richards* v *Delbridge*: the scope of the requirement

Many of the cases first discussed as authorities for certainty of intention are now encountered here as applications of *Richards* v *Delbridge*. This reinforces the point that many cases in which issues of self-declaration of trusteeship arise are also ones in which it must be found that there is actually certainty of intention to create a trust at all. Here, once it is found that a trust is intended, the only realistic way of satisfying the constitution requirement is to find that the settlor also intended to create a trust—in circumstances in which this is not always obviously the case.

For example, on this occasion, *Paul* v *Constance* is authority that in lieu of the settlor actually saying 'I declare myself trustee' (as well as satisfying certainty of intention), the court can infer this from his conduct, or from words that can be construed as equivalent to a declaration of trusteeship, or from a mixture of the two. But just as *Paul* v *Constance* was considered a borderline case as far as certainty of intention was concerned, the same critique can be made of its ability to satisfy *Richards* v *Delbridge* requirements, on the basis of what was said and done by Constance. As Scarman LJ said, 'there must be clear evidence from what is said or done of an intention to create a trust or ... "an intention to dispose of a property or a fund so that somebody else to the exclusion of the disponent acquires the beneficial interest in it"', but at the same time as concluding that there was sufficient evidence of this, Scarman LJ also considered this a 'borderline case, since it is not easy to pin-point a specific moment of declaration'.

What was said and done in *Paul* v *Constance* may not obviously seem equivalent to a declaration of trusteeship, but surely what Constance was really saying is that although (because the bank manager advised it) legal title to the money would be vested in him, the money in fact belonged to both of them. Since Constance had legal title, it could be only the equitable title that was shared, so actually these words are exactly appropriate for a declaration of trusteeship. And, as we will discover in Chapter 8, many declarations of trusteeship are made *very* informally.

Chapter 3 did discuss extensively the significance that Scarman LJ attached to a specific moment of declaration, in light of the fact that trusts are, in principle, irrevocable, and these considerations apply here, albeit that they are now focused on what is required to effect a self-declaration of trusteeship. And in this respect, despite being a borderline case from which it is difficult to make generalizations, *Paul* v *Constance* is authority that words and/or conduct of a simple and unsophisticated nature will, in appropriate circumstances, be regarded as being equivalent to saying 'I declare myself trustee'. Much of its import *can* be seen replicated in *Rowe* v *Prance* [1999] 2 FLR 787.

Paul v *Constance* suggests that some manifestations of this will be more convincing than others, but inherent in Sir George Jessel's judgment is that whilst some words or conduct (or combinations of the two) will be regarded as being equivalent to saying 'I declare myself trustee', other words or actions will fall short of this. It is to illustrate this that other cases considered in the context of certainty of intention also now find their way into discussion of what is required to satisfy *Richards* v *Delbridge*, by virtue of being equivalent to saying 'I declare myself trustee'. In this respect, *Re Kayford Ltd* [1975] 1 WLR 279 and *Re Chelsea Cloisters Ltd* [1980] 41 P & CR 98 are examples of where what is done is regarded as being equivalent with saying 'I declare myself trustee'; *Re Multi Guarantee* [1987] BCLC 257 is authority that words and/or conduct can also fall short of achieving this. However, the *Kayford* cases have been criticized by Michael Bridge [1992] 12 OJLS 333, and it is not actually that clear that they do take us any nearer to understanding what the courts will regard as being equivalent to the words 'I declare myself trustee'.

Paul v *Constance* and the *Re Kayford* line of cases do suggest that what makes the difference between whether what is said and/or done is regarded as being equivalent to 'I declare myself trustee' turns on the same matters as establishing certainty of intention— that is, intention to create a permanent and irrevocable arrangement, which will deprive the original owner-cum-settlor of all beneficial interest in the property, and which will also create responsibilities for it. Once this has been established, the courts seem then to subsume into this a settlor's intention also to become trustee under this arrangement, where it is clear that no one else is being considered for the role.

All of these cases show that the courts *are* mindful of the *nature* of the trust when considering whether what is said and done can actually be equated with saying 'I declare myself trustee'. This is manifested in the extensive references that can be found to the trust as an arrangement that, once put in place, is permanent and irrevocable. And this is very important for proposing that the courts will infer this far less readily on the part of the owner of property than that he intended an out-and-out gift.

Are the courts paying enough attention to 'trusteeship' in self-declarations of trusteeship?

This does also, of course, chime with the highly onerous and burdensome nature of trusteeship itself, which would also explain why the courts are happier to infer that an owner of property is seeking to give it away rather than to make it subject to a trust.

Whilst no one would doubt the importance of establishing certainty of intention to create a trust in determining whether a settlor also intends to act as trustee, should this actually be *sufficient* as well as *necessary*? If there is more to ascertaining whether someone has done something that is equivalent to saying 'I declare myself trustee', the cases do not seem to be very effective at identifying this as a distinct and separate quality. In this regard, although the nuances of trusteeship are evident in the cases, more direct reference to the *nature of trusteeship* is something that the courts *should* be emphasizing much more explicitly alongside the emphasis that *is* being given to the *nature of the trust* itself.

This suggests that the courts really ought to be paying more attention to the implications of a valid trust when determining equivalence with saying 'I declare myself trustee'. This is so in any case, and perhaps especially where, in context of 'trusts from failed gifts', there could be more judicial clarity on keeping the creation of trusts much more conceptually separate from making gifts. Bringing together both of these factors, we now consider *Choithram (T) International SA* v *Pagarani* [2001] 2 All ER 492 as an authority on how a settlor can validly constitute himself trustee under *Milroy* v *Lord*. In this context, *Choithram* suggests that the courts are attaching less significance to finding that a trust has been created, rather than more, when determining *whether* a trust has been constituted. Instead, they seem to take an interest in whether it would be unconscionable to find that the trust had not been effectively constituted. Once again, this seems to be calling into question the continuing relevance of *Milroy* v *Lord*, and it is far from clear how this approach is supposed to satisfy the requirements of *Richards* v *Delbridge*.

Choithram actually suggests that a settlor can do something that is equivalent to saying 'I declare myself trustee' by saying nothing more than 'I *give* my property' to another. As the Privy Council explained, although the wording was what one might expect in the case of a gift, it could instead be construed as a declaration of trust. In Lord Browne-Wilkinson's view, at [11], this novel case was in fact consistent with, and did not contravene the requirements of, *Milroy* v *Lord*:

> Although the words used by [the donor] are normally appropriate to an outright gift—'I give to X'—in the present context there is no breach of the principle in *Milroy v Lord* if the words of [the] gift (to the foundation) are given their only possible meaning in this context. The foundation has no legal existence apart from the trust declared by the foundation trust deed. Therefore the words 'I give to the foundation' can only mean 'I give to the trustees of the foundation trust deed to be held by them on the trusts of the foundation trust deed'. Although the words are apparently words of outright gift they are essentially words of gift on trust.

The observation on how it is necessary to avoid the officious defeat of a gift has already been made, but this case does point to a very high likelihood that it will always be unconscionable to deprive a recipient of the benefit of property. On this approach, it is likely that any words or actions of a donor will be taken as equivalent to saying 'I declare myself trustee'. We can see that this is difficult to square with certainty-of-intention requirements, which demand that an intention to secure a benefit for a recipient will not suffice unless it is clear that this is intention to secure a benefit by way of a trust. And in terms of the additional requirements that are supposed to apply to self-declarations over and above this, it is very difficult to see how much actually remains of the *Richards* v *Delbridge* requirement, as far as making a self-declaration of trust is concerned, in the light of *Choithram*.

5.15 *Richards* v *Delbridge* and business dealings: self-declarations of trust in the commercial context

We have just looked again at the *Re Kayford* cases as illustrations of *Richards* v *Delbridge* requirements of doing something that is equivalent to saying 'I declare myself trustee' for the purposes of constituting a trust, and thereby making it a valid trust. In doing this, it was suggested that it is difficult to see how any of the cases get us closer to understanding what will make the difference between something that is said or done being regarded as equivalent to saying 'I declare myself trustee', and what will fall short of this. This is because these cases are so closely bound up with establishing certainty of intention that what makes them authority that an owner of property is seeking to create a trust and also to act as trustee is not that readily apparent. This is a valid criticism for *Paul* v *Constance* (which was considered a 'borderline' situation in any case) and also *Rowe* v *Prance*, which applied it, but we will now consider the *Re Kayford* cases for exploring whether we can get a sense of how the courts approach establishing equivalence to 'I declare myself trustee' outside interpersonal dealings between private parties, who are often also family members. This follows on from our examination of establishing certainty of intention in the commercial context in Chapter 3.

In Chapter 3, it was suggested that the courts may well be taking different approaches to establishing traditional validity requirements as trusts start to appear in settings that are different from the ones that underpinned the emergence of modern validity requirements. We learned at that point that, even in the 1970s and in *Re Kayford* itself, there was an awareness of distinguishing arrangements concerning private individuals who deal with commercial concerns and those between commercial parties dealing 'at arm's length'. The Law Commission asserted, in its report *Trustee Exemption Clauses* (Law Com No. 301) in 2006, that generally trusts are increasingly becoming instruments of choice for parties who are quite different from traditional trust actors. With most emphasis on the settlor in this context, the Law Commission did observe more generally that settlors in the business context are repeat players of equal strength in known dealings. So how might this affect how the courts approach questions of whether what was said or done is or is not to be regarded as equivalent to saying 'I declare myself trustee'? And it was noted in Chapter 3, in the discussion of the significance of *Pearson* v *Lehman Bros Finance SA* [2010] EWHC 2914 (Ch), that what is required generally for trust formation might well be (or might well be becoming) differently configured as between trusts arising in the commercial context and for traditional interpersonal, or familial, relations. And as we noted in Chapter 3, this core idea has been developed further in *Crossco No. 4 Unlimited* v *Jolan Limited* [2011] EWCA Civ 1619. This line of thought is itself developed further in Chapter 18.

Is a self-declaration of trust treated as a supplemental question?

In *Re Kayford* itself, where intention to create a trust was found, there was certainly suggestion that a different result might well have arisen had those standing to lose out been commercial creditors rather than ordinary members of the public. Because the cases are not very direct about the supplemental issue of self-declaration of trust, which should operate on top of satisfying certainty of intention, we might assume that Megarry J's views also apply to making a self-declaration of trust in addition to establishing certainty of intention. This suggests that the court might not so readily have concluded equivalence to saying 'I declare myself trustee' for the benefit of commercial creditors, before account was taken of *Re Multi Guarantee* [1987] BCLC 257, in which there was not scope for establishing the all-important permanent and irrevocable decision concerning the money in the bank account. In the case of the slightly different *Quistclose* arrangement, the position that the existence of a trust is determined by *Twinsectra* v *Yardley* observations on what a creditor intended (*Twinsectra* v *Yardley* [2002] 2 WLR 802, as considered in Chapter 18), which might suggest that commercial dealings—and even informal ones—are actually quite different from those arising from private, and often familial, relations.

Might self-declarations of trusts be victims of policy considerations?

The way in which both *Re Kayford* and also *Quistclose* arrangements are most commonly found in the context of financial distress adds a further gloss on how differently the courts might regard equivalence to saying 'I declare myself trustee', and both types of arrangement have been criticized at various points for providing secured credit without taking security for creditors of businesses. The decision in *Re Farepak* [2007] 2 BCLC 1 suggests that, in tough economic times, there is judicial reluctance to find that anyone is privileged in the event of an insolvency—even those whom Sir Robert Megarry in *Re Kayford* would have regarded as ordinary members of the public. It has already been suggested that *Farepak* should have succeeded in *Re Kayford* principles, and that one explanation of this is a rigid adherence to insolvency law as a tough response to tough economic times. If this is the case, then it suggests at the very least that it might become more difficult to establish equivalence to saying 'I declare myself trustee' in such arrangements. It might also suggest a paradigm shift towards a more 'arm's length' approach for all who are dealing with businesses, whether they are commercial creditors or not, on the ground that there is a range of persons who can be affected by business failure and that it is bad policy to create a privileged position for any one group in absence of the clearest evidence of an intention to do so. This would suggest that the courts are increasingly mindful of the scope for the creation of trusts in commercial dealings. It also suggests that they view such arrangements as ones that require different 'validity considerations' from the type of arrangements that have been paradigms for the modern law on validity. This is considered in Chapter 18.

 Revision Box

1. In understanding the significance of *Milroy* v *Lord* (1862) 4 De GF & J 264 in transfers of property from one person to another (intended as outright transfers or transfers of nominal legal title to a trustee), consider the key decisions in *Jones* v *Lock* (1865) LR 1 Ch App 25 and *Richards* v *Delbridge* (1874) LR Eq 11.
   (a) Look at the facts surrounding the two cases and the reasons for the decisions reached.
   (b) Ensure that you understand why their outcomes followed from application of *Milroy*.
   (c) Relate the results and their reasonings back to the proposition that equity functions so as to provide flexibility and to prevent injustice, and also to protect and support legal rights.
   (d) Respond to the proposition that, in the course of carrying out these functions, tensions can arise between supporting the supremacy of legal rights and achieving justice for a claimant.

→

→

2. To be sure that you understand the mechanics of a self-declaration of trust and also its implications, after reading the judgment in *Pennington, Choithram (T) International SA v Pagarani* [2001] 2 All ER 492, read Rickett (2001) 65 Conv 515.
   (a) Explain in your own words what you understand to be Rickett's views on this decision, indicating whether or not you agree, and why.
   (b) Consider whether, in your studies of equity's role in transfers of property, you have encountered any evidence that equity has ever striven officiously to defeat a gift.
   (c) Consider whether *Jones* and *Richards* could be seen as examples of where equity *has* officiously striven to defeat a gift, or whether you think that these outcomes were the only possible result in the circumstances.
   (d) Explain, giving reasons for your views, whether you think the courts should adopt a more cautious approach or a more liberal approach to finding that a trust has been constituted.
3. Consider whether you think there are any dangers in adopting an approach that treats making gifts and express trust creation as 'the same' (or substantially the same), indicating what these might be.

FURTHER READING

Bridge (1992) 'The *Quistclose* trust in a world of secured transactions' 12 Oxford Journal of Legal Studies 333.

Garton (2003) 'The role of the trust mechanism in the rule in *Re Rose*' 67 Conveyancer 364.

Halliwell (2003) 'Perfecting imperfect gifts and trusts: have we reached the end of the Chancellor's foot?' 67 Conveyancer 192.

Lowrie and Todd (1998) '*Re Rose* revisited' 57 Cambridge Law Journal 46.

Luxton (2012) 'In search of perfection: the Re Rose rule rationale' 1 Conveyancer 70.

Millett (1985) 'The *Quistclose* trust: who can enforce it?' 101 Law Quarterly Review 269.

Rickett (2001) 'Completely constituting an *inter vivos* trust: property rules? 65 Conveyancer 515.

Tham (2006) 'Careless share giving' 70 Conveyancer 411.

 online resource centre For summaries of a selection of these articles, please visit <http://www.oxfordtextbooks.co.uk/orc/wilson_trusts11e/>

6

Introduction to resulting and constructive trusts

This chapter flows from the introduction, in Chapter 2, to implied trusts as being different from express trusts. Its two starting points are as follows.

- The first is the fundamental principle of trusts law that emerged from the principle in *Westdeutsche Landesbank Girozentrale* v *Islington London Borough Council* [1996] AC 669 that the basis for all trusts is conscience.
- The second relates to the way in which, up to now, the attention that has been paid to trusts that are *private* (rather than publicly enforceable charitable trusts), has related to trusts that have been termed 'express private trusts'.

This chapter introduces trusts that arise on the basis of conscience, but which are different from 'express trusts' because they arise in ways other than as a result of a settlor's express intention to create a trust. This might seem rather odd, given the attention that has been given to the requirements for creating valid private trusts, and especially the ones relating to certainty (of intention) and the constitution of trusts. But what follows in this chapter is an introduction to trusts that arise, but are not expressly created.

Following this, in Chapters 7, 8, and 9, is an extensive exploration of non-express private trusts, pursued through a number of 'case studies'. These show how non-express private trusts arise in a number of settings in everyday life, and help to explain how they work in these individual settings, as well as more generally. Before any of this can happen, there must be some appreciation of why, having gone to the trouble to formulate the 'requirements for validity', equity permits trusts to arise where they have not been expressly created, and indeed why equity has actually 'relaxed' some of the requirements that are otherwise in place for (express) trusts to be valid.

6.1 Introducing trusts that are 'implied': their significance and rationale

It was made clear at the outset that 'property' is at the heart of equity's development of the trust instrument as it has been represented up to now—as one that reflects the express intention of an owner of property to confer a benefit to another. And the central significance of 'property' can also be found in the way in which equity recognizes trusts that are implied alongside those that are express.

The term 'implied trust' in English trusts law denotes trusts other than those expressly declared by the settlor. But both are premised on the importance of the concept of property in English law more generally. Earlier chapters touched on the importance of 'ownership' in English law, because this provides the basis for the high levels of autonomy enjoyed by an owner of property in his use and application of property. An owner of property can do more or less anything with it; this includes his right to enjoy the property, but also includes the right that he has to confer it, or to *give it*, to another. As the first chapter explained, in English law, ownership is manifested in legal title to property, and Chapters 1 and 2 pointed to the way in which, in relation to the express private trust, there are both 'settlor-oriented' and 'beneficiary-oriented' attractions to creating a trust.

In the development of 'non-express trusts', equity acknowledges that the implications of the ownership of property can be very complex. And in developing trusts that do not have to be expressly declared by an owner of property in order to be valid, it is clear that equity is seeking to respond to the *injustices* that can arise from the ownership of property.

Understanding implied trusts and 'locating' injustice in the ownership of property

To help us to understand why equity might have developed implied trusts as a response to injustices arising from ownership of property, once again reference is made to the very beginnings of this text: Chapter 1 considered the way in which 'rights' to, or 'interests' in, property are characteristically very valuable rights. Here, legal title to property ensures that these rights are sufficiently certain. This is because it is important for the owner of property to be certain that he has the capacity to deal freely with his property from his own perspective, and also given that 'dealings' with property are likely to affect the positions of third parties.

The appearance of so-called constructive and resulting trusts is essentially a response to tensions inherent in property and ownership. This is because property rights are extremely valuable and form the basis of many transactional dealings, and this suggests that the position on who can deal with property should be *certain*. However, there can be circumstances in which this commitment to certainty can cause *injustice* to another party to arise. In other words, recognizing only legal title in circumstances in which no express trust has been declared can lead to the interests of another (namely, not the legal owner) being 'overlooked'. Equity's response to this has been that distinct equitable interest in property (in favour of someone other than the legal, and apparently only, 'owner') can subsist even in circumstances under which no express trust of property has been declared. In short, the study of implied trusts has at its 'core' the tensions between ensuring certainty and achieving justice in relation to property.

Focusing preliminary understanding on the key functions and rationale of implied trusts

Shortly, we will learn that there are two types of implied trust that have been developed by equity, and then we will give detailed consideration to so-called 'resulting trusts' and 'constructive trusts'. At this initial stage, we need to appreciate that the essence of an implied trust is that, in certain circumstances, equity will *imply* that an asset being held by another (evidenced by the location of legal title) is to be held wholly or partly for someone other than the holder of legal title. In these circumstances, equity will *imply* a trust where a trust of that property has not been expressly declared. When working through the book, it should be borne in mind that when equity implies a trust, it does so because the interests of justice are greater than prioritizing the position of 'certainty' that attaches to legal title.

- It will also become apparent that, because these trusts will arise in circumstances under which they are not being declared and parties are often unaware that they have arisen, they are not treated as express trusts in many respects.

- The most important consequence of a trust being implied rather than express is that the former type are exempt from formalities that would otherwise pertain to property in the creation of a trust. We have already touched on the significance of this in the *Re Rose*-type cases in Chapter 5, and will do so again much more extensively in Chapter 8.

Different types of implied trust

To introduce the study of implied trusts, up to now attention has been paid to identifying the concept of a trust that is non-express, and also the *unifying features* shared by trusts not expressly declared, in terms of: their *basis in conscience* (in common with all trusts); *how they arise* (notably, they are not expressly declared); *their rationale* in the context of justice; and how they are not subject to all of the requirements tjat must otherwise be met for a private trust to be valid. What needs to be stressed at this point is that there are actually two different types of implied trust.

While all implied trusts can be seen as a response to equity's concern about justice, the precise nature of the response will depend on the circumstances in which the injustice arises and what is required to address it. This need for different responses to different types of injustice has led to the evolution of the 'resulting trust' and the 'constructive trust'. During this chapter, the following will become clear.

- The *resulting trust* is recognition that ownership in property vests in someone other than the apparent owner (the person who holds legal title to property). Understanding this requires us to look closely at the circumstances in which resulting trusts arise, and to appreciate that a beneficiary under a resulting trust is always the original owner of property (who, when this trust arises because legal title has been transferred to another, becomes the 'settlor').

- The *constructive trust* arises in a wide variety of circumstances and fact situations, and there is a widely held view that, in English law, it arises in response to some kind of 'wrong' that is committed by the holder of legal title to property. Here, a trust is imposed because the holder's conscience is said to be affected by his conduct, and as a result he does continue to hold legal title, but he does so as trustee, and this thus makes his 'title' to the property subject to the interests of another.

6.2 An introduction to resulting trusts

Chapter 2 noted that resulting trusts can be difficult to pin down, and that this is mainly because they can be found in a number of very diverse factual situations. It was also suggested that at the heart of all resulting trusts could be found a fundamental characteristic that overarches all of the different factual manifestations and applications—that is, that the settlor and the beneficiary are *always* the same person.

Settlor and beneficiary are the same person

Whilst legal title will become vested in a trustee, the settlor and the beneficiary will always be the same person, and Chapter 2 signposted that this arises from two broad scenarios:

- a trust for the settlor-beneficiary can arise where he has tried, but failed, to create an express trust in favour of a third party, in which case the equitable interest that is created on the transfer of legal title never actually leaves him; and

- it can also arise where property has been divested from the settlor, but for some reason equitable interest in it is at a later date returned to him, on account of an event that has not been foreseen by the donor and hence (or perhaps because of bad drafting) this 'contingency' has not been provided for.

This latter is explained here, alongside a further situation in which a resulting trust can arise.

Shortly, we will look at the creation of the resulting trust on the basis of the *Westdeutsche* determination that, unless and until there is separation of titles, while one person holds property absolutely no distinct equitable title actually exists, and equitable ownership is instead encompassed within the legal title that is held. It is the position post-*Westdeutsche* that equitable title is actually created, and this occurs when legal title is transferred to another—because the conscience of its recipient is affected. For the sake of simplicity, at this point it is best to try to keep in mind that equitable interest created in property as a result of the transfer of legal title *remains with* the settlor, or it is *returned to* him. In this manner, a resulting trust can be seen to provide the basis of a claim for his recovery of his own property. Understanding this is vital, because what follows is a brief consideration of a number of factual situations to which this 'remains with—or returns to' model can be applied.

6.2.1 **Where and in what situations do resulting trusts arise?**

There is much apparent simplicity in the statement above that the resulting trust is 'recognition that ownership of property vests in someone other than' the person who, by holding legal title, appears to own it. However, resulting trusts can be difficult to pin down further because they are found in numerous fact situations that are actually very diverse. And, from this, they can be more difficult to appreciate than constructive trusts, which are (with a possible limited exception that will be considered in due course) impositions of trusteeship in unconscionable situations.

The starting point for understanding resulting trusts, and appreciating where they arise and why they do so, is that all resulting trusts do have one element in common—that is, that the original owner of property that becomes trust property is actually the beneficiary under a resulting trust. The trust arises because legal title is transferred to another, and so here the owner becomes the settlor, but the circumstances in which this transfer arises will ensure that the settlor will also become the beneficiary under the trust arrangement that now exists. But where do these trusts arise and how are they recognizable?

In short, legal title is vested in a trustee, while the settlor and the beneficiary are actually the same person. Some reference has already been made to this in respect of certainty requirements and the absence of certainty (considered in Chapter 3), and by way of introduction it is important to appreciate, at a basic level, when the resulting trust can arise.

(1) Situations in which a resulting trust can be implied include:

where the settlor has tried to create a trust in favour of a third-party beneficiary and, although legal title has been transferred from him, he has failed to divest himself of equitable interest in the property (in which case, equitable title never leaves him), *or* property has been divested from him successfully initially, but it is for some reason later returned back to him; and

where there has been what is known as a 'voluntary conveyance' of property to another, in which case title to property is transferred to another in circumstances under which no consideration is given. A resulting trust being 'implied' is based on the proposition that, in circumstances under which legal title is transferred to another, it is inappropriate for this to confer upon its new holder all of the entitlements of ownership: this will create a distinct equitable interest that will not 'follow' legal title.

(2) Why are the settlor and beneficiary the same person? Applying these situations to 'trust actors':

where an owner of property attempts to settle property on trust for a third-party beneficiary, but fails to do so, the equitable interest that is created on the transfer of legal title never actually leaves him;

where property has been divested from the settlor, but for some reason equitable interest in it is returned back to him at a later date, equitable interest is said to result to him on account of an unforeseen event not provided for, or through careless drafting of the trust; and

where there has been a voluntary conveyance, the owner of that property becomes settlor when he conveys legal title to the new legal owner, and a beneficiary under the trust is created because it is inappropriate for the new holder of legal title to have the full entitlements of ownership when no consideration has been provided.

6.2.2 **How resulting trusts are classified**

Before engaging in detailed consideration of resulting trust fact situations, we need to give some explanation of the way in which resulting trusts of different types are classified. This is the starting point for understanding the fact situations that will now follow, and it will also reiterate the very first point made in this chapter: that the basis of all trusts is conscience and intention. Authority for this general position is *Westdeutsche Landesbank Girozentrale* v *Islington London Borough Council* [1996] AC 669 and, in this respect, the case has also had an important impact on the way in which resulting trusts are actually classified. Indeed, *Westdeutsche* precipitated a rethinking of their traditional classification as 'automatic' and 'presumed intention' resulting trusts, which was the approach adopted in *Re Vandervell's Trusts (No. 2)* [1974] Ch 269, in which Megarry J distinguished at 294 between presumed and automatic resulting trusts:

(a) The first class of case is where the transfer to B is not made on any trust ... there is a rebuttable presumption that B holds on resulting trust for A. The question is not one of the automatic consequences of a dispositive failure by A, but one of presumption: the property has been carried to B, and from the absence of consideration and any presumption of advancement B is presumed not only to hold the entire interest on trust but also to hold the beneficial interest for A absolutely. The presumption thus establishes both that B is to take on trust and also what that trust is. Such resulting trusts may be called 'presumed resulting trusts'.

(b) The second class of case is where the transfer to B is made on trusts which leave some or all the beneficial interest undisposed of. Here B automatically holds on resulting trust for A to the extent that the beneficial interest has not been carried to him or others. The resulting trust here does not depend on any intentions or presumptions, but is the automatic consequence of A's failure to dispose of what is vested in him. Since *ex hypothesi* the transfer is on trust, the resulting trust does not establish the trust but merely carries back to A the beneficial interest that has not been disposed of. Such resulting trusts may be called 'automatic resulting trusts'.

6.2.3 **Resulting trusts and the *Westdeutsche* reclassification**

More recently, it is clear from the decision in *Westdeutsche* that a similar, although not identical, categorization now characterizes English law. According to Lord Browne-Wilkinson, at 708:

> Under existing law a resulting trust arises in two sets of circumstances: (A) where A makes a voluntary payment to B or pays (wholly or in part) for the purchase of property which is vested either in B alone or in the joint names of A and B, there is a presumption that A did not intend to make a gift to B: the money or property is held on trust for A (if he is the sole provider of the money) or in the case of a joint purchase by A and B in shares proportionate to their contributions. It is important to stress that this is only a presumption, which presumption is easily rebutted either by the counter-presumption of advancement or by direct evidence of A's intention to make an outright transfer; (B) where A transfers property to B on express trusts, but the trusts do not exhaust the whole of the beneficial interest [with *Quistclose* trusts also found classified here].

Lord Browne-Wilkinson continued by insisting that both types of resulting trust are traditionally regarded as examples of trusts giving effect to the intention of the parties. A resulting trust is not imposed by law against the intentions of the trustee (as is a constructive trust), but gives effect to his presumed intention. This is clearly where the *Westdeutsche* categorization departs from that set out in *Vandervell*, with Lord Browne-Wilkinson suggesting that he was 'not convinced' that (category B) resulting trusts would arise 'automatically'. But it is very common still to see reference to so-called 'automatic resulting trusts', with this much in evidence in writing that seeks to theorize resulting trusts and their operation. And closely connected with this, as we work through the text, we encounter some examples of resulting trusts that really do challenge the idea that they have arisen because this was what an owner-cum-settlor intended. This is so even notwithstanding that presumed intention very much operates in the absence of a clear alternative.

6.3 **Category (B) resulting trusts: trusts that are implied from failed attempts to create trusts and from equitable interest being 'returned' at some later date**

6.3.1 **Incomplete disposal of the equitable interest**

The settlor may have made it clear that property is intended to be held on trust and may even have transferred the legal title to the trustee. There may be some reason, however, why the equitable interest is not properly disposed of. Obviously, the trustee cannot keep the trust property for himself, and so he holds it on resulting trust for the settlor; there is nowhere else for the equitable interest to go. This can be seen in the following situations.

Situations arising from difficulties concerning formalities, certainty, and public policy

Sometimes, this can arise for technical reasons. For example, we saw in Chapter 4 that formalities may be required for the disposal of an equitable interest. If these formalities are not complied with, there will be no effective disposal. In that case, the equitable interest never leaves the settlor and there is a resulting trust. *IRC* v *Broadway Cottages Trust* [1955] Ch 20 is authority that this outcome can also be seen where certainty-of-objects requirements are not complied with, as explained in Chapter 3.

A trust can also fail for public policy reasons, for example where equity has not allowed a person to retain the fruits of criminal activities, with *Cleaver* v *Mutual Reserve Fund Life Association* [1892] 1 QB 147, and also *Re Crippen* [1911] P 108 and *Re K (dec'd)* [1985] 2 WLR 262, authority that those who commit homicide will be prevented from benefiting from their victim's property.

Situations arising in which equitable interests are undefined

Another possibility is where property is settled on trust, but details of the trust are left unclear (that is, the terms of the trust fail to provide for the totality of the beneficial interest). Chapter 4 looked extensively at *Vandervell* v *IRC* [1967] 2 AC 291, considering the endowment to the Royal College of Surgeons intended to enable the organization to take the dividends declared on those shares. This case (and Vandervell's liability to surtax on the dividends) depended on whether he had divested himself of his entire interest in both the shares and the option. Because the terms of the trust were found to be insufficiently defined, the option was held on resulting trust for him, along with liability to pay surtax on the dividends. In contrast, following *Re Vandervell's Trusts (No. 2)* [1974] Ch 269, Vandervell had succeeded in divesting himself of the entire interest in these shares (the trusts were precisely defined); it was no longer necessary, for this reason, for the equitable interest to remain in the settlor, and therefore there was no resulting trust.

Situations in which a so-called 'necessary precondition' is absent

There can be other reasons, apart from a defective trust instrument, for a failure to dispose of an equitable interest. One possibility is that the body on which money or property is settled has never existed, or has ceased to exist. If a general or paramount charitable intention is shown on the part of the donor, a cy-près scheme may be applied (considered in Chapter 12 in the context of charitable trusts). Otherwise, the property will be held on resulting trust for the settlor.

Another situation is where money or property is given for a purpose, but the circumstances necessary to achieve the purpose fail to materialize. For example, in *Essery* v *Coulard* (1884) 26 ChD 191, a trust for the parties to an intended marriage, and the issue of the marriage, could not take effect when the parties decided to live together without marrying, so Pearson J held that the property was to be held on resulting trust for the settlor. Given that a subsequent marriage would not legitimate the children who had already been born, the settlor's intention to provide for all of the children had been irrevocably defeated by the failure of the parties to marry, with a similar result also pertaining in *Re Ames' Settlement* [1946] Ch 217 (which would have a different result today on account of changes to the law relating to marriage, and which was distinguished by the House of Lords in *Westdeutsche*).

Situations in which there is a partial disposal of equitable interest

Sometimes, the settlor disposes of some, but not all, of the equitable interest. Usually, this occurs because some contingency is unprovided for, perhaps because it is unforeseen or perhaps because of sloppy drafting. In this case too, the undisposed-of residue 'results' to the settlor. A good example is to be found in *Re Cochrane* [1955] Ch 309, which concerned a marriage settlement of funds for the wife and in which the contingency that occurred had simply not been provided for, so that, for a time, there was no clear disposition of the equitable interest. Not only had it not been provided for, but neither did the deed give guidance to the court as to what could have been intended. Harman J held that, for the unprovided-for period, there was a resulting trust of the income to the settlor.

Situations in which a so-called 'necessary condition' comes to an end

Where the very *raison d'être* of a trust that exists for a time then ceases to exist, there will be a resulting trust of any surplus property, as illustrated in *Hussey* v *Palmer* [1972] 1 WLR 1286. Here, a payment of £607 for improvements to property to enable a widow to live with her daughter and son-in-law was held on resulting trust for her when differences arose and she had to leave the house. In this situation, there will only ever be a resulting trust for any amount that is left over, or 'surplus', when the 'necessary condition' comes to an end. But this will not happen at all where the donor is said to have made an unconditional gift.

This arises where the donor did not intend to retain any interest in the surplus should the necessary conditions for the gift cease. In *Re the Trusts of the Abbott Fund* [1900] 2 Ch 326, a fund was collected for the relief of two deaf-and-dumb ladies (who had been defrauded out of their rights under an earlier settlement). No provision was made for disposal of the fund on the death of both of the beneficiaries. A surplus of some £367 remained when they died and Stirling J held that this should be held on resulting trust for the contributors to the fund. This is like *Re Cochrane* (see 'Situations in which there is a partial disposal of equitable interest') in that the contingency of the death of the ladies had not been provided for, but in *Abbott* it was held that the ladies themselves never became absolute owners of the fund, and neither did the trustees: once the purposes are accomplished, no resulting trust occurs if either beneficiary or trustee is intended to take absolutely.

This fund was subscribed to by various friends of the Abbotts, but where the whole of a specific fund is left by a single individual for the maintenance of given individuals, the courts are more likely to construe the transaction as an absolute gift to those individuals, even where the fund is expressed to be left for a particular purpose (although it depends, of course, on the intention of the donor, which is ultimately a question of fact). For example, in *Re Osoba* [1979] 1 WLR 247, a testator left the whole of a fund on trust for the education of his daughter up to university level; on completion of her higher education, she was held by the Court of Appeal to be entitled to the surplus. There was no resulting trust for the testator's estate, and it was found that the educational purpose was merely a statement of the testator's motive to benefit his daughter more generally.

The other possibility is a gift to the trustee. *Re Abbott* applies only where the property was intended to be held on trust, and so does not apply where the intention is to make an out-and-out gift subject to trusts (as opposed to a gift 'on trust', which is subject to the *Abbott* principle). In such cases, the trustee is clearly intended to keep the surplus. An example is *Re Foord* [1922] 2 Ch 519, in which the testator stated in his will 'all my effects including rubber and other shares I leave absolutely to my sister on trust to pay my wife £300 p.a., etc.'.

Situations in which there are anonymous subscriptions to funds

Where money has been given to a fund, say a disaster appeal fund, one might infer the donor's intention from, among other considerations, whether the donation was anonymous (as in the case of small change gathered into box from a street collection). If so, and no means of tracing the donor exists, then the contribution might be construed as an out-and-out gift. Clearly, the donor cannot have intended that any surplus left over be held on resulting trust for him, when he has left the organizers no means of finding him in the event of there being a surplus. If there is a surplus left over after the fund has fulfilled his purposes, therefore, and the fund is not charitable, that part of the surplus attributable to his donation will have no owner. It consequently goes to the Crown as *bona vacantia*.

Where the purpose of the fund is charitable, there will be a different outcome. In this case, a cy-près scheme can be invoked so as to allow the property to be applied to purposes 'as near as possible' to the original purpose. This discussion is therefore confined to funds for non-charitable purposes.

In spite of the general principle suggested, *Abbott* was followed in *Re Gillingham Bus Disaster Fund* [1958] Ch 300 (upheld on a different issue at [1958] 2 All ER 749), and such donations were directed to be held on resulting trust. The case concerned a fund collected to defray funeral and other expenses incurred as a result of a disaster involving the deaths of twenty-four Royal Marine cadets in Gillingham, and also to 'caring for the boys who may be disabled, and then to such worthy cause or causes in memory of the boys who lost their lives, as the mayors may determine'.

Harman J held that this was not a charitable purpose, and that the last purpose was void for uncertainty (on account of the certainty rules considered in Chapter 3). The purposes were therefore taken to be defraying the funeral expenses of the boys who lost their lives and caring for the boys who were disabled, and far more money was collected than was needed for this. So the question arose of who owned the surplus: was it the donors, represented by the Official Solicitor, or the Crown (represented by the HM Treasury Solicitor), as *bona vacantia*? Harman J, following *Abbott*, held that the surplus should be held on resulting trust for the donors, but with the difficulty that many of the donations were made anonymously through street collections. The trustees were compelled to hold the fund on resulting trust for unknown people.

Obviously, this is most inconvenient administratively, and it must surely be that anonymous givers can be assumed not to intend to have their gifts returned (the view taken in *Re Ulverston and District New Hospital Building Trusts* [1956] Ch 622), with an out-and-out gift seeming a far more sensible inference than a gift on trust. But had that latter inference been drawn, then the surplus would have passed as *bona vacantia* and Harman J was, in any case, reluctant to draw the inference that 'the small giver who is anonymous has any wider intention than the large giver who can be named'.

But the part of Harman J's reasoning that rested on resulting trusts arising automatically by processes of law rather than 'any evidence of state of mind of the settlor' cannot survive *Westdeutsche*. And doubt was also cast by Goff J, in *Re West Sussex Constabulary's Widows, Children and Benevolent (1930) Fund Trusts* [1971] 1 Ch 1, on Harman J's inferences about the donor's actual intention, since in the later case the out-and-out gift construction was adopted. The case concerned a fund for widows and dependants, to which the members contributed, but there were also outside contributions raised from:

(a) entertainments, raffles and sweepstakes;

(b) collecting boxes; and

(c) donations, including legacies.

When the fund was wound up at the end of 1967, upon the amalgamation of the constabulary with other police forces, Goff J held that the outside contributions raised from category (c) were held on resulting trust for the contributors. Those raised by categories (a) and (b) were clearly intended to take effect as out-and-out gifts to the fund, and therefore the resulting trust doctrine did not apply to them. It was found that category

(c) donations were indistinguishable from *Abbott Fund*, so the proportion of the surplus attributable to that source was held on resulting trust. But there were also identifiable collections from raffles and sweepstakes (category (a)), which Goff J thought were out-and-out payments subject only to a (contractual) hope of receiving a prize. For category (b) contributions, Goff J declined to follow Harman J's earlier judgment and, because nobody could lay claim to the proportion of the surplus attributable to the last two categories, this passed to the Crown as *bona vacantia*. Notwithstanding that this is a better conceptual approach, it is also clear that the courts generally strive to ensure against the operation of *bona vacantia*, such as, in the context of certainty rules, the apparent rationale for the outcome in *In the Estate of Last* [1958] 1 All ER 31.

6.4 Category (A) resulting trusts: trusts implied from a 'voluntary conveyance'

Broadly, this type of trust arises where there is a voluntary transfer of legal title to property (that is, a transfer that is not one for value). Here, it is provided that *unless* there is a presumption of advancement, the presumption is that equitable title does *not follow* legal title to the transferee, but will instead remain with the transferor. Now, there is a trust: legal title has been transferred to another, but because there has not been a transfer for value, equitable title has not passed to the new legal owner of property.

In other words, where there is a transfer of legal title to property, but the transfer has not been one for value, then although legal title has been transferred, equitable title remains with the transferor. Historically, this has been unless there is a so-called presumption of advancement, which has significantly altered the outcome of a voluntary transfer of legal title by ensuring that equitable title *will* follow legal title.

Authority for the operation of a resulting trust in voluntary conveyances
The presumption of a resulting trust in such situations has a tradition dating back at least as far as the late eighteenth century, with *Dyer* v *Dyer* (1788) 2 Cox Eq Cas 92 being the case most often cited as authority. In this case, Eyre CB remarked that:

> The trust of a legal estate, whether ... taken in the names of the purchasers and others jointly, or in the names of others without that of the purchaser; whether in the name of one or several; whether jointly or successive results to the man who advances the purchase money. This is a general proposition supported by all the cases, and there is nothing to contradict it; and it goes on a strict analogy to the rule of common law, that where a feoffment is made without consideration, the use results to the feoffer [the transferor].

In getting beyond the old-fashioned language, the effect of the presumption of a resulting trust is that equitable title effectively never leaves the transferor—that is, where the presumption is not displaced. As we will discover, equity does not want actually to defeat an owner's intentions to make a gift of his property to another where there is evidence that this is intended. And, in this regard, this position traceable to 1788 was applied much more recently to resolving disputed ownership of a National Lottery win in *Abrahams* v *Trustee in Bankruptcy of Abrahams* [1999] BPIR, 637.

The materials in Chapter 8 show how the category A resulting trust can be applied to determinations of shared home ownership. Cases such as *Stack* v *Dowden* [2007] UKHL 17 show that resulting trusts are still very significant in this sphere, but also how certain aspects of their operation—such as the traditional idea of 'purchase money resulting trusts' and the presumption of advancement—have fallen out of favour in the light of how much has clearly changed in relation to the ownership of real property since *Dyer*.

The presumption of advancement
The presumption of advancement was also mentioned in section 6.2 in both Megarry J's *Vandervell* classification of resulting trusts and also Lord Browne-Wilkinson's reclassification in *Westdeutsche*. It is alluded to in *Dyer* in Eyre CB's articulation of nothing that might contradict the operation of the resulting trust as a result of the rule of common law, whereby if a transfer is made without consideration, it results ('remains with—returns to') the transferor.

6.4.1 The presumption of the resulting trust and presumption of advancement compared

At its most simplistic, historically the operation of the presumption of advancement has produced an outcome that is the complete opposite of that of a resulting trust, ensuring that the recipient of legal title to property will also receive equitable interest in it, because equitable title has followed legal title.

Once again, this concept is rooted in history and in the ideologies of a society very different from that of today. Presumptions of advancement are historically coupled with moral obligation, but as we will see, we must also now prepare to reference the presumption itself as having an operation historically. But in terms of understanding the presumption as it has traditionally operated, the most obvious examples of moral obligations are those that exist in respect of a husband for his wife, and a father for his children, in which instances the existence of such a moral obligation was said to transform the transfer effectively to an out-and-out gift.

As materials on the Online Resource Centre explain, however, in a much fuller discussion of the presumption of advancement and its relationship with the presumption of the resulting trust, this has always been very gendered in its application and operation. Indeed, clearly and paradigmatically, it applies to a father and his children, and—as *Bennet* v *Bennet* (1879) 10 ChD 474 shows—where someone stands *in loco parentis* and thereby has an obligation like that of a parent. However, *Bennet* also shows that this does not extend to a child's mother, with a different approach being developed only recently in *Antoni* v *Antoni* [2007] UKPC 10 and *Laskar* v *Laskar* [2008] EWCA Civ 347. And whilst the presumption has for some time been regarded as a judicial instrument of last resort in cohabitation cases (with *McGrath* v *Wallis* [1995] 2 FLR 114 as authority for this, although also noting its significance in *Laskar*), the presumption has a long tradition in respect of gifts made from a husband to his wife, but it has never applied in the other direction within marriage (and never at all in relationships outside marriage).

6.4.2 Gifts, intention, and modernity and equality

Like its counterpart presumption of a resulting trust, the actual operation of a presumption of advancement in any given situation can be rebutted where there is evidence that this outcome was not intended. In *Marshal* v *Crutwell* (1875) LR 20 Eq 325 and *Re Figgis* [1969] 1 Ch 123, a very old case and a much more recent one make this point. But the value of the presumption of advancement, like all presumptions, is that it provides a way forward for a multitude of scenarios in which people do not make their intentions clear. This is particularly helpful where a donor has died and the presence of a rebuttable presumption is meant to help to clarify any uncertainties surrounding intention.

But the age of the principle, and the very gendered assumptions about property ownership and power within interpersonal relationships embodied in it, have long raised questions about the role of the presumption of advancement. This is so on account of the social and economic transformations that commenced in the second half of the twentieth century. We shall see in Chapter 8 that, for some time now, the presumption of advancement has been treated with considerable judicial dismissal in the context of shared home ownership, and the Equality Act 2010 shows more general concerns about the inequalities embodied in it.

The materials available on the Online Resource Centre also say far more about the Equality Act 2010, which, through the operation of s. 199, seeks to abolish the presumption of advancement. As the materials explain, this has not come into force as yet and will operate only prospectively (and will not apply retrospectively to arrangements subsisting prior to commencement). So the common law, as discussed, will continue to be relevant alongside the statutory provision once this has commenced. And, in relation to the latter, both the Online Resource Centre materials and also the articles that you will find listed in the online 'Reading summary' also point to a body of academic opinion against abolishing the presumption of advancement at all.

6.5 A different type of resulting trust? A final thought on resulting trusts and restitution

The remainder of this chapter considers implied trusts that are constructive, and which provide quite a different type of response to injustices that can arise in relation to property and its ownership. In terms of concluding the study of resulting trusts, it is very significant that the case with which we opened this chapter—*Westdeutsche*—can also be seen as a reference point for how resulting trusts could operate within English law, as well as providing authority for how they do so. In this regard, materials available on the Online Resource Centre explain how a resulting trust mechanism could be applied to reverse an unjust enrichment experienced by a claimant. In looking at Peter Birks' arguments that a resulting trust should arise wherever a defendant is enriched by way of mistake or failure of consideration, for example, there is further opportunity to clarify understanding of how resulting trusts work conventionally in English law.

6.6 Resulting trusts and rebutting presumed intention

This final word on resulting trusts—that is, how they *do* subsist in English law, rather than how they could—is a logical continuation of the discussion of when and where a resulting trust will be presumed. But it also has a wider significance: it can be seen as a measure of *how* comprehensively equity *does* protect property rights of those who—for lots of different reasons—are not the legal owners of the property concerned. The references made to equity *presuming* a resulting trust in particular circumstances means that we have to understand that it will not always be the case that where a resulting trust *can* arise, one actually *will*, as we have already seen in *Re Osoba* [1979] 1 WLR 247. Thus how comprehensively this mechanism is able to protect a donor's potential rights in property that is conferred to another will depend on what exactly is being presumed about the provider's intentions. This can be explored further by introducing *Air Jamaica Ltd* v *Charlton* [1999] 1 WLR 1399 (PC). This case is considered more extensively in Chapter 7, but for present purposes it is the following passage from Lord Millett's judgment that provides interesting insight into what exactly is being presumed about a donor's intentions:

> Like a constructive trust, a resulting trust arises by operation of law, though unlike a constructive trust it gives effect to intention. But it arises whether or not the transferor intended to retain a beneficial interest—he almost always does not—since it responds to the absence of any intention on his part to pass a beneficial interest to the recipient [here, the pension fund trustees].
>
> (*Air Jamaica Ltd* v *Charlton* [1999] 1 WLR 1399 (PC), *per* Millett LJ at 1412)

This means that owners can, of course, choose to give their property to others. Here, the presumption seeks to provide a safety mechanism in circumstances in which an owner will lose the rights and entitlements embodied in ownership without receiving value for this, but ultimately equity will not strive to defeat gifts that are intended. Chapter 7 deals with some of the complexities within this apparently simple position, but this is the position in principle.

6.7 An introduction to constructive trusts

The move from resulting trusts now to constructive trusts reiterates one of the important points made at the beginning of this chapter: while equity's recognition of trusts that are implied alongside those that are express can be explained as responses to 'injustice' arising in relation to ownership of property, in doing so equity has also recognized that not all situations (of injustice) will require the same response.

This accounts for the existence of constructive trusts alongside ones that are resulting, but actually explaining what constructive trusts are and what they do is much more complicated.

There are several factors that make studying constructive trusts challenging. First, they are not to be found easily defined anywhere, and many discussions of constructive trusts are premised on them not being amenable to easy definition and categorization. This is one reason why constructive trusts are also considered very flexible, which in turn means that they can be found across a number of different fact situations. Whilst many see their perceived inherent flexibility as a strength in areas in which they are applied, on account of their being very adaptable and extremely capable of meeting the ever-changing needs of society, this—along with difficulties in pinning down exactly what they are and what they do—is itself regarded with suspicion in some quarters. This has resulted in a vast body of very divided case law and academic commentary on the constructive trust. In some respects, however, they are actually easier to pin down than resulting trusts. This is because however diversely they may be applied in English law, they are widely regarded as being imposed in response to a wrong that has been committed.

In search of definition and illumination of constructive trusts

From this broad consensus that, in English law, constructive trusts arise in situations in which some kind of 'wrong' has been committed, there is also broad acceptance that constructive trusts arise from imposition rather than from presumed intention. On this reasoning, unlike a resulting trust, a constructive trust is imposed on the holder of legal title (characteristically in response to a wrong), and operates independently of (and often contrary to) his intentions.

Beyond this, however, constructive trusts have not proven easy to define. Indeed, in *Carl Zeiss Stiftung* v *Herbert Smith (No. 2)* [1969] 2 Ch 276, at 300, Edmund Davies LJ proposed that:

> English law provides no clear and all-embracing definition of a constructive trust. Its boundaries have been left perhaps deliberately vague, so as not to restrict the court by technicalities in deciding what the justice of a particular case may demand.

Instead, constructive trusts have traditionally been found to exist in a series of disparate and changing situations. This diversity of use and application of constructive trusts is comparable with that pertaining to resulting trusts, but it is also the case that all resulting trusts have the feature of a 'settlor-beneficiary'. Over and above the broad association of the constructive trust with cthe ommission of a wrong, clarifying the meaning of constructive trust has to be considered much more closely in reference to explaining *where* and *how* they arise.

Issues of intention and the courts' 'imposition' of a constructive trust

In working towards this, Edmund Davies LJ's judgment in *Carl Zeiss Stiftung* v *Herbert Smith* also ties into the notions of flexibility and adaptability that were considered at the outset. Similarly, subsequently in *Sen* v *Headley* [1991] Ch 425, Nourse LJ commented that the constructive trust had been a 'ready means of developing our property law in modern times'.

At the heart of discovering what constructive trusts might be and where they can be seen to arise is how, although capable of arising in numerous and diverse circumstances, implied trusts of this nature have a very important fundamental characteristic in common: they are trusts imposed by the courts and they operate irrespective of the actual intention of the owner (of what becomes the 'trust property'). This should be borne in mind in this very brief overview of the different situations in which constructive trusts can arise and the consequences of them doing so.

Circumstances in which a constructive trust arises

Ahead of the extensive and detailed consideration of constructive trusts (along with resulting trusts) in subsequent chapters, examples are now given of situations in which constructive trusts arise. The consequences of this are largely held over for discussion in the dedicated case study chapters.

6.8 Situations in which constructive trusts have been found to exist

Again, like the resulting trust, constructive trusts have come to be applied to numerous and diverse factual situations, from which a number of illustrative examples can be drawn.

(i) The significance of constructive trusts in the application of implied trusts to cohabitation of family homes

In the earlier, and very brief, reference made to the importance of implied trusts for shared family home ownership, it was explained that any detailed discussion would be held over until now, and indeed that much more would follow in the dedicated case study in Chapter 8. But it is appropriate here to signpost that both constructive and resulting trusts are important because of the *general* importance of implied trusts for responding to injustices surrounding disputed home ownership.

In Chapter 8, it will become clear that the constructive trust, particularly, has become central in the 'battleground' of difficulties created where a party who is not the legal owner of property can be left disadvantaged, even where resulting trust principles descending from *Dyer* v *Dyer* will allow those who have made financial contributions to a home that does not belong to them in law to 'retain' a proportionate interest in the home. The resulting trust in this respect represents a 'strict property' approach and what can be recovered is limited *by*, and indeed *to* (in proportionate terms), what is actually contributed.

Because of this, the constructive trust has come to be recognized as a more flexible response to injustice that can be caused to a non-legal owner of property in circumstances in which the parties have reached an agreement in respect of owning their home that is not reflected in legal ownership, or because representations have been made in relation to the property by the person who is its legal owner. The constructive trust can be more flexible because it allows a party who is not the legal owner to acquire a share in the property of another that is not determined by (and thus limited to) the contributions made. Here, the constructive trust will allow a non-legal owner to acquire a share that reflects the agreement reached *with*, or the representations that have been made *by*, the legal owner, by holding the latter to the agreement or representation. The landmark decision in *Lloyds Bank* v *Rosset* [1991] 1 AC 10 shows how central the constructive trust is for the modern law relating to shared beneficial ownership, with this more recently embodied in key decisions of the House of Lords and Supreme Court in *Stack* v *Dowden* [2007] UKHL 17 and *Jones* v *Kernott* [2011] UKSC 53, respectively.

In the period intervening after *Rosset*, strong judicial favour for proprietary estoppel rather than the constructive trust emerged from *Oxley* v *Hiscock* [2004] 3 All ER 703. Authority for applying proprietary estoppel to disputed ownership of family homes actually came from *Rosset* itself and, together with a number of earlier Court of Appeal authorities in the broader sphere of 'land law', *Oxley* had sought to emphasize the points of commonality between constructive trust and proprietary estoppel principles—notably, as mechanisms for holding persons to their representations or conduct—at the same time as suggesting that estoppel would produce a fairer and more appropriate approach, even if the actual outcomes would be the same in a number of cases.

Stack *v* Dowden *and the new significance for implied trusts in the context of shared home ownership*

This text had always suggested that the profound differences between the two doctrines meant that it was difficult to regard them interchangeably. In *Stack*, the prominence of trusts rather than estoppel was placed firmly back centre stage. The House of Lords appeared firmly of the view (for reasons that will be explained in due course) that the trusts approach reflected better the valuable property rights that are at stake in these determinations.

There was less consensus in *Stack* about which type of implied trust should properly apply in these situations. In making the case in favour of the resulting trust, Lord

Neuberger was clearly impressed with its ability to reflect the actual contributions made by a party, with this grounding his view that the courts' starting point should be the resulting trust, and that departure from this in favour of a more flexible constructive trust should occur only where it is evident that (essentially) this was intended.

In this sense, Lord Neuberger was the most conservative judge, and Lady Hale and Lords Hope and Walker were much more in favour of applying a constructive trust approach to reflect the way in which (in Lady Hale's words) the law has 'moved on in response to changing social and economic conditions' from the approach of the resulting trust, which (inappropriately) recognizes only a limited number of contributions (as capable of counting in these situations).

Stack v Dowden *and explaining the significance of the 'ambulatory constructive trust'*

There was also some discussion by their Lordships of the assumptions traditionally built into resolving disputed home ownership, and especially that parties' intentions have been taken to be 'fixed' at the time of acquisition of title (to the property). Lord Neuberger and, especially, Lord Hoffman considered the possibilities of applying a so-called 'ambulatory constructive trust' approach. Essentially, the ambulatory approach is one that recognizes that people's intentions about the ownership of their home often evolve over time in any case, and can be very strongly influenced by the conduct of the parties in relation to the home during their cohabitation of it. For Lords Neuberger and Hoffmann, this would help to respond to the situation in which, for example, the non-legal owner of a home made significant capital improvements to a home owned by another, which significantly increased the value of the property. But we can now see this approach at work in response to a different situation in the Supreme Court ruling in *Jones* v *Kernott*.

(ii) Constructive trusts arising in the creation of 'mutual wills'

Mutual wills arise when two people (usually couples) agree, by the creation of mutual wills, to effect the situation in which, on the death of the first of them, their property shall be enjoyed by the survivor, and thereafter (on the death of the second) pass to beneficiaries who have been nominated. It will become apparent that the constructive trust becomes an issue in response to questions of whether, and to what extent, their original 'mutual' agreement does actually control and even dictate the distribution of their property.

Further discussion of mutual wills in terms of their key issues and their relationship with constructive trusts can be found on the Online Resource Centre materials dedicated to the study of so-called 'equitable fraud'.

(iii) Constructive trusts arising from the commission of crime

There are good reasons of policy that suggest why a perpetrator of a crime should be prevented from benefiting from it. At its most extreme, this would operate to ensure that a murderer is not able to benefit from his killing of a testator under whose will he will benefit. The most famous illustration of this principle is the case of Dr Crippen, whose conduct has already been considered within the material relating to resulting trusts in sections 6.2, 6.3, and 6.4. This case is also discussed in the Online Resource Centre materials on fraud.

(iv) Trusteeship and liability following breach of trust

There are *two broad ways* in which equity's imposition of a constructive trust has become influential in responding to breaches of trust committed by a trustee, with both flowing from breach of trust amounting to conduct disregarding the interests of the beneficiary. They are different because while one responds to this in respect of the trustee who is committing the breach of trust himself, the second acknowledges that a trustee's breach of trust can also involve others who are otherwise unconnected with the trust. This latter situation can itself occur in two recognizable ways: first, trust property might fall into the hands of a third party unconnected with the trust; and second, it may well be that the trustee had help, or 'assistance', in committing the breach of trust. Both of these persons are known as 'strangers' to the trust, because they are otherwise unconnected with it, but they can nevertheless incur liability where there is a breach of trust by a trustee. The connections between constructive trusts and 'stranger' liability are considered after it is explained how constructive trusts are significant in the position of a trustee who makes an unauthorized profit from his position.

Unauthorized profit by a trustee or other fiduciary
The materials in Chapter 13 explain that any occupant of a fiduciary position (including, but not confined to, the trustee) must act unequivocally in the interests of the person in respect of whom the fiduciary position arises. This means that a fiduciary will not be able to keep for his own use property acquired directly or indirectly from his position. Chapter 13 explores how constructive trusts can arise in making a trustee liable 'to account' to the trust for any such 'unauthorized profits', with discussion of *Sinclair Investments (UK) Ltd* v *Versailles Trade Finance Ltd* [2011] EWCA Civ 347 and its favour for a personal liability approach rather than imposing a constructive trust, and the significance of this decision in the light of traditional approaches.

Further, and notwithstanding traditional applications of the constructive trust in the context of unauthorized profit and the very clear applications for constructive trusts for the liability of others following a breach of trust (as we will see next), *Foskett* v *McKeown* [2000] 2 WLR 1299 is authority that the wrongful appropriation of trust property by a trustee should not be viewed not as creating a constructive trust for the trustee himself, but as giving rise to the liability arising from the process of tracing (which is discussed fully in Chapter 17).

Liability of third-party 'strangers' in breach-of-trust situations: the basic idea
Chapter 17 on beneficiary actions considers a beneficiary's position where trust property has been applied by a trustee acting in breach of trust. It will become clear that an area of particular difficulty is the liability that can be incurred by persons other than the trustee who actually commits the breach. It does, of course, follow that the beneficiary should be able to pursue a remedy in respect of trust property against a trustee acting in breach of trust, but it is also the case that persons other than the trustee may come into possession of misapplied trust property, or may even have assisted the trustee's initial breach.

Where persons who are not actually appointed trustees under a settlement find themselves in receipt of trust property (usually on account of it being 'taken' from the trust in breach of trust), or otherwise 'interfere' with the proper administration of a trust, they can be constituted 'constructive trustees'. This forms part of a suite of actions considered in Chapter 17, with emphasis now only on *facilitation* of liability for breach of trust through the machinery of the constructive trust.

Third parties and liability following a trustee's breach of trust
Traditionally, 'stranger liability' has been divided into two categories of 'knowing receipt' (of trust property) and 'knowing assistance' (of a breach of trust). The reason for attaching third-party liability to *receipt of trust property* is explained in Chapter 17

in terms of how it relates to the limitations of the proprietary action of tracing, which requires missing property to continue to exist and to be identifiable to be recoverable. We will learn that tracing *is* sufficiently flexible that the property need not be *physically* identifiable as such, because it may well have been sold; in these circumstances, it may still be possible to trace the *proceeds* of sale, subject to the rules that apply to tracing trust money that has become 'mixed' with other funds.

The value of recipient liability attaches to providing a remedy even where property no longer exists in an identifiable form. So when trust money is spent with nothing identifiable to show for it, a recipient of it can still become a constructive trustee of it where he receives trust property with some degree of knowledge of the trust. There is contention as to the degree of knowledge that is required, but, fundamentally, receipt-based liability is complete *upon* receipt and does not require property to remain in the recipient's hands in order for him to incur liability. Here, constructive trusteeship will arise upon receipt; what happens to the property thereafter is immaterial.

In a similar vein, a stranger to a trust is also able to incur liability on the basis of his *assistance of a trustee's breach of trust*. This was traditionally known as 'knowing assistance', but a new approach now characterizes this as 'accessory liability'. This liability is focused on acting as an accessory to a trustee's breach of trust and has increasingly become associated with an accessory's *dishonesty*, rather than his *knowledge*.

The two species of liability have always differed from one another because it is only a knowing recipient who must actually receive trust property for liability to arise. An assistant, or accessory, is arguably more difficult to fix with trusteeship, because no property is actually received (to which the constructive trust can attach).

Notwithstanding this obvious difference, and on account of their otherwise similar nature in relation to liability, the two categories have generally been treated together and remain so.

They are considered in Chapter 17, in light of leading case law: *Royal Brunei Airlines v Tan* [1995] 2 AC 378; *BCCI v Akindale* [2000] 4 All ER 211; *Twinsectra v Yardley* [2002] 2 All ER 377; *Barlow Clowes International Ltd (in liquidation) v Eurotrust International Ltd* [2006] 1 All ER 333; *Abou-Rahmah v Kadir Abacha* [2006] EWCA Civ 1492; and *Starglade Properties v Nash* [2010] EWCA Civ 1314.

(v) Other situations that can give rise to a constructive trust

These remaining 'other cases' are, like the earlier examples, premised on a common acceptance that constructive trusts all appear to be responses to some kind of 'wrongdoing'. What we seek to do with these two final examples is explore what might actually be meant by 'wrongdoing', and what the limitations of associating constructive trusteeship with imposition of a trust in response to a wrong committed by the legal owner of property might be.

Constructive trusts arising where there is a specifically enforceable contract

A contract is specifically enforceable where (common law contractual) damages would not be an adequate remedy. Although contracts for the sale of personal property are seldom specifically enforceable because of their 'unique' nature, contracts for the sale of land are. How this translates into the creation of a constructive trust is illustrated in *Lysaght v Edwards* (1876) 2 ChD 499. This case proposes that, on account of equity's willingness to enforce such contracts specifically, on the conclusion of the sale the purchaser is considered the owner in equity and, accordingly, the vendor becomes a trustee of the land (property) for the purchaser. The concept of constructive trusteeship arising from specifically enforceable contracts was considered very briefly in Chapter 1. Beyond this very broad proposition, theorization of the way in which specific enforceability engaged a trust situation is not pursued further, save to point out that while there is an element of 'conscience' present, there is arguably a lesser exhibition of improper conduct on the part of the purchaser than in other situations in which constructive trusts are seen to arise.

Does a constructive trust arise where a trust is constituted under the 'rule in Re Rose'?

In Chapter 5, in the discussion on constitution of trusts generally and the 'last act' (of the settlor) doctrine more specifically, it was suggested that there are many questions raised by the decision in *Re Rose, Rose* v *IRC* [1952] Ch 499, and that this is so even if it must be seen as correct and thus as good law (which Court of Appeal endorsement of it in *Mascall* v *Mascall* (1984) 50 P & CR 119 appears to confirm). It was suggested in Chapter 5 that the precise mechanism operating in this case is unclear, but one explanation might lie in the imposition of a constructive trust by equity during the period *after* the transfer had occurred in equity, but *before* it could take place in common law. In the course of making this suggestion, concern was expressed about this as a possibility, because of the apparent inconsistency between the conferment of a gift and the more usual manner in which a constructive trust is invoked in order to impose on the conscience of the legal owner of property on account of his conduct. If this is the case, then the constructive trust in *Re Rose* seems anomalous with the other situations listed so far. Here, the donor clearly had done nothing wrong, and was actively demonstrating generosity in both his intended outright gift and in the express trust that he did seek, although some might consider it unconscionable if the volunteer recipient were to 'miss out'.

6.9 Is the constructive trust too flexible and too adaptable?

The earlier introduction to constructive trusts pointed to the difficulties entailed in defining them. This was aligned very closely with the flexibility of the constructive trust, and pointed to case law suggesting that it was an extremely useful and adaptable instrument. Although there is much intellectual respect for such views within judicial and academic circles alike, it is not a universal view and certainly not one that is beyond question. Indeed, there is a strong view that, during the 1970s and 1980s, the constructive trust became too flexible and Lord Denning's 'new model' constructive trust began to be employed (in his Lordship's own words, in his judgment in *Hussey* v *Palmer* [1972] 1 WLR 1338) 'wherever justice and good conscience require it'. This use of the constructive trust might be regarded as an approach based on outcomes and result, rather than principle or sound theory, as indicated by the statement of Sir Peter Millett (1995) 9 Tru LI 35 that 'the language of constructive trust has become such a fertile source of confusion that it would be better if it were abandoned'. While not all reaction has been so extreme, much academic and judicial commentary has advocated greater employment of the great adversary of flexibility—that is, the need for certainty.

6.9.1 A place in English law for the remedial constructive trust?

The constructive trust in English case law can be seen as a substantive institution that operates to vindicate an existing property right. But this is not the case in many other jurisdictions (including Commonwealth jurisdictions such as Australia, New Zealand, and Canada), which accept also, alongside the *substantive* institutional constructive trust, the existence of a different *remedial*-type constructive trust that, at its most radical, may operate to create a new proprietary interest for the claimant, rather than simply to formalize and provide validity for an interest that already exists and to which the courts will give recognition. While the existence of the remedial constructive trust in English law has been left open, it is clearly a principle that is regarded with suspicion in the highest judicial circles. Indeed, the commentary of Lord Millett (1995) 9 Tru LI 35 suggests that it is a device for which there is no room in English law, and one that is actually capable of causing much mischief:

> In our view it is a counsel of despair which too readily concedes the impossibility of propounding a general rationale for the availability of proprietary remedies. We need to be more ready to categorize wrongdoers as fiduciaries and to extend the situations in which proprietary remedies are made available, but we can still do all this while adhering to established principles.

6.9.2 Trusts, conscience, and the 'overlapping' of resulting and constructive trusts

There is, at present, much confusion in the law between resulting trusts and constructive trusts. Consequently, the theoretical differences between them are not clear-cut and it can be difficult, on particular fact situations, to determine which type of implied trust will arise. This will become particularly plain in our later analysis of trusts arising from cohabitation and family arrangements. But, for present purposes, the way in which confusion is easily reached in an analysis of constructive and resulting trusts is illustrated by reference to an extract from Lord Denning's judgment in *Hussey* v *Palmer* [1972] 1 WLR 1286, at 1289:

> Although the plaintiff alleged that there was a resulting trust, I should have thought that the trust in this case, if there was one, was more in the nature of a constructive trust; but this is a matter of words than anything else. The two run together.

The ways in which this 'blurring' of distinctions can be seen to operate, as well as an assessment of the view that it is a distinction only in rhetoric, shall be carried over into the area in which it can be illustrated most graphically—trusts relating to the family home, considered in Chapter 8.

 Revision Box

1. Drawing on the materials in the chapter and using them as illustration, ensure that you can answer the following questions.
   (a) Why has equity developed implied trusts alongside express ones declared by a settlor?
   (b) Why can the existence of implied trusts be seen as a particularly bold development in the context of the ownership of property?
   (c) Why has equity developed two quite different types of implied trust?

   ➡

➙

2. In relation to resulting trusts, explain the following.
   (a) What key feature underpins all resulting trusts and how does this explain the way in which they operate?
   (b) How can this be illustrated by reference to actual examples of where they can be found?
3. Using the materials above and also textbook accounts of 'constructive trusts', return to *Re Rose, Rose* v *IRC* [1952], and consider whether the trusts that arose from equity's recognition of property transfers that were incomplete at law should be regarded as constructive trusts. Here, you should consider:
   – the basis of constructive trusts strongly apparent from 'constructive trusts theory'; and
   – observations on imposition of constructive trusts made in Lowrie and Todd (1998) 57 CLJ 46.

FURTHER READING

Lowrie and Todd (1998) '*Re Rose* revisited' 57 Cambridge Law Journal 46.

Millett (1995) 'Equity: the road ahead' 9 Trust Law International 35.

Because this chapter was introductory in nature, further reading can generally be found under substantive consideration of resulting and constructive trusteeship in Chapters 7, 8, and 9.

 online resource centre For summaries of a selection of these articles, please visit <http://www.oxfordtextbooks.co.uk/orc/wilson_trusts11e/>

7

Resulting trusts, gifts to non-charitable unincorporated associations, and pension funds

A number of the chapters in this book, which follow previous chapters' introductions to constructive and resulting trusts, are case studies that require us to look at constructive and resulting trusts closely alongside each other. All of the case studies focus on the features and characteristics of constructive or resulting trusts, which were introduced in the previous chapter. The case studies also try to communicate how these instruments work in operation, and consider critically whether, and in what ways, their operation 'in reality' reflects textbook assessments that are made of them. In the same vein, this chapter on unincorporated associations and pension funds follows one introducing constructive and resulting trusts, and as such is a case study on the features and operation of trusts that are 'resulting'. By way of reminder, although resulting trusts arise in a number of different contexts, what is common to all is that, although legal title is vested in a trustee, the settlor and the beneficiary are actually the same person. This position will arise on account of two broad situations:

- it will follow a failed attempt to create a trust in favour of a third-party beneficiary (because equitable interest, which is created upon the transfer of legal title to the trustee, never actually leaves him); or
- it occurs when property is divested from the settlor, but for some reason equitable interest in it returns to him (perhaps on the occurrence of an event that has not been provided for because it was unforeseen or because the trust instrument was poorly drafted).

7.1 The question of ownership: who can 'own' property?

Moving into a more substantive consideration of resulting and constructive trusts, and following on from our earlier discussion of the beneficiary principle and purpose trusts, this chapter considers difficulties that arise where property is conveyed to an unincorporated association—such as a society, a social club, or a religious group. Such associations will exist to use property for a particular purpose. *Unincorporated* associations cannot own property themselves because they lack the legal personality to do so. *Incorporated* bodies, such as companies, do have requisite legal personality, and can thus own property in their own right. The difficulties (and possible solutions) that shall be considered in this chapter will arise only in situations in which the unincorporated body itself is non-charitable. Indeed, as will become apparent when the position of charities is considered later in the text, there is no difficulty when a gift is made to an unincorporated body with charitable purposes, because in these circumstances the association's officers can hold the property as charitable trustees.

Non-lawyers might well be astonished at the legal difficulties to which a transaction as simple as giving property to a club or other unincorporated association gives rise. The problem is that analyses based on trusts do not work very well, whereas a contractual analysis, which can usually be made to work, seems very unfair. In this scenario, the donor of the property has to give up all interest in the gift that he is making. In a contractual analysis, the donor cannot make his gift conditional, nor can he prevent the club members from using the property for any purpose they please, whether or not it is for the original purposes of the club.

Advantages of a Re Denley-*style purpose trust*

At first sight, it might be thought that a *Denley*-style purpose trust (after *Re Denley's Trust Deed* [1969] 1 Ch 37, considered in Chapter 3) might be a good method of allowing property to be conveyed to a non-charitable unincorporated association: the property would be held in trust for the members of the association, for the purposes of the association, and it would be necessary only that the identity of those members was sufficiently certain. This would certainly have advantages for donors, since the property could be constrained to be used for the association's purposes and members would not be able (for example) to dispose of it for their own benefit. If the purposes of the association were fulfilled (for example, if vivisection were abolished, if the association in question were the National Anti-Vivisection Association), or became impossible (for example, if a gun club were prohibited by legislation from carrying out its previously lawful activities), the donor would obtain any property not already used on resulting trust. Unfortunately, however, a gift to members for the time being (that is, present and future, assuming a fluctuating membership) will usually infringe the perpetuity rules (another difficulty in *Leahy* v *Attorney-General for New South Wales* [1959] AC 457, seen in Chapter 3), so the trust solution is not generally appropriate. It should be noted that, in *Denley* itself, the grant was effective only until twenty-one years after the death of the last survivor of a number of specified persons (with a gift over to a hospital), so no perpetuity difficulty arose. There are also, of course, no perpetuity difficulties where the association is charitable.

Traditionally, the premise for this chapter has been strongly tied into the perpetuity difficulties arising from creating trusts that are not charitable, but are ones for purposes rather than people. But because the law on perpetuities has changed, and perpetuity rules are considered much more marginal, the emphasis of this chapter has changed. Some reference was made to unincorporated associations, and their characteristics and legal basis, in Chapter 2; discussion of perpetuity problems associated with a trusts analysis of unincorporated associations—once a mainstay of this chapter—has been relocated to the Online Resource Centre.

In the light of this, this chapter now continues directly from Chapter 2. This chapter's premise is about explaining why unincorporated associations are characteristically structured on contractual principles, rather than a trusts model. This means that whilst there is discussion of how resulting trusts can apply in the setting of unincorporated associations, such a situation is very unusual because the vast majority are based on a contractual model.

7.2 The importance of the contractual analysis

For this reason, gifts to non-charitable unincorporated associations are usually construed as being to existing members only, but subject to their contractual duties as members of the society or club. These will be determined by the rules of the association, but usually a member will be prevented from severing his share and it will accrue to other members on death or resignation. Thus although present and future members of a fluctuating body will benefit de facto, because the gift is construed as one to existing members alone, there is no perpetuity problem.

This was Cross J's analysis in *Neville Estates* v *Madden* [1962] Ch 832, in which he analysed in detail the methods by which property can be conveyed to a non-charitable unincorporated association:

> The question of the construction and effect of gifts to or in trust for unincorporated associations was recently considered by the Privy Council in *Leahy* v *Attorney-General for New South Wales* [1959] AC 457. The position, as I understand it, is as follows. Such a gift may take effect in one or other of three quite different ways. In the first place, it may, on its true construction, be a gift to the members of the association at the relevant date as joint tenants, so that any member can sever his share and claim it whether or not he continues to be a member of the association. Secondly, it may be a gift to the existing members not as joint tenants, but subject to their respective contractual rights and liabilities towards one another as members of the association. In such a case a member cannot sever his share. It will accrue to the other members on his death or resignation, even though such members include persons who became members after the gift took effect. If this is the effect of the gift, it will not be open to objection on the score of perpetuity or uncertainty unless there is something in its terms or circumstances or in the rules of the association which precludes the members at any given time from dividing the subject of the gift between them on the footing that they are solely entitled to it in equity.
>
> Thirdly, the terms or circumstances of the gift or the rules of the association may show that the property in question is not to be at the disposal of the members for the time being, but is to be held in trust for or applied for the purposes of the association as a quasi-corporate entity. In this case the gift will fail unless the association is a charitable body.
>
> (*Neville Estates* v *Madden* [1962] Ch 832, *per* Cross J at 849–50)

Trusts for purpose valid only if charitable

This passage is interesting in a number of respects. Cross J (whose views are technically *obiter*, because the property was in the event held on charitable trusts—see Chapter 11) first sets out the difficulties of construing a gift to an unincorporated association as a gift to the members of the association at the relevant date as joint tenants. Second, he sets out the usual solution to the problem: that of a gift to the existing members not as joint tenants, but subject to their respective contractual rights and liabilities towards one another as members of the association. In that case, he points out that a member cannot sever his share. Third, he reiterates the orthodox position that a trust for purposes is valid only if charitable.

It is also essential to the analysis that the members at any one time own the entirety of the fund—that is, that they can, if they so wish, dissolve the association and divide the property among themselves. Donors can place no conditions on their donation, for fear of infringing the perpetuity rules (and remember that *Neville Estates* was decided prior to the Perpetuities and Accumulations Act 1964). In *Re Lipinski's Will Trusts* [1976] 1 Ch 235, Oliver J gave effect to a gift to the Hull Judeans (Maccabi) Association to be used solely for construction and improvements of the association's buildings, despite having rejected charity arguments, but only by striking out the condition relating to buildings, and holding that the present members of the association were absolutely entitled and could use the property in any way they liked. He could thus bring the case within the second *Neville Estates* category.

The limits of the contractual analysis became apparent from Brightman J's judgment in *Re Recher's WT* [1972] Ch 526. The testatrix left some of her residuary estate to a non-charitable unincorporated association, which, on the construction of her will, was identified as the London and Provincial Anti-Vivisection Society. By the date of the will, however, that society had ceased to exist, but had amalgamated with the National Anti-Vivisection Society. The question was whether the gift could take effect in favour of the National Anti-Vivisection Society.

Brightman J held that the gift could not be construed as a trust for the purposes of the National Anti-Vivisection Society. It would have been possible to construe the gift, on the basis of Cross J's views in *Neville Estates*, as a gift to the members of the London and Provincial Anti-Vivisection Society, subject to the contract towards each other to which they had bound themselves as members, had the Society been in existence at the date of the testatrix's will. By then it had been dissolved, however, and the contract between the members terminated. The gift could not be construed as a gift to the members of a different association (that is, the National Anti-Vivisection Society) and, accordingly, failed.

Re Grant: *division between local and national control*

A slightly different difficulty arose in *Re Grant's WT* [1980] 1 WLR 360, in which a grant to the Chertsey and Walton Constituency Labour Party (CLP) failed. The difficulty in *Re Grant* was that the members of the CLP did not have control over their own property, because they were also bound by the rules of the Labour Party nationally. Thus a gift to the CLP could not be construed as a gift to the members of the CLP beneficially, since they could not direct that the bequest be divided among themselves as beneficial owners. The gift could take effect, if at all, only as a private purpose trust, in which case it infringed the rule against perpetuities.

This merits further examination, since the relationship between national and local Labour parties was unusual, in that the local association appeared to have virtually no control over its own funds. Indeed, the national party could itself take direct control of the local party's funds, and it is not at all surprising, therefore, that Vinelott J held that the funds were owned by the national rather than the local party. However, it does not follow that gifts can never be made to local branches of federated societies. In *News Group Newspapers Ltd v SOGAT 1982* [1986] ICR 716, the local branch of the Society of Graphical and Allied Trades (SOGAT) could unilaterally secede from the national union and was therefore held still to control its own property. Presumably, therefore, it would have been possible to make a donation to the local branch. Many federated societies adopt an intermediate position under which, although the local branches cannot unilaterally secede, the national society has no direct control over the local funds, the local society instead paying an annual membership subscription and agreeing to be bound, to a greater or lesser extent, by national rules. It is uncertain whether the reasoning in *Re Grant's WT* applies in this situation.

It is clear, then, that there are serious limitations on the contractual analysis. Trust analyses were even more fraught with difficulties, mostly because of the common law rule against perpetuities, as considered on the Online Resource Centre.

7.3 **Winding up unincorporated associations**

The correct analysis of a gift to an unincorporated association, such as a club or society, also controls the distribution of its assets when it is wound up, since that question depends on who are the owners of the fund.

When is a fund wound up?

It is necessary first to consider when a fund may be wound up. According to Brightman J in *Re William Denby & Sons Ltd Sick and Benevolent Fund* [1971] 1 WLR 973, winding up of a fund is not at the discretion of the treasurer or trustees of the fund, but may occur only when:

(a) the rules allow for dissolution; or

(b) all interested parties agree; or

(c) a court orders dissolution; or

(d) the substratum upon which the fund is founded is gone (such as in *Re St Andrew's Allotment Association* [1969] 1 WLR 229, in which an allotment association was wound up when the land for allotments was sold to developers for £70,000).

Many of the cases arise when the club or association has simply been inactive for a number of years, but no positive moves have been made to wind it up. The courts are reluctant in these circumstances to infer that the substratum has gone. In *William Denby* itself, the substratum had not disappeared, although after an industrial dispute many of the company's employees left and, for some time (about four-and-a-half years), nobody had contributed to the fund. But before the dispute, the fund was viable, and indeed increasing, and mere inactivity by the members did not necessarily lead to the conclusion that they had acquiesced in the dissolution of the fund, since a less drastic interpretation was possible—namely, that they had acquiesced in the temporary suspension of contributions and grants.

A similar dispute arose in *Re GKN Bolts and Nuts Ltd Sports and Social Club* [1982] 2 All ER 855, noted at [1983] Conv 315, in which Megarry V-C allowed what he called 'spontaneous dissolution'—that is, the winding up of a club without any resolution or court order to that effect. He observed, however, that mere inactivity is not enough, unless it is so prolonged that dissolution is the only reasonable inference. A cataleptic trance, he said, may look like death without being death, and suspended animation may be continued life, not death. Here, however, spontaneous dissolution had occurred, but it required a positive act—in this case, a resolution to sell the club's only remaining asset, the sports ground.

The basis on which funds are held

The types of fund with which this section is concerned are members' clubs or friendly societies, which are unincorporated associations. As it has been suggested, the property of unincorporated associations is not normally held in trust for the members; instead, the relationship between the members is contractual. Members' contributions or subscriptions are regarded as out-and-out gifts, each member retaining contractual rights (based on the rules) to use the property of the club or society. On resignation from the club or society, although the gift of the subscriptions remains (otherwise a retiring member could claim back a share of these), the retiring member gives up any contractual claim on the property of the association.

It ought to follow, therefore, that when such an association is wound up, only existing members have a right to claim any part of the fund. The basis of their claim is a contractual right to share in the property, and the method by which the division is calculated is considered in section 7.4.

It is nevertheless possible, in theory, for funds to be held by trustees on trust for the members, even though this is rare in practice. The main difficulty was always the rule in perpetuities, because, with memberships likely to fluctuate, dispositions in favour of future members might fall outside the perpetuity period. This was not traditionally a problem where the fund is intended only for the benefit of existing members or is of short-term duration (for example, it is limited to twenty-one years from the death of the last survivor of a number of specified persons, like the trust in *Re Denley's Trust Deed* [1969] 1 Ch 373, considered in Chapter 3), though it is very unusual to find this.

7.4 Surplus contributions and the operation of a resulting trust

If such a fund is dissolved, the *surplus of the contributions themselves* will be held on resulting trust. All contributors, including those who have ceased to contribute, will be entitled to a share, and division will be in proportion to the *total amount* that they have contributed. Thus, assuming that everyone pays subscriptions at the same rate, a person who has contributed for ten years is entitled to twice as much of the share of the proceeds as someone who has contributed for only five.

This was the basis of division in *Re Hobourn Aero Components Ltd's Air Raid Distress Fund* [1946] Ch 86, affirmed at [1946] Ch 194. From 1940 to 1944, employees of a company in Coventry made weekly contributions to a fund to assist employees who had suffered damage as a result of air raids. Only contributors to the fund could benefit. The fund was closed in 1944, and the question arose as to what to do with surplus moneys. The Crown did not claim the fund as *bona vacantia*. The contributors wanted the surplus back. The Charity Commissioners wanted to adopt a cy-près scheme, which they could do only if the fund were charitable (see Chapter 12).

At first instance, Cohen J held that the purposes of the organization were not charitable, since there was an insufficient element of public benefit. It followed that a cy-près scheme could not be directed. That being so, the contributors were entitled to distribute the fund among themselves, in proportion to the total amount that each had contributed, on resulting trust principles: '[The] basis on which the contributions are returned is that each donor retained an interest in the amount of his contributions except so far as they are applied for the purposes for which they were subscribed.' In other words, a proportion of the *total* contribution of each individual contributor is held on resulting trust, the assumption being that he retains an interest in his contribution. On a contractual analysis, however, anyone ceasing to contribute to the scheme loses any benefits that they had under the scheme and also loses any property interest in the fund. All those who are still contributors at the date of closure of the fund are usually entitled to an *equal* share in the surplus, not a share that is based on their past contributions (see further section 7.4.1).

The Crown, in *Hobourn Aero*, appealed on the issue of the charitable status of the fund alone, and the Court of Appeal upheld Cohen J's decision (on which aspect of the case, see further Chapter 11). However, nothing was said in the Court of Appeal about the distribution of the funds.

One of the problems with Cohen J's analysis is that the rule against perpetuities appears to be infringed unless either the fund is expressly limited in duration or there are no fluctuations in membership. Arguably, the fund in *Hobourn Aero* did not infringe the rule, although there were fluctuations in the identity of the individual contributors, because of its essentially temporary nature. Presumably, however, nobody knew how long the fund would continue at its inception, and no express limit appears to have been put on its duration.

Re West Sussex *and the analysis in* Re Bucks

In *Re West Sussex Constabulary's Widows, Children and Benevolent (1930) Fund Trusts* [1971] Ch 1, there was an extensive discussion of *Hobourn*. Goff J noted that there were no contractual benefits in *Hobourn*, so that the usual contractual analysis may well not be applicable—but that does not in any way answer the perpetuity difficulties inherent in Cohen J's analysis.

It is thus respectfully suggested that Cohen J's analysis is wrong. At any rate, the case cannot be regarded as laying down any principle applicable to the majority of fund cases, since their duration is not limited and fluctuating membership is assumed.

Walton J's analysis in *Re Bucks Constabulary Widows' and Orphans' Fund Friendly Society (No. 2)* [1979] 1 WLR 936 will usually be more appropriate. The case involved a fund that was made up of voluntary contributions from its members, for the relief of widows and orphans of deceased members of the Bucks Constabulary. In April 1968, the Bucks Constabulary was amalgamated with other constabularies to form the Thames Valley Constabulary; in October 1968, the society was wound up. The trustee applied to the court to determine how the funds were to be distributed. Walton J thought that the members' rights to share in the fund were governed by their contractual rights and duties *inter se*, and that, in the absence of evidence to the contrary, members who resigned lost all claim on the fund. Therefore division should be made among only those who were still members at the time of the dissolution of the fund and, in the absence of evidence to the contrary, they were entitled to an equal share in the fund. Accordingly, he held that the surplus should be held by the trustees for the members at the time of dissolution in equal shares.

7.4.1 **Contractual vs resulting trust analyses: final resolution?**

It cannot be assumed, however, that the courts have finally resolved the issue in favour of a contractual basis for the holding of funds. In *Re West Sussex Constabulary's Widows, Children and Benevolent (1930) Fund Trusts* [1971] Ch 1, Goff J held that the proportion of the surplus attributable to identifiable donations and legacies was held on resulting trust. He thought these indistinguishable from *Re the Trusts of the Abbott Fund*. Presumably, then, before the dissolution of the constabulary, the donations and legacies had been given to the association on trust. The problem is that this is not at all like *Re the Trusts of the Abbott Fund* (considered in Chapter 3), which concerned a trust for two identifiable ladies, living at the time the trust was set up. There could not possibly be any perpetuity problems with such a trust. It is suggested that neither could there be in *Re Gillingham Bus Disaster Fund* [1958] Ch 3000, in which the purposes (or, at any rate, the valid purposes) were taken to be defraying the funeral expenses of the identifiable boys who had just died and caring for those living who, as a consequence of the disaster, were left disabled. But if there were a trust of donations in *Re West Sussex Constabulary's Widows, Children and Benevolent (1930) Fund Trusts*, the beneficiaries would have been a fluctuating body of present and future members, and exactly the same perpetuity problems would arise as in the *Hobourn Aero* case.

Introduction to pension funds: Davis *v* Richards and
Wallington Industries Ltd

Similar reasoning was adopted by Scott J in *Davis* v *Richards and Wallington Industries Ltd* [1991] 2 All ER 563, which concerned the winding up of a pension fund. The *ratio* of the case was that distribution of the assets was by a definitive deed that was executed by the trustees, but Scott J went on in his judgment to consider what would be the position if he were wrong. Employers, employees, and money transferred from other funds were the three main sources of contributions to the fund. Scott thought that the employers' contributions should be held on resulting trust for them, on account of their similarity with the *West Sussex* legacies. There was no reason to rebut the conclusion that there was a resulting trust. But the problem is exactly the same as we have just considered: what was the trust upon which the funds were held prior to the winding up of the fund? It must have been a trust for a fluctuating body of individuals and, once again, this will raise perpetuity difficulties. *Re Bucks Constabulary Widows' and Orphans' Fund Friendly Society (No. 2)* was not mentioned by Scott J, although, according to the report, the case was cited and there was some consideration given to a contractual analysis (at 589–90). No obvious reason was given for the rejection of this latter analysis. It is suggested, however, that in such a situation (which is distinct from the more general position of pension funds) a trust analysis simply cannot work. It is greatly hoped, therefore, that the courts will adopt the analysis of Walton J in *Re Bucks Constabulary Widows' and Orphans' Fund Friendly Society (No. 2)*.

7.4.2 Conclusion: the general position of unincorporated associations and support for the contractual basis for the calculation of shares

Notwithstanding the alternative approaches considered in relation to the general position of unincorporated associations, it is suggested that a contractual basis for the division of funds is the only tenable mechanism. This is, of course, the solution provided for by the *Re Bucks Constabulary* case. In this situation, if the rules provide for the contingency of dissolution of the fund, division will be according to the rules, because they will form the basis of the contract.

Often, the rules do not so provide, however, and in this event the courts are left to imply terms. In accordance with normal contractual doctrine, this will be on the basis of inferred intention and, since this is largely a question of fact, no rigid rules of law can be stated. Nevertheless, certain presumptions appear to apply, as follows.

(1) Only existing members can claim, because it is assumed that past members gave up all claims on the fund on resignation (*Re Bucks Constabulary Widows' and Orphans' Fund Friendly Society (No. 2)* [1979] 1 WLR 936). Sometimes, the rules expressly so provide, as in *Re West Sussex Constabulary's Widows, Children and Benevolent (1930) Fund Trusts* [1971] Ch 1.

(2) Generally speaking, in the case of members' clubs, division is equally among existing members. In mutual benefit or friendly society cases, the prima facie rule also appears to be equal division (*Bucks Constabulary*), although there have also been cases in which division has been proportional to total contributions— which seems appropriate where the benefit contracted for while the fund subsists is also proportional to total contributions. In *Re Sick and Funeral Society of St John's Sunday School, Golcar* [1973] Ch 51, there were two distinct classes of membership, one of which (adults) paid and received twice the benefit of

the other (children). Division was such that adults received twice as much as children. It must be emphasized, however, that inferred intention is a question largely of fact, and that it would be a mistake to deduce rigid principles of law from these cases.

(3) If the assumption can be made that a contributor has made an out-and-out gift of his contributions, retaining no rights in the fund at all, then the property will go to the Crown as *bona vacantia*, because nobody has a claim on it. This conclusion has sometimes been drawn where only third parties could benefit from the fund (as in *Cunnack v Edwards* [1896] 2 Ch 679, in which only the widows of contributors were entitled to benefit). The same result was reached in the *West Sussex* case: Goff J thought that the contributors had parted with their property out-and-out, and had retained no interest in the fund, since it was held for the benefit of third parties (the widows and dependants of the deceased members), but on this point the case was criticized in the *Bucks Constabulary* case. In the later case, Walton J observed that merely because the members have contracted between themselves to provide benefits for third parties does not mean (in the absence of a valid trust in favour of the third parties) that they have relinquished their property in the fund. They can still, after all, collectively agree to distribute the fund among themselves, or to vary the benefits under the scheme. The position is essentially analogous to *Beswick v Beswick* [1968] AC 58, in which, although two parties had contracted to provide a benefit for a third party, they could at any time agree to vary the benefit to be provided for the third party and the third party had no enforceable claim against either of them. If they had set up an enforceable trust in favour of the third party, of course, the position would be different, but in that case the third party would have the beneficial interest in the surplus. In neither case should the property go to the Crown as *bona vacantia*.

7.5 Resulting trusts and pension funds

As we learned in Chapter 2, the rise of the pension fund in recent times has ensured that issues of operation and regulation have come sharply into focus on a number of social, economic, and legal fronts. The discourses that have taken place in furtherance of creating a workable legal framework for the operation and safeguarding of pension assets demonstrate clear favour for the trust as the most appropriate mechanism for ensuring this. The favourable view of the trust was confirmed in the *Report of the Pension Law Review Committee* (1993, Cmnd 2342), chaired by Sir Roy Goode. The Committee's recommendations resulted in the passage of the Pensions Act 1995. The 1995 Act sought to reflect the importance of rigorous regulation and supervision of pension schemes, and one of its principal tenets was its accommodation of the reality that the beneficiaries under a pension scheme differed from the normal trust position of volunteers; indeed, the entitlement of beneficiaries under a pension scheme could be seen to arise from contractual origins (provided by their contracts of employment). This aside, the trust was the device that was strongly favoured in the promotion of the expedient and safe use of such schemes. Here, even perpetuities difficulties, which are usually fatal in other examples of unincorporated associations, do not arise, thanks to specific consideration made in pensions legislation.

As a result of this topical interest in pension funds and the primacy of place given to the trust, it is perhaps not surprising that academic commentators are enthusing in the way that is evident in the article by Charles Harpum (2000) 64 Conv 170. Harpum suggests that these are most interesting, and even exciting, times for trusts lawyers and pensions lawyers alike.

One source of this excitement can be attributed to a theme that runs throughout this text: hailing the trust as one of the most flexible and adaptable, and also most useful, instruments in English law. Much is made of the way in which its application cuts across domestic and commercial contexts, providing certainty and protection in relation to property rights in commercial relationships as much as private familial ones. The use of the trust instrument in the context of pensions operation and pensions law also indicates something in addition to this, and which has up to now been implied rather than made explicit. The issue of pensions and their operation in contemporary society is one of the most important socio-economic issues of today. To recap, with the combination of a declining birth rate, longer life expectancy, and a broader global context signalling the dismantling of the welfare state, the focus on privately funded pensions outside state provision have come increasingly to the fore. Today's issues arise very strongly from the need to plan for tomorrow, and private pension schemes (occupational and otherwise) are very much concerned with planned long-term personal asset management.

Indeed, it has already been suggested that while the trust's traditional associations are strongly with wealth and its preservation, it is nevertheless significant that it is these age-old principles that are envisioned as the blueprint for this personal asset management into the twenty-first century. This is a testament to the trust's versatility, adaptability, and also its endurance. This is so notwithstanding that demonstrating how pension funds are modelled on the trust instrument will reveal some crucial departures from 'ordinary' trust principles.

Clearly, the huge shifts in social and economic demography have contributed to the rise of the pension fund, but it is the very characteristics that provided the introduction to this subject right at the outset of this book that form its backbone. It is those fundamental principles of fiduciary responsibility and (from the beneficiaries' perspective) the proprietary rights conferred upon the equitable owners of property that have ensured that the trust has shaped the pension fund, and will remain central to its evolution.

7.5.1 Trust actors and pension situations

The term 'trust actor', in this context, is used to illustrate how the parties that are central to the trust—as understood by this text—can be applied to the pensions scenario. In this situation, the trust is a pension scheme and trust property arises in the form of contributions made to it, which ultimately become payable under it. In this respect, the term 'trust party' is used to 'locate' the settlor, the trustee, and the beneficiary (parties central to the trust's operation) in the pension context. It does not, of course, refer to parties *to* the trust, because the beneficiary of a properly constituted trust has rights to enforce the trust, but is not party to its creation. But the settlor, the trustee, and the beneficiary are all central to the operation of a private trust, and will now be explained in the operation of the pension trust.

In the case of an occupational pension trust, the employer is the settlor and the members of the scheme—typically employees and their dependants—occupy the position of beneficiaries. The scheme will have trustees, which may well include the employer and other key organizational figures from the particular occupational culture concerned (for example, from the board of directors), or appointed from a separate specialist trustee company. The involvement of the employer in the scheme confers even greater (theoretical, at least) power than would subsist in the employer–employee relationship alone, in a 'structural' power sense. But in addition to this, more abstract, sense of power (which *is* regarded as a significant consideration and is reflected as such in the Pensions Act 1995's provision that a proportion of trustees are to be nominated by members of the scheme), the position of the employer as trustee will vest in him *trust* powers in a real sense under the scheme. A glance back to the work on certainty and the introduction to the nature of trusts in Chapter 2 will provide a reminder of the nature of powers; clearly, the powers conferred to trustees of such a scheme will be fiduciary powers and will include the power to appoint any surplus (in the fund).

7.5.2 Duties and powers of trustees under a pension scheme

Just as in the case of any express private trust, trustees under a pension scheme are duty-bound to protect the trust assets and to administer the trust in accordance with its terms. This is a gross oversimplification, because there are a number of legal considerations reflecting the differences between pension funds and other trust instruments. In terms of protecting the trust assets, the trustees must ensure that settlor contributions falling due under the scheme are paid to it. Duties arising from administration are more complicated, and different issues will arise according to whether the scheme continues to operate and is due to remain operational, or whether it is being wound up. Other factors that will affect the administration of pensions trusts flow from the way in which they are likely to be operational for a long duration of time. On one level, this would give rise to important perpetuity implications were it not for the way in which the 1995 Act exempts 'approved schemes' from perpetuities provisions. On another, the long-term management of assets that is required has resulted in pension trustees having powers of investment that are wider and more delegable than would normally be the case. Investment policy is also required to be formalized through the production of a formal statement of investment strategy. Statutory requirements exist, requiring trustees to select investments, to diversify portfolios and to observe their operations, and to take advice and review them. The trustees of a pension scheme are also under a duty to seek recovery of funds where pension funds become 'lost' (usually on account of a breach of trust), with potential implications flowing from liabilities of fellow trustees and previous ones, and where property applied in breach of trust has come into the hands of third parties.

Members as beneficiaries and key entitlements
It is the members of the pension scheme (along with their relatives and dependants) who are its beneficiaries. And, in terms of being 'beneficially entitled' to the fruits of the fund, the members of the pension scheme are no different from the beneficiary under an ordinary private trust. As we have already noted, the key crucial difference lies in the contributions that comprise the basis of the pension entitlement. Contributions of this nature will include ones made by the beneficiary himself, directly and also indirectly. This is not the position in many ordinary private trusts, and in this respect the beneficiary has provided consideration for the benefit ultimately due under the scheme. However, this does not necessarily give the beneficiaries any additional rights to be informed about decisions taken by trustees (in respect of their own, rather considerable, obligations arising) regarding the fund, and the 'normal' position on this is considered below in the discussion of trusteeship. It is also the case that the remedies available to the pension fund beneficiary against trustees and strangers (those not parties to the

trust) are identical to those arising in any other private express trust—as explained in Chapters 16 and 17.

Workable resulting trusts: Davis v Richards and Wallington

At this point, you might wonder how this view of the trust can be squared with the analysis given of *Davis*, and indeed the important pensions case *Air Jamaica* v *Charlton* (considered next) does distinguish *Davis*. Furthermore, it is especially important to note at this stage that the scheme in *Davis* was unusual, in as much as such schemes will normally provide for the allocation of surplus assets on the winding up of such a fund. This was not the case in *Davis*, and this is what triggered the operation of the general law relating to unincorporated associations (and the conclusion offered that the correct analysis to be applied was the one in *Re Bucks Constabulary*).

7.6 The resulting trust in action: *Air Jamaica* v *Charlton*

Air Jamaica v *Charlton* [1999] 1 WLR 1399 (PC) concerned a contributory pension fund, which was started in 1969. The fund was wound up following the company's privatization, upon which all of the employees were made redundant. Many employees were re-engaged, but under new pension arrangements. The (original) scheme (and subject of the litigation) had been funded from (compulsory) deductions made from employees' salaries, and from matching payments that had been made by the employer. However, whereas each employee became a member of the pension scheme by virtue of his employment, his entitlement to a pension arose under the trusts of the scheme and not under his contract of employment.

The case concerned two key provisions relating to the scheme. The first was clause 4 of the trust deed. This provided, inter alia, that: 'No moneys which at any time have been contributed by the Company under the terms thereof shall in any circumstances be repayable to the [airline] company.' The second was s. 13 of the pension plan, which authorized the airline to amend the plan or to discontinue it, but not in a way that was incompatible with the exclusive use of the fund for the members, and their families and dependants also entitled under it. The fund was to be used for making annuity purchases for existing and future beneficiaries, and any surplus was to be directed to the provision of additional benefits for dependant beneficiaries following a member's death (to be applied to them at the discretion of the trustees).

7.6.1 *Air Jamaica* and a familiar problem: disputes arising from distributed funds

The litigation concerned the issue of the disposition of the large balance in the original fund when the company was privatized in 1994. As a result of new conditions of employment, no further contributions were made to the original fund, nor deductions made from the members of the scheme. The sum remaining was US$400 million, and was surplus (that is, not subject to any liability under the scheme). The members of this pension plan sought declaration that the plan had been discontinued and, in accordance with s. 13 of the plan, that the balance of the fund should be distributed for the benefit of the intended beneficiaries (the employees and their dependants). Almost immediately, the airline sought to amend the trust deed and to plan to try to ensure that the surplus subject of the beneficiaries' claims would return to it, rather than be distributed among the beneficiaries. A 'royal lives' clause (as discussed in the Online Resource Centre materials on perpetuities) was introduced to try to counter claims that the scheme (and its underlying trusts) was void for perpetuity. Meanwhile, the Attorney-General alleged that the scheme was void for perpetuity and that the surplus funds should pass to the Crown as *bona vacantia*.

Distribution of the fund and direction of distribution: three parties in dispute

In the Privy Council (following a decision in the Jamaican Court of Appeal that the rule against perpetuities did not apply to the scheme, which, arising out of the contract of employment, was correctly the province of the law of contract), the Board concluded that the scheme had been established as a trust fund. It was found that membership of the scheme had arisen from the contract of employment, but entitlement to it flowed from the trust nature of the scheme. The scheme was subject to the rule against perpetuities and was found to be in infringement of the common law perpetuity rules. The Perpetuities and Accumulations Act 1964 does not form part of the law of Jamaica, so the common law perpetuity rules applied. This meant that there was no 'wait and see' facility, and the effect of this on the operation of the 'class gift' (in favour of members, their widows, and their dependants) was that this would be governed by common law. Under this scheme, this meant that some (of the class) were not 'lives in being' at the time of the settlement and it followed that there was the possibility that the gift might vest outside the perpetuity period (twenty-one years after the death of a member).

Partial failure, distribution, and operation of the resulting trust

As a consequence of the partial failure of the trusts, determination had to be made about the surplus and to whom it must be directed. It was held that there was a resulting trust in operation in favour of the member contributors and for the airline (on account of its 'matched employer' contributions under the scheme). The share to be returned to the members on resulting trust was to be on a pro rata basis, according to the contributions that individual members had made, but without reference to the time (dates) on which contributions had been made or any benefits received under the scheme.

This case, its decision, and its reasoning can be summarized as follows.

(1) Although the common law perpetuity period applied to this scheme, it did not follow that it was altogether void. The view of the Law Commission, expressed in its 1998 report entitled *The Rules against Perpetuities and Excessive Accumulations* (Law Com. 251), para. 353, was adopted. The trusts took effect as separate settlements entered into by each employee. Each separate settlement comprised the contributions made in respect of the employee, either by him or by the employer. This would satisfy the common law rule with the employee as the 'life in being'.

(2) The pension plan was discontinued when the employer ceased to deduct contributions from its employees and to pay matching contributions to the trustees.

(3) The surplus was held on resulting trust, being treated as provided as to one half by the employer and one half by the employees. Clause 4 did not negate the inference of a resulting trust; it is a failure of the company to dispose of the funds similar to *Vandervell* v *IRC* [1967] 2 AC 691. As for the employees' contributions, *Davis* v *Richards and Wallington Ltd* [1991] 2 All ER 563 could be distinguished, since here they had not received all they had bargained for, but in any case the inferences as to intention drawn in *Davis* were disproved.

7.7 The regulation of pension trusts: the Pensions Act 2004

The foregoing material has provided a brief introduction to the special features that pertain to pension trusts and the special rules that apply to them as a reflection of this. Indeed, in due course (in Chapter 16), you will come across the reference made by the Law Commission, in its 2006 report on *Trustee Exemption Clauses* (Law Com. 301, Cm. 6874), to pension trusts as ones that are 'to a great extent a law unto themselves'. By way of brief explanation, the Law Commission suggested that such trusts are 'conceptually different from other types of trusts and operate in a distinct manner', and note has already been made of the way in which they are quite unlike other trusts in many respects, including the relationships between the parties and the way in which beneficiaries under such trusts are not volunteers, for example.

In many respects, the Pensions Act 2004 is best understood by reference to the Pensions Act 1995 as legislation enacted to protect the position of beneficiaries in light of the possibilities for maladministration and fraud, and also insolvency. In this respect, requirements that trustees must keep proper records, that contributions received by them must be placed in a separate account within an authorized institution, and that an offence can be committed where an employer fails to pay over contributions that have been deducted from members, are well established in the framework of modern pension trust law. However, this legislation also sought to 'unpack' still further, and to respond to, the rather unusual position of pension trusts, and the different 'interests' and relationships that arise between the key parties.

The 2004 Act introduced a number of changes, and detailed discussion of this and subsequent legislation (primarily the 2008 Act) is beyond the scope of this text, which is why the consideration given to pensions trusts is very brief and basic. However, it is probably worthy of note that the background to the 2004 Act was one of numerous perceived shortcomings in the 1995 Act, both in terms of its scope and utility, and also in the nature of its operation. Thus very brief reference will be made to the provisions for funding requirements under the Act, and also to those relating to enhanced professionalism among the trustees of pension funds. It is also the case that the 2004 Act has created the office of Pensions Regulator.

The 'special nature' of trusteeship under pension funds

The 'special nature' of pension trusts and the trusteeship that arises from them is recognized in the provisions of the 2004 Act that relate to enhanced expectations of trustees. Under the new provisions, a trustee must (pursuant to s. 249) have the requisite degree of knowledge and understanding to enable him to exercise his functions in accordance with the scheme of which he is a trustee. Accordingly, in *general*, trustees must have knowledge and understanding of the law relating to pensions and trusts, and the principles of scheme funding and investment. In furtherance of ss. 247 and 248, trustees must also be conversant with a number of key matters relating to their *specific* scheme—namely, the trust deed itself and rules of the scheme in question, the scheme's statements of investment and funding principles, and any documents recording policy adopted by the trustees relating to the scheme.

Pension trusts and their new regulator

In the spirit and direction of the 2004 legislation—to continue to emphasize the importance of protecting pension trusts and to recognize shortcomings in the regime provided by the 1995 Act—the new Act has created a new office of the Pensions Regulator. The Pensions Regulator now holds all of the powers that were originally vested in the Occupational Pensions Regulatory Authority by virtue of the 1995 Act. As you will see from looking at the Regulator's website (<http://www.thepensionsregula-tor.gov.uk/doc-library/guidance.aspx>), pensions are in a state of rapid and extensive change, and for this reason the office of Pensions Regulator is also highly dynamic. In such times of rapid change, it is possible only to outline the key functions of the Regulator.

As the website suggests, the Pensions Regulator is the UK's regulator of work-based pension schemes. It derives its powers from the Pensions Acts of 2004 and 2008, and has the following goals:

- to protect members of work-based pension schemes;
- to promote and improve understanding, and the good administration, of work-based pension schemes;
- to reduce the risk of situations arising that may lead to compensation being payable from the Pension Protection Fund (PPF); and
- to maximize employer compliance with employer duties (including the requirement to enrol eligible employees automatically into a qualifying pension provision with a minimum contribution) and with certain employment safeguards.

In classifying its powers as falling within one of three headings, 'Investigating Schemes', 'Putting Things Right', and 'Acting against Avoidance', the Pensions Regulator has very wide powers to ensure that pension schemes are operated properly. These include a range of powers to ensure that those who are trustees are 'fit and proper' persons, who can demonstrate their competency through reporting requirements, etc., and who will be replaced if necessary. There are also a number of powers that support the statutory requirements relating to the schemes themselves. This is because assets within pension funds need considerable protection from inadequacies in funding that might otherwise arise in this very complex and, in many respects, highly intangible 'long-term' trust arrangement, as well as from the heightened risk of trustee impropriety in this context. Ultimately, the Regulator has the power to wind up the scheme if it considers it to be inadequate in any of these regards.

 Revision Box

1. Using the decisions in *Hobourn Aero Components Ltd's Air Raid Distress Fund* [1946] Ch 86, aff'd [1946] Ch 194, *West Sussex Constabulary's Benevolent Fund Trusts* [1971] Ch 1, and *Re Bucks Constabulary Fund Friendly Society (No. 2)* [1979] 1 WLR 93, identify and explain the following.
   (a) What is meant by the term 'unincorporated association'?
   (b) What issues arise in the operation and 'winding up' of unincorporated associations?
   (c) What is the competing 'basis' for responding to the needs of unincorporated associations to be found in the law of trusts and contract law?
2. In relation to pensions, explain the reasons why trusts are considered such an appropriate mechanism for structuring pension arrangements and how this reinforces the understanding that you have gained about trust arrangements thus far.

→

3. From reading the decision in *Air Jamaica* v *Charlton* [1999] 1 WLR 1399 (PC), ensure that you understand why:
 – the contributory pension fund was being *wound up*;
 – the fund was deemed to be *in surplus*;
 – there were *three competing viewpoints* on what should happen to the surplus; and
 – the Privy Council ultimately ruled as it did.

FURTHER READING

Gardner (1992) 'New angles on unincorporated associations' Conveyancer 41.

Harpum (2000) 'Perpetuities, pensions and resulting trusts' 64 Conveyancer 170.

Warburton (1985) 'The holding of property by unincorporated associations' Conveyancer 318.

online resource centre For summaries of a selection of these articles, please visit <http://www.oxfordtextbooks.co.uk/orc/wilson_trusts11e/>

8

....

Beneficial interests in the family
home: a case study

This chapter is a central reference point for several key themes covered so far in this text. Initially, Chapter 1 introduced the nature of the trust, and its respective treatment of beneficial interests and legal title, and it was noted that trusts are widely used across human interactions—increasingly in the commercial sphere, while for a long time they have arisen in relation to family property and financial arrangements. This latter theme continued in Chapter 2, which signposted cohabitation of the 'family home' directly. In respect of both these initial chapters, discussing ownership of family homes directly now brings sharply into focus the everyday significance of trusts and trusts law, and in a context to which almost everyone can relate directly or indirectly. Fundamentally, this is through consideration of central issues flowing from legal ownership of a home, and of how equity will treat ownership of property in ways that are both similar to, and also different from, approaches taken by law.

Thus the materials in this chapter also resonate with discussion of constituting trusts in Chapter 5. As we progress, it will become very clear how that study of the way in which property becomes trust property by being vested in a trustee, who then holds it subject to another's entitlements, is very significant here. And thereby we will also find connections with questions of formality requirements considered in Chapter 4, which noted that differences were drawn between trusts depending on whether or not they are 'express'.

This chapter also follows on directly from Chapters 6 and 7. In Chapter 6, we learned that constructive and resulting trusts can be found under the unifying heading of trusts that are 'implied' by equity in response to some kind of injustice that would otherwise arise in relation to ownership of property. Chapter 7 developed this by offering a case study of the operation of resulting trusts, through examining unincorporated associations and also pension funds. This case study of the family home is mostly a study of constructive trusts, because we find trusts imposed against the will of the trustee, but there is also scope for applying resulting trusts.

8.1 A case study in the working of constructive and resulting trusts

We do also find express trusts in this study, but it remains centrally a study of implied trusts. In following key aspects of Chapter 6, we can now start to understand in a more contextual way just how important implied trusts are, as devices that allow us to circumvent the formality requirements in place for express trusts. Centrally, this is a study of how trusts arise as a response to injustice, and particularly it helps us to understand how the constructive trust will have all of the features an express trust, except for the statutory requirement of formality that the declaration of trust is manifested and evidenced in writing (s. 53(1)(b) of the Law of Property Act 1925). This is a study of how proprietary interests in shared homes arise informally, within which we shall also consider how implied trusts measure up alongside a different mechanism that equity has developed to achieve this—that is, proprietary estoppel—and look at the interplay that can be seen between them.

8.2 Appreciating the significance of the family home for exploring resulting and constructive trusts: a case study and a hypothetical model

We shall see in this chapter just why family homes have become such a central reference point for understanding implied trusts in their everyday setting. Given that the origins of the trust lie in the complexities that can arise in the ownership of property, today the family home can be seen as a contemporary setting for appreciating the injustices that can arise from ownership of property and the ways in which equity responds to them.

In this setting, the tensions to which equity is seeking to respond reflect the way in which recognizing legal title alone in the context of ownership is important for achieving certainty in relation to valuable property rights, because legal rights are universal and inflexible, and thus certain. Alongside this, equity appreciates that acknowledging only the interests of a legal owner can also lead to injustice when the interests of another are overlooked. As we shall see, some claimants are actually legal owners of their property, albeit that this is unusual. And if there is an overarching rationale for equity's application of an implied trust in situations of shared home ownership, it is equity's recognition that, in the sphere of domestic relationships, proprietary interests in family homes can arise very informally. Although equity provides the facility for those who might be victims of injustice to avoid this through the existence of an express trust, equity also recognizes that, where ownership arises informally, it is unlikely that an express trust has been declared in a claimant's favour. Equity's response to this was to develop the facility for a trust to be implied into situations in which a claimant should have a proprietary interest in the home, but cannot secure this by formal means. In relation to property that is land, for an express trust to arise, a declaration of trust evidenced in writing is required, and so equity has provided that a trust that is implied does not have to satisfy formality ordinarily required.

The consequences of equity being prepared to imply a trust

Where equity is prepared to find that a trust exists without one being formally created, this has the effect of transforming property that appears to be property owned outright at law into trust property. This means that a legal owner of property is not actually an owner who has all of the rights of ownership, including the right to deal freely with his property. This situation means that a legal owner is, in fact, a trustee, whom equity will require to use the property to benefit the party who has a proprietary interest in it. A trustee in this type of arrangement will not be subject to all of the duties and responsibilities that we will find out (in Chapters 13 and 14, and 16 by way of example the extensive responsibilities relating to investment) attach to express trusteeship. But, in an implied trust arrangement, a legal owner must accept that his property is, in fact, owned by someone other than himself, as well as by him. This is an example of the situation that we first encountered in Chapter 1, where it was explained that the same person will be a settlor and a trustee, and also a beneficiary. In turn, this will affect what he can do with the property, which must be dealt with to reflect these other entitlements, so that this other is not disadvantaged.

Before progressing any further, this rationale is central to understanding that two key hypothetical models relating to the location of legal title to property dominate the nature of perceived injustices that can arise in relation to the family home, as follows.

- *Injustices that can arise from situations in which a family home is actually owned in law by one of the parties* This situation arises where although the property is a shared family home, it actually has only one legal owner. Here, legal title is vested solely in one party, and this is the most common traditional reason for equity's concern for achieving justice in circumstances in which, despite this, the non-legal owner should have entitlements to it.

- This has traditionally been the dominant situation in disputes relating to the ownership of shared homes, and indeed it has been the (one) hypothetical model that has been used in previous editions of this text. In this situation, typically, an unmarried couple purchase a home in which they intend to live together, but legal title is conveyed to one party alone for some reason. The issues raised here concern whether the party who is not a legal owner of the property can nevertheless acquire a proprietary interest in the property. Because only one party holds legal title, the nature of any proprietary interest acquired by the other must be one in equity. And it is in these circumstances that equity is concerned with avoiding injustices that are possibly hidden behind sole legal ownership. This raises questions of what conditions must be present for a party seeking an equitable interest in the property to be able to do this, and if this can be shown, there are further questions of size and extent—namely, how large the interest will be.

- *A different type of situation? The emergence of the* Stack v Dowden *injustice* Although the traditional context is very much 'one party' legal ownership disputes, *Stack* v *Dowden* [2007] UKHL 17 marked the arrival of disputed home ownership arising from joint legal tenancy. Here, the family home is actually legally owned by both parties, and so here equity's concern is different and responses for avoiding injustices must address the situation in which, although both parties are holders of legal title to the property, the matter of who actually owns the equity in the home (the valuable part) has not been made clear in this formal arrangement.

- In this situation, *Stack* is authority that having legal title to a property ensures an interest in this in equity, immediately making this situation different from the 'one legal owner' scenario, because here existence of an interest in equity is established by virtue of legal ownership. The key issue here is how large this interest will be and whether the size of the equitable interest will reflect the legal equality between the parties.

Recent authority that disputes between joint legal owners raise different questions from those encountered involving a home owned by one party only is provided by *Jones* v *Kernott* [2012] UKSC 53, in which, in the Supreme Court, the joint lead judgment of Lady Hale and Lord Walker makes direct reference to their different premises, or 'starting points'.

8.3 Understanding the injustices themselves: how do they arise and how are they manifested?

As suggested, injustices arising in this context to which equity seeks to respond have traditionally focused on the sole legal ownership of one party. In *this* setting—and in contrast with joint legal ownership—equity recognizes the following two broad injustices that justify recognition that a claimant has a proprietary interest in the home and that a trust should be implied to reflect this:

- a non-legal owner has contributed to the purchase of the property, which actually belongs in law to another person; or
- the parties have formed an agreement relating to their home, or the legal owner has made a representation to the effect that ownership of the home is to be shared, and this is not mirrored in legal ownership.

In contrast with equity's concerns (for apportionment) where legal ownership is actually already shared, in situations of sole legal ownership, while apportionment is significant, there is fundamentally a question of *whether* an interest should arise at all. In these circumstances, questions relating to contributions made by the parties, and any agreement to which they might have come in relation to beneficial ownership, will come to the fore.

Shared homes, disputes, and establishing 'injustices'
However, it is important to note at this stage the significance of the wording used in the foregoing, indicating how this chapter is essentially a study of the way in which 'equity is concerned with avoiding injustices that are possibly hidden behind legal ownership'. We need to emphasize the significance of 'possibly', which signals that home ownership—and even disputed home ownership—will not always harbour injustices. And it will become apparent that while this area of law shows that equity is willing to respond to injustices that arise, it is equally the case that equity will not read injustice into every case in which a home is being 'shared' by the parties. It will become apparent that equity's jurisdiction here is strongly based on reflecting the parties' intentions regarding ownership of their property, and in this regard important distinctions are drawn between intention to share actual ownership of property and an intention to share (instead) its occupation and enjoyment.

8.4 The context for these disputes and the significance of formal partnerships

When we consider how the courts have become involved at all in questions of disputed home ownership, we can see that, in many cases, this will be because of a dispute between two parties in a relationship that has broken down. Within this, we shall see that a large number of these concern parties whose relationship was, before it broke down, an informal partnership, which is often termed 'cohabitation'. The reason for this is that there are special provisions that apply where the relationship breakdown has occurred within a formal partnership recognized by law. Here, we find that there are statutory provisions where a marriage or a registered civil partnership between same-sex couples is brought formally to an end, and which apply as between these parties in acknowledgement of this. These are found, respectively, in the Matrimonial Causes Act 1973 (as amended by the Family Law Act 1996) and the Civil Partnership Act 2004. More is said about these mechanisms in the materials available on the Online Resource Centre, and their essence is a discretion-based jurisdiction within which the importance of the prior property interests of the spouses is reduced.

What needs to be stressed at this point is that the general hypothetical examples given in this chapter now apply only to unmarried couples and same-sex couples who have not registered a civil partnership.

So where does the 'general law' apply?

From this discussion of the special provisions that govern married couples and same-sex couples who are registered civil partners, it should be clear that the general law always applies to cohabitants outside these formal partnership models and any others who are in unconventional living arrangements. The general law will also, by virtue of living arrangements that are unconventional, apply to shared living arrangements between family members, and also 'companion' living, in which ownership of a shared home is called into question.

It is also the case that the scope of these special legislative provisions for formal partners will apply only in the context of relationship breakdown. Where ownership is disputed without there being a breakdown in the parties' relationship, then recourse will be to the ordinary law. As *Lloyds Bank* v *Rosset* [1991] AC 107 illustrates, issues about who has a beneficial interest in the home can arise where the home has been used as security for a mortgage and then, upon default of payment, the lender seeks to realize its security.

8.5 The reasons underlying the hypothetical model and current policy movements

It is, of course, possible for the parties themselves to avoid disputes concerning home ownership, with *Stack* v *Dowden* being one of the more recent periodic statements made by the courts of their frustration that, when homes are shared, more thought is not given to questions of beneficial ownership, and their call for title to shared property to include an express declaration of trust accordingly. But the courts themselves have been criticized for responding to the way in which comparatively few parties who share homes do make their intentions clear in this formal way. The Law Commission is a long-standing critic of the courts in this regard, as seen in its 1995 statement that 'the present legal rules are uncertain and difficult to apply and can lead to serious injustice' (*Sixth Programme of Law Reform*, Law Com. 234, item 8). This sentiment was reiterated in its 2002 discussion paper *Sharing Homes* (Law Com. 278, Cm. 5666), suggesting that new approaches were needed to reflect the rich variety of interpersonal living arrangements, whilst urging the courts to adopt an altogether fairer approach to determining home ownership. The cohabitation project generated by the then government's instruction to the Law Commission in 2005 to 'examine the options for reforming the law that applies to cohabiting couples on separation or death' has not precipitated reforms hoped for by many, but it shows once again the extent of the Law Commission's criticism of judicial approaches.

Discussion now focuses on exploring the law as it is, rather than as it might be or even should be. And while most earnest encouragement is being given by the courts, and also in policy discourses, for parties to make their intentions relating to ownership of property clear, this chapter is a testament to the way in which equity has been left to respond to prevent injustice precisely because the parties have not done so. And because the Law Commission project did not precipitate law reform, the courts are destined to remain the gatekeepers of disputed home ownership.

8.6 An introduction to key issues and concerns arising in the general law

In a direct continuation of these suggestions, the importance of this study flows from understanding that shared occupation of a home does not necessarily amount to shared *ownership of* a home. Indeed, *Goodman* v *Gallant* [1986] Fam 106 provides authority pre-dating *Stack* v *Dowden* by a decade that even where legal title to property is vested in both parties, documents of title to land relate to its legal ownership only and not to the apportionment of the equity in the property. Where there is a declaration of beneficial interests (declaration of trust) contained in the documents of title, this will be conclusive, as recently restated by the Court of Appeal in *Pankhania* v *Chandegra (by litigation friend)* [2012] EWCA Civ 1438. But it is still very common for legal title in the family home to be vested in the name of one party alone, and there is often no declaration of the parties' interests in the property beyond this.

As authority that where there is a written declaration of trust, the courts will enforce it, *Goodman* v *Gallant* becomes significant in due course, when reference is made to what the parties might feel about the contributions that they actually make to the property. While the Law Commission has recommended that express declarations of trust should be made, and HM Land Registry rules now require this where legal title is jointly held, this is prospective and rarely happens other than when so required.

We know that, traditionally, disputes arose from sole legal ownership of family homes and, as we will discover, there are a number of reasons why *Stack* v *Dowden*-type joint legal ownership disputes are likely to remain more unusual. In the first situation, appeal must be made to equity precisely because the claimant has no rights to the property that law will recognize; in the second, equity wishes to respond to the substance of ownership behind the formality of title ownership of the property at law. In turn, equity has recourse to the implied trust because there is no express declaration of trust. We know that the courts have been heavily criticized in this regard, and other noteworthy initial points include the following.

- *Disputes relating to home ownership most commonly arise as disputes as between couples.* There are cases that arise from time to time in which disputed ownership occurs as between family members, or more exceptionally between non-related 'companions' who share living arrangements, but which almost always arise between what, in everyday language, we would term a 'couple' or, in the language used by the Law Commission in its 2006–07 publications on cohabitation, persons in an 'intimate and exclusive' relationship. The significance of distinguishing ownership of a shared home from its occupation as a core element in these disputes has been noted and will be very significant throughout this chapter, and it helps us at the outset to understand why virtually all of these cases concern couples.

More recently, *Stack* v *Dowden, Fowler* v *Barron* [2008] EWCA Civ 377, and now the Supreme Court *Jones* v *Kernott* [2012] UKSC 53 recognize that those who live in a couple arrangement will typically regard their relationship as a joint venture, which is characterized by 'classic pooling of resources'. Because of this, most couples will make assumptions that shared occupation does amount to shared ownership. So while you might *hope* for this if you were to live with your mother, aunt or brother, or even a lifelong friend, you would be more likely to *expect* this as part of a couple without feeling that you have to raise the issue. This is likely to be so in any case, but it becomes an even stronger assumption where a couple has children, which will frequently mean that primary childcare responsibilities become those of one of the parties.

- *These situations arise because parties in a relationship frequently do not discuss the beneficial ownership of their home.* This might sound bizarre, but it happens a lot and for a number of different reasons. But, like the cases illustrating certainty of intention and also arising in relation to the constitution of trusts, this is an example of people not making intentions clear. And if we consider the 'couple' example, this is because a large number of persons in such living arrangements will read such an intention into the sum of their 'joint venture'.

- *These issues will often be considered only when a relationship is breaking down, or has already done so.* The judge-made property law thus applies potentially to all types of party sharing a home, and the most common context for this is the breakdown of the relationship between the parties. The special statutory provisions for spouses and civil partners have ensured that most 'ordinary trusts law' cases concern cohabiting unmarried couples. However, the 'signature event' on which disputes concerning home ownership will become exposed will not always be relationship breakdown. This is significant because it will very often be only on the occurrence of a signature event that the parties will confront the realities of sharing ownership, and not simply occupation of a home, because they are forced to do so. As the Law Commission's 2006–07 work on cohabitation reminds us, this can also be the death of a partner. But for our present purposes, the signature events we encounter are relationship breakdown and also the situation like that in *Lloyds Bank* v *Rosset* [1991] AC 107 in which the potential loss of a home forces the parties to consider their interests beyond being able to enjoy occupying it.

- *The context of relationship breakdown makes determinations of shared ownership particularly problematic for the courts.* However, because much of the case law reflects relationship breakdown, we see the courts having to make these determinations in very unsatisfactory circumstances. At best, these are parties who were once very intimate and who are now not so, but relationship breakdown can be very acrimonious. It is also the case that the courts must look at the history of a relationship over a long period of time to consider whether there is actually an injustice to which equity should respond.

- *Traditionally, the emphasis of this has been ordinary trusts law, but in the past decade there has been a marked trend in the courts taking a distinctive approach based on proprietary estoppel.* In common with the trust, proprietary estoppel is an equitable doctrine, and in some respects at least it serves functions that are very similar to implied trusts. But it will become clear that, in other ways, its approach is different from that of the trust, and that judicial favour is currently now strongly for the trust.

Questions to be asked and questions to be addressed

As a 'wrap' for this general introduction and in anticipation of the material to follow, it now becomes clear that judicial approaches to any case of disputed home owner-ship are underpinned by two questions. This is the case whether the courts show a preference for trusts or estoppel, but reiterating that the current approach is now a trusts one.

Traditionally, there have been two questions that needed to be *addressed*. But it is now more accurate to identify two questions that need to be *asked*. Traditionally, these questions to be addressed have been, first, *can* the party who is claiming an interest in the property actually establish that he or she has a beneficial interest in the home, and second, if he or she can do so, *what size* should that beneficial interest be?

We shall look more closely at the change to this traditional formulation in more detail in due course, but to clarify things at this juncture, the essence of this traditional two-question formulation does still apply to the vast majority of cases. The only cases to which it will not apply are *Stack* v *Dowden*-type situations in which both parties are legal owners. This suggests that the first question to be *asked* is whether the claimant holds legal title to the property. If the answer to that question is 'yes', then there is only one question to be *addressed*. In these circumstances, in order to provide justice, equity is concerned only with how much of a share each legal owner acquires, because *Stack* is authority that holding title at law assumes some sharing in equity. For *Stack* cases, the only issue to be addressed is the 'how much?' question.

In focusing on the general law, the two-question formulation to be addressed still applies where the answer to the question of 'does the claimant hold legal title?' is 'no'. Understanding that this has been the norm traditionally provides the basis for appreci-ating the modern law, and how it has emerged and been shaped.

8.7 Uncertainty in the law, dissatisfaction, and the significance of *Lloyds Bank plc* v *Rosset*

Even at this early stage, we are already aware that the courts have received much criti-cism for responses to disputed home ownership, and it will become clear how much this has influenced new approaches. But first, in linking traditional judicial approaches with the Law Commission's association of this with 'injustice' for claimants, we shall note that the law was particularly unsatisfactory prior to 1991. At this point, it was vir-tually impossible to make any kind of statement on what the law was with any kind of certainty, let alone clarity. Here, 1991 is seen as a key date on the basis that this is when the House of Lords stepped in with a remarkably clear statement of law, courtesy of Lord Bridge, in *Lloyds Bank plc* v *Rosset* [1991] 1 AC 107.

However, before introducing *Lloyds Bank* v *Rosset* as a very clear statement of the law, we will need some background on why this clear statement actually appeared at this point in time. The first thing to explain is that it was, in many respects, a response to inconsisten-cies in the case law. These inconsistencies had themselves emerged through very different responses to the tension between certainty and justice during the 1970s and 1980s. In this sphere, the tensions between certainty and justice—which provide the setting for implied trusts—had created a body of highly inconsistent case law for a number of reasons.

This became very strongly associated with considerable disagreement about the appro-priate use and application of the constructive trust in cases of disputed home ownership.

Significantly, much of this stemmed from the way in which applying the other response to injustice in these circumstances—the resulting trust—was proving to be very limited in scope.

8.7.1 The growth of the use of constructive trusts and the problems created by this

In Chapter 6, we learned that the resulting trust is a mechanism for recovering one's own property, with *Dyer* v *Dyer* [1788] 2 Cox Eq Cas 92 illustrating how the so-called 'voluntary conveyance' resulting trust would ensure that property belonging to one person could be retained by him even if legal title was then transferred to another. This means that, in circumstances under which a non-legal owner of a property has made no contribution of his own property to the home, he will be unable to recover any on the basis of a resulting trust. In short, the resulting trust will only ever address situations in which money has *actually been provided* in the acquisition of a home at all. And even in this latter situation, the mechanics of recovering 'one's own property' will 'limit' the amount recoverable in respect of this to the amount that has actually been provided, or, more accurately, the proportion of the *value* of the home that this amount represents.

In these circumstances, it is not surprising that the more flexible and adaptable constructive trust has become highly influential. It is not premised on recovering property and so its remedial properties are not limited in this way. Instead, the constructive trust is premised on reasons of imposition on conscience and, for disputed home ownership, this has become attached to reasons of conscience pointing to why the parties *should* share ownership. It will become clear that, in turn, this has become strongly attached to the way in which the parties appear to have agreed to share ownership, notwithstanding the location of legal title and that the agreement should accordingly stand. It has also become attached to situations in which the legal owner has made some representation to the effect that ownership is to be shared by the parties, and the way in which he should accordingly be held to what has been said.

In seeking to draw together these key elements of the rationale for the constructive trust, it has become recognized as a mechanism to give effect to the parties' 'common intention' that ownership in their home is shared, manifested in a conventional agreement, or an understanding arising from the legal owner's representations. *Both* are linked by the way in which equity imposes a constructive trust because it would be unconscionable for a legal owner of property not to be held to the agreement reached or representation made. We shall also see how the constructive trust has also become used in situations beyond this in which there is no agreement to share ownership.

Although this narrative does explain how the constructive trust has become so influential in determinations of disputed home ownership, it can also help to explain why a number of difficulties have arisen and why uncertainty came to characterize the approaches adopted by the courts. This is because applying the constructive trust to shared home ownership has been problematic, as evidenced by the very divided case law that was in evidence prior to *Rosset*.

8.7.2 Difficulties arising in the application of constructive trusts to disputed home ownership: divided case law and the context for *Rosset*

During the 1970s and 1980s, case law reflected the way in which the constructive trust was becoming the mechanism of choice for resolving disputed home ownership, and also inconsistencies in situations in which it was being implied by equity in order to address an injustice. This occurred along the fault line of finding evidence of a common intention to share ownership in a home, which resulted in two types of response situation in which common intention could not be ascertained.

Ascertaining beneficial interests in the absence of common intention

Strict property principles should apply where a common intention to share ownership beneficially of a home belonging only to one party at law could not be found. *Burns* v *Burns* [1984] Ch 317 illustrates the principle that mutual intention regarding the sharing of their lives together and occupying the property together did not amount to mutual intention to share beneficial ownership in the property. In that case, Fox LJ stated that 'The mere fact that parties live together and do the ordinary domestic tasks is, in my view, no indication at all that they thereby intended to alter the existing property rights of either of them'. *Gissing* v *Gissing* [1971] AC 866 insisted that a constructive trust could only ever be applied in response to the parties' common intention and that, in the absence of this, strict property principles applied, and at the heart of any interest arising would be financial contributions made by the claimant.

Ascertaining beneficial interests based on criteria of fairness and justice

Alongside the strict property principles that were being adopted in absence of common intention, an alternative approach based on 'conscience and justice' started to appear. This reflected the belief that too little weight was being attached to indirect contributions, and that the courts should be more flexible in looking at the conduct and intentions of the parties after acquiring the property, as well as upon it. Lord Denning pioneered this, and key cases including *Eves* v *Eves* [1975] 1 WLR 1138 and *Hussey* v *Palmer* [1972] 1 WLR 1286 were being based upon a new model constructive trust, which could be imposed 'whenever justice and good conscience require it'.

Thus, in many respects, the case study of disputed home ownership can be seen as a microcosm of the tensions that have subsisted in constructive trust theory, which were identified in Chapter 6. These cluster differing views on whether, in English law, the constructive trust is more appropriately viewed as a substantive institution that formalizes an existing proprietary entitlement, or is capable of subsisting as a more radical 'remedial' type, which is capable of actually creating a proprietary entitlement for the claimant.

8.8 The context for *Rosset*: clarification and restatement—and finality in law?

Because of the very divided views on applying constructive trusts coming across in the case law pre-*Rosset*, the law in respect of the position of non-legal owners of property became very difficult to state with any degree of certainty. Cases could easily go 'either way' with very little indication and, in a number of cases, a great deal appeared to 'turn' on very little. This was increasingly deemed as being unsatisfactory, because property rights are valuable and the function of equity is to manage the tensions that arise from ownership of property, not to disregard them.

In this respect, Lord Bridge's judgment in *Rosset* was seen as providing a very clear statement of the law and, for this reason, it will be the starting point for the substantive consideration given to the law shortly. However, in still having much to say by way of introduction, we must also be aware that, notwithstanding its apparent clarity and definitiveness, the law post-*Rosset* became unsettled and uncertain once again. Much more recently, and certainly since 2007, more certainty has returned to the law, but there are still very significant issues that remain unclear. And this new phase of the law has also, in some respects, seen *Rosset*'s significance eclipsed by the House of Lords' decision in *Stack* v *Dowden* [2007] UKHL 17, with much of the ground for this being prepared by the Court of Appeal's decision in *Oxley* v *Hiscock* [2004] 3 All ER 703.

As we shall discover, the influence that these cases have brought to bear on the law can be seen as unsettling and the cause of uncertainty, because they do show some very marked differences from Lord Bridge's very clear statement of law, which we will see was regarded by him as restating, rather than rewriting, the law. Crucially, both *Oxley* and *Stack* are authority that the fundamental distinction that Lord Bridge drew between 'two types of case'—in addressing the two key questions at the heart of any dispute—have been blurred to some degree. However, as will become apparent, it is not clear to what degree this has occurred. It certainly has so in the question of quantifying beneficial interests that have been found to exist, but it is far from clear that there has been any departure from the approach adopted in *Rosset* for determining whether a beneficial interest actually exists. As we will see, there was talk in *Stack* about 'moving the law on' from *Rosset* in this latter regard, but it is not clear that this has happened: *Oxley* was more circumspect about this, and in any case observations made on establishing an interest in both of these authorities (and also several decisions which have followed since) are *obiter*, because all of these cases concerned situations in which existence of beneficial interest was not in dispute and so they concerned only the question of *quantum*.

Four key cases: setting out the facts by way of introduction

This suggests that *Rosset* remains very important as a matter of law, as well as being very convenient for structuring these materials. Its value in both of these regards follows from understanding why it was such a significant case in 1991. Ahead of this, though, and in recognition that today it is one of three very significant cases, it might be helpful to set out the facts of each of these cases as a way in to understanding the legal issues that they raised, and the legal authority that they actually provide for how the courts approach questions of shared home ownership. Once we have an idea of the stories behind these cases, we will return to using them to analyse the law, and this will commence with looking at how and why *Rosset* was such a significant case in 1991.

- In *Lloyds Bank* v *Rosset* [1991] 1 AC 107, a married couple decided to purchase a semi-derelict farmhouse for £57,000. Mrs Rosset understood that the entire purchase money was to come out of a family trust fund, and the trustees' insistence that the house be conveyed in Mr Rosset's sole name appeared to be the only reason why this occurred. The house required renovation, and it was intended that this should be a joint venture. The vendors allowed Mr and Mrs Rosset to enter the property a number of weeks before completion in order to begin repairs and to render the house habitable. During this period, Mrs Rosset spent a lot of time at the house, urging on the builders and attempting to coordinate their work (until her husband insisted that he alone should give instructions), going to builders' merchants to obtain material required by the builders, and delivering the materials to the site. She also assisted her husband in planning the renovation and decoration of the house (she was a skilled painter and decorator), wallpapering two bedrooms, arranging the insurance of the house, arranging a crime prevention survey, and assisting in arranging the installation of burglar alarms. Unknown to his wife, Mr Rosset had needed further funds to make the purchase and obtained an overdraft of £18,000 from Lloyds Bank on the date of completion of the purchase, secured by a legal charge on the property. He later defaulted on the repayments; when the bank sought possession, Mrs Rosset claimed a beneficial interest in the property, binding the bank by virtue of her actual occupation as an overriding interest under the Land Registration Act 1925, s. 70(1)(g). In the Court of Appeal, most of the discussion revolved around whether Mrs Rosset was in actual occupation when the charge was created, in order to be able to rely upon s. 70(1)(g). The House of Lords was able to avoid all discussion of s. 70(1)(g), simply holding that Mrs Rosset had no beneficial interest. There was no evidence of any agreement between the parties to share the beneficial interest, and the wife's contributions were regarded as *de minimis* on the principles discussed thus far.

- *Oxley* v *Hiscock* [2004] concerned a home shared by the claimant and her former partner, the defendant. Initially, the parties lived in a council house occupied by the claimant and her children from a former marriage; in September 1987, the claimant exercised her right to buy the council property. This purchase was funded by the defendant from proceeds of the sale of his property; in 1991, a larger house (the disputed property) was purchased using £61,500 from the sale of the original former council house, a further £35,500 from the defendant, and a mortgage loan of £30,000. The new property was registered in the defendant's name despite the claimant's solicitor advising her to secure her position through joint registration. Thereafter, both parties contributed towards the maintenance and improvement of the property, and pooled resources more generally in the belief that each had a beneficial interest. By 2001, the mortgage had been paid off, but the parties' relationship had broken down and the home was sold. The claimant sought a declaration that the proceeds of sale of the property were held on trust for both parties in equal shares, and at first instance this was upheld. On appeal, it was found that, in the absence of 'evidence of any discussion between the parties as to the amount of the share each was to have', the fairest outcome would be a 40:60 per cent split in favour of the defendant, with the observation made that ordering an equal distribution would be unfair to the defendant.

- The facts of *Stack* v *Dowden* [2007] UKHL 17 concerned a relationship that commenced in 1975, when the parties were teenagers; subsequently, Ms Dowden became the legal owner of a property (10 Purves Road) costing £30,000, which she shared with Mr Stack. The purchase was funded with £8,000 from Dowden's building society account (it is not clear whether Stack made any contribution to this fund), and £22,000 by way of a mortgage executed in Dowden's sole name and for which she took sole responsibility—something that she also did in relation to all main outgoings (in the form of utility bills and council tax, etc.). Considerable improvements were made to the property by both parties and, in time, the couple had four children; throughout, Dowden earned almost double the amount earned by Stack. In 1993, the family purchased a new home, which was conveyed into the parties' joint names, but no declaration was made in respect of beneficial ownership. The purchase was made with consideration coming from the following sources: £128,813 from Dowden (from her building society account and from the proceeds of sale of the property in Purves Road); and £65,025 provided by way of a joint bank loan. Stack paid all mortgage interest payments and joint endowments, and the capital that was repaid on the property was in the following amounts: by Stack, £27,000; and by Dowden, £38,435. Once again, the utilities arrangements were all made in Dowden's name, and the parties kept separate accounts, savings, and investments. The parties separated in 2002 and, at first instance, an equal distribution was ordered, based on the nature of the partnership underlying the parties' relationship and focusing on their entire course of conduct together. Distribution on this basis would also have split the proceeds of sale from the Purves Road house had the relationship ended at that stage, but the Court of Appeal found that there was no basis on which Stack could show that it was intended that he should have an interest at this stage, on the view that he could not be shown to have contributed to the building society account from which the initial payment of the original home was paid. Dowden appealed against this and the Court of Appeal upheld this, making an award of beneficial interests amounting to a 65:35 per cent split in Dowden's favour. Stack appealed to the House of Lords, claiming an additional 15 per cent of proceeds, worth approximately £112,000, which would significantly represent a 50 per cent share; his appeal was dismissed.

- The parties in *Jones* v *Kernott* [2012] UKSC 53 started cohabiting in 1983; in 1985, a property was purchased in joint names, using the proceeds of sale from Jones' home and taking out a joint mortgage for the balance. They lived there together until they separated in 1993, when Kernott moved out and purchased another property. Kernott made no further contribution to the payment of the mortgage, or to the upkeep of the jointly owned property or to the outgoings in respect of it. In 2006, he sought to realize his share and, in 2008, severed the joint tenancy. Jones issued proceedings to determine the parties' respective beneficial interests, which resulted in an apportionment of 90:10 per cent in Jones' favour, because the parties' common intention had changed over time in the light of the circumstances, which found Jones to have made a much greater contribution to the property following Kernott's cession of contribution to it. This finding was overturned by the Court of Appeal, following the principle set out in *Stack* v *Dowden*—that is, that the presumption of equal sharing in equity had not been displaced by the subsequent inequality in actual contribution. In the absence of evidence of changed intentions relating to the extent of ownership, it was not possible for the Court to infer *changed* intentions regarding ownership of the home from the parties' conduct since separation. In the judgment handed down on 9 November 2011, the Supreme Court unanimously allowed the appeal and restored the order of the county court that Kernott's withdrawal from any contribution to the home for over fourteen years entitled the Court to conclude that the parties' common intention had actually moved away from that of equal sharing, which it was accepted subsisted up to the point of separation.

With the facts of the four key cases now set out, we return to why *Rosset* was such a significant case in 1991.

8.9 *Lloyds Bank* v *Rosset*: certainty and restatement articulated through two different types of case

Given the inconsistencies in applying the constructive trust to cases of disputed home ownership, the case law had become very divided and uncertain. *Rosset* was regarded at the time as an important statement of certainty in the law. Interestingly, as Lord Bridge himself saw things, it was actually a *restatement* of existing law rather than a *statement* of a new legal position. It was clearly intended to be an authoritative statement, and even a definitive statement. In Lord Bridge's view, it was a restatement of the way in which the constructive trust subsisted to give effect to the parties' common intentions surrounding ownership of their home; where a common intention to share ownership could not be found, beneficial interests would be determined by property-based principles (reflecting the parties' contributions of their own assets). Accordingly, the constructive trust was not a device for ensuring 'justice' by reading an injustice into every case of disputed ownership, and if a party were to contribute nothing of his own to the home of another, then he would not acquire an interest in it by virtue only of the fact that he had shared its occupation.

In taking this position (and, as he believed, restating the correct position of the law), Lord Bridge identified two types of case in which a common intention to share the ownership of a home could be found, and thus two broad types of situation that were capable of establishing a proprietary interest in a home belonging to another. As will become clear, for Lord Bridge, although both these case types were capable of establishing proprietary interests, they were actually very different. These types of case were to be ascertained from a 'first and fundamental question which must always be resolved'. For Lord Bridge, this would be central to distinguishing the two types of case, as follows:

> The first and fundamental question which must always be resolved is whether, independently of any inference to be drawn from the conduct of the parties in the course of sharing the house as their home and managing their joint affairs, there has at any time prior to acquisition, or exceptionally at some later date, been any agreement, arrangement or understanding reached between them that the property is to be shared beneficially. The finding of an agreement or arrangement to share in this sense can only, we think, be based on evidence of express discussions between the partners, however imperfectly remembered and however imprecise their terms may have been. *Once a finding to this effect is made it will only be necessary for the partner asserting a claim to a beneficial interest against the partner entitled to the legal estate to show that he or she has acted to his or her detriment or significantly altered his or her position in reliance on the agreement* in order to give rise to a constructive trust or proprietary estoppel.
>
> (*Lloyds Bank* v *Rosset* [1991] 1 AC 107, *per* Bridge LJ, at 132, emphasis added)

Lord Bridge continued, at 132, by explaining that:

> In sharp contrast with this situation is the very different one where there is no evidence to support a finding of an agreement or arrangement to share, however reasonable it might have been for the parties to reach such an arrangement if they had applied their minds to the question, and where the court must rely entirely on the conduct of the parties both as the basis from which to infer a common intention to share the property beneficially and as the conduct relied on to give rise to a constructive trust. In this situation *direct contributions to the purchase price by the partner who is not the legal owner, whether initially or by payment of mortgage instalments, will readily justify the inference necessary to the creation of a constructive trust. But, as we read the authorities, it is at least extremely doubtful whether anything less will do.*
>
> (Emphasis added)

This speech identified *two types of case*, which have since been referred to as '*Rosset* category 1' and '*Rosset* category 2'.

- *Rosset* category 1 cases arise where there is evidence of agreement to share the property beneficially. In these circumstances, the non-legal owner of property can 'claim' an interest in the property in equity by virtue of this agreement. In these circumstances, it is the agreement that is central in establishing the beneficial interest, with contributions made being central to invoking this by way of a constructive trust (to avoid s. 53(1)(b) requirements).

- *Rosset* category 2 cases are ones in which there is no 'independent' evidence of agreement to share the property beneficially and in which the only means that the court has of inferring this is from the contributions that the non-legal owner of property has made to the property. This means that the contributions that are made by the non-legal owner are the only means available to establish that the claimant has a beneficial interest in the home.

Applying constructive trusts to Rosset's two categories

Lord Bridge suggested that the beneficial interest being sought could be 'claimed' by the non-legal owner by virtue of constructive trust or proprietary estoppel. For some time after *Rosset*, the courts had a distinct preference for the constructive trust rather than the estoppel approach, which is also an equitable doctrine (but with a different premise and a response oriented towards achieving fairness, as we will note briefly in due course), and this position was reaffirmed by the House of Lords in *Stack* v *Dowden*. The two *Rosset* categories can be mapped onto the constructive trust as follows.

- Rosset *category 1* The express common intention constructive trust is based on an 'agreement or understanding reached between them that the property is to be shared beneficially' that was reached 'independently of any inference to be drawn from the conduct of the parties in the course of sharing the house as their home and managing their joint affairs'. As Lord Bridge envisioned the law, this type of constructive trust will arise from showing detrimental reliance on this agreement.

- Rosset *category 2* In the case of the inferred common intention constructive trust, there is no independently subsisting agreement and the court must rely 'entirely on the conduct of the parties', both as the basis on which to infer a common intention to share the property beneficially and as the conduct relied on to give rise to a constructive trust.

The situation arising in category 2 has also been analysed as an orthodox presumed resulting trust, rather than a constructive trust, in *Oxley* v *Hiscock* [2005] Fam 211 and *Stack* v *Dowden* [2007] UKHL 17. This is given some consideration in due course, where it will be suggested that Lord Bridge's analysis of the mechanism at work as a constructive trust, rather than one that is resulting, was actually quite deliberate.

8.10 *Rosset* and 'common intention' to share ownership of a home beneficially

According to Lord Bridge in *Rosset*, shared beneficial *ownership* in a family home by way of a constructive trust will only occur where it is the parties' common intention to share their home in this way. The significance attached to this by Lord Bridge reflected that, for some considerable time, the parameters of the law had been set by the proposition that *shared occupation* did not amount to *shared ownership*. Distinguishing this intention to share ownership then provides the justification for equity imposing a constructive trust on the legal owner of the property, whilst in absence of this intention there would be no justification for equity to do so.

In terms of appreciating the differences between the two types of case as Lord Bridge saw things, the key factor distinguishing them was the presence or absence of an agreement to share the property beneficially. The existence of an agreement (or understanding) between the parties would provide the clearest justification for a proprietary interest (here, ownership in equity) for the claimant to arise, but to qualify as such it appeared that this must be based on express discussion between the partners (about which more is said shortly). More importantly still, for Lord Bridge, this agreement must be independent of the contributions that the parties actually make (referred to as the 'conduct' of the parties), and this suggested that it would be the agreement rather than contributions made that would ultimately determine how much of a share in the home's ownership the claimant would be able to secure. This is significant because, although this is what the case law prior to *Rosset* suggested, this latter idea has undergone some significant change under the influence of *Oxley* v *Hiscock* and *Stack* v *Dowden*, whereby much more significance is now attached to what the parties have *actually contributed*.

Returning again to how Lord Bridge saw things, rather than how things might have changed in the aftermath of *Rosset*, the second type of case is where there is no evidence subsisting independently of the conduct of the parties (such as contributions to the home) of any such agreement. *Rosset* itself was such a case. Here, if any inference is to be drawn of an intention to share the beneficial interests, it can be drawn only on the basis of the contributions themselves. Thus the contributions are used to establish the existence of the beneficial interest 'owned' by a non-legal owner of property and, because there is no evidence other than this, they also appear to represent the means by which it would actually be quantified. It is important to appreciate at this point that Lord Bridge's opinion was that, in this type of situation, it was likely that only direct contributions to the purchase price by the partner who is not the legal owner would suffice, and that this could be manifested by way of initial deposit money or subsequently in mortgage repayments, and that nothing else would suffice. More will be said about this shortly, especially given the way in which Lord Bridge's strict approach to establishing an interest through conduct has been criticized, most recently in *Stack* v *Dowden* and in the decision of the Privy Council in *Abbot* v *Abbott* [2007] UKPC 53.

As Lord Bridge saw things in *Rosset*, the conduct of the parties was also to be relevant in the first type of case, but of far less importance than in the second type; in cases in which there was an agreement concerning ownership (in category 1 cases), it was not necessary for the claimant to have made any direct contributions to the purchase price. This is because the agreement to share is shown independently of the parties' conduct, and for Lord Bridge it appeared that the only function of the conduct is to get around the formality requirements of s. 53(1)(b) of the Law of Property Act 1925. This allows the inference to be drawn that the legal owner has declared himself trustee for himself and the other party. To be valid, such a declaration would need to be in signed writing (by virtue of s. 53(1)(b)) unless there is an implied, resulting, or constructive trust, in which case, by virtue of s. 53(2), the provisions of s. 53(1)(b) do not apply. There will be a constructive trust if the claimant has acted to his detriment or significantly altered his position in reliance on the agreement. Traditionally, contributions made in these circumstances have thus been regarded as conduct showing detrimental reliance, which will then allow formality requirements to be circumvented. This is because, as explained by Lord Bridge in *Rosset*, for a claimant who can establish that he has altered his position in reliance on an agreement 'an enforceable interest ... by way ... of a constructive trust' can arise.

On this analysis, it follows that no detrimental reliance is required if the agreement is in writing—for example, where the parties communicate by signed letters—and that it will not be required where the property is not land (for example, a caravan or houseboat). As we will discover, however, this very functional view of contributions made in the context of category 1 agreements has been challenged by *Oxley* v *Hiscock* and *Stack* v *Dowden* (as already intimated, and as considered further extensively and across several sections within this chapter).

The modern law and the significance of Rosset, as it was intended by Lord Bridge

In trying to get a measure of the significance of the decision in *Rosset*, it was considered a landmark on two counts, which were closely related to one another. First and foremost, it reasserted that the proper role for the constructive trust was to give effect to the parties' intentions relating to ownership of shared homes; second, in making this clear, distinction was drawn between two types of case, which, although both capable of giving rise to an equitable interest in a home belonging to another, operated in very different ways. The decision made a distinction between cases in which evidence of agreement between the parties concerning sharing of beneficial interests existed and cases in which there was no independent evidence of this. In making an analysis of the case law, with *Rosset*'s classification at heart, two points of focus are central. We have already been introduced to these, and essentially these can be understood as questions of what must be shown in order for a party who is not a legal owner to establish the existence of a beneficial interest, and, once this has been shown, how the courts will decide how sizeable this interest should be.

Rosset was intended to be important clarification of the position of establishing a beneficial interest in property. However, even in respect of the position of a non-legal owner of property who is seeking to establish that shared occupation *does amount to shared ownership* (either on the basis of express agreement, or conduct-based evidence of agreement through making contributions), the position post-*Rosset* has become confused and unsettled in a number of ways. Key reasons for this are now explained in brief, but will make much better sense when read alongside the material relating to the later application of *Rosset*. For now, you need simply to be aware that difficulties in applying *Rosset* post-*Rosset* have emerged from:

- a *blurring of distinction* between category 1 cases and category 2 cases, in that (small direct) contributions made in absence of express agreement started to produce very similar results to those that Lord Bridge stressed were permitted in the presence of an express agreement to share (category 1), the most striking example of this being *Midland Bank* v *Cooke* [1995] 4 All ER 562;
- the courts having *regard to indirect financial contributions* in absence of express agreement to share (such as in *Le Foe* v *Le Foe* [2001] 2 FLR 970), contrary to Lord Bridge's statement in *Rosset*;
- the difficulties raised by *any* contributions that arise *after the home is acquired* (acquisition is *Rosset*'s point for ascertaining the parties, intentions regarding ownership), including very significant improvements to homes that are capable of adding significant capital value;.
- the *rise and fall* of the trusts-based analysis of beneficial ownership in the family home, with *Oxley* v *Hiscock* [2005] Fam 211 being a high watermark for the courts in applying an estoppels-based analysis to quantifying shared interests in family homes;

- instances in which, according to *Oxley* v *Hiscock*, 'each party is entitled to that share which the *court considers fair* having regard to the "whole course of dealing" between them in relation to the property' (including indirect contributions and 'later' contributions);
- the rise and fall *and rise again* of a trusts-based analysis of beneficial ownership evidenced in *Stack* v *Dowden* [2007] UKHL 17, in which, while in favour of *Oxley*'s holistic 'whole course of dealings' approach, the House of Lords criticized the emphasis on the courts' assessment of fairness, because the focus should be on what the parties *intended*, making reference to the need for the courts to infer parties' intentions rather than to impute them, and that a trusts approach was a better reflection overall of the valuable property rights that were at stake.

In addition, both *Stack* v *Dowden* and *Oxley* v *Hiscock* appeared to leave unchanged a fundamental part of Lord Bridge's requirements in *Rosset*—that any claimant must establish an interest in the home. Thus, in the essence of *actually establishing* this agreement to share, the approach adopted in *Rosset* as to how this is shown (through reference to category 1 and category 2 cases) stands. Here, *Oxley* and *Stack* are both best analysed as *quantification* cases, with *Rosset* remaining the leading case on establishing the existence of a beneficial interest, although both cases were very critical of the strict approach adopted in *Rosset* concerning 'acceptable contributions'. The same can now be said about *Jones* v *Kernott*, with this now appearing to provide Supreme Court authority for the continuing application of *Rosset* in sole legal ownership disputes, certainly in essence.

Stack v *Dowden* has resolved a number of these difficulties and also the uncertainties that started to emerge or reappear post-*Rosset*. This will be noted as we consider the application of *Rosset* in the modern law, at the pertinent times. However, before this happens, it is also worth noting that *Stack* v *Dowden* has precipitated recognition that, in the absence of an express declaration of trust, even jointly held legal title in a family home does not necessarily reflect the parties' intentions regarding the shared home.

The next section provides the foundations for understanding what has happened to *Rosset* since 1991. In due course, this becomes focused on how the important statements made in *Rosset* concerning how a claimant can establish an interest in a shared property, and thereafter how its size will be determined, have fared since *Rosset*. We now consider each of these questions as they were approached in *Rosset* itself, looking at both categories of case identified by Lord Bridge.

8.11 Establishing an interest in a shared family home under *Rosset*

Unless the parties both hold legal title to the disputed home, this is the first question that must be asked in all cases of disputed home ownership, and it is one that must be addressed in any claim for a beneficial interest in a home that belongs in law solely to someone other than the claimant. And, in making a fundamental distinction between two categories of case, it becomes very quickly apparent from *Rosset* that Lord Bridge envisaged this question being addressed very differently under each one.

8.11.1 **Establishing an interest as a *Rosset* category 1 claimant**

For Lord Bridge, the essence of the agreement that he described as characterizing category 1 cases is that this subsists independently of any contributions that are made.

What follows now is an examination of the key elements in this formula for establishing an interest, relating to actually forming an agreement and what is required. Notwithstanding that Lord Bridge suggested that interests in property arising in this category could do so by virtue of constructive trust or proprietary estoppel, *Stack v Dowden* [2007] UKHL 17 suggested that a trust was a better mechanism for determining the valuable property rights that underpinned beneficial ownership of homes. This is very significant, because it contrasts with the approach taken in *Oxley v Hiscock* [2005] Fam 211, and with the long-standing criticism of this book that a superficial equation of two doctrines that might have some similarities actually overlooks the their fundamental differences in operation and actual outcome.

Lord Bridge and the similarities, and differences, between trust and estoppel
Given that Lord Bridge insisted that a category 1 claim could arise by way of a constructive trust or proprietary estoppel, this text has always explained the similarities between the two doctrines, as clearly envisioned by Lord Bridge. Both are concerned with ensuring that parties who represent a particular position cannot then assert one that is different from this, with both arising from a claimant's reliance on what is represented. The text has also put much stress on their differences, suggesting that Lord Bridge too readily concluded that trust and estoppel were straightforward 'either/or' mechanisms. As we know, a trust is premised on an irrevocable commitment, and the significance of this becomes clearer as we look at *how* estoppel operates to ensure that a party who has misled another is not permitted to go back on his word and *what* it can deliver for a claimant.

An estoppel requires that one party has been misled by another, but demands nothing more than that the claimant has relied to his detriment on what has been represented. This means that, unlike in the case of a trust, there are no express communication requirements for an estoppel to arise, and so this might seem more flexible than requiring 'express communication' (which Lord Bridge did, in fact). But estoppels are also more limited in terms of what is capable of being recovered by the claimant, with this being measured by, and limited to, the extent of the encouraged reliance. Further to this, the guiding maxim for what a claimant is entitled to is the 'minimum equity to do justice'. Thus this text has always maintained that the consequences of applying a trusts or estoppel analysis can affect the size of the share received by the party establishing the interest in the shared home.

The popularization of the estoppel approach in *Oxley v Hiscock* was itself very strongly influenced by a number of Court of Appeal authorities relating to interests in land generally, including, centrally, the decision in *Yaxley v Gotts* [2000] Ch 162, in which Walker LJ suggested that, in many cases, operation of a trust and estoppel principles would produce similar results. However, shortly prior to this and mirroring the views of this text, in *Hyett v Stanley* [2003] EWCA 942, Sir Martin Nourse's views were that the two doctrines were quite different in effect, as well as in operation. In *Stack v Dowden*, the House of Lords did reaffirm the view that the trust mechanism does provide a better reflection of the valuable nature of beneficial interests in family homes. As part of this, it is interesting to see Lord Walker's reflections of his own views (as Walker LJ) in *Yaxley v Gotts*, and his acceptance of the differences in the two doctrines.

In the light of *Stack* v *Dowden*, it is no longer necessary to consider the application of proprietary estoppel to shared home ownership, and thus this analysis of category 1 cases is concentrated on how Lord Bridge's requirements apply to category 1 claims secured by way of a constructive trust.

Express discussion is required for an agreement to arise

From Lord Bridge's judgment, it is clear that, to amount to an agreement for the purposes of a category 1 case, the agreement to share ownership (the basis of the common intention) must be direct and must actually amount to *express discussion* between the parties. Lord Bridge was more flexible in other respects, and suggested that this could occur at *any time prior to the* acquisition (and even conceded that, in exceptional cases, it could arise 'at some later date'). It is also clear from Lord Bridge's speech that the agreement reached does not have to be perfectly remembered or even very precise. Nevertheless, to amount to an agreement, some actual discussion is necessary. Authority for this can be found in *Springette* v *Defoe* [1992] 2 FCR 561 and *Savill* v *Goodall* [1993] 1 FLR 755, both of which concerned the significance of discounts obtained by council tenants under 'right to buy' schemes in determinations of shared home ownership.

In *Springette* v *Defoe*, the parties purchased a house at a price discounted by 41 per cent on account of Springette's entitlement under 'right to buy'. The property was conveyed into joint names, but there was no determination made about beneficial ownership. Both were liable for mortgage repayments and both contributed equally to this. Both parties also provided other moneys, making Springette's overall financial contribution (including her discount value) about 75 per cent and Defoe's 25 per cent. When the relationship broke down, Springette insisted that she was entitled to 75 per cent, reflecting her contributions, while Defoe sought a 50 per cent share by virtue of being a *Rosset* category 1 claimant. The Court of Appeal rejected his claim, because there was no evidence of any express discussion between the parties and, in the words of Steyn LJ, '[o]ur trust law does not allow property rights to be affected by telepathy'. This meant that the actual common intention that Defoe alleged could not be established, and one could be inferred only from his conduct through contributions; in other words, he was a category 2 claimant rather than one in category 1.

Shortly afterwards, a different result was achieved in *Savill* v *Goodall*, in which a 42 per cent discount entitlement of the defendant was put towards a house purchase for which the remainder of funds came from a mortgage that Mr Savill accepted liability to repay. This property was also transferred into the joint names of the parties, but on this occasion the Court of Appeal held that the express discussions between the parties that beneficial interests should be divided equally, when combined with Mr Savill's agreement to repay the mortgage capital and costs of redemption, meant that beneficial interest subsisted equally between them. Prior to *Stack*'s ruling on sharing in equity by joint legal owners, the only substantive difference between *Springette* v *Defoe* and *Savill* v *Goodall* was the absence of any discussion in the former and its presence in the latter case.

Although the need for express discussion was thrown into doubt subsequently in *Midland Bank* v *Cooke* [1995] 4 All ER 562, Lord Bridge's insistence on requiring express discussion was quite deliberate. For Lord Bridge, this was a better basis for creating valuable property rights than the kind of assumptions about this that will commonly be read into couple partnerships. In this respect, while in *Cooke* Waite LJ might have been correct in saying that the parties in *Springette* were a middle-aged couple whose domestic arrangements should not be subject to the same levels of formality as a commercial partnership, he also overlooked some of the vital underpinnings of this area of law in trusts law.

The basis of a constructive trust is that, where one is found, it would be unconscionable for the legal owner to deny the rights of the other party, which in category 1 cases is where a claimant is said to have relied on what amounts to a declaration of trust by the legal owner. For this, it follows that something has to have been said for there to have been a declaration, because, as we know from Chapter 3, although the courts will accept conduct in lieu of words in principle (as illustrated in *Re Kayford Ltd* [1975] 1 WLR 279), this has to be appropriate in the circumstances. There is also the way in which a declaration of trust is an irrevocable and onerous commitment of property that has implications for its legal owner, and is also capable of binding third parties. This suggests in favour of requiring actual communication of an intention to share ownership to the other party (unless there is evidence that the parties are able to communicate by telepathy!).

Can an unconventional 'agreement' amount to an agreement?

The express discussion between the parties in *Savill* points to an agreement in the conventional sense of the word, but Lord Bridge alluded to an 'agreement or understanding' that beneficial ownership should be shared. Here, *Eves* v *Eves* [1975] 1 WLR 1338 and also *Grant* v *Edwards* [1986] 1 Ch 638 (both Court of Appeal cases) show how representations made by the legal owner of the property concerning its ownership can amount to being an agreement or understanding between the parties, even where what the claimant is being told is untruthful. In *Rosset*, both cases were explained as authorities that the express common intention at the heart of category 1 cases could be manifested in representations made, as well as by more conventional agreement. This was so on the basis of the inferences that could be drawn from them by the claimant, and the way in which this was, in turn, capable of influencing subsequent conduct of the party to whom the representation was being made.

Eves and *Grant* concerned very similar situations in which both female parties were given excuses as to why legal title to the homes that they shared with their partners would have to be vested in the male partner alone. Linda Grant was told that this was to prevent prejudice in her divorce proceedings, whilst Janet Eves was told that it was not possible for her to hold title at law because she was under 21 years old. In both situations, these were simply cover stories for their partners who did not want to share ownership, and the claims of both were upheld, with Grant being awarded a 50 per cent beneficial share and Eves securing one of 25 per cent; in *Rosset*, Lord Bridge said of both that they were 'outstanding examples ... of cases giving rise to situations in the first category'.

In *Grant* v *Edwards*, the reasoning was explicitly that the excuse could be construed as a common intention to share beneficial ownership of the home, on which Grant had relied to her detriment, so that she was entitled to a half-share by way of a resulting or constructive trust. When we look at category 2 cases, it will become manifestly clear that, under *Rosset* itself, Grant's actual contributions—which were not particularly significant or extensive—would not have given a half-share in absence of Edwards' representation, and that this 'reason' why the claimant's name could not be reflected in the legal documentation was the crucial element for the case. But how was this statement that was a *lie* ever construed as providing evidence of common intention? At first sight, we can see that Edwards had intentions very contrary to this, but what he said was interpreted by the Court as meaning 'Your name would go on the title, but for the fact that it would prejudice your matrimonial proceedings'. This was because, had Edwards intended to say 'The house is to be mine alone', there would have been no need for an excuse. By this tortuous reasoning, the Court was able to infer, independently of her contributions, a common intention that Grant was to have a half-share, and the case depended on this.

We can see the same principle at work in *Eves* v *Eves*, but this is not the way in which Lord Denning reasoned the outcome of a 25 per cent beneficial share for Janet Eves. We have already met *Eves* as an example of the wayward constructive trust application of which Lord Bridge was very critical in *Rosset*, and Lord Denning's view was that this outcome arose because it was a just one in the circumstances and that equity's capability to evolve to meet the needs of justice meant that the Court had discretion to depart from strict property principles. *Rosset* sought to restate strict property principles in applying a constructive trust, and so *Eves* was upheld as a category 1 case on *Grant* v *Edwards* reasoning, whilst Lord Bridge dismissed the Denning reasoning for its outcome.

But *Grant* v *Edwards* reasoning has been criticized for being entirely fictional on the basis that the male parties in both *Grant* and also *Eves* clearly did not intend for their partners to have any interest in the property. This has been noted by Simon Gardner (1993) 109 LQR 263, 265:

> If I give an excuse for rejecting an invitation to what I expect to be a dull party, it does not mean that I thereby agree to come: on the contrary, it means that I do not agree to come ... It is hard to think that the judges concerned really believed [in the fallacious reasoning].

Gardner's objections do have force if we take a *subjective* view of intention. But if we think back to Chapter 5, we already know from work on self-declarations of trusteeship that such are determined by examining what an owner-cum-settlor has said or done. We can also now analyse that this is determined objectively, with the obligation of the courts to give words their proper meaning being stressed in both *Richards* v *Delbridge* (1874) LR Eq 11 and *Re Kayford Ltd* [1975] 1 WLR 279. Indeed, at first instance in *Eves* v *Eves*, Brightman J remarked that 'The defendant clearly led the plaintiff to believe that she was to have some undefined interest in the property, and that her name was only omitted from the conveyance because of her age'.

Glover and Todd [1995] 5 Web JCLI suggests that Gardner's reasoning is misplaced on account of the merits of (and indeed the pedigree for) an objective approach where parties expressly, or more implicitly, invite others to rely on what they say or do. Once it is established that an objective approach is taken, by saying 'Were it not for your matrimonial proceedings, title to this home would be vested in you', the import was that the home would, in reality, belong to them both, without which there would be no reason for the excuse. In these circumstances, what Edwards actually thought is not relevant and what he can be taken to have meant is actually a very clear declaration of trust.

8.11.2 The significance of the 'agreement' and how a constructive trust arises from it

When we first encountered Lord Bridge's explanation of a category 1 claim, it is clear that he did not only identify an agreement to share, but also insisted that this needed to be relied upon by the claimant. This can be seen from both *Eves* v *Eves* [1975] 1 WLR 1338 and also *Grant* v *Edwards* [1986] 1 Ch 638, which show that when an equitable interest in a shared home does arise, it does so because a constructive trust is imposed on the holder of legal title as a result of what is said. However, the agreement or representation will not *of itself* give rise to an interest by way of constructive trust, and this must be coupled with detrimental reliance. For Lord Bridge, this is what invokes s. 53(2) of the Law of Property Act 1925, which allows the law to treat the trust as a constructive one rather than one that is express, which would be subject to s. 53(1)(b). This works because the claimant's reliance on what is said to him would make it unconscionable for the legal owner not to be held to what he has said. This is why, for Lord Bridge, contributions were very important, even in the presence of an agreement, because they provided evidence of reliance.

Establishing detrimental reliance, what is required, and what is difficult to show

In *Grant* v *Edwards*, detrimental reliance was established from the way in which Grant had made some repayments on a second mortgage taken out, and made substantial contributions towards general household expenses, provided housekeeping, and brought up the children. In *Eves*, Janet Eves' detrimental reliance involved participating in the extensive refurbishment of the disputed home by famously wielding a 14 lb sledgehammer to break up the concrete in the front garden so that it could be levelled and turfed. In *Ungurian* v *Lesnoff* [1990] Ch 206, the claimant gave up her flat in Poland and her career to cohabit with the defendant in London, following a whirlwind meeting and his assurances of making her secure and happy. And in *Hammond* v *Mitchell* [1991] 1 WLR 1127, Vicky Mitchell's reliance on Hammond's assurances about the property did give rise to a half-share in it.

In terms of what actually amounts to detrimental reliance, in *Grant* v *Edwards*, Nourse LJ explained this as 'conduct on which the claimant could not reasonably have been expected to embark unless she was to have an interest in the house'. The difficulties that can arise here include establishing that conduct actually is detrimental reliance rather than acting 'ordinarily' on account of love and affection. We can explain this by thinking back to how so many of these disputes arise. Earlier, it was explained that this is because couples will commonly make assumptions about ownership of their home on the basis of a belief that their relationship is a joint venture; in these circumstances, it will be very difficult for a claimant to show that he or she acted in reliance of acquiring an interest in the home rather than in furtherance of the partnership—and indeed out of love and affection.

This means that, perversely, showing this is especially difficult for parties in very close relationships with others, and it is with this in mind that we can start to understand how the approach taken in *Grant* v *Edwards* was developed and refined in *Wayling* v *Jones* [1993] 69 P & CR 170 and also *Ottey* v *Grundy* [2003] EWCA Civ 1176. In *Ottey* v *Grundy*, the test adopted to establish detrimental reliance was, according to Arden LJ, not to be that 'the claimant would have left the maker of the assurance if the promise had not been made, but only that he would have left the maker of the assurance if the promise had been withdrawn'. This was the test adopted in *Wayling* v *Jones*. Under *Wayling*, once the claimant shows that a promise was made, the burden of proof falls upon the maker to show that the claimant did not, in fact, rely on the promise and acted as he or she did for different reasons—which, in a number of close relationships, could so easily be out of love and affection. This shows that the courts do very clearly understand the implications of the close and often intimate relations between the parties. It also shows the courts seeking actively to manage these by trying to ensure that a defendant cannot unfairly exploit the closeness of the partnership in order to be free from the promise that he or she appears to have made.

8.12 *Rosset* category 2: establishing an equitable interest in property by way of an inferred common intention constructive trust

There are a large number of cases in this category that arise precisely because so few people actually discuss ownership of their homes and, where disputes arise, it will be left to the courts to come to a view on whether or not there was a common intention to share ownership of the home beneficially. Because there is no 'independent' evidence of agreement in these circumstances, any contributions that have been made by the parties provide the only means by which the courts can *infer* the existence of a common intention to share ownership (rather than occupation or enjoyment) of the property, or conclude that such a common intention does not exist. For Lord Bridge, in this type of case, contributions would play a central role, unlike their more ancillary function in category 1 cases. And, in turn, Lord Bridge's determination of which contributions would suffice was very strict, mirroring closely the strict property approaches found in pre-*Rosset* case law, evidenced in cases such as *Gissing* v *Gissing* [1971] AC 866 and *Pettit* v *Pettit* [1970] AC 777. According to Lord Bridge:

- contributions must be directly referable to the *initial* acquisition of the home— and, in this category, deposit monies or mortgage repayments will readily justify the inference necessary for creating a constructive trust; and
- contributions that will *not* suffice were all others that did not relate 'directly to the purchase of the home'.

It will become apparent that it is in regard to category 2 that most change to the law post-*Rosset* can be seen in the light of *Oxley* and *Stack*. However, the exact scope of this is not clear, whilst it *is* clear that the way in which *Stack* reinforced *Oxley* has manifestly changed the way in which beneficial interests are quantified from that envisioned by *Rosset* (as we will consider in due course). It is far from clear that *Rosset*'s position in respect of establishing an interest has been altered at all. But before considering either of these propositions, we shall take a look at how Lord Bridge envisaged that a category 2 claimant would be able to establish an interest through the parties' common intention to share ownership of the home being inferred by the court.

8.12.1 Contributions that *are* capable of raising the inference of ownership

Here, the spotlight is on contributions actually made by a claimant precisely because there is no independent evidence of his intention, and the significance of this requires us to understand that, in Lord Bridge's view, he was restating the law rather than re-writing it. Given that it was only proper to impose a trust over a shared home where the parties are said to have a common intention to share ownership of the home, and not simply its occupation, it should not be too surprising that Lord Bridge insisted that only some contributions were capable of raising the inference of common intention that ownership should be shared. This meant that there would be a limited number of acceptable contributions, and whilst Lord Bridge suggested that deposit money and mortgage repayments would readily 'raise the inference' that ownership was to be shared, it is also possible to conclude from this that these were likely to be the *only* contributions that were *acceptable*. Lord Bridge explained his view as being the way in which he understood the earlier authorities, and such a view is, of course, entirely consistent with *Rosset*'s apparent basis in strict property reasoning.

What can be added to this is the position of so-called 'discounts' attaching to right to buy, rather than actual cash, as seen in *Springette* v *Defoe* [1992] 2 FCR 561. *Springette* was decided after *Rosset*, but clearly such contributions are direct, in as much as they do directly inform the purchase price; in that respect, they are also clearly referable to the acquisition of the home and were accepted as such in what was a category 2 case. It is not clear that, for Lord Bridge, anything else would suffice, and there are a number of contributions that do arise which we can definitely say would be outside the scope of permissible contributions, on the basis that Lord Bridge would consider them *de minimis*.

8.12.2 Contributions definitely outside the second category according to *Rosset*

Lord Bridge insisted that he was restating the law, and that his views on contributions were derived from the authorities as he understood them. Here, we can see that Lord Bridge's perspective was clearly influenced by *Gissing* v *Gissing* [1970] AC 886, *Pettitt* v *Pettitt* [1971] AC 777, and *Burns* v *Burns* [1984] Ch 317. All of these cases point to the way in which, for cases within category 2 (where common intention regarding ownership is being inferred without evidence of an agreement), no value is accorded to contributions falling short of deposit money and mortgage repayments. In *Gissing* v *Gissing*, Mrs Gissing failed to establish an interest in the home owned at law by her husband notwithstanding sixteen years of marriage, because this was one of the strict property authorities pre-dating *Rosset*. An attempt at a more flexible approach towards contributions was made by Lord Denning in *Eves* v *Eves* [1971] 1 WLR 1138, reasoning that equity was 'not past the age of child bearing' and thus not incapable of providing more flexibility, but the inflexible view on indirect contributions was reiterated in *Burns* v *Burns* before it was restated in *Rosset* (as Lord Bridge saw things).

Burns v *Burns* had very similar facts to those of *Gissing*, except that the parties remained unmarried notwithstanding living together for nineteen years (seventeen of which in the disputed property itself). The house had been purchased in the name of Patrick Burns alone, who also paid the entire purchase price and subsequent mortgage repayments. The claimant—Valerie Burns—made no financial contributions, but had brought up their children, performed domestic duties, and recently contributed from her own earnings towards household expenses. She also bought various fittings and a washing machine, and redecorated the interior of the house. When the relationship broke down, Valarie Burns was unable to establish a beneficial interest in the home, because this would have to be determined by orthodox property principles (the by-then-enacted Matrimonial Causes Act 1973 could not apply because the parties were not married) and in the absence of financial contribution that could be related to the acquisition of the property (or even an identifiable financial contribution enabling Patrick Burns to pay the mortgage instalments), which approach was upheld in *Winkworth* v *Edward Baron Development Co. Ltd* [1988] 1 WLR 1512.

This orthodox position was then taken by Lord Bridge as the authoritiative position in *Lloyds Bank plc* v *Rosset* [1991] 1 AC 107. The cases culminating in *Rosset* suggest that what is required for beneficial interest to be acquired in this type of case (under category 2) is that the contributions being relied upon must not only be significant (and not *de minimis*), but also must be referable to the *initial* acquisition of the property. There is no such requirement under the first category in *Rosset*, where there is independent evidence of the intentions of the parties. In many ways, taking a very strict view on permissible contributions could mean that the realities behind shared home ownership can be too easily ignored, and can even lead to perverse outcomes in disputed home ownership; in reasserting strict property principles, it is likely that, in *Rosset*, Lord Bridge's statement of permissible contributions was considered exhaustive and intended to be so.

Criticisms of the category 2 approach, strict property principles, and the 'family economy'

The cases within category 2 have traditionally stood as authority that other contributions are not valued for the purposes of a claimant acquiring a proprietary interest in a home belonging to another. Ones that are very striking in this latter category are those associated with what was subsequently termed 'the family economy' in *Le Foe* v *Le Foe* [2001] 2 FLR 970, such as child rearing, payment of the household expenses, or providing furniture and domestic services, and even quite significant decorating and maintenance of the property. Generally speaking, these are contributions more typically made by the woman living in a home, and the law's approach of attaching value only to 'hard cash' contributions such as deposit money and mortgage repayments has long been criticized as operating to the disadvantage of female homemakers. Criticisms of this nature are most commonly attached to *Burns* v *Burns* [1984] Ch 317 in pre-*Rosset* case law, and this case was used by the Law Commission in its 2007 report on *Cohabitation* (Law Com. 307, Cm. 7182) as illustration of the injustices that have arisen from judicial approaches to shared home ownership.

It is also the case that pre-*Rosset* case law suggests that it is not only in respect of contributions associated with 'homemaking' that the courts could be criticized, and this is evident from the treatment of capital improvements made to homes owned by others. It is not clear whether Lord Bridge wished specifically to exclude the way in which improvements made by one party can dramatically increase the capital value of a home, and one view is that *Rosset* simply ignored this in discussions of contributions capable of raising the inference of ownership. However, capital improvements do raise potential difficulties from how Lord Bridge did express acceptable contributions, and it is clear that they caused some difficulty in the pre-*Rosset* case law.

Capital improvements and Rosset's inferred common intention constructive trust

In *Pettitt* v *Pettitt* [1971] AC 777, a cottage was purchased in the name of the wife, Mrs Pettitt, who provided the entire purchase price. The husband significantly improved the property, using his own labour and money, and claimed an equitable interest in the property on account of this; his claim was rejected in the House of Lords, where it was held that he had no interest in the cottage. However, this was solely on the ground that his improvements were actually only ones that were short-lived and not of a substantial character. In these circumstances, it was not reasonable for him to obtain a permanent interest in the house in return for making improvements of this nature, and instead what was done was construed as a gift made to the legal owner. This case precipitated enactment of the Matrimonial Proceedings and Property Act 1970 and the Law Reform Miscellaneous Provisions Act 1970, giving the courts discretion to vary beneficial interests in respect of spouses and fiancées on account of 'contributions in money or money's worth to the improvement of real or personal property in which ... both of them has or have a beneficial interest'.

It is also the case that, in *Pettitt* itself, there were marked differences between the views expressed in the individual judgments themselves: whilst Lord Upjohn was equivocal, Lord Reid expressed some enthusiasm for the idea that improvements could be capable of establishing interests in property in principle. However, the same result—that of no interest—occurred in what was clearly a much stronger case in *Thomas* v *Fuller-Brown* [1988] 1 FLR 237, in which the male partner in a relationship was unable to establish an interest in the home owned by his partner notwithstanding that, in the view of Slade LJ, the work undertaken was 'obviously quite substantial'.

The finding that the work was intended as a gift for the legal owner was even more contentious than in *Pettitt* because it was so extensive; *Cooke* v *Head* [1972] 2 All ER 38 provided authority for a different approach whereby improvements were capable of substantiating proprietary interests, with passages of Fox LJ's judgment in *Burns* v *Burns* also appearing to support this position. One possible explanation of why *Rosset* did not address this issue was so that the problems created by improvements could be ignored. A simpler one might be that it is because this was not an issue in the case itself (with Mrs Rosset's contributions being on the *de minimis* end of things rather than the added capital value end). In this light, what was said by Fox LJ in *Burns* v *Burns* [1984] Ch 317 about variety in contributions (which became very central to the approach developed in *Le Foe* v *Le Foe* [2001] 2 FLR 970 a decade later, and considered shortly) might be significant—especially given the significance accorded to *Burns* in *Rosset*.

Difficulties of clarifying improvements in the light of Rosset's silence
There is also the very real difficulty that even very significant capital improvements will fail to be directly referable to acquisition because they will arise after acquisition. This will be the case even if they are 'paid for' in capital terms by the claimant (rather than achieved through contribution of his labour), because, once again, improvements are likely to arise at some point *after* acquisition. The difficulty with following this reasoning is that, by virtue of it, even very substantial improvements that can increase a home's capital value do not appear to be capable of establishing an interest in the property. This is problematic given that there are improvements that would be capable of being a greater capital contribution than acceptable deposit money or mortgage repayments, such as building an extension. For these reasons, it is conventionally suggested that *Rosset* ignored improvements rather than intended to exclude them.

It will become clear that much has happened to question Lord Bridge's views on contributions on account of the Court of Appeal case in *Oxley* v *Hiscock* and the House of Lords' decision in *Stack* v *Dowden*. But to appreciate how they might have changed the law, it is necessary to understand the law as was intended under *Rosset*. What remains for this is to consider how quantification of beneficial interests was envisaged under *Rosset*.

8.13 Traditional approaches to quantification: quantification envisioned under *Rosset* category 2 cases

When we considered establishing an interest, we could see that, according to Lord Bridge, there were two factors that would be crucial: first, the existence or otherwise of an agreement or understanding; and second, the contributions made to the acquisition of the home by the claimant. If we think back to how this was established for category 1 and in turn category 2 cases, we can see that the importance of an agreement and the significance of contributions played a role in establishing whether a claimant could establish an interest. We can also see that the role of each one of these was different in the two categories, and so it is suggested that what is required in each of these cases is an evaluation of the relative significance of an agreement and the contributions made.

Here, we learned that the agreement to share ownership was the centrepiece of a category 1 claim and that, whilst contributions would be important, they were so for establishing the detrimental reliance in order to invoke a constructive trust. In contrast, in category 2, because there is no agreement to share ownership, the contributions made by the claimant are the only means by which the court can infer ownership.

Once a claimant can establish a beneficial interest in a shared home, this theme of the relative significance of the agreement to share ownership and a claimant's contributions continues to be significant as we consider how the size of this share will be quantified. From earlier 'signposting' of what has happened since *Rosset*, we have a sense that there has been a marked change in approaches to quantification, but in order to appreciate this we need to consider how quantification was envisaged under *Rosset*.

This latter phrase is used quite deliberately, because we do not actually know how quantification under *Rosset* was intended to work from *Rosset* itself. This is because *Rosset* did not consider quantification at all: the House of Lords found that Mrs Rosset could not establish an interest. In absence of an express agreement to share ownership of the home, Mrs Rosset would be able to raise only the inference of ownership on the basis of contributions that she made to the acquisition of the home, which Lord Bridge found to be *de minimis*. As a matter of practicality, this means that we have to try to extrapolate how *Rosset* might have envisaged quantification from what was said, bearing in mind that, as a matter of law, any observations that might have been made in this regard are also technically *obiter*.

8.13.1 Quantification under *Rosset* category 1 as a reflection of relative significance given to contributions made and the 'agreement' to share ownership

From what we have learned about the relative significance of contributions and the agreement between parties that is present in category 1 cases, we now need to understand how quantification of a beneficial interest under this heading might look. We know that, for establishing an interest under a category 1 claim, Lord Bridge considered that contributions served the ancillary function of establishing detrimental reliance (which invokes a constructive trust), whilst the agreement actually established the interest. The relative significance of the agreement or understanding continues in how we understand quantification would be calculated under *Rosset*, because the 'independent' *agreement to share* remains critical for *quantifying the size* of the interest. This can be seen in a number of cases that attest to how parties who have done very little, but have done this in reliance on an agreement, will acquire significant shares in a property belonging in law to another, and indeed as much as a half-share in the property.

This is so precisely because it is the agreement or representation that measures the interest (unlike category 2) rather than the contributions, and this can be seen in the outcomes of *Eves* v *Eves* [1971] 1 WLR 1138 and *Grant* v *Edwards* [1986], and also *Ungurian* v *Lesnoff* [1990] Ch 206 and *Hammond* v *Mitchell* [1991] 1 WLR 1127. These cases also give us further insight into how quantification was envisioned under *Rosset* in two ways that are closely related. It is suggested that, because Lord Bridge saw *Rosset* as a restatement of law, his approval of *Eves* v *Eves* and particularly *Grant* v *Edwards* as category 1 authorities would extend to their illustration of the general approach adopted by the courts to questions of quantification. Here, both cases illustrate that, prior to *Rosset*, questions of quantification in what became classified as category 1 cases—ones of express common intention—were approached with the presumption of an equal share for both parties. This was reasoned as the most appropriate reflection of common intention, but because it was a presumption, it could be rebutted with evidence of a contrary intention. This explains the difference between the half-share awarded to Linda Grant and the 25 per cent share awarded to Janet Eves in the pre-*Rosset* case law, and why a half-share was awarded to Vicky Mitchell post-*Rosset*.

However, there are other cases pointing to different approaches at work. *Stokes* v *Anderson* [1991] 1 FLR 391 and *Passee* v *Passee* [1988] 1 FLR 263 are authority that, even in the traditional approach, contributions *can* matter for quantification in category 1 cases. However, in keeping with the traditional approach, these cases both suggest that this will arise only in circumstances under which the parties have agreed that what they actually contribute will determine the size of interest that each one will acquire. A more interesting and, at first glance, quite different approach can be seen in *Drake* v *Whipp* [1996] 1 FLR 826. This is the so-called 'broad brush' approach to quantification, in which the courts look at the *contributions actually made* rather than the *presumption of a half-share*. Here, Mrs Drake was awarded a third share, with Peter Gibson LJ observing that, 'in constructive trust cases, the court can adopt a "broad brush" approach to determining the parties' respective shares'. However, Whipp's intention was not actually clear from his declaration, and Mrs Drake's share appears to have been determined from all of the evidence, including the respective contributions of the parties. Since she actually claimed only 40 per cent, it would clearly have been reasonable to rebut the half-share presumption in the light of contrary evidence. The parties' entire course of conduct together was considered relevant, and this can be explained by showing similarities with *Stokes* v *Anderson*, in which case *Drake* v *Whipp* is not authority for a different approach.

8.13.2 Quantification in category 2: the (continuing) significance of contributions in absence of an agreement

For understanding how beneficial interests in category 2 cases were intended to be *quantified under Rosset*, we need to appreciate that these are situations in which there is no evidence of an express agreement between the couple to share ownership of their home. Such a claimant can establish an interest only if the contributions that he makes are capable of raising the inference of common intention to share ownership, and the logic here is that contributions represent not only the only means for *inferring the existence* of an agreement to share ownership, but also the only means for determining *the size* of any interest that can be inferred. This meant that acceptable contributions, such as deposit money, mortgage repayments, and 'discounts' (and possibly capital improvements), were actually the measure of a beneficial interest and will limit its size to what is actually contributed, because the courts simply have nothing else to take into consideration when determining 'how much'.

So this tells us what is taken into account for the purposes of quantification, but it does not tell us how it works as far as how the calculations are made. This is because, whilst Lord Bridge suggested that direct contributions to the purchase price by the partner who is not the legal owner 'will readily justify the inference necessary to the creation of a *constructive* trust', it is also the case that this does look like a straightforward application of a resulting trust according to *Dyer* v *Dyer* (1788) 2 Cox Eq Cas 92.

In some respects, analysing contributions as a straightforward 'voluntary conveyance' resulting trust does work, and seems to question why Lord Bridge should have termed the mechanism at work as a constructive trust. We can find evidence in support of an orthodox resulting trust analysis much more recently in the Court of Appeal's decision in *Oxley* v *Hiscock* [2004] 3 All ER 703 and the House of Lords' decision in

Stack v *Dowden* [2007] UKHL 17. Alongside this, strong intellectual support for this view comes from the way in which Chapter 6 explained that a voluntary conveyance resulting trust arises to enable an original owner of property to retain beneficial interest in it when legal title to it passes to someone else. Here, the property would be a shared home, which is owned legally by someone other than the claimant. The simplest illustration for this would be where the claimant *has* ownership of the property, but passes legal title to another, and will retain equitable interest on *Dyer* principles, meaning that what has been transferred elsewhere is bare legal title. This is what did happen in *Hodgson* v *Marks* [1971] 1 Ch 892, but this is not what happens in a typical *Rosset* situation.

Applying a resulting trust analysis to 'acceptable' category 2 contributions

We can see how a resulting trust can arise from contributions to the purchase money made by the party who is not the legal owner on principles set out, if in turn the money is referable to the acquisition of property. The claimant must start off by having legal title to some property (under which all rights and entitlements are subsumed). This scenario envisions that legal title to this property is then transferred to another, who, in this context, will be the person who is or becomes the legal owner of the disputed home. Where this concerns deposit money, this would have the effect that, on its acquisition by the legal owner, the equitable 'interest' owned in the property by the party who does not have title at law (which remains with him) is converted into an interest in the property. Alternatively, if both parties make separate payments to the vendor, then the vendor becomes trustee of the money for both parties in the proportions in which they have paid it, until such time as the property is conveyed, when again the equitable interests are converted into interests in the property.

For these purposes, the origin of the money advanced by the non-legal owner is irrelevant, as shown in *Huntingford* v *Hobbs* [1993] 1 FCR 45.

However, although the resulting trust reasoning works for deposit money and mortgage repayments in principle, this does not map onto the way in which mortgages are actually administered and structured in practice, where early repayments are disproportionally appropriated to administration and then interest rather than actual capital, which will produce perverse results where a couple has intended a share on a 50:50 basis.

This is problematic, given that mortgage contributions were paradigm contributions for Lord Bridge, and a resulting trust analysis does not work at all for *Springette* v *Defoe* [1992] 2 FCR 561 'discounts', which were accepted as a permissible category 2 contributions for the purposes of establishing an interest under category 2. *Springette* discounts could be seen as arising from a legal chose in action enforceable against the council, legal title to which was then transferred, but this will not explain *Marsh* v *Von Sternberg* [1986] 1 FLR 526.

Did Lord Bridge appreciate the limitations of the resulting trust?

Even without direct reference to 'discounts', it may well be that Lord Bridge understood the practical *limitations* of the resulting trust for recovering one's own property, whilst, of course, buying in very strongly to the principle of providing one's own property in order to be able to raise the inference of ownership. So he might well have appreciated the practical difficulties arising from any kind of credit purchase of property, which is the norm for many, if not most, and might account for his preference for a more flexible constructive trust once it could be seen that the claimant had actually made contributions in 'hard cash' or its 'chose in action' equivalent.

Together with the obvious limitations of the resulting trust, Lord Bridge could well have been mindful that the voluntary conveyance resulting trust traditionally operated, which would also potentially cause complications and which was, in the 1990s, seen as an instrument of last resort (*McGrath* v *Wallis* [1995] 2 FLR 114, although noting *Laskar* v *Laskar* [2008] EWCA Civ 347, considered in Chapter 6).

Was the category 2 trust a constructive one by conscious design?

We can say for certain that, unlike some of his brethren during the 1970s and 1980s, Lord Bridge clearly was not seduced by the flexibility of the constructive trust for widening the scope of category 2 claims beyond hard cash or its equivalent. This is so given the conservative nature of his judgment and its intended effect as a definitive statement of law founded on strict property principles. But there is one reason why Lord Bridge might have made a conscious election in favour of the constructive trust: from Lord Bridge's perspective, cases such as *Gissing* v *Gissing* had shown that, some twenty years earlier, constructive trust reasoning *was* compatible with strict property principles, and moreover that the constructive trust was a better conceptual match with the issues arising from shared ownership than a resulting trust. This is because the constructive trust became a device for reflecting the intentions of *both* parties, even if the practical result of this was that a constructive trust was imposed on property belonging (in law) to only one of them.

As we know from Chapter 6, once we allow for the way in which constructive trusts are imposed often against intention, like all trusts, ones that are resulting are based on intention. However, unlike constructive trusts, a resulting trust would appear to reflect the intentions of only one of the parties—namely, the party who retains equitable interest in the property, notwithstanding losing legal title to it. In Chapter 6, we learned that, in the aftermath of *Westdeutsche Landesbank Girozentrale* v *Islington London Borough Council* [1996] AC 669, all resulting trusts are based on the presumed intention that an owner of property who loses legal title to it retains beneficial interest in it. This would not obviously satisfy the common intention requirement, because it does not take into consideration the position of the other party. It may account for his conscience being affected, because he knows that a contribution is actually from property belonging to someone else, meaning that he holds it as trustee rather than as owner. A much less convoluted reasoning for this is that equity imposes a trust because otherwise it would be unconscionable for the legal owner of property to treat the property as his own in these circumstances, which is essentially how a substantive institutional constructive trust works.

8.14 The fate of *Rosset* post-*Rosset*: what has happened since 1991?

We do already have a sense from what has been said up to now that whilst Lord Bridge regarded *Rosset* as a clear and definite statement of law (which was a restatement of existing law), *Rosset* did not actually provide the 'last word'. It was suggested almost at the outset that, not long in the aftermath of *Rosset*, the law became unclear and uncertain once again, and this was fleshed out a little in section 8.10, which introduced *Rosset* as Lord Bridge intended it. We now know that there were a number of things on which *Rosset* did not provide a clear statement, because it was silent on particular things or its statements were *obiter* on account of the particular facts in *Rosset* itself. Taking this together with Lord Bridge's intention that *Rosset* would provide a clear statement of law, we might conclude from this that lack of clarity post-*Rosset* could have concerned these matters. However, if we look back to the overview of things that have happened post-*Rosset*, we can see that some developments have actually contradicted Lord Bridge's supposedly very clear statement of law.

As it happens, the most significant developments have occurred in the sphere of quantifying beneficial interests on which *Rosset* was silent. However, it will also become apparent that, as the law has developed here, it has made some inroads into core *Rosset* principles. This is where we need to be aware of the other two very significant cases that sit alongside *Rosset*, and which have been responsible for some quite considerable changes to what Lord Bridge originally intended. It is also the case that, as far as quantification is concerned, the most significant changes can be seen in relation to category 2 claims. Just to reiterate, this is the more common claim type, because comparatively few couples do discuss ownership of their home, and it is on this type that much of the accusation that the courts are failing to achieve justice for claimants can be found concentrated. This is because, as *Burns* v *Burns* [1984] Ch 317 illustrates for us, the courts are most prescriptive about contributions that are capable of giving the inference of common intention to share ownership—and this has knock-on effects for lack of flexibility for quantification purposes.

In this regard, serious inroads into *Rosset*'s authority came with the decision in *Midland Bank* v *Cooke* [1995] 4 All ER 562, in which, in the absence of any discussion at all, direct contributions amounting to 6.74 per cent of the purchase price of the property resulted in a half-share for the non-legal owner. Waite LJ insisted that, once the claimant had established an interest by direct contribution (a permissible contribution under *Rosset*), the court was then able to take the conduct of all of the parties into account in determining quantum of interest. Despite this reasoning, it did appear very much at the time to be confusing category 1 and category 2 outcomes, which, with the benefit of hindsight provided by *Oxley* and *Stack*, can be explained differently. But before these two cases, the approach in *Cooke* was adopted in *Le Foe* v *Le Foe* [2001] 2 FLR 970, which we have already referenced as drawing attention to the concept of the 'family economy', and about which we will now say more.

In *Le Foe*, it was suggested that family economies were complex because they depended on a number of contributions, and not simply the more visible direct financial ones championed by Lord Bridge in *Rosset*. These indirect contributions, according to *Le Foe*, could be seen manifested in indirect financial contributions such as payment of utilities and council tax, and other household bills and expenses, as well as more familiar non-pecuniary ones associated with homemaking and particularly childcare. There was, it was suggested, a particularly complex interaction between so-called indirect financial contributions and the all-important (certainly as far as establishing a category 2 claim was concerned) direct financial ones, in as much as these could commonly be seen as being essential for freeing up other assets (typically those of the other party) for the payment of the mortgage. In this light, it was manifestly unfair that only the highly visible direct payments were taken into consideration, and that recognizing these contributions alone would frequently conceal the financial realities within a living arrangement. Instead, these contributions were of utmost importance, which in turn suggested that they should be relevant in the exercise of determining the parties' beneficial interests in a home.

In 1984, over fifteen years before *Le Foe*, we can see appreciation of the family economy, and even of the close dependence between direct contributions and ones that are indirect, in passages of Fox LJ's judgment in *Burns* v *Burns*. However, while this did not have direct impact at the time, the spirit of *Burns* v *Burns* was very much in evidence in the Law Commission's 1995 pronouncement on the considerable scope for claimant injustices in the sphere of shared home ownership. And in 2006–07, *Burns* became the flagship for the Law Commission's attack on continuing injustices arising in shared home ownership in its cohabitation project. Moreover, in the immediate aftermath of

Le Foe, the Law Commission urged the courts to adopt its regard for a wider range of acceptable contributions. In its discussion paper on *Sharing Homes* (Law Com. 278, Cm. 5666), published in 2002, the Law Commission had concluded that it would be virtually impossible to devise a framework for determining property entitlements across the diversity of living arrangements that could be found in the United Kingdom. The Law Commission thus urged the courts to do what they could to promote justice for claimants, and in 2004 this became embodied in the 'whole course of dealings' approach adopted in the Court of Appeal in *Oxley* v *Hiscock*. In turn, *Stack* v *Dowden* [2007] UKHL 17 supported the view that wider approaches to quantification should be adopted (apart from Lord Neuberger in respect of indirect contributions, which his Lordship considered to be household expenses), and broadly adopted *Oxley*'s approach in so doing.

As the material on *Stack* v *Dowden* on the Online Resource Centre notes, where the House of Lords did not take up *Oxley*'s approach, this was because their Lordships evidenced a preference for the trust rather than for proprietary estoppel, and insisted that it was for the court to give effect to the parties' agreement rather than to impose an outcome that the courts considers fair. Beyond this, *Oxley*'s 'whole course of dealings' approach was adopted in *Stack* v *Dowden*, and so we now need to find out more about what *Oxley*'s approach here actually amounted to.

8.15 Quantification as it appeared to be in the aftermath of *Oxley* v *Hiscock*

Following on from the facts of *Oxley* v *Hiscock* [2004] 3 All ER 70 set out under 'Four key cases: setting out the facts by way of introduction', it was found at first instance that, in absence of express agreement, both parties had evinced an intention to share the benefits and burdens of the property jointly and equally, and the claimant was awarded a half-share. On appeal, the defendant claimed that, because there had been no discussion about the parties' respective beneficial interests at the time of the purchase, while the property was held on trust for both parties, this was in beneficial shares proportionate to their contributions. In concluding that an agreement to share the property beneficially *could* be found, Chadwick LJ nevertheless insisted that 'it does not follow from the fact that the parties live together in a house they both regard as their home that they share the ownership of that house equally'. In ordering a 40:60 per cent share in favour of the defendant in the absence of 'evidence of any discussion between the parties as to the amount of the share each was to have', Chadwick LJ suggested that declaring that the parties were entitled in equal shares would be 'unfair to Mr Hiscock'. This was so notwithstanding the 'classic pooling of resources' by the couple found by the judge at first instance, and was founded upon Hiscock's contribution of £60,000 being significantly greater than the £36,500 made by Oxley (with the couple being treated as having made roughly equal contributions to the discharge of the mortgage).

8.16 The position of the law in the aftermath of *Oxley*

The aftermath of *Oxley* appeared to be characterized by a number of key matters, which must now themselves be reconsidered in the light of the House of Lords' decision in *Stack* v *Dowden*. But, in terms of how the law looked in light of *Oxley*, there are a few things to note. First, *Oxley* appears to acknowledge the continuing significance of *Rosset* in this area. This can be seen in respect of the continuing significance of agreement to share through finding common intention, and also the continuing significance of the existence of the two categories of case set out in *Rosset*. In relation to the first—finding between the parties a common intention that their home should be shared beneficially—the continuing significance of this core element of *Rosset* can be seen in Chadwick's explanation of primary and secondary questions arising from beneficial home ownership. Chadwick LJ suggests that his reading of Lord Bridge's references to common intention is that this applies only to the primary question of *whether* there was 'a common intention that each should have a beneficial interest in the property', thereby leaving it open for a more flexible (and also court-determined) view on the secondary question: 'What was the common intention of the parties as to the extent of their beneficial interests?' Although *Stack* v *Dowden* did make some modification of this approach, as far as *Oxley* (and thus the Court of Appeal) was concerned *Rosset* continued to govern initial determination of whether an equitable interest in property can be established.

Oxley *v* Hiscock *and establishing an interest in a shared home*
The acknowledgement of two categories of case is a further testament to the continuing authority of *Rosset*, and Chadwick LJ makes direct and explicit reference to them in saying that:

> In many such cases—of which the present is an example—there will have been some discussion between the parties at the time of the purchase which provides the answer to that question. Those are cases within the first of Lord Bridge's categories.

> (*Oxley* v *Hiscock* [2004] 3 All ER 70, *per* Chadwick LJ at 68)

He continues:

> In other cases—where the evidence is that the matter was not discussed at all—an affirmative answer will readily be inferred from the fact that each has made a financial contribution. Those are cases within Lord Bridge's second category.

This suggests that, as far as *Oxley* was concerned, the authority of *Rosset* continued by providing the framework for determining the existence of a beneficial interest, which was the prerequisite for any consideration of quantification.

Oxley *v* Hiscock *and approaches to quantification*
However, beyond this broad acknowledgement that two categories of case remain, there are a number of observations that can be made about approaches to quantification that *Oxley* was seeking to adopt. Clearly, the thrust of *Oxley*'s approach to quantification was the whole course of dealings—that is, the 'whole course of dealing between [the parties] in relation to the property'—at the heart of which was taking up the entreaty of the Law Commission from 2002 and giving authority to the *Le Foe* proposition of 'family economy dynamics' for the recognition of a wider range of contributions for category 2 cases. Here, *Oxley* is authority that, once a beneficial interest is established (the primary question), the courts will have regard to a wider range of contributions for the purposes of quantification (the secondary question) than would be permissible under *Rosset*. In this regard, the whole course of dealings would be a holistic assessment of the parties'

contributions overall and would involve having regard to indirect financial contributions, such as the payment of significant bills and other household expenses, including those arising from decorating, alongside traditional ones. In this regard, *Oxley* also confirmed that capital improvements would count in this calculus as far as quantification was concerned, which provided a clear authoritative position that improvements would no longer be looked upon as a gift to a legal owner.

It has already been suggested that the volume of litigation in category 2 cases reflected the way in which questions of ownership are frequently not discussed by the parties, and that the problematic quantification in category 2 follows naturally and foreseeably from this in many respects. In this vein, it is not surprising that the injustices caused by failing to acknowledge key contributions would be more keenly felt than in category 1, in which cses very little that is done by a claimant will suffice where this is done in reliance of an agreement. However, it is clear from *Oxley* that the need for quantification with 'equalising effects' was not seen to be confined to category 2. *Oxley* is authority for judicial perception that, historically, principles of quantification have treated category 1 claimants far too generously.

Oxley's *approach to quantifying shares of category 1 claimants*

We learned earlier on in the chapter that quantification, as envisaged under *Rosset*, was likely to reflect pre-*Rosset* precedents, which presumed equal shares on account of the common intention that was said to subsist between the parties in order for an equitable interest to arise at all. At that point, it was clear that this could be rebutted with evidence of contrary intention, but that it was not unusual for a claimant to obtain a half-share and that this was often on the basis of very little in the way of contribution, with Lord Bridge's own approach extending not a great deal further than requiring some express discussion. *Oxley* is authority against this approach to quantification, and it is now clear that some category 1 cases will be subject to the 'whole course of dealings between the parties' approach. In these circumstances, a category 1 claimant could acquire significantly less than a half-share, which is a significant departure from quantification as envisioned under *Rosset*.

This is where we see that *Oxley* sought to subdivide category 1 cases into two different types. Here, *Oxley* distinguishes between category 1 *Rosset* cases in which the agreement to share a property beneficially will also determine the size of the parties' respective interests. This is because the couple will agree (prior to the sale of the property or the breakdown of their relationship) that the property will be shared, and will also agree that it is to be shared in a particular way (whether equally or in specified proportions). In absence of this, even within category 1 cases, there could be no presumption that the parties intended beneficial interests to be shared equally, and for cases in which *quantification* is not fixed in advance of the sale of the property or the breakdown of the parties' relationship (Chadwick LJ pointed explicitly to *Stokes* v *Anderson* [1991] 1 FLR 391, and it has been suggested that *Passee* v *Passee* [1988] 1 FLR 263 appears to be another example) and a remedy is sought, *quantum* will be determined by the 'whole course of dealing between them in relation to the property'.

So, in many ways, what was proposed by *Oxley* was a significant departure from the letter and the wider intended import of *Rosset*, notwithstanding that, in other respects, *Oxley* did provide a significant restatement of *Rosset*'s authority after a period of uncertainty surrounding its continuing significance. But in emphasizing that new approaches were needed in order to promote fairness and justice, Chadwick J acknowledged that the cases in the area had shown that 'the courts have not found it easy to reconcile that final step [of awarding a share considered to be fair in all of the circumstances] with a traditional property-based approach'. This is probably on no small account because this 'final step' makes category 2 cases, as envisioned by Lord Bridge, virtually indistinguishable from all but the most clear and unambiguous cases in category 1.

Stack *v* Dowden *and quantification*

However, this displacement of traditional approaches in category 2 cases is technically *obiter*, because *Oxley* itself was actually a category 1 case; the House of Lords in *Stack v Dowden* endorsed much of *Oxley* wholeheartedly. This was especially so with *Oxley*'s accommodating views on a range of contributions, which could be applied across category 2 cases and all but the most clear ones in category 1 (in which the express agreement actually quantifies the interest). In this respect, and certainly in relation to quantification questions, *Oxley* ensured that a range of contributions beyond deposit money and mortgage repayments, and including household bills and expenses, could provide a much better reflection of the realities of shared living, and thus much more scope for justice for claimants.

However, the House of Lords did not endorse all of *Oxley*'s framework, because, whilst for *Oxley* this was a determination of what the *court* considered fair in the light of the whole course of dealings, *Stack* insisted that the focus should be doing so in light of what the parties *themselves* intended. Although much of the language surrounding intention of the parties used by the House of Lords in *Stack* itself (and subsequently in *Abbott* v *Abbott* [2007] UKPC 53, and in the judgments of Lady Hale in particular) is a bit woolly and imprecise, for Lord Neuberger in *Stack* this amounted to distinguishing between intention that was inferred and that which was imputed. And while it was permissible for the court to infer the parties' intention from the course of their dealings with one another, it was not appropriate for the court to impute intention on the part of the parties.

Beyond putting the parties to the dispute back at the heart of its resolution, the only disagreement about the merits of a broad range of contributions for inclusion under the heading of 'whole course of dealing' as far as quantification was concerned came from Lord Neuberger, who suggested that such expenses were ones more properly associated with occupation and not ownership.

8.17   *Stack* v *Dowden* as a clear statement of law: was it a *Rosset* of its time?

Given that *Stack* was the first time that such a case had reached the House of Lords since *Rosset*, some attention is now paid to its significance beyond endorsing a more flexible approach to quantification across categories 1 and 2, and one that is clearly articulated through promoting justice and being prepared to move away from strict property principles in this respect. In these circumstances, one would have hoped for a very thorough consideration of this area of law given its troubled history and its long-standing unsettledness. And in this regard there are a number of interesting observations that can be made on it.

8.17.1   Quantification in the case of a jointly held legal title to a shared home

Remaining for now in the sphere of quantification, *Stack* is authority that, although once the province of 'sole legal owners vs non-legal owners', disputed home ownership is capable of arising even where couples are joint legal owners of their home. We can see from *Stack* that, in these circumstances, disputes will concern where beneficial ownership lies as a result of this, and the point was made at the outset that legal title is concerned with ownership as formal entitlement to property and not with the equities arising from shared ownership. The view of the House of Lords was that where there is such a legal joint tenancy, it should be assumed that some sharing of beneficial interest is intended by this, *and furthermore that* ordinarily it should be assumed that the beneficial interest should reflect this position through *equal* beneficial sharing. This is an application of the maxim of 'equity follows the law', and the principle that a very high burden should be placed on any party seeking to establish that the legal position is not also the equitable position.

In *Stack* itself, the House of Lords also commented that this was a very unusual case, because it was not common for couples who had lived together for so many years and had children together to keep their affairs so rigidly separate. However, on these facts, the couple had kept their personal affairs entirely separate, and Stack's contributions overall were much less extensive than those made by Dowden. After *Stack*, *Fowler* v *Barron* [2008] EWCA Civ 377 is authority that it will be very difficult for joint legal owners to show that this position is not mirrored in equity, and that departure from the presumption of equality will occur only in circumstances that are very exceptional.

Fowler is authority that this will require more to be shown than simply stark inequalities in contributions made. There were stark inequalities in contributions made by the parties, but because, unlike those between the parties in *Stack*, who—notwithstanding a relationship spanning twenty years and rearing four children together—had kept their financial affairs rigidly separate, all of the evidence pointed to Fowler and Barron pooling their assets, derived almost entirely from income. Thus in the absence of any evidence of rejecting an intention to share beneficial interests equally in the face of considerable financial inequalities subsisting between them, there was no ground for displacing the presumption of equal sharing in equity.

An important 'gloss' is now clear from *Laskar* v *Laskar* [2008] 2 FLR 589, which is authority that *Stack* v *Dowden*'s presumption of equal beneficial share will apply only in situations in which there is a joint tenancy as between a couple in an 'intimate' relationship. Lord Neuberger refused to read this presumption into a joint tenancy between family members, and so this must be assumed to be the case in relationships outside those between couples.

Jones v *Kernott* [2012] UKSC 53 is now authority that presumed equal sharing as between a couple who are joint legal tenants can be displaced when the parties' (one time) intention to share equally has changed subsequently. In *Jones* itself, evidence that equal sharing was no longer intended was found in Kernott's complete withdrawal from contributions for a period of fourteen years. This is clearly a further chapter in the 'Stack story' on departing from the presumption in 'exceptional circumstances'.

It is also an interesting illumination of the idea of the 'ambulatory constructive trust', explored by Lords Hoffmann and Neuberger in *Stack* itself as a device for managing intentions that change over time. This is considered more extensively in materials available on the Online Resource Centre, but essentially in *Stack* this was discussed as a mechanism for responding to intentions to share ownership much more equally emerging over time because of changing circumstances. *Jones* now shows how this reasoning can be applied to intention to share ownership receding over time and with changing circumstances.

More generally, the *Stack* approach to quantification can be found summarized in Lady Hale's lead judgment in that case, at [69], with the premise that 'context is everything' and that each case will turn on its own facts. But, in anchoring this to an identifiable approach, Lady Hale continued by stressing that 'Many more factors than financial contributions may be relevant to divining the parties' true intentions'. She continued by illuminating that:

> ... any advice or discussions at the time of the transfer which cast light upon their intentions then; the reasons why the home was acquired in their joint names; the reasons why (if it be the case) the survivor was authorised to give a receipt for the capital moneys; the purpose for which the home was acquired; the nature of the parties' relationship; whether they had children for whom they both had responsibility to provide a home; how the purchase was financed, both initially and subsequently; how the parties arranged their finances, whether separately or together or a bit of both; how they discharged the outgoings on the property and their other household expenses. When a couple are joint owners of the home and jointly liable for the mortgage, the inferences to be drawn from who pays for what may be very different from the inferences to be drawn when only one is owner of the home. The arithmetical calculation of how much was paid by each is also likely to be less important. It will be easier to draw the inference that they intended that each should contribute as much to the household as they reasonably could and that they would share the eventual benefit or burden equally. The parties' individual characters and personalities may also be a factor in deciding where their true intentions lay. In the cohabitation context, mercenary considerations may be more to the fore than they would be in marriage, but it should not be assumed that they always take pride of place over natural love and affection.
>
> (*Stack* v *Dowden* [2007] UKHL 17, *per* Lady Hale at [69])

With much of this clearly focused on joint legal tenant claimants, Lady Hale also nodded to more general application in endorsing Chadwick LJ's view in *Oxley* 'that regard should be had to the whole course of dealing between them in relation to the property'. It is now also the case that this approach has itself been reformulated in *Jones*.

8.17.2 *Stack* v *Dowden* quantification as formulated in *Jones* v *Kernott*

How the courts respond to questions of quantification can now be found in *Jones* v *Kernott* [2012] UKSC 53, with the following 'five-point formulation' taken from the combined leading judgment of Lady Hale and Lord Walker, at [51], presented as 'the principles applicable in a case ... where a family home is bought in the joint names of a cohabiting couple who are both responsible for any mortgage, but without any express declaration of their beneficial interests':

> (1) The starting point is that equity follows the law and they are joint tenants both in law and in equity.
> (2) That presumption can be displaced by showing (a) that the parties had a different common intention at the time when they acquired the home, or (b) that they later formed the common intention that their respective shares would change.
> (3) Their common intention is to be deduced objectively from their conduct: "the relevant intention of each party is the intention which was reasonably understood by the other party to be manifested by that party's words and conduct notwithstanding that he did not consciously formulate that intention in his own mind or even acted with some different intention which he did not communicate to the other party" (Lord Diplock in *Gissing* v *Gissing* [1971] AC 886, 906). Examples of the sort

of evidence which might be relevant to drawing such inferences are given in *Stack v Dowden*, at para 69.

(4) In those cases where it is clear either (a) that the parties did not intend joint tenancy at the outset, or (b) had changed their original intention, but it is not possible to ascertain by direct evidence or by inference what their actual intention was as to the shares in which they would own the property, "the answer is that each is entitled to that share which the court considers fair having regard to the whole course of dealing between them in relation to the property": Chadwick LJ in *Oxley v Hiscock* [2005] Fam 211, para 69. In our judgment, "the whole course of dealing … in relation to the property" should be given a broad meaning, enabling a similar range of factors to be taken into account as may be relevant to ascertaining the parties' actual intentions.

(5) Each case will turn on its own facts. Financial contributions are relevant but there are many other factors which may enable the court to decide what shares were either intended (as in case (3)) or fair (as in case (4)).

Jones and quantification in the context of sole legal ownership

This statement deals very comprehensively with determining quantification in the context of a joint legal tenancy and explains how the courts will address departures from presumed equal sharing. It is also obvious from it that this does not cover quantification outside this context and that, as explicitly noted, it does not apply to a family home in 'the name of one party only'. The very next paragraph states that, for such cases, '[t]he starting point is different. The first issue is whether it was intended that the other party have any beneficial interest in the property at all. If he does, the second issue is what that interest is'. In clarifying that there is no presumption of equal sharing, or indeed *any* sharing, Lady Hale and Lord Walker explain that, where common intention to share ownership can be deduced objectively from conduct, but this does now show what size shares are intended, 'the court will have to proceed as at para 51(4) and (5) above'.

So what does *Jones* have to say about actually establishing this common intention at all?

8.17.3 The primary question of shared home ownership: *Jones* and establishing a beneficial interest

We can now add *Jones* to *Oxley* and *Stack* as a corpus of quantification cases—ones in which the size of a beneficial interest was in dispute, but not its actual existence. Given this, it is not surprising that all of these decisions have been very strongly oriented towards issues of quantum. But this is not the totality of what was discussed in any of them, and we have already seen references made to establishing an interest in *Oxley*, in which it appeared that Chadwick LJ accepted the continuing authority of *Lloyds Bank* v *Rosset* for what he termed 'primary questions of common intention'. We have already encountered some suggestion of the continuing significance of common intention in *Stack* and now *Jones*, and we now need to look at requirements for establishing an interest in a home belonging to another more closely.

Stack *v* Dowden *and capital improvements*

Following *Oxley*'s acceptance of capital improvements as part of the whole course of dealings between the parties, the House of Lords in *Stack* appeared to remove the ambiguity surrounding whether they are actually capable of raising the inference of shared home ownership in favour of such contributions, with support for this coming particularly form Lords Hope and Neuberger. This puts capital improvements into the category of acceptable contributions, alongside deposit money and mortgage repayments, but the House of Lords also indicated that Lord Bridge's requirements for establishing an interest might be too strict to meet the needs of justice in current times, and that the interests of justice would be better served if, as in relation to quantification, the law might 'move on' in the direction of allowing a wider range of contributions to be capable of establishing a beneficial interest.

Although *Stack* (like *Oxley* before it and also *Abbott* in its aftermath) was a quantification case (in which existence of an interest was not being ascertained), which would have made any discussion of this nature *obiter*, it is a pity that fuller discussion did not take place around Lord Bridge's requirements in *Rosset* beyond the opinion of all (apart from Lord Neuberger) that disallowing indirect financial contributions altogether was an approach that was too strict.

Following *Stack*, a number of cases—centrally, *Abbott* v *Abbott* [2007] UKPC 53, *James* v *Thomas* [2007] EWCA Civ 1212, *Parris* v *Williams* [2008] EWCA Civ 1147, and *Thomson* v *Humphreys* [2009] EWHC 3576—all suggested caution in concluding that much had changed as far as actually establishing an interest in a shared home was concerned. Indeed, contrary to some readings of it, *Abbott* appears to suggest little more than that permissible contributions *may* have been widened slightly beyond deposits, mortgage repayments, and (now, thanks to clarification in *Stack*) capital improvements. But in any case this is *obiter*, because existence of an interest was not being disputed and the claimant could establish a claim on the basis of contributions that would have been acceptable for Lord Bridge.

Alongside that, *James* and *Parris* provide Court of Appeal authority suggesting that, in the absence of an express agreement, parties who make no direct contributions (and, on account of *Stack*, almost certainly capital improvements) will continue to have greatest difficulty in establishing an interest in equity (with *Parris* referencing explicitly detrimental reliance). These cases also show continuing commitment from the appellate court to the *Rosset* framework.

Further affirmation of this position can now be drawn from *Jones'* insistence that a 'different starting point' subsists for cases in which homes are in the name of one party only, in which 'The first issue is whether it was intended that the other party have any beneficial interest in the property at all', and this sounds very much in the vein of *Rosset*.

These cases suggest that central to the question of whether the law 'moves on' is the extent to which indirect financial contributions might ever become applied to determining the existence of a beneficial interest in a shared home. This has real scope to alter radically the law as it was envisaged by Lord Bridge in *Rosset*. For many members of the judiciary and academic commentators, this is what should happen on account of changing needs of justice, but the cases themselves suggest that this is genuinely an 'open' question. This is because *Jones* does continue to emphasize contributions that are financial alongside utterings of modernization, whilst discussions of indirect contributions both financial and non-financial remain open-textured rather than concretized.

8.17.4 *Jones* v *Kernott*: changing ideas of justice and establishing a beneficial interest

The issues associated with indirect contributions are discussed further in materials available on the Online Resource Centre, and they are likely to remain at the forefront of the law in this sphere. Because the reforms recommended by the Law Commission are now unlikely to transpire (also considered online), the courts will remain gatekeepers of justice in determinations of home ownership.

In terms of assessing the significance of *Jones* v *Kernott* in this story, it did make important observations on the primary question of establishing an interest, which the Supreme Court termed a question that would merit careful thought. This text had considered the decision in *Stack* a rather cautious offering on determinations of whether an interest actually exists, notwithstanding its soundings about the needs of justice in the twenty-first century, and attributed the House of Lords' trepidation to the concurrence of the Law Commission's cohabitation project. While it is clear that this will not produce law reform in the foreseeable future, and that *Jones*' observations on establishing an interest are technically *obiter*, are open-textured, and are short on detail, the judgment does seem to have a bolder tenor than *Stack*. Perhaps this reflects judicial acknowledgement that the courts will continue to be gatekeepers of justice for the foreseeable future.

The most significant part of the Supreme Court ruling is that which acknowledges that finding common intention will remain central, and this is how *Jones*' observations on actually finding intention are now presented.

Jones v Kernott: *ruling on intention through imputing intention*
In terms of assessing the overall coherence of the Supreme Court decision, Lord Collins insisted that any differences in the reasonings given by their Lordships were 'largely terminological and conceptual and are likely to make no difference in practice'. Whilst Lord Kerr agreed with this broad assessment of differences of reasoning between the brethren, he insisted that he was 'less inclined to agree, however, that the divergence in reasoning is unlikely to make a difference in practice'.

This was attached directly to the Supreme Court's finding that the parties' intentions might be imputed (to them) by the Court if they could not be inferred. This has been a matter of great interest to this text's analysis, because of the decision in *Abbott* in which Lady Hale appeared to be collapsing together and equating quite different non-express manifestations of intention of the parties relating to the disputed home. This text had suggested that considerable differences subsisted between intention that was inferred and that which was imputed, and precisely so on account of factors that now have judicial recognition from Lord Kerr. Lord Wilson considered that, on the facts of *Jones*, it was impossible to infer the intentions of the parties, and the Court could impute to the parties only an intention that the house be held in fair proportions along the lines of those set out by the county court judge. This has considerable significance for disputes concerning non-legal owner claimants and, of course, the ongoing uncertainty surrounding the scope of 'acceptable contributions'.

How is intention ascertained? *The role of imputing intention in dispute resolution*
The starting point here, in many respects, can be found within Lord Wilson's judgment in *Jones*, in which he sets out at 78 the nature of the difficulties presented for the courts and also their source:

> In the light of the continued failure of Parliament to confer upon the courts limited redistributive powers in relation to the property of each party upon the breakdown of a non-marital relationship, I warmly applaud the development of the law of equity, spearheaded by Lady Hale and Lord Walker in their speeches in *Stack v Dowden* [2007] 2 AC 432, and reiterated in their judgment in the present appeal, that the common intention which impresses a constructive trust upon the legal ownership of the family home can be *imputed* to the parties to the relationship.

On the fundamental nature of imputed intention itself, Lord Kerr suggested that whilst it may well be that 'the outcome in many cases will be the same, whether one infers an intention or imputes it', this does not mean that 'the process by which the result is arrived at is more or less the same'.

Interestingly, his Lordship added that the Court should strive wherever possible to ascertain the parties' intention, but it should not be reluctant to recognize, when it is appropriate to do so, that inference of an intention is not possible and that imputation of an intention is the only course to follow. However, when this was the case, it seemed to him that a 'markedly and obviously different mode of analysis will generally be required'. Indeed, as Lord Kerr explained at 74:

> The reason that I question the aptness of the notion of imputing an intention is that, in the final analysis, the exercise is wholly unrelated to ascertainment of the parties' views. It involves the court deciding what is fair in light of the whole course of dealing with the property. That decision has nothing to do with what the parties intended, or what might be supposed would have been their intention had they addressed that question. In many ways, it would be preferable to have a stark choice between deciding whether it is possible to deduce what their intention was and, where it is not, deciding what is fair, without elliptical references to what their intention might have—or should have—been. But imputing intention has entered the lexicon of this area of law and it is probably impossible to discard it now.

There is much in the speeches of Lords Kerr and Wilson suggesting regret for the use of imputed intention alongside discussions of its necessity, and how different it is from intention that is inferred. And Lord Kerr did stress that, contrary to views in some quarters, Lady Hale's discussion of intention in *Stack* and *Abbott* did not signal her own intention to 'recognise a power to impute a common intention at all'.

This assessment of the particular character of intention that is imputed to parties has to be correct. It also reinforces a very important point that continues to pervade this area of law, notwithstanding the increasing dominance of joint legal title amongst disputes pitching legal owners against non-legal owner claimants, and also the facility for making express declarations relating to beneficial ownership in the context of registration of title.

There is recognition within the Supreme Court that imputing intention should arise only when there really is no alternative. This does make *Jones* a decision that is satisfying from the perspective of clarifying that inferences of intention and imputations of it are quite different 'animals'. But this is itself a most regrettable reflection of the way in which parties themselves do not address their minds to questions of ownership when confronted with registration of title.

In this regard, *Jones* takes its place as part of the cautionary tale of parties not making their intentions concerning ownership clear, and of not doing so before they experience the difficulties that will actually 'trigger' questions of who owns what. Where this does arise, it is clear that the status of indirect financial contributions, and also non-financial contributions, are likely to remain at the heart of the battleground for achieving justice for claimants in the twenty-first century, in the context that ownership will be deduced 'objectively from conduct'. As such, these contributions will continue to cause the most trouble for the courts. More immediately, very shortly after the Supreme Court decision, *Jones* can be applied in *Aspden* v *Elvy* [2012] EWHC 1387 (Ch). *Aspden* is specifically an application of *Jones'* findings on the ability of the court to impute intention where inferring the parties' intentions regarding respective shares is impossible. This marks the beginning of 'fleshing out' this framework. Also, very significantly, although its facts were 'in any view unusual, *Aspden* also illustrates *Jones'* application to cases where the starting point is different because there is a single legal owner.

Revision Box

1. Explain why trusts law has become so significant in determining questions of disputed home ownership.
2. Explain why the resulting trust might actually be a very limited way of establishing a proprietary interest in a shared home for someone without legal title, using the theoretical basis for this type of implied trust to do so.
3. Explain the restrictions placed on the use of constructive trusts in establishing a beneficial interest that can be seen embodied in *Lloyds Bank* v *Rosset* [1991] AC 107.
4. What does the Supreme Court decision in *Jones* v *Kernott* [2012] UKSC 53 say about establishing an interest for:
   (a) those who hold joint legal title to a home?
   (b) the situation in which a claimant is not the home's legal owner?

FURTHER READING

Dixon (2007) 'The never ending story: co-ownership after *Stack* v *Dowden*' 71 Conveyancer 456.

Etherton (2008) 'Constructive trusts: a new model for equity and unjust enrichment' 67 Cambridge Law Journal 265.

Etherton (2009) 'Constructive trusts and proprietary estoppel: the search for clarity and principle' 73 Conveyancer 104.

Ferguson (1993) 'Constructive trusts: a note of caution' 109 Law Quarterly Review 114.

Gardner (1993) 'Rethinking family property' 109 Law Quarterly Review 263.

Gardner and Davidson (2012) 'The Supreme Court on family homes' 128 Law Quarterly Review 178.

Glover and Todd [1995] 'The myth of common intention' 5 Web Journal of Current Legal Issues.

Harding (2009) 'Defending *Stack* v *Dowden*' 73 Conveyancer 309.

Hayton (1990) 'Equitable rights of cohabitees' Conveyancer 370.

Hughes et al. (2008) '"Come live with me and be my love": a consideration of the 2007 Law Commission proposals on cohabitation breakdown' 72 Conveyancer 197.

Lee (2012) ' "And the waters began to subside": imputing intention under *Jones* v *Kernott*' 5 Conveyancer 421.

Mee (2007) 'Joint ownership, subjective intention and the common intention constructive trust' 71 Conveyancer 14.

Mee (2012) 'Ambulation, severance, and the common intention constructive trust' 128 Law Quarterly Review 500.

Panesar (2012) 'Quantifying beneficial interest in joint ownership disputes: is the constructive trust changing?' 17 Coventry Law Journal 59.

Pawlowski (2002) 'Beneficial entitlement: do indirect contributions suffice?' 32 Family Law 190.

Powlowski (2012) Imputed intention and joint ownership – a return to common sense: Jones v Kernott 2 Conveyancer 149.

 online resource centre For summaries of a selection of these articles, please visit <http://www.oxfordtextbooks.co.uk/orc/wilson_trusts11e/>

9

Secret and half-secret trusts (and constructive and resulting trusts)

As Chapter 4 explained in relation to *inter vivos* transactions, there are formality requirements where property is left by will. To be valid, under s. 9 of the Wills Act 1837 (as amended by s. 17 of the Administration of Justice Act 1982), wills have to be made in writing, and must be properly signed and witnessed. Within Chapter 4, the essence and significance of 'formality' was presented very much in the light of preventing secret dealings with property. The concept of secret trusts, and the law that facilitates and governs their operation, flows from this particular requirement of formality relating to the validity of wills.

9.1 What are secret and half-secret trusts?

As suggested, then, even understanding what a secret trust might be requires us to understand first what must be satisfied for a will to be valid. Thus the full text of s. 9 of the Wills Act 1837, as amended, is as follows:

> No will shall be valid unless—
>
> (a) it is in writing, and signed by the testator, or by some other person in his presence and by his direction; and
>
> (b) it appears that the testator intended by his signature to give effect to the will; and
>
> (c) the signature is made or acknowledged by the testator in the presence of two or more witnesses present at the same time; and
>
> (d) each witness either—
>
>   (i) attests and signs the will; or
>
>   (ii) acknowledges his signature, in the presence of the testator (but not necessarily in the presence of any other witness),
>
> but no form of attestation shall be necessary.

If the provisions of s. 9 are not complied with, the will is completely void and any trusts that it purports to create will also be invalid. As will be seen, however, a secret or half-secret trust may take effect on the death of the testator without any need to specify the terms of the trust in the will, or even to reveal its existence.

The purpose of s. 9 (as amended) is to prevent fraud; formality requirements are meant to prevent this, and to reflect the way in which making a will is a major transaction and the result of deliberate action. As in other areas, however, formalities can sometimes encourage fraud, but 'equity will not permit a statute to be used as a cloak for fraud', and the doctrines of secret and half-secret trusts have evolved in this area to prevent this.

9.1.1 Reasons for testators wishing to avoid formality requirements

There are at least two reasons why a testator may wish to avoid formality provisions (see, for example, Sheridan (1951) 67 LQR 314). First, he may wish the identity of the beneficiary to remain secret. This was especially common in the nineteenth century, if a gift of land to a charity was intended, when the Statutes of Mortmain (which prevented testamentary gifts of land to charities between 1736 and 1891) were in force. Another common situation was (and still is) where the beneficiary is to be a lover or mistress, or illegitimate child. Possibly the need for secrecy in this situation has diminished since 1969, because until then there was a presumption that a gift to 'children' in a will excluded illegitimate children. Thus it was necessary to identify them to include them. That presumption was reversed in 1969, so that a gift to 'children' on its own now includes illegitimate children (the relevant provisions being found in the Family Law Reform Act 1987). Even so, secrecy may still be desired if the testator wishes to keep their very existence secret.

Second, the testator may simply not have made up his mind at the time of making the will about the details of all of the dispositions. It has been argued (for example, by Watkin [1981] Conv 335) that whereas the law should indulge secrecy, it should discourage indecision; to at least a partial extent, it has taken this line.

9.1.2 Methods of avoiding formality provisions of the Wills Act

There are two methods by which the Wills Act can effectively be avoided.

- A can leave property by will to B, in a manner that complies with the provisions of the Act, but having come to an (unwritten) understanding with B that he is merely trustee of it in favour of C. The understanding does not, of course, comply with the formality requirements of the Act. This is called a *fully secret trust*.

- Alternatively, A can leave property by a valid will 'to B on trust', but where the beneficial interest under the trust (for example, in favour of C) is undeclared. This is called a *half-secret trust*, because, while the details of the trust are secret, it is made clear that B holds as trustee and not beneficially.

For clarity, 'A', 'B', and 'C' will be used in this fashion throughout this chapter.

In general, the principles for the enforcement of fully secret and half-secret trusts are probably the same (although some argue otherwise). Thus most of what follows in the next section (on fully secret trusts) applies equally to half-secret trusts. However, because it is necessary to refute arguments that their basis of enforcement is different, and because there are respects in which half-secret trusts are treated differently, there is also a separate section on half-secret trusts.

9.2 The enforcement of fully secret trusts

Subject to the constraints on the doctrine outlined in the remainder of this section, fully secret trusts will be enforced by the courts: C can enforce the trust against B. The question therefore arises: on what basis does equity allow the clear provisions of the Wills Act to be avoided?

9.2.1 **Fraud theory**

The leading authority on fully secret trusts is the House of Lords' decision of *McCormick* v *Grogan* (1869) LR 4 HL 82, which clearly states that the basis of their enforcement is fraud. The precise nature of the fraud is discussed shortly, but, at the very least, if it would be fraudulent for B to take beneficially, he will be required to enforce the trust in favour of C. This would be the case, for example, if the only reason why the property was left to B in the will was because of the unwritten understanding that he would hold it on trust for C.

The facts in *McCormick* v *Grogan* were that, in 1851, the testator had left all of his property by a three-line will to his friend Mr Grogan. In 1854, he was struck down by cholera. With only a few hours to live, he sent for Mr Grogan. He told Mr Grogan, in effect, that his will and a letter would be found in his desk. The letter named various intended beneficiaries and the intended gifts to them. The letter concluded with the words: 'I do not wish you to act strictly on the foregoing instructions, but leave it entirely to your own good judgment to do as you think I would, if living, and as the parties are deserving.' An intended beneficiary (an illegitimate child) whom Mr Grogan thought it right to exclude sued.

The House of Lords held that, although in principle the courts will enforce secret trusts, the terms of the letter in this particular case were not such that equity would impose on the conscience of Mr Grogan and the secret trust alleged would not be enforced.

9.2.1.1 *McCormick* v *Grogan*: different facts and a different result

Although in *McCormick* v *Grogan* itself it was held that no secret trust was created in favour of C (an illegitimate child), but merely a moral obligation imposed on B, the court made it clear that, had the facts been different, a fully secret trust would, in principle, have been enforceable by C, in spite of the provisions of the Wills Act. In fact, the principles of enforcement of secret trusts go back at least as far as *Thynn* v *Thynn* (1684) 1 Vern 296.

It is by no means self-evident that equity should uphold a trust despite a clear statutory provision to the contrary. In *McCormick* v *Grogan*, Lord Hatherley LC and Lord Westbury emphasized that the justification for the doctrine is personal fraud. In several places in his speech, Lord Westbury in particular emphasized the need for a *malus animus* to be 'proved by the clearest and most indisputable evidence' (at 97):

> the jurisdiction which is invoked here ... is founded altogether on personal fraud. It is a jurisdiction by which a court of equity, proceeding on the ground of fraud, converts the party who has committed it into a trustee for the party who is injured by that fraud. Now, being a jurisdiction founded on personal fraud, it is incumbent on the court to see that a fraud, a *malus animus*, is proved by the clearest and most indisputable evidence.
>
> (*McCormick* v *Grogan* (1869) LR 4 HL 82, *per* Lord Westbury at 97)

9.2.1.2 Fraud and a deliberate intention to deceive

On one view, this means that a deliberate intention to deceive must be shown on B's part (for example, where B had deliberately induced the testator to leave the property to him in the will, on the clear representation that he would hold it in trust for C), and it could also be argued that the standard of proof is as in common law fraud—in other words, a very high standard indeed is required. It may well be that this was what

Lord Westbury meant. However, the statement has recently been explained in different terms. As will be explained, *malus animus* may mean no more than the state of mind required for equity to impose a constructive trust on B's conscience—a very different proposition from common law fraud. Further, 'clearest and most indisputable evidence' may mean no more than the standard of proof that the court will require before rectifying a written instrument. This is, at any rate, how the passage was interpreted by Brightman J in *Ottaway* v *Norman* [1972] Ch 698, discussed briefly in Chapter 6 and more extensively in materials available on the Online Resource Centre.

9.2.1.3 How 'fraud enforcement' might work

The fraud basis of enforcement could operate in one of two ways: either equity imposes upon the conscience of the secret trustee, B, and forces him to hold the property received under the will on constructive trust for the secret beneficiary, C; or secret trusts are express trusts to which the Wills Act 1837 does not apply, because equity will not allow a statute intended to prevent fraud to be used as a cloak for fraud (see the equitable maxims in Chapter 1). The question whether secret or half-secret trusts are express or constructive is considered shortly.

9.2.2 **Why no resulting trust?**

The principles enunciated in *McCormick* v *Grogan* (1869) LR 4 HL 82 raise an important question: if the only basis of the doctrine is to prevent B from fraudulently keeping the property for himself, why is it necessary to enforce the trust in C's favour? If the defeat of the intended trustee's (B's) fraudulent profit is all that was desired, surely it should be sufficient merely to compel him to hold the property on a resulting trust for the testator's estate? This solution would deprive B of his personal gain and the policy of the Wills Act 1837 would appear to be effected. Why should equity further disregard the requirements of the Wills Act 1837 to the extent of giving effect to the testator's oral instruction that the property should go to someone not named in the will?

Clearly, however, the House of Lords in *McCormick* v *Grogan* would have been prepared to enforce a secret trust on its terms (although, on the facts, no trust was held to have been created). Indeed, even long before *McCormick* v *Grogan*, it was clear that the courts did not favour the resulting trust solution and that equity would enforce the trust in favour of C. There are, in fact, three answers to the resulting trust argument.

9.2.2.1 The residuary legatee argument

A historical reason why a resulting trust would not have provided a satisfactory solution is that, prior to the Executors Act 1830, an executor was entitled to take as residuary legatee all property not specifically disposed of in the will. If, as might well happen, the intended trustee (B) was also the executor, a resulting trust would merely have the effect of granting him indirectly what the court refused to allow him to take directly.

An early example is *Thynn* v *Thynn* (1684) 1 Vern 296. The testator (A) had made his wife sole executrix. The son (B) persuaded the wife to make him sole executor instead, upon a completely fraudulent pretext. The Lord Keeper held that the property must be held in trust for the wife (C). If the court had not enforced the trust, but had allowed the property to result to the estate, the fraudulent son B (as executor) would himself have benefited from that as residuary legatee, and indeed would have taken beneficially. Clearly, therefore, this solution would have been inappropriate and the only way in which to prevent personal fraud was to enforce the secret trust.

9.2.2.2 *McCormick* v *Grogan* and the significance of the Executors Act 1830

By the time *McCormick* v *Grogan* was decided, the Executors Act 1830 had altered the rule. Nowadays, the effect of a resulting trust in favour of the testator's estate will be to pass the property to the person named as residuary legatee, or, if there is none, to those persons (usually close relatives of the testator) who are entitled to take in the event of his total or partial intestacy.

Hence, were the same facts to have arisen today as in *Thynn* v *Thynn*, B may not have personally benefited in the same way from a resulting trust. Yet *McCormick* v *Grogan* applied the same principles to a case under the Wills Act 1837. This appears to go further than necessary and to defeat the intention behind the Act. There can still be similar problems today, as in *Re Rees* [1950] Ch 204, in which the intended trustee, B (the solicitor who had drafted the will), was also the *named* residuary legatee. Where B is named as residuary legatee, the arguments advanced in *Thynn* v *Thynn* retain their full force. Any argument favouring a resulting trust must therefore, at any rate, make an exception to cover this situation.

9.2.2.3 The policy argument

It is also possible to justify enforcing the secret trust on policy grounds. A common reason for setting up a secret trust is the desire to benefit someone whose existence the testator would prefer to keep hidden from his family, such as a mistress or, as in *McCormick* v *Grogan*, an illegitimate child. A resulting trust in favour of the estate would divert the property to the very last people whom the testator wished to benefit (his legitimate family).

But if the court is to give weight to this sort of consideration, it must accept that the testator's wishes are of sufficient importance to justify ignoring the clear terms of a statute in order to enforce the trust. The policy argument alone cannot justify enforcement, as opposed to a resulting trust, although if there are other justifications as well, it is a significant additional factor.

9.2.2.4 The nature of the fraud

More importantly, however, we must examine the nature of the fraud upon which the doctrine is based. Just because Lord Westbury insisted on an element of intention to deceive, it does not follow that the nature of that deceit rests only in the personal gain of B.

Hodge [1980] Conv 341 has a different explanation. It should be remembered that the gift to B depended, in the first place, on B's promise to carry out the wishes of the testator. Hodge argues that the nature of B's fraud lies not simply in keeping the property personally, but in the fact that it was the promise to carry out the testator's wishes *in their exact terms* that induced him to leave his property to the intended trustee. It is the intended trustee's (B's) failure to do this that makes the fraud, not the element of greed.

B's fraud then, in equity, lies in the defeat of the testator's wishes, not necessarily in his own personal gain. He would be just as fraudulent with regard to the testator's confidence if he were to give the property to a charity as he would be if he were to keep it for himself. And the testator would be no less defrauded if the intended trustee were (say) to hand over the gift intended for the testator's mistress to his innocent and long-suffering wife. A deception practised out of high moral principle is still deceit.

Therefore nothing less than the enforcement of the testator's wishes will suffice to avert a fraud in this situation.

9.2.2.5 *McGormick* v *Grogan*: the consequences if the circumstances had suggested fraud

On this argument, had the facts in *McCormick* v *Grogan* suggested fraud, it could have been resolved only by the enforcement of the trust in C's favour; a resulting trust would not have sufficed.

This line of reasoning is not universally accepted, but is clearly the basis on which, at any rate, *Blackwell* v *Blackwell* [1929] AC 318 was decided in the House of Lords (see section 9.2.3.2). A similar statement can be found in Lord Sterndale's judgment in *Re Gardner* [1920] 2 Ch 523, at 529: 'The breach of trust or the fraud would arise when [the secret trustee] attempted to deal with the money contrary to the terms on which he took it.' It is not necessary for him to attempt to keep it beneficially, and indeed, in *Re Gardner* itself, he had no intention of so doing.

9.2.3 Developments since *McCormick* v *Grogan*

Lord Westbury's requirement in *McCormick* v *Grogan* was for a *malus animus* to be proved by clearest and most indisputable evidence. This seems to suggest that a deliberate intention to deceive must be shown on the legatee's part (for example, where he had deliberately induced the testator to leave the property to him in the will on the clear representation that he would hold it in trust for the secret beneficiary). It also appears that the standard of proof is as in common law fraud—that is, that a very high standard indeed is required.

There is limited authority that, since *McCormick* v *Grogan* (1869) LR 4 HL 82, their Lordships' stringent requirements concerning *malus animus* have been relaxed. Before considering the law itself, however, which is not yet clear, it is useful to consider why Lord Westbury was so concerned to limit the doctrine as he did and what has altered since 1869.

McCormick v *Grogan* concerned an attempt to make a secret gift in favour of an illegitimate child. Secret trusts were also frequently used, however, in providing for charity. Testamentary gifts of land in favour of charities were, at that time, void. The practice therefore grew up whereby A left property to B, who was a trusted friend, on the understanding that he would later give the property to the charity (C).

It must be appreciated that it was not the intended beneficiary (C) in these cases who brought the action; rather, it was A's family, who attempted to show that the secret trust was enforceable. This can be seen from *Wallgrave* v *Tebbs* (1855) 2 K & J 313, in which the secret trust failed for reasons discussed in section 9.3.

The reason for this extraordinary state of affairs was this: if the secret trust was unenforceable, B took the property beneficially, and he could be relied upon, as a friend of the testator, to carry out A's wishes. If, however, it was enforceable, then, by virtue of the Statutes of Mortmain, it was void. Thus there would be a resulting trust to the estate (that is, A's family). This accounts for the surprising circumstance that it was the very last people who might, at first sight, be expected to benefit from the secret trust being enforceable who argued that it was. On the other hand, it was in the interests of the charity for it not to be enforceable, because the charity could rely on B carrying out A's wishes.

9.2.3.1 *McGormick* v *Grogan*: its strict limitations

It is likely that the House of Lords in *McCormick* v *Grogan* did not wish to allow gifts to charities to be defeated in this way. On the other hand, if B had procured a bequest dishonestly, their Lordships did not wish to see a mistress or illegitimate child deprived of his or her rightful interest because of the provisions of the Wills Act 1837. In the first case, B was far from being fraudulent—indeed, he wished only to carry out the trust. In the second case, he was. Hence the stringent limits placed on the doctrine in that case.

The position changed in 1891, and the last vestiges of the Mortmain legislation disappeared in 1960. Only the second type of secret trust remains today as a consequence. Arguably, their Lordships' limits to the doctrine are no longer appropriate. Their status is, of course, *obiter*, albeit from the House of Lords, because in the event C lost on other grounds and there is some authority that the limitations will no longer be stringently applied.

9.2.3.2 Equitable fraud and 'other' fraud

For example, although it seems that the basis of enforcement is still based on fraud, in so far as equity will not allow a statute intended to prevent fraud to be used to perpetrate fraud, it is possible that fraud in equity is nowadays a wider concept than it was in 1869. Today, there is some authority that it bears little relation to the common law or criminal law concept of the same name. It imposes on B's conscience, but may not necessarily demand the same degree of *mens rea* as fraud in the common law or criminal sense. Because of this, it may also demand a lower standard of proof.

Lord Westbury's remarks were not essential to the decision in *McCormick* v *Grogan*, and indeed seem not to have been adopted in later cases. For example, in the later House of Lords' authority, *Blackwell* v *Blackwell* [1929] AC 318, Lord Buckmaster thought that all that was required to show a fraud was:

(a) the intention of the testator to subject the intended trustee to an obligation in favour of the intended beneficiary;

(b) communication of that intention to the intended trustee; and

(c) the acceptance of that obligation by the intended trustee, either expressly or by acquiescence.

Blackwell v *Blackwell* concerned a half-secret trust, but it is clear that the reasoning was intended to apply equally to fully secret trusts.

9.2.3.3 *Ottaway* v *Norman*

In *Ottaway* v *Norman* [1972] Ch 698, Brightman J enforced an oral secret trust of land without any suggestion that the intended trustee (B) had procured her prior life interest by deceit. Miss Hodges' (B's) employer, Mr Ottaway (A), left her his bungalow in his will, on terms that she would leave it by her own will to Mr Ottaway's son (C). Brightman J was prepared to enforce that agreement by imposing what he described as a constructive trust upon the bungalow in the hands of Miss Hodges' executor (she having later changed her mind and left her property to a cousin).

At the time of the arrangement between Miss Hodges (B) and the testator, Ottaway (A), she clearly intended to carry out her promise to leave the land to Ottaway's son (C) in her own will. Although she later changed her mind, there was no evidence that she had procured the bequest by deceit: certainly, the evidence was insufficient to surmount the stringent standard of proof required for common law fraud. Her failure in the event to carry out her promise is clearly a fraud, in the sense that it defeats the intention of the testator, but no question of *malus animus* arose. Far from requiring fraud in the sense required by Lord Westbury, Brightman J held that enforcement of a secret trust in C's favour depended only on those criteria derived from *Blackwell* v *Blackwell*. Brightman J also thought that it was immaterial whether these elements precede or succeed the will. This seems correct in principle: if acceptance of an obligation by B persuades A not to revoke an existing will in B's favour, for B to break this obligation is quite as clearly a fraud on A as it would have been had A been persuaded by B's acceptance of the obligation to make a will in his favour.

Nor did Brightman J see any reason to depart from the ordinary civil standard of proof—that is, the balance of probabilities.

Blackwell v Blackwell *and the imposition of a constructive trust*

Brightman J called the trust that he imposed upon the legatee of the (by then deceased) trustee a 'constructive' trust. This is a description of the mechanism by which secret trusts are enforced, not the basis of their enforcement. The constructive trust is simply a device of equity to protect beneficiaries where trust property has found its way into the hands of someone who, even if personally innocent, cannot assert a better right to that property.

The fact that the trust (of land) was oral was not a bar to its enforcement, despite the Law of Property Act 1925, s. 53(1)(b), because the executor was held to be a constructive trustee of the bungalow. In principle, a fully secret trust of land should be enforceable despite the absence of writing. This is so either based on the assumption that such trusts are to be regarded as constructive since they are imposed on the ground of conscience, or because equity will not allow a statute intended to prevent fraud to be used as a cloak for fraud.

So much for the trust of land in *Ottaway* v *Norman*. According to the evidence given by the son and his wife, Miss Hodges also undertook to leave them the furniture and other contents, including her money. Brightman J accepted that the secret trust comprised such furnishings and fixtures as Miss Hodges had received under Mr Ottaway's will, but not that it included all of Miss Hodges' other property and cash from whatever source.

In respect of the last, it seems that Brightman J was not convinced that so far-reaching an obligation had, in fact, been envisaged in the agreement, but if the intended trustee (B) had clearly accepted such an obligation, it would appear, based on analogy with mutual wills (on which, see Chapter 6 and the Online Resource Centre), that this obligation also could be enforced against her estate.

What is the status of the Ottoway trust?

This raises the issue of the status of the trust during Miss Hodges' lifetime. In *Ottaway* v *Norman*, Brightman J employed the concept of a 'floating trust', derived from the Australian case of *Birmingham* v *Renfrew* (1937) 57 CLR 666, which would remain in suspense during the life of the trustee and crystallize on her death, attaching to whatever property was comprised within her estate. This, as the learned judge noted, would seem to preclude Miss Hodges from making even a small pecuniary legacy in favour of her relatives or friends. This reasoning is similar to that of Nourse J in *Re Cleaver* [1981] 1 WLR 939 in the context of mutual wills.

9.2.3.4 *Re Snowden*

Sir Robert Megarry V-C partially dissented from Brightman J's view in *Re Snowden* [1979] Ch 528. He thought that a higher standard of proof was required where fraud (which he seemed to view in the narrower Lord Westbury sense) had to be proved, as was necessary for some, but not all, secret trusts. In other words, in his view, there are two classes of secret trust, some of which require a more stringent burden of proof than others. Unfortunately, he did not go on to elaborate on the distinction, which appears to have been a desperate attempt to reconcile Brightman J's views with the apparently irreconcilable views of Lord Westbury, but perhaps he had in mind that if the only way in which a would-be beneficiary can assert the existence of a trust in his favour is to allege facts that necessarily impute fraud to the alleged trustee, then the higher standard of proof applies. If the three elements listed in section 9.2.3.2 can be shown without proof of fraud, however, presumably he may succeed on the ordinary civil standard of balance of probabilities.

In the event, it was not necessary for Sir Robert Megarry V-C to elaborate, because there was really no evidence at all on which a secret trust could be established. His views are therefore *obiter*. In any case, if the criteria in *Blackwell* v *Blackwell* and *Ottaway* v *Norman* are sufficient, it is difficult to see why it is ever necessary to allege fraud in the Westbury sense, in which case the higher standard ought never to be required. If, on the other hand, Lord Westbury is correct, it is difficult to see why the higher standard is not always required.

9.3 **Limitations on enforcement of secret trusts**

The limitations on the enforcement of half-secret trusts are mainly concerned with the time of communication of the terms of the trust. It appears to be necessary for the existence of the secret trust to be communicated to the trustee before the death of the testator, and there is some authority that the terms also have to be communicated before the testator's death. Whether or not these communications precede or succeed the date of the *will* is irrelevant to the enforcement of a fully secret trust (although it is probably different in the case of half-secret trusts). The authorities are *Wallgrave* v *Tebbs* (1855) 2 K & J 313 and *Re Boyes* (1884) 26 ChD 531.

9.3.1 *Wallgrave* v *Tebbs*

Whether the stringent limitations of *McCormick* v *Grogan* (1869) LR 4 HL 82 still apply or whether the law was correctly stated by Brightman J in *Ottaway* v *Norman* [1972] Ch 698, it is clear that, once B has received a gift absolutely, any subsequently imposed obligations cannot deprive him of that gift. Apart from the principle that gifts are irrevocable, there is no reason, in such a case, to impose on B's conscience.

Thus, in *Wallgrave* v *Tebbs* (1855) 2 K & J 313, the existence of the secret trust in favour of a charity was not communicated to B until after A's death. B was entitled to the property absolutely. The testator had left property to close friends (B) without informing them in his lifetime that he wished the land to be used for a religious charitable purpose (that is, in favour of C). The court held that the friends (B) were entitled to the property beneficially—a decision that, surprisingly enough, was most likely to give effect to the wishes of the testator, since if a secret trust had been found to exist, it would have been void under the (now repealed) Statutes of Mortmain.

As it was, the friends were free to carry out the testator's wishes. If, as the testator's relatives had argued, a secret trust had been created, they would have had to hold the property on resulting trust *for those relatives*, the purpose of the trust being unlawful. Hence the surprising situation that the very last people who might be expected to argue for a secret trust (the relatives) did so in that case, and in other cases to which the Statutes of Mortmain applied.

The case is authority for the proposition that, for a fully secret trust to be enforced, the intended trustee must be told of the existence of the trust before the testator's death. There is no particular difficulty in justifying the decision in *Wallgrave* v *Tebbs*, since if the intended trustee knew nothing about the trust until after the testator's death, there could have been no fraud in the procuring of the bequest, and thus no reason for the court to compel the intended trustee to do anything in particular with what was now his own property.

Another justification is that any other decision would have permitted the testator (A) to derogate from his grant. A bequest ought not to be 'snatched back' after it has been made, any more than a birthday present could be later reclaimed.

9.3.2 *Re Boyes*

A more difficult case is *Re Boyes* (1884) 26 ChD 531, in which the intended trustee (B) was told of the existence of the trust before the testator's death, but was not told its terms until after the death of the testator.

A legacy was given to the testator's solicitor, who was told, before the testator's death, that he was to hold the residuary estate upon trust. However, he was not told its terms until a letter was found, after the death of the testator, which directed him to hold the residuary estate on behalf of a lady who was not the testator's wife. The solicitor wished to carry out the testator's wishes, but the validity of the trust was challenged by the testator's family. Kay J held that the solicitor held the property as trustee, but on resulting trust for the testator's estate.

If *Re Boyes* is correct, then not only the existence, but also the terms, of a fully secret trust must be communicated to the trustee before the death of the testator. Kay J said, at 536:

> If the trust was not declared when the will was made [that is, a fully secret trust], it is essential in order to make it binding, that it should be communicated to the devisee or legatee in the testator's lifetime and that he should accept that particular trust.

This is a difficult case to fit into the general scheme of things, and the result was arguably a fraud on the testator, because A obviously did not intend the property to go to his estate, but it is clear from Kay J's judgment that his understanding of the basis of enforcement was substantially that outlined in the previous sections: 'The essence of [the early cases on secret trusts] is that the devisee or legatee accepts a particular trust which thereupon becomes binding upon him, and which it would be a fraud in him not to carry into effect.'

9.3.2.1 Fraud and the knowledge of the intended trustee

There is nothing in the fraud basis of enforcement, however, which would require that an intended trustee must know the terms of the trust *by the time the will is executed*. There is no real difference between making a bequest on the strength of the intended trustee's promise and leaving that bequest unrevoked on the strength of his later assurance. So there is no reason to refuse to enforce the trust where the intended trustee becomes aware of its terms only after the execution of the will. All that is necessary is that he should be aware of them, or where they are to be found, before the bequest takes effect—that is, *upon the testator's death*.

Further, in *Re Boyes*, the intended trustee (B) was willing to carry out those terms. It seems that the case must be explained as one in which the scope of any possible fraud was limited to denying the existence of the trust. The intended trustee could hardly be said to have procured the bequest by a promise to adhere to its terms, since he did not know them; all he knew was that the testator wished him to take the property in the capacity of trustee and not beneficially, so by compelling him to hold as trustee, the court had done all that it needed to in order to make him comply with the terms on which the bequest had been granted.

There may also be sound policy considerations for not enforcing a trust on its terms in a *Re Boyes* situation, sufficient to outweigh the argument for enforcement of the trust in C's favour. In particular, to enforce the trust would sanction indecision by A, which is arguably bad policy, since to allow a testator to establish a trust the terms of which he may change from moment to moment is to permit the very luxury of indecision that the Wills Act 1837 sought to circumscribe. Furthermore, the court has to set a limit on the time for which trustees are required to hold property without knowing who the objects are, and it is a reasonable solution to insist that they know from the outset— although this may be not until the estate has been administered (that is, later than death), so arguably this, rather than death, should be the deadline.

9.3.2.2 Is *Re Boyes* correct?

Another possibility is that the case is simply wrong: it is, after all, only a High Court case, which has not been followed. It is suggested that *Re Boyes is* correct, however, and is explicable on one or both of the foregoing grounds.

It is enough, incidentally, for the intended trustee (B) to be aware of where the terms of the trust could be found (for example, if the terms of the trust are to be placed in a sealed letter to be opened only after the testator's death); then it could be said that he accepted those terms and was bound by them. In this situation, he would hold the property on the terms of the secret trust (*Re Keen* [1937] Ch 236, 242). Further, although B is not informed of them until after A's death (as in *Re Boyes*), the policy reasons discussed in the foregoing against enforcing the secret trust in C's favour do not apply: A is not being indecisive and B is not being asked to hold property for any length of time as trustee without knowing the identity of the objects of the trust.

9.4 **Half-secret trusts**

Half-secret trusts are also valid in principle and, like secret trusts, can be enforced by the intended beneficiary. The leading House of Lords' authority is *Blackwell* v *Blackwell* [1929] AC 318. The justification for enforcement of half-secret trusts is exactly the same as that for fully secret trusts: that equity imposes upon the conscience of the secret trustee for the prevention of fraud. This is clear from the speech of Viscount Sumner in *Blackwell* v *Blackwell*, at 335–6:

> For the prevention of fraud equity fastens on the conscience of the legatee a trust, a trust, that is, which otherwise would be inoperative; in other words it makes him do what the will in itself has nothing to do with; it lets him take what the will gives him and then makes him apply it, as the court of conscience directs, and it does so in order to give effect to wishes of the testator, which would not otherwise be effectual.

From the quotation, three propositions can be gleaned.

(1) The reason why equity fastens on the conscience of the legatee is for the prevention of fraud.

(2) The effect of the trust is to make the legatee 'do what the will in itself has nothing to do with'; in other words, the trust operates independently of the will.

(3) In order to prevent fraud, equity directs the legatee to give effect to wishes of the testator.

This last point is of some importance. The fraud the commission of which is being prevented is not the taking of the property beneficially by the legatee, but, having taken it, not giving effect to the wishes of the testator.

The facts of *Blackwell* v *Blackwell* were that, by a codicil to his will, a testator transferred £12,000 to five trustees, to apply the income 'for the purposes indicated by me to them', with power to pay over the capital sum of £8,000 'to such person or persons indicated by me to them'. He had given detailed oral instructions on the codicil to one of the trustees, and all five knew the general object of the codicil before its execution. The trustees accordingly proposed to pay the income to a lady who was not the testator's wife. The testator's legitimate family challenged the validity of the half-secret trust. The House of Lords held that the half-secret trust was valid.

9.4.1 Fraud theory

It is sometimes argued that the fraud theory ought to draw a distinction between fully and half-secret trusts, on the ground that there is no possibility of an intended trustee of a half-secret trust claiming the property for himself, since the fact of the trust is plain from the will. All that is needed to avert fraud, therefore, is to compel him to hold on resulting trust for the testator's estate.

Some writers have argued that fraud cannot be the justification, because B cannot, in any event, take beneficially himself, whereas he could if fully secret trusts were not enforced. This is because half-secret trusts differ from the fully secret variety, in that the will makes it clear that B takes as trustee only. So if half-secret trusts are not enforced, B holds the property not beneficially, but on resulting trust for the residuary legatee. Therefore there is no possibility of personal gain by B (unless, of course, B is also residuary legatee).

It is no answer to say that a resulting trust would be a fraud on C, the intended beneficiary. As an argument in favour of enforcement, the reasoning is circular, because if a half-secret trust is not enforceable, there is no beneficiary to make the argument work. C is a beneficiary only if the conclusion has already been reached that half-secret trusts are to be enforced.

The answer to the resulting trust argument, however, is exactly the same as that for fully secret trusts: the resulting trust is a fraud on the testator (A), and the property has been given to B only because of an express or implied promise made by B to A. This is clear from the facts of *Blackwell* v *Blackwell* itself. A intended to benefit his mistress and illegitimate son. A resulting trust would have given the property to his wife and legitimate child—indeed it was they who argued for a resulting trust. Clearly, A did not intend that they should benefit. He would not have settled the property on B had he thought that the result would be a gift in favour of his wife and legitimate child. B's acceptance of the property would have been a fraud on A unless the trust were enforced in favour of C. The justification for the enforcement of half-secret trusts, therefore, is exactly the same as that for fully secret trusts.

It is, in any case, clear from Viscount Sumner's speech that the basis of the enforcement of half-secret trusts is fraud, and that the fraud lies not in the personal gain of the intended trustee (B), but in not giving effect to the promise made to the deceased testator.

The case also contains statements to the effect that the law does not distinguish between the enforcement of fully secret and half-secret trusts.

9.5 Limitations on the enforcement of half-secret trusts

9.5.1 *Re Keen*

It appears, however, that half-secret trusts differ from their fully secret cousins in one respect: it is necessary, for their enforcement, for B to have accepted the obligation before the will is made. This distinction is difficult to justify in principle, because a will is a revocable instrument having no legal status until death. And if it is argued that the contrary result allows the testator to alter the identity of the beneficiaries every day, at any time up to his death, then why not have the same rule for fully secret trusts?

Nevertheless, there are dicta that appear to support the distinction in *Blackwell* v *Blackwell* itself, in which Viscount Sumner observed:

> A testator cannot reserve to himself a power of making future unattested dispositions by merely naming a trustee and leaving the purposes of the trust to be supplied afterwards, nor can a legatee give testamentary validity to an unexecuted codicil by accepting an indefinite trust, never communicated to him in the testator's lifetime.
>
> (*Blackwell* v *Blackwell* [1929] AC 318, *per* Viscount Sumner at 339)

9.5.1.1 What do the dicta in *Re Blackwell* stand for?

It is possible that Viscount Sumner meant no more here than to restate the general principle that there must be acceptance by the secret or half-secret trustee, and that such acceptance must take place within the lifetime of the testator, but this passage clearly can be taken to support the distinction made in the previous paragraph. *Blackwell* v *Blackwell* was used as authority for that distinction in *Re Keen* [1937] Ch 236. It is arguable that the time of communication was not the true basis of the decision in *Re Keen*, since the alleged communication did not in any way match the description given in the will, but the rule derived from *Re Keen* has since been applied in *Re Bateman's WT* [1970] 1 WLR 1463.

In *Re Keen*, a clause in the testator's will gave £10,000 on trust to two persons, who were directed to dispose of it 'as may be notified by me to them or either of them during my lifetime'. In fact, some months prior to the will, the testator had given one of the two trustees a sealed envelope containing a sheet of paper on which he had written the name and address of the proposed secret beneficiary (a lady to whom the testator was not married).

The Court of Appeal held that no valid half-secret trust had been created, and the £10,000 fell into residue. One reason was that, simply as a matter of construction, the clause in the testator's will referred to a *future* direction, whereas the direction had by then *already* been communicated to one of the two trustees. Therefore the express terms of the will were inconsistent with the terms of the trust being contained in the sealed envelope. Had that been the only ground for the decision, the case would have created no difficulties, and the position for half-secret trusts would have been identical to that for fully secret trusts.

9.5.1.2 *Re Keen* and the timing of the finalization of the trust

Lord Wright MR also said, however, that the testator, having declared the existence of the trust in the will, should not be able to reserve to himself the power of making future dispositions without a duly attested codicil simply by notifying them during his lifetime. If that is correct, it follows that the terms of a half-secret trust must be finalized by the date of the will. In *Re Bateman's WT*, the trustees were directed by a clause in the will to pay the income from the testator's estate 'to such persons and in such proportions as shall be stated by me in a sealed letter in my own handwriting and addressed to my trustees'. As in *Keen*, this refers to a *future* direction, but unlike *Keen*, the trustees in *Bateman* received their instructions by means of a sealed letter after the will, but before the death of the testator. Therefore the express terms of the will were not inconsistent with the timing of the communication.

Nevertheless, the Court of Appeal held that the direction to the trustees was invalid. The only possible explanation for the case, and indeed the one actually adopted by Pennycuick V-C, was that, as a general principle, a half-secret trust is enforceable only where its terms are known at the date of the will.

The distinction drawn in *Keen* and *Bateman* has not been adopted in the Republic of Ireland: in *Re Prendiville (dec'd)*, Irish High Court, 5 December 1990, noted at [1992] Conv 202, the alternative view of the *Blackwell* dicta was adopted.

9.5.2 **Justifications for *Re Keen***

9.5.2.1 Analogy with incorporation by reference

A possible explanation is that there is a second principle at work in addition to the fraud principle already discussed: that where reference is made in a will to a document, that document must already be in existence, otherwise the possibility exists of testators creating unattested codicils. It may be that, of the two principles, the latter prevails where there is conflict.

With fully secret trusts, the question does not arise, because the will is silent. It applies only to half-secret trusts, because the existence of a half-secret (but not fully secret) trust is openly declared in a formal testamentary bequest. The argument proceeds that the testator having availed himself of this luxury, later additions or changes to the statement that the property is to be held on trust must also be made in a properly attested will or codicil. Therefore if the testator chooses to declare the terms of his trust later than the date of executing his will, he is committed to using the correct formalities. Thus the distinction between half-secret and fully secret trusts is justified.

This argument has a superficial attraction, taking account as it does of the fact that the problem of adequate proof is one that bedevils the whole area of secret trusts. If a testator has blandly asserted that property is to be held on trust, it is obviously vital to ensure that any other statements that he may have made regarding the precise terms of that trust are indeed referable to that particular trust and no other. Perrins [1985] Conv 248 explains the timidity of the courts in accepting evidence that postdates the will.

In this, they appear to have been influenced by the probate doctrine of incorporation by reference. This, in brief, permits the incorporation into the will of any document that was in existence at the time that the will was executed, and was referred to as such in the will itself. It is a useful doctrine in that it saves the bother of copying out lengthy trust documents in the will itself merely for the purpose of adding a fresh sum to those trusts by way of bequest. The testator can instead simply refer to those documents and rely on a short declaration that the bequest is to be held on the terms set out in those documents. He cannot, however, incorporate a document that is not yet in existence at the time of making the will: to allow this would be to tempt fraudulent claims that this or that document was the one to which the testator meant to refer.

Policy for the limitations upon half-secret trusts

It is therefore easy to see why the courts, conscious of the wisdom of these limits to the doctrine of incorporation by reference, may have thought it prudent to import those limits into the enforcement of half-secret trusts. But as a principled justification for the communication rules, the explanation has defects.

For example, it is not necessary to the enforcement of a half-secret trust that any document at all should exist to declare the terms of the trust. So long as he communicates the terms before signing his will, the testator is free to rely on a purely oral communication, which must be even more susceptible to later misrepresentation than a document. If the courts are prepared to accept the existence of fully secret trusts on quite slender evidence, such as in *Ottaway* v *Norman*, it would be odd if they were to refuse to accept oral evidence to show the terms of a half-secret trust, where the chance of fraud is, if anything, less.

In any case, to argue that the testator, having once committed himself to formality, remains bound by the need for further formality if he wishes to expound the terms of his trust later than the date of making his will is merely to penalize him for partial compliance with the Wills Act 1837, while allowing the testator who ignores that Act entirely (by creating a fully secret trust) to have his wishes enforced. This therefore seems to fall short of being a rational justification.

9.5.2.2 The policy against indecision

Another, related argument, which was stated in *Blackwell* v *Blackwell* and repeated in *Re Keen*, is that to permit a testator simply to state the existence of a trust and to communicate its terms at his leisure would be to permit a will to be freely altered by unattested dispositions, thus defeating the policy of the Wills Act 1837.

Thus, for example, Watkin [1981] Conv 335 argues for the *Bateman* position on policy grounds—namely, that whereas the law should not, and does not, object to secrecy, it should not encourage indecision. A testator should have made up his mind by the time the will is made.

The argument reflects a respect for the policy of the Wills Act 1837, and the logic of this reasoning (if correct) also applies to fully secret trusts. Indeed, Watkin argues that they should be brought into line by statute. This, it is argued, would allow the testator who has made up his mind where he wants his property to go, but wishes its destination to be secret, to fulfil his desires by making his communication prior to the will, while defeating the testator who is merely indecisive and wants the luxury of changing his will without the trouble and expense of making fresh testamentary provisions. As Watkin acknowledges, however, the practice of permitting indecisive behaviour via a fully secret trust is so firmly entrenched that a statute would be required to effect the change.

9.5.3 **Codicils**

It has been seen that half-secret trusts must be communicated prior to, or contemporaneously with, the execution of the will. Suppose that the trusts are communicated after the date of the will, but before a later codicil: this raises the question of the effect of the codicil. Another issue is whether additional property can be added to an existing secret or half-secret trust by codicil.

In *Blackwell* v *Blackwell* [1929] AC 318 itself, the gift that was subject to the half-secret trust was contained in a codicil, but in that case the gift was created for the first time by the codicil and the trustees had been duly informed in advance. Suppose, however, that the half-secret trust is originally created earlier, in the will, and the intended trustee (B) has not been informed in advance. There is no direct authority whether the later reference to that trust in the codicil will suffice, first, to create the trust contained in the will and, second, to add extra property to this trust.

In favour of allowing the trust, it can be argued that the policy of the *Re Keen* rule is merely to ensure that the trust is communicated prior to some properly executed testamentary disposition, which indicates its terms, and that therefore the mention of the trust in the codicil should be good enough. A codicil has the effect of republishing a will; in other words, it is as though the will itself had been made at the date of the later codicil.

The position is different where additional property is added by the codicil, since the trustees may not have accepted any obligations regarding the additional property. In *Re Colin Cooper* [1939] Ch 811, a testator had left £5,000 to trustees on half-secret trust in his will, having duly informed them in advance and obtained their agreement, and later added a further £10,000 to this trust in a codicil. The Court of Appeal held that only the first amount mentioned in the will could be subject to the half-secret trust and that the amount added by the codicil fell into residue. In *Re Colin Cooper*, the trustees had agreed to hold £5,000 and that was the limit of their obligation, since they never knew of the further obligation imposed in the codicil. As Sir Wilfred Greene MR said, at 818, 'it was not with regard to any sum other than the £5,000 that the consciences of the trustees (to use a technical phrase) were burdened'. He seemed to envisage, however, that if the agreement had been that the trustees would hold £5,000 or whatever sum the testator finally chose to bequeath, it would have been enforceable on those terms. This also accords with the view taken by the courts that a sealed envelope may be sufficient communication, despite the fact that the terms are, *ex hypothesi*, unknown to the trustee, who assents to carry them out whatever they might turn out to be.

9.6 **Secret and half-secret trusts take effect independently of the will**

It is also clear from *Blackwell* v *Blackwell* that secret and half-secret trusts operate independently of the will. It is possible that they operate as express trusts created *inter vivos* by the agreement reached between the testator and the intended trustee, the function or relevance of the will being to vest the property in the intended trustee at the agreed time for the assumption of his office. From the passage in Viscount Sumner's speech, however, to which allusion has already been made (at section 9.4), it seems more likely that, after the will has transferred legal title to the legatee, the court fastens on the conscience of the legatee by imposing on him a trust. This is probably best analysed as a constructive trust, imposed in order to prevent fraud.

A similar analysis was adopted by Lord Westbury in *McCormick v Grogan* (1869) LR 4 HL 82, at 97:

> The court of equity has, from a very early period, decided that even an Act of Parliament shall not be used as an instrument of fraud; and if in the machinery of perpetrating a fraud an Act of Parliament intervenes, the court of equity, it is true, does not set aside the Act of Parliament but it fastens on the individual who gets a title under that Act, and imposes upon him a personal obligation, because he applies the Act as an instrument for accomplishing a fraud.

Whichever analysis is correct, whether secret and half-secret trusts are express *inter vivos* trusts or constructive trusts imposed once the legatee has received the property (at which we will look further shortly), the will does no more than constitute the trust, transferring the legal property to the secret trustee. It seems likely that the trust could also be constituted by intestacy, in the absence of any will, if the settlor refrains from making a will in the knowledge that the property will pass to the intended trustee by virtue of the Administration of Estates Act 1925, rather than using a more usual form of transfer for an *inter vivos* trust.

It is sometimes argued that if secret and half-secret trusts are ordinary *inter vivos* trusts, the Wills Act has no application to them. If this is so, then fraud ought not to be strictly necessary for their enforcement; the mere fact of an existing trust should be enough for equity to intervene to enforce it, irrespective of any *malus animus* on the part of the trustee.

Yet while it is undoubtedly correct to say that the *mechanism* by which secret and half-secret trusts are enforced has nothing to do with the will, merely to describe the mechanism is not the same thing as to provide a reason for their enforcement. The reason that equity imposes on the conscience of the legatee is fraud, and the mere fact that the mechanism operates independently of the will in no way affects that requirement.

The operation of secret and half-secret trusts independently of this will does have other consequences, however. In *Re Young* [1951] Ch 344, a half-secret trust was enforced despite the fact that the beneficiary had witnessed the will, which, under s. 15 of the Wills Act 1837, would normally have the effect of invalidating the gift to the witnessing beneficiary. Since he took outside the will, however, this rule did not apply. Danckwerts J commented, at 350:

> The whole theory of the formation of a secret trust is that the Wills Act has nothing to do with the matter ..., since the persons do not take by virtue of the gift in the will, but by virtue of the secret trusts imposed upon the beneficiary, who does in fact take under the will.

In *Re Gardner (No. 2)* [1923] 2 Ch 230, a secret trust in favour of a beneficiary who had predeceased the testator was upheld. It is not possible to leave property to a dead person by will, and it is difficult to justify this decision even on the basis that the will has nothing to do with the matter. The usual analysis is that, at the very least, the will constitutes the trust by transferring legal title to the secret trustee, but Romer J saw no reason why a declaration of trust by the secret trustee should not have occurred at the moment of communication of the trust to him, saying at 233:

> The rights of the parties appear to me to be exactly the same as though the husband [secret trustee], after the memorandum had been communicated to him by the testatrix …, had executed a declaration of trust binding himself to hold any property that should come to him upon his wife's [settlor's] partial intestacy upon trust as specified in the memorandum.

If Romer J's view is correct, then the consequences are not limited to an ability to make a secret or half-secret trust in favour of a beneficiary who predeceases the testator. If the trust comes into force from the moment of communication, then it must also follow that it is irrevocable from that moment, and that neither the testator nor the secret trustee would be able later to change his mind. This would be an unfortunate consequence if the communication were made many years before the testator's death and circumstances had changed radically in the meantime. Suppose, for example, that the secret beneficiary had run off with the secret trustee's wife: could not the secret trustee inform the testator that he was no longer prepared to accept the property on the original terms? Or, if he were no longer able to get in touch with the testator, could he not refuse to take the property under the will? One would have thought that, in principle, he should be able to change his mind, but if Romer J is right and the trust is created from the moment of communication, then it may well be that he cannot.

Romer J's view is, in any case, inconsistent with views expressed in the Court of Appeal in *Re Maddock* [1902] 2 Ch 220, to the effect that the trust becomes binding only once the legatee accepts the legacy. For example, Collins MR said, at 226:

> But the right of the [beneficiary] is wholly dependent on whether the legatee accepts the legacy with knowledge of the mandate, and no right for them arises at all unless and until the legatee has, with notice, accepted the legacy.

Cozens-Hardy LJ took a similar view, at 231:

> Now, the so-called trust does not affect the property except by reason of a personal obligation binding the individual devisee or legatee. If he renounces and disclaims, or dies in the lifetime of the testator, the persons claiming under the memorandum can take nothing against the heir-at-law or next-of-kin or residuary devisee or legatee.

These statements clearly imply that the trust is not constituted until the testator has died and the legatee has accepted the trust property.

There is another difficulty with Romer J's analysis: the secret trustee must be declaring himself trustee of after-acquired property, since only on the testator's death is legal title vested in him. The conventional view is that trusts of future property are void, and the orthodox view is that *Gardner (No. 2)* is wrong.

9.7 **Express or constructive trusts: does it matter?**

It has been seen that the basis of enforcement of both fully secret and half-secret trusts is B's fraud, defined in a wide equitable sense. Additionally, both varieties implement the express intentions of the testator, even though those intentions may not be expressed correctly, in writing, signed and attested, etc. Each takes effect outside the will. It is said that it matters whether they are classified as express or constructive trusts because the formality requirements of the Law of Property Act 1925, s. 53(1) (see Chapter 4), apply to express, but not (by virtue of s. 53(2)) constructive trusts.

Section 53(1)(b) requires express trusts of land to be declared in writing, yet a fully secret trust of land was enforced in *Ottaway* v *Norman* [1972] Ch 698 despite being oral. Further, that case ostensibly rested on constructive trust principles. This is therefore apparently authority that fully secret trusts at least are constructive. Yet some writers distinguish between the two varieties, and argue that *Ottaway* v *Norman* applies only to fully secret trusts. Indeed, *Re Baillie* (1886) 2 TLR 660 suggests that writing is required for half-secret trusts of land, although perhaps not too much emphasis should be placed on cases prior to *Blackwell* v *Blackwell*, and there can be no justification for the distinction if the basis of enforcement of half and fully secret trusts is the same.

It is suggested that writing is never required for any secret trust of either variety. The mechanism appears to be that B obtains property under the will, and that equity, operating outside the will, imposes on his conscience and requires him to hold as constructive trustee for C. On this basis, both fully and half-secret trusts are constructive.

It is also suggested that the issue is wholly academic and of no practical importance whatsoever. The classification is relevant only to the formality requirements of s. 53. Yet the validity of half-secret and fully secret trusts depends on a principle of equity, which is not defeated by s. 9 of the Wills Act 1837. Surely it will also not be defeated by s. 53 of the Law of Property Act 1925, or any other statutory formality provision intended to prevent fraud? If equity will not permit a statute intended to prevent fraud to be used as an instrument for fraud, there is no reason why it should distinguish between statutes for these purposes. The principle applies as much to the Law of Property Act 1925, s. 53, as to the Wills Act 1837, s. 9. This will be so however secret trusts are classified, because it is not therefore necessary that they fall within the s. 53(2) exception to avoid the requirements of s. 53(1). (For more on this point, see Perrins [1985] Conv 248, 256–7.)

Further support for the view that s. 53(1)(b) is treated in a similar fashion to the Wills Act itself can be found in *Sen* v *Headley* [1991] Ch 425.

The conclusion is, then, that whether secret and half-secret trusts are express or constructive, they are not affected by any statute requiring formality.

 Revision Box

1. Ensure that you can explain what is meant by a 'secret trust' and what its origins are.
2. Explain what the law relating to secret trusts can reveal about:
   (a) the significance of formality in the creation of trusts; and
   (b) the significance of implied trusts for addressing injustices arising from property and its ownership.
3. Explain what is meant by 'fraud enforcement'.
4. Explain what the decision in *McCormick* v *Grogan* (1869) LR 4 HL 82 reveals about resulting trusts in the context of secret trusts.

FURTHER READING

Hodge (1980) 'Secret trusts: the fraud theory revisited' Conveyancer 341.

Kincaid (2000) 'The tangled web: the relationship between a secret trust and the will' 64 Conveyancer 420.

Meager (2003) 'Secret trusts: do they have a future?' 67 Conveyancer 203.

Perrins (1985) 'Secret trusts: the key to the "dehors"' Conveyancer 248.

Sheridan (1951) 'English and Irish secret trusts' 67 Law Quarterly Review 314.

Watkin (1981) 'Cloaking a contravention' Conveyancer 335.

online
resource
centre

For summaries of a selection of these articles, please visit <http://www.oxfordtextbooks.co.uk/orc/wilson_trusts11e/>

10

....

Introduction to charity and charity law

In many respects, the law relating to charity is anomalous with the general law of trusts, because it has grown up around trusts that are publicly enforceable. This is in stark contrast with private trusts, which are enforceable only by beneficiaries. It is also the case that this is central to why charity law is such an important inclusion for a text on the law relating to trusts. This is because charity law illustrates a perspective on using property that is quite different from the paradigmatic 'benefit for another' express trust. In doing so, we can see that, in much the same way as the increasing presence of trusts in commercial dealings might be drawing commercial lawyers in to trusts law, charity law is likely to appeal to those who would not otherwise be drawn to trusts law. Given how charity operates publicly in a number of spheres of what might be termed 'public policy', charity law is often a matter of interest for those who concern themselves with legal relationships between the state, public bodies, and individuals. Here, we can see how public lawyers might become interested in trusts law on account of the significance of charity in a number of public operations, such as housing policy, child protection, and environmental concerns.

This chapter marks the beginning of an extended treatment of English charity law, and it seeks to introduce the fundamentals of 'charity law' ahead of its substantive study in the next two chapters. These three chapters are more accurately described as extended, rather than extensive, because charity law is actually a sizeable body of law with a number of different dimensions, and space does not permit an extensive study of the law in this text. In this regard, the material of this text has traditionally made extensive reference to specific periods in the history of the law in order to contextual-ize the next chapter, which provides an overview and analysis of the legal definition of 'charity'. However, on account of constraints in space, as well as possibly declining immediate relevance, coverage of it is now much reduced. Instead, this introduction to English charity law will now concentrate on explaining the origins of English charity law only in so far as this is necessary to signpost its core institutions and its key consid-erations of policy, and also the significance of current law.

The current law is embodied in the Charities Act 2011, which came into force in March 2012.

10.1 The emergence of English charity law and the significance of the trust

The connection of charity with 'trusts' is an interesting one, because although a number of charities today do exist in the form of a trust, this is not the case for all, and histori-cally the law has recognized charity for longer than it has recognized the trust itself. So how has charity law ever become part of what we might regard as 'trusts law', albeit a part that is regarded as anomalous?

What we would today recognize as charitable organizations actually date from medieval times, when they were regarded as part of the province of the medieval church, and from this the responsibility for supervising this activity lay with the ecclesiastical courts. Things started to change in Tudor times, when increases in donations to charitable activities occurred at a time when 'the Use' was providing considerable impetus for the emergence of the Court of Chancery. Donations to charitable activity increased at this time because, as economy and society started to transform from medieval into early modernity, it started to become apparent just how much poverty persisted in society. This meant that donations to charity became increasingly separated from donations to the church, and charity became adopted by the burgeoning Court of Chancery. Here, generosity underpinning charity appealed to equity's own developing sense of good conscience, and at this time the Chancellor was himself an ecclesiast.

With a coalescence of all of these factors, the Chancellor started to use the Use as a way of enforcing gifts to so-called 'pious purposes' at the same time as the Use appeared in relation to land. As the Use developed into the trust, because of its intrinsic simplicity and the effectiveness of remedies that had grown up around it, it became the mechanism of choice for those who were inclined to dedicate their property to worthy causes.

10.1.1 Charitable trusts compared with other types of trust

Trusts that are recognized by equity as 'charitable trusts' are quite unlike other trusts of property, because they are not ones that are seeking to provide benefits of property for individuals, but rather trusts for public benefit. They are actually what can be termed 'purpose trusts'. When we looked at purpose trusts in Chapter 3, we learned that it is very unusual for a private trust to be valid if it is one for purposes rather than for individuals, and that attempts to create such a trust will fail under *Re Astor's ST* [1952] Ch 534 unless it can be brought within the 'anomalous exceptions', which the Court of Appeal suggested in *Re Endacott* [1960] Ch 232 should not even obviously be followed. By contrast, charities that are trusts are always purpose trusts, and we had an introduction to this when we looked at the position of private purpose trusts.

You might remember that *Morice v Bishop of Durham* (1804) 10 Ves 522 is authority that, in order to be valid, a private trust must have a human beneficiary who is in a position to enforce it, which could then be read alongside *Bowman v Secular Society Ltd* [1917] AC 406. In this latter case, Lord Parker decreed that 'A trust to be valid must be for the benefit of individuals ... or must be in that class of gifts for the benefit of the public which the courts in this country recognise as charitable'. This provided a preview of the way in which charitable trusts are always purpose trusts. As Lord Parker tells us, they are ones that exist for public benefit and not to benefit individuals. As we will discover, whilst private trusts are always subject to perpetuity rules, these never apply to charitable trusts, because dedicating property to charity indefinitely is considered a good thing, rather than not, because these are purposes for public benefit.

For present purposes, this view of charitable trusts tells us that they are not subject to the beneficiary principle. Even if we can explain why perpetuity rules have no application for charitable trusts, how can we explain that trusts can be valid without a beneficiary? We can see the rationale for this in that 'charitable purposes' are purposes that are for the public good, but given that normally it is only a beneficiary under a private trust who is in a position to enforce it, how does a trust ever work without a beneficiary?

Again, because charitable trusts have a public focus, they are actually publicly enforceable trusts, and so there is no need for a beneficiary for this purpose. Historically, this public enforcement role was held by the Attorney-General on account of his *parens patriae* role—that is, his role as guardian of public interest. But from the late nineteenth century (which is actually a very significant time for the development of modern charity law), this role has increasingly been taken up by what is today known as the Charity Commission. As we will discover, this is the body now responsible for the registration and regulation of charitable activity, which emerged from the Charity Commissioners, who were involved in the administration of charity law since the nineteenth century.

10.1.2 Charity, the trust, and other 'choices of charitable form'

Although not all charities exist in the form of a trust, the trust is still a very common medium of charity today, both in terms of the quantity of trusts in existence and in terms of the value of their funds. The trust seems to be most favoured, on the one hand, by private individuals, and, on the other, by the largest and wealthiest of charitable enterprises, the foundations of which often originate within international commercial corporations. We have already seen an example of this in Chapters 3, 4, and 5, which all discussed *Choithram (SA)* v *Pagarani* [2001] 1 WLR 1.

From the perspective of a private donor, the trust form is simple to create and sufficiently flexible to allow for a degree of individuality to be expressed in its provisions. For a large and well-funded organization, the trust form offers the opportunity to maintain large capital funds producing high levels of income, which can be distributed on a discretionary basis. For these reasons, the trust will probably remain the most usual form of charitable enterprise and charity law will continue to take its direction from the doctrines developed in equity. Indeed, the courts have always shown a preference for treating all charities as having the nature of a trust, on account of the historical association between these two institutions, even where actual institutional arrangements are quite different from this.

In respect of this, we do now need to explain that charitable organizations may exist in a number of 'organizational forms'. They can be unincorporated associations, companies, or a new form, established by the Charities Act 2006, called a 'charitable incorporated organization'. What all charitable organizations experience in common, regardless of their precise form, is that responsibility for their governance and administration rests with their trustees, and that this in turn is overseen by the Charity Commission.

Incorporated and unincorporated charities, and the new charitable incorporated organization

An increasing number of charitable ventures nowadays operate within a corporate structure, and this form is particularly well suited to collective, active enterprises. A corporate charity will usually be a company limited by guarantee and will usually have a constitution forbidding the distribution of profit among its members. Otherwise, the establishment of a company limited by guarantee is broadly similar in terms of formality to the setting up of an ordinary commercial company. As with a commercial company, the liability of the charity is limited to its assets, thus protecting its members from unlimited personal liability in the event of the charity becoming insolvent. The advantage of corporate status is that the charity can operate as a legal person. So it has the capacity to make contracts, to incur liabilities, and to hold property in its own right without the need to involve trustees. Also, it does not need to effect alterations in the documents of title to its property at every change in personnel. Corporate status is therefore well suited to charities that undertake extensive long-term operations. These often have considerable assets, sufficient to make the expense of incorporation worthwhile.

Charities can also exist as unincorporated associations, which provide a less rigid framework, and can be very attractive for those wishing to undertake charitable work in a more flexible and perhaps more democratic way. Because the arrangement is more flexible, it allows better 'real-time' adjustment to changing circumstances. In this situation, control of the organization and its funds, if any, will typically be vested in a committee of managers, who will probably be elected in conformity with the wishes of the current membership. The reason for this is that, because the organization is unincorporated, it cannot hold property in its own right, which might be perceived as an advantage or a disadvantage, and individuals will not be protected from personal liability in the event of the organization's indebtedness.

Long before the newly created charitable incorporated organization, English law recognized the charitable corporation, which is also distinct from the traditional 'incorporated body' charity (organizations of this nature typically being 'guarantee companies'). The charitable corporation form has traditionally been illustrated by universities, hospitals, and establishments such as the British Museum; they are established either by charter from the Crown (known as a 'royal charter', as is the case with universities) or else by legislation (such as the Charitable Trustees Incorporation Act 1872 and the British Museum Act 1963). The character of these institutions has been diverse with no standard form, with each endowed with a constitution specific to its own requirements. These charities are generally considered to enjoy high prestige by virtue of their unique character, and represent something of an elite category within the range of charitable organizations.

Whatever their precise form, all of these organizations fall under the general jurisdiction of charity law, which is considered a branch of trusts law. This also applies to the charitable incorporated organization (CIO), which was a new type of charitable organization vehicle introduced by the Charities Act 2006. As the Charity Commission information dated May 2008 makes clear (<http://www.charitycommission.gov.uk/Start_up_a_charity/Do_I_need_to_register/cios/default.aspx>), this new legal form was designed specifically for charities. As the information explains, the CIO reflects that whilst there are advantages to incorporation for charities, much of the framework of the company structure, designed primarily for commercial organizations, may mean that it is not always a suitable vehicle for charities, in which commercial dimensions are actually very restricted. The new form embodies a single registration procedure (requiring registration only with the Charity Commission), and reporting and accounting requirements that are less onerous than would be required otherwise, and also less rigid ones relating to changes in constitutional and governance arrangements.

The law relating to CIOs is now to be found in s. 204 *et seq* of the Charities Act 2011, and regulations on how CIOs must be established and must operate will be produced by way of secondary legislation. The CIO became available in October 2012, and the Charity Commission 2008 document *Choosing and Preparing a Governing Document* (available online at <http://www.charity-commission.gov.uk/Library/guidance/cc22text.pdf>) provides information on the current structures open to charities. The CIO is available for *ab initio* charitable organizations, with the facility also for any existing charitable company and charitable industrial and provident society to convert, simply by re-registering as a CIO.

10.2 Legal regulation of charities: the consequences of charitable status

Before considering the legal definition of 'charity' in the next chapter, some attention needs to be given to the consequences that flow from charitable status. For the consequences outlined to apply, it is necessary to show that the property is to be held beneficially for charitable purposes. As *Liverpool City Council* v *Attorney-General*, The Times, 1 May 1992, establishes, it is not sufficient for the recipient merely to covenant to use the property for purposes that happen to be charitable purposes. However, once it has been established that property is held beneficially for charitable purposes, a number of legal consequences come into play. These have already been noted as indefinite existence and public enforcement. Both are considered extensively throughout this study of charity, in discussion of the role of the Attorney-General, the Charity Commission, and also the courts in achieving this. References to the indefinite existence of charitable organizations and the indefinite settlement of property to them will be closely tied in with explaining why charity is such a significant institution in English society and culture.

What follows now is explanation that securing charitable status will also confer tax advantages for the organization concerned and any property that it acquires. There will then be an introduction to the way in which securing charitable status also ensures that, once property is given to charity, this is an indefinite gift, even where property given cannot be applied to the actual charitable purposes for which it was dedicated by being cy-près or 'as close as possible'. All of this taken together is directed towards thinking about why there is a distinct body of trusts law called 'charity law', and how the policy of charity law has always been to ensure that only those organizations that should achieve charitable status are able to do so. This becomes very significant in the next chapter's discussion of the legal definition of 'charity', which is concerned entirely with ensuring that only those organizations that should have charitable status will be able to acquire it. This shows us how the law has sought to develop this limited access historically. At this point, we will need to reflect on what 'charity' means in English society and culture in the twenty-first century, and whether the Charities Act 2011 reflects that maintaining this limited access has required reinforcing traditional ideas on how to achieve this, or has required the law to move in new directions.

10.2.1 The fiscal advantage of charitable status and the significance of taxation

A full inventory of tax advantages arising from property that is held beneficially for charitable purposes can be found in the 2007 Charity Commission publication *Trustees, Trading and Tax: How Charities May Lawfully Trade* (<http://www.charitycommission.gov.uk/library/guidance/cc35text.pdf>). Charities enjoy exemption from income tax on all income, rents, dividends, and profits, provided that these are applied for charitable purposes, and may reclaim from HM Revenue and Customs (HMRC) any income tax already paid prior to receipt of the income. No income tax is chargeable on the profits of any trade carried out by the charity, so long as these are applied for charitable purposes only, and the trade is either exercised in carrying out the primary purposes of the charity or the work is carried out mainly by its beneficiaries (such as workshops for the disabled). Charitable corporations are exempt from corporation tax. Gifts to charity are largely exempt from inheritance tax, and capital gains tax is not payable where gains are applied to charitable purposes. All charities are exempt from 80 per cent of council tax falling due on premises occupied in connection with the charity, including charity shops, and premises used for religious purposes are entirely exempt from rates. In addition, there is now the 'gift aid' scheme for donations made to charity (which is in any event tax-exempt) by a person who is a taxpayer: in these circumstances, the charity can also claim from the tax authority the amount that would be the basic rate of tax on the amount donated. Generally, charities do pay value added tax (VAT) on goods and services, but certain goods, such as some equipment for the disabled, are zero-rated.

As a matter of social policy, tax concessions for charitable activity have a long history, which is connected with why the ecclesiastical courts, and then the Court of Chancery, were so keen to recognize and enforce giving to worthy causes. More will be said about this at times in the next chapter, but essentially, in pre-welfare-state times, responsibility for ensuring what we would call 'social welfare'—that is, caring for vulnerable members of a community, the upkeep of roads and bridges, etc.—would fall to local communities. So those who wished to give to worthy causes were looked on very favourably by everyone, and where it appeared that those who had died wished to benefit the community in this way, the Ecclesiastical Court and then the Court of Chancery were very keen to facilitate this.

Charitable activity, social benefits, and taxation
Some conception of the importance of the taxation consequences of charitable status may be gleaned from the number of cases considered in the next chapter involving the Inland Revenue (now HMRC). This shows us that much can ride on whether a disposition made in favour of an organization is a charitable bequest. The way in which it is the function of the UK tax authority to try to maximize what can be 'claimed' from individuals for the public (living and deceased alike) for the public purse also provides a way into appreciating how contentious the tax advantages enjoyed by charitable organizations can be. The basic premise for this on a structural 'societal' level, in the operation of the modern state, is that tax concessions given to one sector in society will have knock-on effects for other social sectors, which will have one of two broad consequences. One result of this is that there is higher taxation of other sectors of society, in order to ensure that there is no decline in social utility—that is, services that come from public funding, such as health care and education. But because high (or even higher than necessary) taxation is unpopular, the only other option when some are paying less tax than they could is an overall reduction of social utility.

As well as taxation being generally a touchy subject in English society and culture on account of the fact that this is a low taxation society, providing tax concessions for the charitable sector generally creates scope for individuals to be displeased should causes that they would not wish to support be given public support at all. This is magnified if it is seen as the reason why everyone else has to pay more tax than is actually necessary, and any enforced individual support of particular charitable activity of which an individual disapproves will operate on top of this still further. Getting accurate figures on how this impacts financially across the ambit of society's interests is not easy, but tax concessions to charity are thought to cost each individual in the United Kingdom as much as £100 per year.

10.2.2 The fiscal advantages of charitable status cy-près

The doctrine of cy-près is a key embodiment of the way in which, once property is given to charity, this is a once-and-for-all dedication of that property to charitable purposes. We know that, for this to happen, the bequest must actually have been made, and not simply covenanted, but that, once it has been, this is 'once and for all'. In this, we can see the opposite policy at work from that which explains the perpetuity rules, which allow property that is settled on trust to be tied up in trust only for so long on the basis that preventing free dealings with property over extended periods of time can have a negative impact on economy and social opportunity far into the future. The reforms to the perpetuity rules courtesy of the Perpetuities Act 2009 suggest that, while that might once have been the case, the scope for private trusts to influence economy and society has reduced significantly on account of general trends of growth in economic complexity, and also increasing globalization, and so there is a much longer perpetuity period for private trusts now in force. However, all private trusts do remain subject to perpetuity limitations, whilst property dedicated to charity has never been subject to this limitation.

This reflects significantly the special status of charity within English society and English legal culture, and as we discover more about charity law, we will see just what a significant 'social good' charity is considered to be. Historically, this is on account of how everyone in a community, as administered through the church-originated parish system, would benefit from those who gave to 'worthy causes' as individuals or as institutions (such as religious groups who were willing to provide education or welfare provision for orphans and widows, etc.). And, in due course, it will be suggested that, today, charity actually provides a very effective mechanism for providing high levels of social utility without those in society having to pay 'real costs' for the benefits of medical research, for example. In this light, it is not difficult to see why dedicating property to charity emerged as something that should be indefinite, because this was in the interests of society as a whole, rather than something that would detrimentally affect society.

The cy-près doctrine has emerged as a supporting mechanism for this position in as much as where a charitable organization ceases to operate because it is being wound up altogether, or because its activities have merged with other similar organizations, issues arise regarding to what to do with property that has been given to it. The cy-près doctrine allows for property that is given to a particular charitable organization to be considered an indefinite bequest to charitable purpose, because it allows for property to be given to a purpose that is as 'close as possible' to the original one for which it was given, if what was arguably intended cannot be carried out. This is the translation of cy-près, which is an Anglo-Norman term, and we will learn more about the different ways in which the cy-près doctrine works in Chapter 12.

10.3 Regulation by the Charity Commission

Much of what follows in this chapter and in the next flows from the significance that modern charity law attaches to the registration of charitable organizations. We shall see that the legal definition of charity that underpins charitable status, and thus the recognition of purposes as charitable purposes, is ultimately a question for the courts, and is strongly oriented towards obtaining formal recognition of charitable status through registration. The process of inclusion on the register of charities is central in 'gatekeeping' the advantages of charitable status. This works for charities that must by law be registered, apart from those deemed by law to be exempt from registration. Although current rules on registration were introduced by the Charities Act 2006, they are, like the other key provisions discussed in this text and much current charity law beyond this, now governed by the Charities Act 2011. Any charity must be registered with the Charity Commission if it has an income of more than £5,000 a year, or has the use or occupation of any land or buildings, or has assets that constitute permanent endowment, unless it is *exempt from* registration. Those organizations that are exempt are typically universities and other 'educational' establishments. But being exempt is a process of recognition of status like registration itself. And obtaining tax advantages depends on being recognized through the process of registration, or by being exempt from it. (More information about this can be found on the Charity Commission's website.)

10.3.1 The regulation of charitable activity through the regulation of *charitable status*

Registration is perhaps the key component in the way in which charity law regulates charitable activity, but the Charity Commission has a number of other regulatory functions, some of which are new under the Charities Act 2006 and others of which date back much further than this. We have suggested that securing charitable status is very strongly tied up in the process of registration, and that inclusion on the register of charities is overseen by the Charity Commission. However, until 2006, an organization seeking charitable status would have applied for registration to the Charity Commissioners, who have traditionally had the power to grant or withhold registration according to their view on whether the purpose is one that the law would regard as charitable. This office was created in 1853, but at that point had much more limited powers than it has today, and until 2006 the powers vested in the office of Charity Commissioner were held by its individual occupants. The 2006 Act created the Charity Commission of England and Wales as a body corporate with a distinct existence from those individuals who serve it, and with the status of a non-ministerial government department. The Charity Commission now has responsibility for registration of charities and other administration of charity law, such as monitoring accounts, supervising the running of charities, and advising charitable trustees. In addition, the Charity Commission has taken an increasing role in enforcing charitable organization. As suggested, traditionally, this has been the role of the Attorney-General; increasingly, it is one in which the Charity Commissioners (and now the Charity Commission) take an active part.

10.3.2 The Charities Act 2006 and creation of the Charity Commission, and the Charities Act 2011

The register of charities is to be kept by the Commission by virtue of s. 29 of the Charities Act 2011, and the way in which the Charity Commissioners have traditionally undertaken the role of enforcing charitable trusts alongside the Attorney-General is widely regarded as the reason why there is comparatively little litigation on charity, and particularly on the scope of charity and its legal boundaries. What we have in charity law is instead a handful of 'test cases', which raise significant issues of law. And it is indeed the case that, in reaching their decisions, the Commissioners (and now the Commission itself) may consult with other bodies, such as HMRC, the interest of which in the validity of claims to be treated as a charity has spawned some, but not all, of English law's most prominent 'charitable status' litigation.

Refusal by the Charity Commission to register an organization
and the new Charity Tribunal
Refusal by the Commissioners to register an organization has traditionally given rise to a right of appeal (to the Board of Charity Commissioners under s. 4 of the Charities Act 1993), and through the courts (initially through the High Court, and from there to

the Court of Appeal and House of Lords, now the Supreme Court). However, the 2006 Act introduced a new mechanism for ensuring critical appraisal of Charity Commission decisions on registration: the role of the Charity Tribunal, known formally as the First-Tier Tribunal (Charity), is explained in the 2012 Charity Commission guidance entitled *Dissatisfied with One of the Commission's Decisions? How Can We Help You?* (<http://www. charity-commission.gov.uk/library/about_us/decision_review.pdf>) as an independent legal body that has the power to look again at some of the decisions made by the Charity Commission and the power to quash, change, or add to them. The guidance also provides practical information application and likely time frames for decision-making. The law relating to the Tribunal is now located in Pt 17 of the 2011 Act, in ss 314 *et seq*. Interestingly, the guidance on the Tribunal also stressed that, in some cases, the Tribunal may direct the Charity Commission to take further action or to rectify a decision made. This did actually happen in 2011, when the Commission was forced to withdraw 'those aspects of our public benefit guidance that require rewriting to ensure that the guidance is consistent with the Upper Tribunal's decision'. This followed an action brought by the Independent Schools Council, which is discussed further in the following chapter, and in materials located on the Online Resource Centre. Where a matter is before (or on appeal from) the Tribunal, the Attorney-General has power to intervene to represent any wider public interest in the public good performed by the charity concerned.

10.3.3 The requirement to keep the register of charities, and new functions for the Charity Commission

The current requirements relating to keeping the register of charities introduced by the 2006 Act are closely connected with current favour for the growing supervisory role of the new Commission. This can, in turn, be understood from linking the way in which, while charitable status can bring with it considerable advantages for an organization, it also invites scrutiny relating to curbing abuse of charitable status and maladministration. And it will become ever more apparent as the material progresses that, in the early years of the twenty-first century, this increasingly became associated with perceived declining public confidence in the charitable sector. Politically, this manifested in growing criticism of charities law for some time, with the process of law reform leading to the Charities Act 2006 formally set in motion in 2002 by the publication of the Prime Minister's Strategy Unit document entitled *Private Action, Public Benefit: A Review of Charities and the Wider Not-For-Profit Sector*.

Regulation by the Charity Commission, and the significance of 'exception' and 'exemption' in registration requirements
More will be said on this shortly, but these issues—clustering political responses to perceived public discomfort about charitable status—are clearly at the heart of a more prescriptive approach to applications for charitable status, the reviewing of charitable status, and ultimately the removal of 'unsuitable' organizations from the register of charities. This is also the rationale for another new and distinct policy of the 2006 Act, now reflected in s. 30 of the Charities Act 2011: the general principle that every charity must be registered (in the register of charities). Certain exceptions and exemptions characteristic of traditional approaches have been maintained, but these are clearly intended to be much narrower and more tightly controlled than has traditionally been the case. The key difference between charities that are exempt and those that are excepted is that, in the case of the latter, exception to registration is granted by order of

the Charity Commission or by regulations (rather than under statute), with key provisions here to be found in ss 30 and 31. However, the reference to gross income of not exceeding £5,000 (by virtue of s. 30) introduced by the 2006 Act as a threshold for registration was actually an increase in threshold, and reflective of a further policy in current thinking of charity law—namely, to 'release the smallest charities … from the registration requirement'.

The Charities Act 2006 and a new key supervisory function for the Charity Commission

A key 'supervisory function' of the Charity Commission under the Act, and a close companion of registration, is requirements that the Act has put in place for the Commission relating to 'public benefit'. In the next chapter, we shall see how this is linked with s. 4 of the 2011 Act, which stipulates the public benefit requirement and consolidates the 2006 Act, which first placed this traditional requirement of charity law on a statutory footing. While the substance of the requirement is found in s. 4, the Commission has a central role in setting out how this requirement is satisfied. This is reiterated in s. 17, which explains what the Commission *must* do here and what it is *permitted* to do. This, along with s. 4, is discussed extensively in the following chapter.

10.4 The historical foundations of modern charity law and current developments

The combined effect of the courts generally wanting to give effect to the wishes of owners of property with the appreciable benefits to society for those wishing to give to worthy causes has led to a tendency for the legal definition of 'charitable purpose' to be broad rather than narrow. However, contention generated by tax concessions has created tensions in determining what is or is not a charitable activity, and has become part of the character of charity law and indeed a central aspect of its function. Contention of similar magnitude has also been generated by tensions subsisting between the promotion of worthy causes and the grievances of families who believe that 'charity begins at home'. Indeed, whilst some litigation has clearly been spawned by the interest that the 'public purse' has in disputing charitable meaning and status, a far greater volume has been generated by disgruntled relatives. This reflects that where the charitable status of a bequest is successfully challenged, the property will be returned to the donor, or his estate, by way of a resulting trust, as illustrated in the next chapter (and more extensively in Chapter 17), with reference to *Chichester Diocesan Fund* v *Simpson* [1944] AC 341.

As we work through the material, it will become ever more clear that this function of 'charity law' is to ensure that only those purposes that should be deemed charitable are in fact so deemed. And it will also become clear how these difficulties, which emerging charity law has sought to manage, can help to explain the somewhat haphazard development of the law. In ways that are both related to these issues and distinct from them, it is also the case that, at various points in time, charity has been viewed in equal measure with considerable favour and extreme suspicion. This was so particularly by the medieval church, on the basis that donations to charity outside 'church auspices' allowed for the beginnings of a secular organ of governance to develop to protect the interests of society: this was, of course, 'the state'. From a different perspective, and much later in the eighteenth and nineteenth centuries, the Mortmain legislation 1736–1891 reflected concerns that the growing popularity of testamentary gifts to charity was responsible for taking away the rightful expectations of heirs. The Mortmain legislation operated to widen the legal definition of what was considered charitable, but this was for the somewhat perverse reason of seeking to ensure that such gifts to worthy causes would be invalid and so would be rightfully claimed by heirs.

As we shall discover, in the earliest years of the twenty-first century there were concerted state-originated efforts to reinforce charity as a force for public good, and this spirit has become embodied in the Charities Act 2006. But in terms of understanding the mixture of motivations that has given us our modern charity law, the Statute of Elizabeth 1601 is a very significant reference point. The lasting significance of this legislation can be seen from the way in which, until the Charities Act 2006, the Preamble from the long-out-of-force statute had considerable significance for the development of charity law. It provided the basis for the modern classification of charitable purposes embodied in *Commissioners for Special Purposes of the Income Tax* v *Pemsel* [1891] AC 531, and was central in the recognition of new charitable purposes thereafter. However, its origins are complex.

10.4.1 Charity law emerging from Elizabethan times to the eighteenth century

The decline of the influence of Catholicism, combined with population growth, difficulties with food production, and a fragile fledgling 'modern' economy, meant that, in Elizabethan times, poor relief became a problem for the emerging 'state'. From this came statutory provision for the poor, to be administered by the parish and paid for out of local rates, which was introduced in 1572, and comprehensive Poor Codes were enacted in 1597 and 1601. Under these auspices, the parish became the key reference point not only for religion, but also for religious instruction and poor relief. Alongside this, it was in the interests of the state to encourage those who had property to give it to worthy causes in order to reduce the burden of poor rates. The development of charity law at this time, therefore, was geared primarily towards relief of poverty in numerous and various forms, which was administered closely alongside religious activity. We can see the prominence of poor relief, and also religion and education (arising from religious instruction), in the Preamble to the Statute of Elizabeth 1601, which has acquired a life of its own beyond this piece of legislation:

> Whereas Lands, Tenements, Rents, Annuities, Profits, Hereditaments, Goods, Chattels, Money and Stocks of Money, have been heretofore given, limited, appointed and assigned, as well as by the Queen's most excellent Majesty, and her most noble Progenitors, as by sundry other well disposed persons; some for Relief of aged, impotent and poor People, some for the Maintenance of sick and maimed Soldiers and Mariners, Schools of Learning, Free Schools, and Scholars in Universities, some for the Repair of Bridges, Ports, Havens, Causeways, Churches, Sea-Banks and Highways, some for the Education and Preferment of Orphans, some for or towards Relief, Stock or Maintenance for Houses of Correction, some for the Marriages of Poor Maids, some for Supportation, Aid and Help of young Tradesmen, Handicraftsmen and Persons decayed, and others for the Relief or Redemption of Prisoners or Captives, and for Aid or Ease of any poor Inhabitants concerning Payments of Fifteens [a tax on moveable property], setting out of Soldiers and other Taxes; which Lands, Tenements, Rents, Annuities, Profits, Hereditaments, Goods, Chattels, Money and Stocks of Money, nevertheless have not been employed according to charitable Intent of the givers and Founders thereof, by reason of Frauds, Breaches of Trust, and Negligence in those that should pay, deliver and employ the same: For Redress and Remedy whereof, Be it enacted ...

However, the primary purpose of this Act was to provide for commissioners to be appointed to investigate the administration of charities, and in particular the misappropriation of (trust) property, which was already becoming a problem.

As far as influencing the development of modern charity law is concerned, the Preamble was intended to be a comprehensive statement of worthy causes considered to be charitable at the time. It was, in many respects, strongly focused on the relief of poverty—broadly configured—but it embraced very divergent charitable purposes, and thereby became most useful for expansions of the definition of charity during the eighteenth and nineteenth centuries. This was also a time of changing conceptions of public benefit: originally, a purpose had to benefit the poor in order to be charitable; but nineteenth-century influences from philanthropic thoughts and emerging middle-class values suggested refocusing charitable activity on those who were deserving, rather than necessarily destitute. This era would start to raise questions about the significance of charitable provision alongside the development of increased welfare provision, which have become magnified over time on account of the development of the modern welfare state. It was also during the later nineteenth century that ties between charitable status and tax concessions started to emerge. In this regard, in *Commissioners for Special Purposes of the Income Tax* v *Pemsel* [1891] AC 531, which formed the basis for the *modern definition* of 'heads of charity', it became clear for the first time that relief from taxation might be tied in to the definition of charity. This case can be seen as a significant milestone, albeit that the judges themselves do not appear to have appreciated the importance of the connection.

10.4.2 The modern classification of charitable purposes and its wider significance

As it will become clear shortly, Lord Macnaghten's *Pemsel* classification remained unchanged until the statutory definition of charitable purposes under the Charities Act 2006 came into force in April 2008. But there has long been a sense that the definition of charity was not static. Just as *Pemsel* was a conscious attempt to classify purposes that were either in the Preamble of the Statute of Elizabeth or developed from it organically subsequently, in *Scottish Burial Reform and Cremation Society Ltd* v *Glasgow Corporation* [1968] AC 138, Lord Wilberforce stressed that the legal definition of charity was evolving, and would be reflective of both current needs of society and also changing ones:

> But three things may be said about [the *Pemsel* classification], which its author [Lord Macnaghten] would surely not have denied: first that, since it is a classification of convenience, there may well be purposes which do not fit neatly into one or other of the headings; secondly, that the words used must not be given the force of a statute to be construed; and thirdly, that the law of charity is a moving subject which may well have evolved even since 1891.
>
> (*Scottish Burial Reform and Cremation Society Ltd* v *Glasgow Corporation* [1968] AC 138, *per* Lord Wilberforce at 154)

10.4.3 Charity law for the twenty-first century: the Charities Acts 2006 and 2011

Charity law that evolves as society evolves

Similar statements were also expressed subsequently in the House of Lords in *IRC* v *McMullen* [1981] AC 1. But the key development for understanding charity law as it currently is was the policy movement leading to the Charities Act 2006, which was anchored to two key documents: the 2002 Strategy Unit of the Cabinet Office publication *Private Action, Public Benefit;* and the government's responses to its recommendations, *Charities and Not-for-Profits: A Modern Legal Framework—The Government's Response to 'Private Action, Public Benefit'*, published in 2003. These reveal how much the impetus for reform of the law was grounded in modernization and effectiveness, transparency, accountability, and regulation, which in turn helps us to understand the changes introduced by the Charities Act 2006, now embodied in the Charities Act 2011.

The scope of concerns for charity law

Charity law has always been a reference point for policy designed to encourage the support of worthy causes by those who own property. It has also been concerned with how charitable organizations could become embroiled in 'political' struggles for social control (and especially in ones along the fault line between religion and secular approaches), and ones about how they should respond in times of economic unrest and hardship. Significantly, charity law has always been concerned about the opportunities for the misappropriation of property by those responsible for delivering its benefits to worthy causes. From the nineteenth century, we can add to this heady mix the tensions that have emerged over time about the generous tax treatment of those activities deemed to be charitable purposes.

Much of the impetus for the Charities Act 2006 can be seen in the light of all of these factors. The charitable sector is the recipient of much societal generosity: tax concessions are the obvious one and, as we saw with the *Vandervell* litigation in Chapter 4, this generosity extends beyond the organizations themselves, to those who are actually donors. There are other advantages too, such as the facility for public enforcement, and the operation of the cy-près scheme to ensure that any property dedicated to charity always remains able to further charitable activity, even when a particular organization is unable to carry this out.

At the heart of conferring much generosity to charitable activity is recognition of the publicness of charitable activity, which is in turn reflective of *credo* within the English psyche that charitable activity is activity for the public good. The function of charity law has always been to ensure that only those organizations that should be charitable are so, but equally to ensure that those that are so can secure the advantages that flow from being regarded as activity 'for the public good'. For these reasons, charity law as we know it has always required that, for an organization to be charitable, its purposes must be 'charitable' and must benefit 'the public', as defined by charity law.

Charity and its evolution, and the nature of current concerns of charity law

The reform movement leading to the Charities Act 2006 suggested that charity law needed to be much more effective in both of these two key regards. That charity law needed to be much more effective in ensuring that only organizations that should be charitable would be so was evident from government recognition that public confidence in charity was not as good as it should be. Alongside this was recognition of public perception that charitable status was awarded too easily on the basis of too little evidence for unsuitable purposes. Such concerns are particularly strongly attached to reforms relating to public benefit requirements, and which are intended to achieve and sustain what then Minister for the Cabinet Office Hilary Armstrong MP explained in Parliament in June 2006 as 'high levels of public confidence in charities', which are to be achieved through 'effective regulation'.

Charity law in the twenty-first century: regulation—and liberalization

This tells us that achieving (through restoration and then continued sustenance) high levels of public confidence was central to the reform movement leading to the Charities Act 2006. But it does not actually tell us why achieving this was so important, and the reasons for this are complex and intricate. In the reforms around public benefit considered in the next chapter, we can see that, in one respect, reforming charity law has sought to restore confidence in charity by seeking to place restrictions on purposes deemed to be for the public good. But we can also see a different approach at work. In reforms relating to classifying purposes as charitable, we can also see the intention to expand the definition of purposes with charitable character, so that more purposes can potentially be charitable. Alongside the essence of effective regulation, in parliamentary discussion Hilary Armstrong echoed the widely held view that charities 'play a fundamental role in the fabric of our society' because they 'provide a vital service to individuals and communities'. Thus a key policy of charity law, alongside regulation and accountability flowing from the special status of charity, must be to 'break down the barriers that face the charitable sector', itself central to raising the profile of charity, and thereby to increase its scope for further 'public good'.

There are two key elements behind this insistence that the importance of charity in society needs to be promoted: the first is clearly a perception of loss of public confidence in charity; the second is belief that there is actually a need to restore confidence in charity because charity is so important for society. This latter proposition is the part that needs explaining. The reason why it is important for charity to be able to increase its potential for further public good is that, whatever individual feelings are about particular charities or even charity as a concept, society as a whole benefits from supporting charitable activity.

This is much less tangible than it will once have been in pre-welfare-state times, when local inhabitants would have been able to experience first-hand reductions in rates payable on account of the philanthropic activities of others. But it is also the case today that charitable activity enables much higher levels of social utility and general civility than would be possible if we all had to pay for certain 'public goods' that we utilize. Medical research is a good example of this, because much of what we can benefit from under National Health Service (NHS) treatment (and indeed private medical health care) is made possible by work carried out through charitable organizations, rather than more directly financed through taxation. Thus giving tax concessions to charitable activity can be a more cost-effective way of securing high levels of civility and social benefit than asking citizens to pay higher taxes, and it also one that is considered more socio-politically acceptable. This is why charity is marketed so strongly as being for the public good, and why it is claimed that society as a whole loses out from lack of 'public confidence' in charity, which then affects *inter vivos* donations and bequests, whilst tax concessions felt to be underserved cause considerable resentment.

10.4.4 Charity law for the twenty-first century: the Charities Act 2011

There are counter-arguments for these perspectives considered on the Online Resource Centre. But as far as understanding the reform movement is concerned, this is why it had to concentrate so much on restoring high levels of public confidence in charitable activity.

In the next chapter, we shall find out how these twin strategies of enhancing the regulation and accountability of charitable organizations, whilst at the same time providing a regime for defining charitable purposes that is capable of growing the sector considerably, can be found represented in the law. The Charities Act 2006 has itself now been substantially replaced by the Charities Act 2011, of course. But, in acknowledging this, it is also important to understand that the 2011 legislation had a very different impetus and underlying rationale. In distinguishing the origins of the two Acts, the view of this text was always that the Charities Act 2006 could be seen as a project of continuity and change—in its recognition that, to make charity law fit for purpose in the twenty-first century, new directions would be required, but also that the new law would take much of its inspiration and even its letter from the way in which charity law has always sought to reflect the public good associated with charitable activity. In contrast, the 2011 Act is actually consolidating legislation that does not alter the changes introduced by the Charities Act 2006. Whilst the 2006 Act represented a very significant milestone for English charity law, its enactment resulted in a statutory regime of charity law spanning four Acts: the 2006 Act; the Recreational Charities Act 1958; and the Charities Acts 1992 and 1993. As the Charity Commission explains, the 2011 Act is 'intended to make the law easier to understand by replacing four Acts of Parliament with one. It doesn't make any changes to the law'.

In this regard, sweeping changes *were* made by the 2006 Act, both to the letter of charity law and its underpinning policy. But, in other respects, the 2006 Act does appear to retain much of the spirit and actually letter of traditional law. And in alluding to the practical significance of the 2011 Act, the Charity Commission conceded that accommodating its enactment has required the updating of nearly 500 web pages and PDFs on its website, just to reference the new legislation. All of this, taken together, indicates that the law relating to charity is vast. And as we discover in the next chapter, even focusing this entirely on the legal definition of charity is no small task, given the references that must now be made to the 2011 Act and also the significance of the 2006 Act.

This is because directions that were new in 2006 need to be explained and this, as well as its points of continuity, require extensive reference to 'traditional' charity law. This is the principal reason why the coverage of charity law by this text is so extended. But it is also the case that, alongside the consolidating effect of the 2011 Act, the substance of charity law introduced by the Charities Act 2006 has actually been under review, with the final report of Lord Hodgson's Review of the Charities Act published in July 2012. This is likely to impact significantly on future coverage of charity by this text.

This now leads us straight into the legal definition of charity in the next chapter.

 Revision Box

1. Ensure that you can identify the key stages in the development of English charity law from 1601 to the present, and from this answer the following questions.
   (a) What does each stage in this 'history' reveal about the relationship between property and its ownership, and the support of worthy causes?
   (b) Why did equity become involved in charitable giving?
   (c) What are the two key sources of litigation in the sphere of charitable giving and what are the reasons behind each?
   (d) What is the 'twist' in the operation of the Mortmain legislation?
   (e) Explain the long-standing significance of the Statute of Elizabeth 1601.
   (f) Explain the combined significance of *Commissioners for Special Purposes of the Income Tax* v *Pemsel* [1891] AC 531 and *Scottish Burial Reform and Cremation Society Ltd* v *Glasgow Corporation* [1968] AC 138.
   (g) What are the key advantages flowing from charitable status?
2. Ensure that you can explain the background to the reform of charity law by the Charities Act 2006, and the similarities and key differences between this and the enactment of the Charities Act 2011.

FURTHER READING

Because this chapter was introductory in nature, references for further reading can be found at the end of Chapter 11, which studies the legal definition of 'charity'.

11

The legal definition of 'charity'

Following on from the previous chapter, this one is focused on the legal definition of 'charity' itself. In making this point, we need to appreciate that, in seeking to achieve the effective regulation of charities whilst also seeking to bolster the charitable sector, the reach of charity law now embodied in the Charities Act 2011 is much more extensive than the coverage given to it in this text. There is much more to achieving the effective regulation of charity whilst also seeking to strengthen the influence of charity in society by growing the sector than provisions relating to the legal definition of charity.

This is evident when we look at reforms relating to public benefit, for example, where it will become apparent that a core tenet in achieving both of these aims is policy for drawing distinction between different charitable organizations on the basis of size, with the most liberal 'administrative' demands associated with registration and compliance being applied to the smallest charities, and much more onerous demands being made of much larger organizations, which hold sizeable assets. In this context, size is being very strongly determined by an organization's assets and the scope of its activities, and it is good to be aware of this given that there are a number of ways in which current thinking on charity law at the heart of the Charities Act 2006 (as now consolidated in the 2011 Act) reflects this policy, notwithstanding that there is little coverage of it in this text. Similarly, the Act is also concerned with governance requirements for organizations, expectations of charitable trustees, and demonstrating compliance with the regulatory regime—but such matters are largely beyond the scope of this text.

However, there is some considerable merit in considering the legal definition of 'charity', which is elemental to an organization's recognition as one that is charitable, and which makes considerations of governance and compliance ones that are secondary. And, in this regard, some of the key issues not relating to the new statutory definition of charity under the 2006 Act (and now the 2011 Act) can be found discussed within material available on the Online Resource Centre.

Focusing on the legal definition of charity

What this chapter is concerned with is how an organization becomes subject to 'charity law' at all—that is, how it becomes subject to this special body of trusts law, which entitles it to tax concessions in a number of respects and which allows generous treatment of donations made to it, from the perspective of donor as well as recipient. This special body of law also facilitates the effective use of property that is considered dedicated to charitable purposes once and for all once it has been donated, and underpins all of this with 'public enforcement'.

Notwithstanding that the statutory basis for English charity law is the Charities Act 2011, this is consolidating legislation, and therefore the Charities Act 2006 remains a central reference point for understanding how charity is to be defined in the twenty-first century, because it does represent a very determined attempt to make the requirements for obtaining charitable status more rigorous, whilst also being more facilitative. These are not obviously compatible aims, and the ambition of the new regime can be seen in the way in which the legislation seeks to achieve a number of divergent objectives.

It has already been suggested that the 2006 Act recognized that charity law needs to facilitate a vibrant and sizeable charitable sector. It has also been stressed that charity law is equally determined that governance requirements and levels of accountability need to reflect the power that the charitable sector could have if it were to achieve this potential in terms of size and vibrancy. In another respect, the legislation is seeking to try to match governance and accountability requirements with size of organization, but equally it is committed to the principle that, for all charitable organizations, securing charitable status is to be continuing rather than a 'one-off' application for registration.

We will be able to consider most of these key points in this chapter as we explore how the legislative regime under the new Charities Act 2011 defines 'charity'. This is the key to all of these objectives, given that an organization will fall subject to the privileges of charitable status, and also to its responsibilities, only on being found to be what the law will recognize as charitable. This makes how 'charity' became defined under the Charities Act 2006 (now located in the Charities Act 2011) very significant for understanding how charity law will become shaped in order to be fit for purpose for the twenty-first century. However, it is also the case that, notwithstanding the current trend towards codifying charity law, what will be termed 'traditional law' remains very significant.

The Preamble to the Charities Act 2011: the Charities Act 2006 as a product of continuity and change

The combined effect of the sheer volume of English charity law and its scope for governing charitable activity ensures this chapter is one of the most substantial within the text, even in being entirely focused on the legal definition of charity. This, in turn, ensures that it is possible to make only a brief study of even the legal definition of charity (and not looking at charity law any more widely than this). This involves understanding how purposes are recognized as 'charitable', why they must be for public benefit and how this is determined, and what can disqualify a purpose from being considered charitable. However, this is far from straightforward. Notwithstanding that it has already been replaced by the Charities Act 2011, it remains far from clear how much of the statutory footing for the legal definition of charity created by the Charities Act 2006 amounted to new approach and how much amounted to a restatement of traditional charity law. In accepting that there are still more questions than answers at this stage, it might be helpful to keep a few considerations in mind, as follows.

- The Charities Act 2011 seeks to consolidate the law, making it clearer and more accessible, and does not alter the law or policy of the regime under the Charities Act 2006. Indeed, Lord Hodgson's review of whether the legal framework provided by the 2006 Act 'is fit for purpose now and in the future' continued to its conclusion in July 2012, notwithstanding the new Act.
- The rationale for the Charities Act 2006 can, in many respects, be understood in relation to concerns about perceived lack of public confidence in charitable activity.
- The 2006 Act can be seen to reflect a political rationale to restore confidence in charitable activity and underpinning charity law on account of a strong belief that charitable activity is beneficial for, and is in the interests of, society generally.

- In this regard, the approach of the 2006 Act can be seen to manifest new law, which draws much inspiration and direction from traditional approaches that have always sought to be stringent for purposes seeking charitable status, and which is also mindful that affirming public confidence in charity requires some new direction and ideas.

In this respect, the Charities Act 2006, as enacted, can be seen to be an important project of continuity *and* change in English charity law. Whether it is found to be fit for purpose remains to be seen, but in explaining the essence of continuity and change, it might be helpful to have in mind that the Charities Act 2006 (as enacted):

- appears in many respects to be law that is a 'restatement' of traditional charity law; and
- can also be seen to depart from traditional approaches in order to bolster public confidence with requirements that are more stringent still.

Exploring and examining the Charities Act 2006

With Lord Hodgson's Review of the Charities Act 2006 only recently concluded and its report, *Trusted and Independent: Giving Charity back to Charities*, published in July 2012 (<http://www.cabinetoffice.gov.uk/sites/default/files/resources/Review-of-the-Charities-Act-2006.pdf>), exploring the law put in place by the Charities Act 2006 remains an interesting task. Centrally for this chapter's examination of the legal definition of charity, it is still unclear how much of the new law is actually traditional law placed on a statutory footing and what might actually be a new direction. In some instances, this is clear; in others, it is less so, and so the sensible starting point remains 'traditional' charity law. Looking at law dating from *Comm for Income Tax* v *Pemsel* [1891] AC 531 will be helpful in evaluating clear points of departure or change in the new regime, and what might be intended continuity with traditional approaches. So references to the new regime will be woven into material setting out traditional law that emerged from the application of *Pemsel*, and some tentative assessment of the new provisions will follow this, with reference also to key policy literature both underpinning the changes and, in other respects, implementing them.

In terms of understanding what was new and different in the legislation, this reference to 'intended continuity' is quite deliberate. This is because, when we look at the provisions and the policy material underpinning the 2006 Act, it becomes clear that the influences of then 'existing law' are very strong. Whilst any assessment that is made is, of course, subject to the findings of Lord Hodgson, we will encounter matters that were believed were in need of new approaches at the time that the 2006 Act was conceived, because then-existing law was not deemed fit for purpose in securing high levels of public confidence in charity and achieving effective regulation of the sector. However, we will also find evidence of determined efforts to import existing law into the new regime. And, regardless of Lord Hodgson's conclusions, this had to signal belief that aspects of traditional charity law *were* considered fit for purpose and should remain a part of defining charitable purpose into the twenty-first century.

Defining 'charity': the statutory definition and references to 'traditional' law

What this text refers to as 'traditional' law is actually what the 2006 Act legislation and its companion Explanatory Notes termed 'existing charity law'. This can now be found termed 'old law' by the Charities Act 2011, with s. 2 (4) explaining that this references 'the law relating to charities in England and Wales as in force immediately before 1 April 2008' (the date on which the provisions in the 2006 Act relating to the legal definition of charity came into force).

Except when quoting the legislation verbatim, this chapter uses the term 'traditional law' to denote what is now 'old law' for the purposes of the Charities Act 2011. Interestingly, the 2011 Act makes much fewer references to 'old law' than the 2006 Act made to 'existing law', perhaps indicating a perception that the latter statutory regime is starting to embed itself. But it is also hard to ignore the position that, whilst the 2006 Act did inculcate some very important new policy directions in charity law, these new definitions of charity derived much of their direction and authority from traditional law.

Notwithstanding that Lord Hodgson's conclusions will require some extensive and ongoing assessment, there is also a further dimension for this analysis to consider beyond the extent to which the current statutory regime is a project of change, or one of continuity. This is whether, and to what extent, the regime under the 2011 Act will provide simplification, clarification, and increased accessibility to English charity law.

11.1 Features of 'traditional law' as an introduction to approaches taken in the Charities Act 2006, and now the Charities Act 2011

For all of these reasons, it is important that we understand how charity law has been traditionally configured and especially that, certainly from its modern formulation dating from the nineteenth century, it has been concerned to ensure that only those worthy causes that should be recognized as providing a public good would actually be recognized as being charitable.

A charitable trust must have charitable aims and objectives ('purposes'), as established by law, and this has traditionally been determined by the Charity Commission on application for registration. The tests that have been devised to determine whether purposes are charitable can be classified as representing three key requirements, as follows.

- *Determining whether the character of the purposes is charitable* The key reference point for this in the modern law was the classification of charitable purposes set out by Lord Macnaghten in *Commissioners for Special Purposes of the Income Tax* v *Pemsel* [1891] AC 531. This was a scheme that provided four 'heads' for classifying charitable purposes:
  - (1) purposes for the relief of poverty;
  - (2) purposes for the advancement of education;
  - (3) purposes for the advancement of religion; and
  - (4) other purposes that are beneficial to the community.

This classification was based on those purposes specified within the Preamble of the Statute of Elizabeth 1601, and in this regard what is known as '*Pemsel* head 4' was regarded as a general location for everything that was considered charitable, but which could not be accommodated under one of the first three specific heads. However, it was also the case that, following *Pemsel*, a number of purposes came to be recognized as charitable notwithstanding being absent from the Preamble, which was explained in *Scottish Burial Reform and Cremation Society Ltd* v *Glasgow Corporation* [1968] AC 138 as the courts having regard to what has become known as the 'spirit and intendment' of the Preamble. This case also made the very significant point that charity law evolves because charity in society evolves. This means that, although *Pemsel* is regarded as the modern classification of charitable purposes, we shall also see how the Preamble remained very significant for the development of head 4. However, it will also become clear that, notwithstanding Lord Wilberforce's suggestion that the *Pemsel* classifications should not prescribe the development of charity law, the *Pemsel* classification only became displaced at all by the introduction of the Charities Act 2006—and there are very real arguments for suggesting that this displacement is largely one of form on account of the continuity agenda of the new law.

- *Determining whether the purposes meet the requirement of 'public benefit'* The previous chapter introduced the public nature of charitable trusts, identifying them as purposes that are publicly enforced and controlled, and which have certain tax concessions. This means that, in order to be charitable, modern charity law has always required that a purpose with charitable character must also confer a public benefit. We shall see that this requirement has traditionally been manifested in two key tests, which must both be satisfied in order for a public benefit to subsist. We shall also see that these two key tests have been applied quite differently under the different *Pemsel* heads, and this is very significant for considering how public benefit might be approached post-2006.

- *For purposes meeting both the requirement of 'charitable purpose' and 'public benefit', it must be established that there are no factors that will prevent it from qualifying as charitable* For purposes that are capable of being accommodated under one or more of the *Pemsel* heads, and which satisfy the public benefit requirements in place, to securing charitable status, one remaining hurdle asks whether there is anything about the purpose that will disqualify it from being charitable. There are a number of factors that have traditionally operated to disqualify potentially charitable purposes from achieving charitable status, with the most important being: that the purpose is not 'exclusively charitable', because it advances charitable aims and ones that are not so; that the purpose is profit-making; and that the purpose has political objectives. There is also the general principle, which applies to all trusts: that those that are unlawful or contrary to public policy will not be permitted.

The role of the courts: who is involved with enforcing trusts and litigating charity law?

Because charity law has, up to now, been developed mainly through case law, these tests have been developed by the courts and applied where the matter is litigated. In explaining how these issues are actually generated for the courts to consider, we can see the courts being required to consider 'concerns' about a charity or its activities that the Attorney-General encounters as public enforcer of charities. This will become apparent when we look at organizations that appear to have political objectives, which are inconsistent with charitable status.

As suggested, there are also two further significant catalysts for litigation in which the courts will have to make rulings on how charity is defined as a matter of law. The first is the interest that the UK tax authority takes in organizations seeking charitable status, or in the status of gifts made to particular purposes, as explained in the previous chapter, because of the consequences of charitable status for what can be collected for the 'public purse'. We can see this in operation in litigation in which the tax authority—whatever its name at the time—is a party in the action being brought.

But most litigation surrounding the legal definition of charity has been brought by 'next of kin'. These are the disgruntled relatives of those who are deceased, who have been so inconsiderate as to favour worthy causes over flesh and blood: those who have clearly forgotten that charity begins at home—and preferably stays there! Thus much litigation is concerned with disputing the validity of gifts supposedly made to charity, remembering that (as explained in the previous chapter), upon a successful challenge to the charitable nature of a gift, this will be returned to a donor or his estate by way of a resulting trust.

In now setting out traditional approaches to defining charity in English law, the materials help us to appreciate whether the statutory regime now under the Charities Act 2011 can be analysed as a project of continuity and change. And, as academics and practitioners work through Lord Hodgson's findings, this text aims to provide a glimpse at whether the regime put in place by the Charities Act 2006 is likely to provide charity law that is fit for purpose in the twenty-first century, through delivering its aims of effective regulation of the charitable sector, and will facilitate its growth in size and in social significance.

Part I Traditional English charity law

We know from the foregoing general introduction that understanding the modern law does not require us, to any significant degree, to think further back than to the late nineteenth century. What follows now is that each of the three traditional elements for satisfying the legal definition of charity is considered in turn. This commences with explaining purposes with charitable character from their classification in *Pemsel*, which involves looking in some detail at the case law that has emerged from this. This will then move to satisfying the public benefit requirement, and then observing the significance and operation of factors that, if present, will disqualify a purpose from being recognized as charitable.

This examination of defining purposes with charitable character takes each *Pemsel* head in turn and sets out the core elements of judicial approaches to it.

11.2 Charitable purposes under traditional law

11.2.1 Purposes for the relief of poverty

The courts have not attempted to define 'poverty' in precise terms (which would align this with a particular level of income, for example), but it is clear that this has been influenced by notions of 'the deserving poor'. Hence 'poverty' is not as extreme a concept as 'destitution' (reflecting that people can be poor, yet not destitute) and it varies depending on a person's status in life. People who are sufficiently well off to be able to live without state aid can be regarded as being poor for these purposes. Paradoxically, it is nowadays very difficult to relieve poverty among the poorest sections of society, because a claimant of state benefits can suffer a reduction in that benefit if he receives more than a small donation from charity.

It is also clear from *Re Coulthurst* [1951] Ch 661 that poverty under *Pemsel* was to be considered a relative term and is aligned with having to 'go short' in the light of what would be usual. For this reason, the courts have permitted as charitable trusts those provided to assist social categories of person such as 'distressed gentle folk' (as in *Re De Cartaret* [1933] Ch 103), and foundations for those falling on 'hard times' have achieved registration as charities (such as that for investors in the successful *AITC Foundation Application for Registration as a Charity* [2005] WTLR 1265)).

In 2008, the Charity Commission defined 'people in poverty' as including those who are destitute, but also those 'who cannot satisfy a basic need without assistance', and, anchored to this, those who lack what is necessary to achieve 'a modest, but adequate standard of living'. This also signposts the traditional requirement that, for the purposes of this head, only the poor can benefit; whereas a trust under any of the other three heads can be charitable even where affluent people can enjoy its benefits, a trust that may benefit rich persons as well as poor will fail under this head. This is the reason why disaster fund appeals are often not charitable, but in any case those who are rich must usually be expressly excluded, because the courts have been very reluctant to infer their exclusion even where the nature of the benefit is unlikely to make it attractive except to the destitute. This is evident in the outcomes of *Re Gwyon* [1930] 1 Ch 255, and *Re Drummond* [1914] 2 Ch 90, with judicial persistence with this requirement evident in *Re Sanders's WT* [1954] Ch 265. In terms of how gifts are actually expressed, a gift for 'deserving' persons, or 'those in need of financial assistance' suffice, but 'indigent' and 'needy' can be regarded as synonyms for poverty. Poverty can also often be implied in the case of gifts to elderly or disabled recipients.

Construction: the trend against hard-and-fast rules

While the courts are reluctant to infer exclusion of the rich in the absence of an express limitation to the poor, they will do so on occasions. This can be seen in *Powell v Attorney-General* (1817) 3 Mer 48, and *Re Niyazi's WT* [1978] 1 WLR 910, notwithstanding that *Re Niyazi's WT* is probably more or less confined to its facts because the amount of money left for the purpose was relatively small and the word 'hostel', rather than 'dwelling', was able to suggest very inferior accommodation. Thus settlors would be wiser in expressly limiting benefit to those who are poor.

Methods of relieving poverty

The measures must actually relieve poverty, so merely providing amusement for the poor will not suffice under this head, although it might under the second head, if educational. It used to be thought that relief of poverty had to be ongoing, rather than by way of an immediate distribution of property (thought to be indistinguishable from an ordinary private bequest), but *Re Scarisbrick* [1951] Ch 622 establishes that poverty can be relieved by way of one-off payment or distribution.

It is also not necessary for relief to be direct handouts of money, goods, or services, and can be allowing access to necessary amenities at reduced cost. This can be seen in *Joseph Rowntree Memorial Trust Housing Association Ltd v Attorney-General* [1983] Ch 159, in which the sale of homes to elderly persons at 70 per cent of cost was charitable, even though recipients had to 'bargain their bounty'.

11.2.2 Purposes for the 'advancement of education'

The scope of educational activities accepted as charitable at common law was surprisingly wide, and this does not seem to have arisen from the perverse operation of the Mortmain legislation, because this did not really affect educational charities, which were mainly incorporated by royal charter. The Preamble to the Act of 1601 speaks only of 'schools of learning, free schools, scholars in universities', and the 'education and preferment of orphans', but in modern times this category has grown to cover a very wide range of educational and cultural activities extending far beyond the administration of formal instruction.

A comprehensive statement on 'education today' can be found in the Charity Commission's supplementary guidance, published in 2008, on *The Advancement of Education for the Public Benefit* (<http://www.charity-commission.gov.uk/Library/guidance/pbeductext.pdf>), but in terms of locating the law prior to 2006, schools and universities have always been charitable; increasingly, so have nursery schools, adult education centres, and societies dedicated to promoting training and standards within a trade or profession. Indeed, education has never been limited to teaching, and learned societies that bring together experts in a field to share and exchange knowledge may be charitable. Museums, zoos, and public libraries may be educational to the public at large, quite apart from their research activities. Even cultural activities such as drama, music, literature, and fine arts can come within this head, on the ground that they have a role in the cultivation of knowledge and taste. As with other heads of charity, it is essential that the organization should not be profit-seeking and the purposes must be exclusively charitable. Thus a trust for 'artistic' purposes may be too wide (see *Associated Artists Ltd* v *IRC* [1956] 1 WLR 752).

Education must be advanced

To be charitable, a purpose for education also had to advance education. This means that although research can be charitable, it probably will not be if it is 'top secret', for example. Scholarship for its own sake is also not charitable, and this is one of the reasons why researching the advantages of a new forty-letter alphabet was held to be non-charitable by Harman J in *Re Shaw* [1957] 1 WLR 729.

Learned societies are charitable, and professional and vocational bodies that advance education, such as the Royal College of Surgeons, are also charitable, even though one of the ancillary purposes is the protection and assistance of its members. Other examples include the Royal College of Nursing, the Institution of Civil Engineers, and the Incorporated Council of Law Reporting; indeed, in *Incorporated Council of Law Reporting for England and Wales* v *Attorney-General* [1972] Ch 73, the Attorney-General tried unsuccessfully to argue that the citation of law reports in court could not be educational, because judges are deemed to have complete knowledge of the law. Bodies the chief purpose of which is to further the interests of the members and to promote the status of the profession will not, however, be charitable, as illustrated by *General Nursing Council for England and Wales* v *St Marylebone Borough Council* [1959] AC 540.

Issues arising from physical education

It will shortly become apparent that physical activity that is of a purely recreational nature was not charitable at common law, and would not be so unless it fell within the provisions of the Recreational Charities Act 1958. Games and other leisure-time pursuits can be charitable under this head, however, if educational. Thus, in *Re Marriette* [1915] 2 Ch 284, a gift to provide squash courts at a public school was held to be charitable, Eve J remarking that the playing of games at boarding schools was as important as learning from books, and that the proper education of young people can include 'development of the body' as well as that of the mind. On the same principle, the provision of toys for small children can be charitable (the National Association of Toy Libraries is a registered charity), as are youth movements, such as the Boy Scout Movement, or trusts to provide school outings. In *Re Dupree's Deed Trusts* [1945] Ch 16, a chess contest for young men in the Portsmouth area was held to be charitable, although Vaisey J left open the question of less intellectually demanding pursuits such as stamp collecting and birds' egg collecting, and even some games. These cases were approved and followed by the House of Lords in *IRC* v *McMullen* [1981] AC 1, a case involving the playing of football at schools and universities, which also insisted that the legal conception of charity was not static, but changed with ideas about social values.

All of these cases concerned the education of children or young persons. There is no reason, in principle, why adult education should not also be charitable, but a different approach seems to be taken to adult *physical* education: we shall find out that a police athletic association was held not to be a trust for recreational purposes, and therefore not charitable. This reasoning suggests that driving schools or flying schools would also not be thought to be charitable on account that they are educational.

Education for the purpose of defining charity, and the role of 'value judgements' and a focus on 'outcomes'

Inevitably, with a wide definition of educational purposes, the courts and the Charity Commission may be involved in subjective value judgements as to whether a particular purpose falls within or outside the definition. There appear to be two separate issues: first, does the activity have any educational value at all; and second, in the case of research, based on the assumption that any discoveries made will be of value, to what extent should the courts take account of the likelihood of finding nothing? It is clear that the courts are prepared to embark upon value judgements on the first question. The views of the donor will, of course, not be conclusive, and expert evidence will be admitted in order to assist in evaluating the merit of artistic and cultural work.

In *Re Pinion* [1965] Ch 85, for example, the testator left his 'studio' for the purposes of a museum to display his collection of what were claimed to be 'fine arts'. However, expert witnesses assessed paintings as 'atrociously bad' and the collection was dismissed by Harman LJ in the Court of Appeal as 'a mass of junk'. In *Re Delius* [1957] Ch 299, a trust for the appreciation of the composer's works was held charitable, but Roxburgh J insisted that the same view would not be taken of a composer who lacked the obvious merits of Delius.

Where research is concerned, the courts will also presumably assess the value of the ultimate aim of the project, but, given the very essence of research, it is often not possible to ascertain in advance the value of research. Determinations of charitable character appear to be mindful of this, as evident in the decision in *Re Hopkins* [1965] Ch 669, in which a bequest to the Francis Bacon Society for the purposes of finding the Bacon–Shakespeare manuscripts was upheld as charitable. The discovery was accepted as being very unlikely, but if made would likely be 'of the highest value to history and to literature'. This view does illustrate that value judgements are very difficult to operate when the outcome of the quest is uncertain, as will usually be the case when genuine research is concerned.

Education and political purposes

A trust for the advancement of political purposes will not be charitable, but it is also the case that education can undoubtedly cover political theory and philosophy. The borderline appears to fall at the point where partisan propaganda is seen to be masquerading in the guise of instruction. In *Re Hopkinson* [1949] 1 All ER 346, a trust for adult education in socialist principles fell foul of this division of acceptable from that which is not. The political angle was another reason why the trust in *Re Shaw* [1957] 1 WLR 729 failed. But a different outcome arose in *Re Koeppler's WT* [1986] Ch 423, which we will consider when we look more closely at the problem of political purposes generally for qualifying as charitable.

11.3 Purposes for the 'advancement of religion'

In understanding how charity and religion interact, the first thing to note is the traditionally highly tolerant approach of law towards religion, and also its neutral stance as between different religions. This is explained by Cross J in *Neville Estates* v *Madden* [1962] Ch 832, in which a trust for the members of the Catford Synagogue was held charitable: 'As between different religions the law stands neutral, but it assumes that any religion is at least likely to be better than none.'

This sense of neutrality can be seen half a century earlier than *Neville Estates* in the decision in *Bowman* v *Secular Society Ltd* [1917] AC 406. We have already encountered this case in Chapter 3, when we discussed private purpose trusts, and in this context the part of Lord Parker's judgment that is relevant is that where he submits that a trust for the purpose of any kind of monotheistic theism would be a good charitable trust.

However, it would be a mistake to assume from this that there is a long history to this tolerant approach, and the only reference to religion in the Statute of Charitable Uses 1601 is to the repair of churches. The rise of predisposition towards religion may be one example of how a perverse result of the Mortmain legislation in force from 1736 to 1891 was actually widening of the legal definition of charity (considered briefly in Chapter 10, with further material explaining this available on the Online Resource Centre), albeit that this was actually a device to effect striking down of testamentary gifts. Examples of cases that can be explained in this way include *Thornton* v *Howe* (1862) 31 Beav 14, in which charitable status was given to promoting the writings of Joanna Southcote, the head of a small, but fervent, sect in the West of England, who had proclaimed that she was with child by the Holy Ghost and would give birth to a second Messiah. More recently, in *Re Watson* [1973] 1 WLR 1472, charitable status was upheld, notwithstanding the limited theological merits of religious writings of a retired builder.

Thus the charitable character of a number of non-Christian religions—such as Jewish, Sikh, Hindu, and Muslim faiths—has been accepted, and *Re Le Cren Clarke* [1996] 1 WLR 288 is authority that faith healing can be charitable. However, the limits of this traditional tolerance can be seen in *Re South Place Ethical Society* [1980] 1 WLR 1565, in which Dillon J clarified that religion must concern man's relations with God, and so it was, therefore, that belief in some kind of God (or gods) was a requirement. The Society was held not to be a religious charity, because although its objects included 'the study and dissemination of ethical principles' and 'the cultivation of a rational religious sentiment', its beliefs were non-theistic, and instead concerned ethics, which related to 'man's relationship with man'.

Similar reasoning can be seen at work in the Privy Council decision in *Yeap Cheah Neo* v *Ong Cheng Neo* (1875) LR 6 PC 381, which concerned the worship of ancestors and not a higher being. These cases must now be looked at differently in the light of the Charities Acts 2006 and 2011, but at common law, to be charitable under this head, purposes must be exclusively religious; for this reason, gifts for 'missionary work' or 'parish work' could experience difficulty, unless, as in *Re Simson* [1946] Ch 299, a gift to a named clergyman 'for his work in the parish' is held to be impliedly confined to his religious duties. Buddhism did present a problem in this context, and it was not entirely clear why it was deemed charitable traditionally, and was thus widely regarded as an exception. Similar difficulties would also pertain to any 'human deity'.

Purposes must advance religion

At common law, it was not sufficient for religion simply to be practised, but it must actually be *advanced*. As with education, the means by which religion may be advanced may be many and various. Apart from the provision and maintenance of churches, and provision of or for the benefit of clergymen, such matters as church choirs, Sunday school prizes, and even exorcism have all been held to advance religion. It is also clear from *United Grand Lodge of Ancient Free and Accepted Masons of England and Wales* v *Holborn Borough Council* [1957] 1 WLR 1080 that some action is actually required. In explaining why the freemasons were not advancing religion, Donovan J said, at 1090, that:

> There is no religious instruction, no programme for the persuasion of unbelievers, no religious supervision to see that its members remain active and constant in the various religions they may profess, no holding of religious services, no pastoral or missionary work of any kind.

Here, religion may have been a necessary qualification for membership of the lodge, as it might be for a church squash club, for example, but the lodge did not advance religion any more than a church squash club would.

Is some religion always better than none? Religion, anxiety, and law reform

Given what has been said in about the neutrality of the law as regards different religions, the White Paper *Charities: A Framework for the Future* (May 1989, Cmd 694), which led to the Charities Acts 1992 and 1993, considered whether the law in this area should be altered. It looked at whether religion itself was increasingly becoming a source of social concern, noting 'anxieties' about the destructive influences of some organizations. Certainly, some distrust of religion has arisen from an increasing and general secularization of society, but some religious activities were causing policymakers some concern about the continuing status of religion in charity law. In some ways, the Charities Act 2006 actually increased the scope of interactions between law and religion, and so radical proposals to remove charitable status from all religions, and also to embargo registration of new religious charities have not come to pass. And, prior to 2006, it was felt that the Charity Commission could address concerns about the conduct of certain organizations through 'gatekeeping' registration. Much of the concern expressed in 1989 was being directed towards Scientology, and the Charity Commission did indeed refuse it registration in 1999 (see Charity Commissioners for England and Wales, *Application for Registration as a Charity by the Church of Scientology (England And Wales)*, 17 November 1999, available online at <http://www.charitycommission.gov.uk/Library/start/cosfulldoc.pdf>).

There are also concerns that this 'gatekeeping' role is being directed towards the suppression of religion more generally. This can be seen in reactions to the Charity Commission's denial of charitable status to a group of the Plymouth Brethren in November 2012, on the basis that the regulator was 'unable to conclude that the organisation is established for the advancement of religion for public benefit within the relevant law'. This reflected the organization's ability to restrict access to Holy Communion, but has sparked accusations of a conscious policy of 'active suppression' of religion in the UK and, according to Charlie Elphicke MP, 'particularly the Christian religion'.

11.4 'Other purposes beneficial to the community'

The analysis that follows of the final *Pemsel* category shows how, as its 'title' suggested, it provided a residual category of charitable purposes prior to 2008 when the Charities Act 2006 came into force. This is where a vast number, and very diverse purposes, could be found 'grouped', and as a reflection of this it became a classification almost impossible to define clearly. The first point to note here is that not every purpose that might, by common consensus, be considered beneficial to the community was capable of being charitable within this head. What determined its charitable character was instead governed by the general statement of charitable purposes that was set out in the Preamble to the Statute of Charitable Uses 1601. Indeed, this is where Lord Macnaghten classified all of the purposes recognizable as charitable within the Preamble, but which could not be accommodated under the three specific heads relating to poverty, education, and religion. Although the 1601 Act has long been repealed, until the Charities Act 2006 the courts continued to rely on its Preamble in making rulings on the charitable character of novel purposes. For such a purpose to be charitable, the question was not whether it is beneficial in some general sense, but whether it fell within the spirit and intendment of the Preamble, or could be regarded as analogous with it on principles developed through the cases.

Purposes specifically included in the Preamble

The Preamble makes specific mention of the relief of 'aged', 'impotent' (meaning disabled), and 'poor' people, and it has never been necessary to show that the recipients possess all three characteristics simultaneously. Trusts to assist the elderly are common, as are trusts for the disabled, and no further requirement of poverty in the recipients is imposed. In other words, this head is wider than the relief-of-poverty head. It must be the case, however, that the proposed purpose will offer some relief to the recipients. Since many of the disadvantages that accompany age or general disability can, in fact, be eased by material provision in the form of money or special equipment, this general requirement was usually easily satisfied. Even here, however, a gift of money that was wholly confined to wealthy elderly or disabled people would probably have failed, because it would be unable to relieve the disadvantage of their condition and would also not satisfy the public benefit requirements considered shortly.

At common law, *trusts for the benefit of the sick* were prima facie charitable, and before the introduction of the National Health Service (NHS) in 1946, charitable gifts were the main source of provision for those needing hospital care, but unable either to afford it or to insure against illness or injury. At common law, gifts to private hospitals were regarded as charitable, on the controversial justification that they help to ease the pressure on public services, as suggested in *Re Resch's WT* [1969] 1 AC 514. For being charitable, it was permissible for such hospitals to be of direct benefit to those who are relatively rich, although, as with under other heads of charitable purpose, a purely profit-making institution will not be charitable.

There is no need to confine the benefits of the trust directly to the patients, and gifts that improve the efficiency of the service by providing homes for nurses, or accommodation for visiting relatives, are included under this head. Even organizations offering help with family planning, and those that seek to promote health by encouraging temperance, have been accepted for registration, but difficulties have been experienced in relation to fringe methods of healing not widely recognized by the medical profession (as noted in the Charity Commissioners' Annual Report 1975, para. 70). However, methods that are widely recognized, such as acupuncture, osteopathy, and even faith healing (with *Funnell* v *Stewart* [1996] 1 WLR 288 as authority for this), are acceptable, but in other cases some evidence of effectiveness would be demanded.

'Trusts for the benefit of soldiers', as referenced in the Preamble, has become extended to include the well-being and morale of the forces, or specific units thereof, charities for ex-servicemen, and the promotion of the efficiency of the police and the maintenance of law and order. Gifts to the Inland Revenue (now HM Revenue and Customs, or HMRC) and for 'my country England' have been held charitable (*Re Smith* [1932] Ch 153), but gifts expressed to be for 'public' or 'patriotic' purposes have failed, as being too wide and not exclusively charitable.

Anomalies: purposes in the Preamble without modern counterparts at common law

Gifts for the 'repair of bridges, ports, havens, causeways, sea-banks and highways' were included in the Preamble; now that the state assumes responsibility for such matters, this category has grown to include such miscellaneous amenities as the National Trust, museums, art galleries, parks, and community centres. In *Scottish Burial Reform and Cremation Society Ltd* v *Glasgow Corporation* [1968] AC 138, a crematorium was held charitable. And while it was not charitable for a person to erect a monument to himself at common law, as in of *Re Endacott* [1960] 232, the commemoration of significant people or events (such as war memorials) did qualify.

Old ideas and modern applications: bringing the Preamble up to date

The 'preferment of orphans' mentioned in the Preamble has its modern counterpart in the provision of orphanages and local authority homes, but in *Re Cole* [1958] Ch 888 a majority of the Court of Appeal held non-charitable a trust for the general welfare and benefit of children in such a home. This was out of fear that this might permit the provision of amenities not of an educational nature, such as radios or televisions, and this decision was followed in *Re Sahal* [1958] 1 WLR 1243. Thus purposes were unlikely to succeed under this head unless they also succeeded under the educational head.

Trusts to aid the *rehabilitation and reform of prisoners* have been accepted as charitable since the nineteenth century, but a more interesting example perhaps can be seen in the reference in the Preamble to 'ransom of captives'. In one respect, it might be easy to dismiss this idea as a relic from the past, and there is certainly the sense that, in many respects, society has become safer (and increasingly civilized), and that, accordingly, it is unlikely to find captives being held for ransom. However, this could perhaps apply in the light of today's heightened concerns about terrorism, and more still the growing threat of 'deep sea' piracy associated with the Indian Ocean.

A gift for the *benefit of a locality such as a town, county, or parish*, or for its inhabitants was capable of being charitable at common law, even though, for reasons to which we will come, this looks as though it should have been caught by failure to specify exclusively charitable purposes, or on the ground that there is an insufficient public benefit. The explanation may lie in an analogy with gifts to local authorities. These have long acted in the capacity of trustees of various charities and so such gifts may be *impliedly* confined to charitable purposes. In any event, gifts to localities were probably within the spirit of the reforms of 1601 historically, because these reforms were largely directed towards easing the burden of local poor rates. To be valid, such a provision must have been cast in terms of benefit for an area or its residents for the time being (not, for example, a trust for expatriate Welshmen, unless the purposes were charitable for some other reason).

The significance of animal charities

Animal charities are amongst the most popular charitable purposes today, but their inclusion within this head of charity owes nothing to the Preamble to the Statute of Charitable Uses 1601, and instead rests upon reasoning by analogy. As with religious toleration, the motive for recognizing purposes relating to animals as having charitable character may well have been to invalidate charitable gifts under the Mortmain legislation, but precedents of that period remained central for the common law. In *London University* v *Yarrow* (1857) 1 De G & J 72, a trust to study the diseases of animals useful to mankind was held charitable, but this would probably have been a valid educational charity anyway. A more general authority is *Tatham* v *Drummond* (1864) 4 De GJ & Sm 484, in which a bequest for the relief and protection of animals taken to be slaughtered was held charitable, so that the gift failed under the Mortmain legislation. Romer J also held a gift to a named lady to aid her work in caring for cats and kittens to be charitable in *Re Moss* [1949] 1 All ER 495.

In understanding why animal charities have been found within the spirit and intendment of the 1601 purposes, it is not benefits for animals themselves that provided principled justification for their inclusion under this head at common law; instead, it is in respect of humans that the benefits of recognizing kindness to animals are directed. This is because such purposes encourage 'feelings of humanity and morality generally', as explained in the judgment of Swinfen-Eady LJ in *Re Wedgwood* [1915] 1 Ch 113, at 122. This provided the basis for a very large number of organizations, including the Royal Society for the Prevention of Cruelty to Animals (RSPCA) and the People's Dispensary for Sick Animals (PDSA) to be charitable, and actually militated against charitable status in *Re Grove-Grady* [1929] 1 Ch 557. Here, the Court of Appeal found that a sanctuary in which animals would be protected from all human intrusion could not be charitable. The same logic would apply to protecting humans from animals that endanger man, but both scenarios could be valid as educational charities if their purposes were suitably drafted to include a conservation element.

Purposes beneficial to the community: Pemsel *and continuing evolution*

Long before the Charities Act 2006 came into being, tasked to increase the size of the charitable sector, Lord Wilberforce had remarked in *Scottish Burial Reform and Cremation Society Ltd* v *Glasgow Corporation* [1968] AC 138 that the nature of charity in society was dynamic and that charity law must reflect this. In this respect, it is not surprising that much of this growth of charitable purposes at common law occurred through the 'catch-all' *Pemsel* head. This can be illustrated by a number of examples in which the Charity Commission has made determinations on such 'topical' issues, with a brief discussion of some key areas also helping to signpost how a number of newer charitable purposes have become embodied in the new statutory definition of charity.

Prior to 2006, a number of *trusts for the relief of unemployment* (directly, rather than through the traditional routes such as the alleviation of poverty) to provide training and business start-ups, etc. had been recognized. This development of charitable purposes through the 'other purposes' head can also be seen in the recognition of trusts for *urban and rural revival*, in circumstances under which the organization seeking charitable status could demonstrate that it sought to improve 'physical, social and economic infrastructure', and would assist in alleviating disadvantage that has arisen on account of social and economic circumstances. This could include financial assistance for or the promotion of improving standards in housing and education, providing public amenities and maintenance of places of interest, and also infrastructure, etc. (with this latter being a modern counterpart for the Statute of Elizabeth's reference to 'repair of bridges etc'.). The Charity Commission also recognized trusts for the *preservation of national heritage and the environment*, as seen in the National Trust's long-standing charitable status, which also illustrates the 'public access' requirement for such purposes. In a rather different vein, recognition has also been given to purposes that *promote the incorporation of ethics into their business practice*, and which provide advice or protection for employees faced with ethical difficulties encountered in their work, and trusts for the *promotion of fair trade* have been recognized as charitable since the 'Fair Trade' mark received charitable status in 1995. The Charity Commission also recognized a number of purposes for the relief of poverty in the developing world under this head, and ones relating to 'humanitarian' purposes.

Recreational purposes, legislation, and the Charity Commission

Until the 1950s, it was assumed that, while some *recreational purposes*, such as boys' clubs, women's institutes, and parish halls, were potentially charitable, sporting facilities were not, unless they were either educational or promoted efficiency in the armed forces. A series of cases in the 1950s, however, suggested that no recreational purpose would be charitable at common law, precipitating the addition by statute of a fifth (limited) head of recreational charities. This had arisen from the way in which charitable status was denied in three key cases—*IRC v Glasgow Police Athletic Association* [1953] AC 380; *Williams' Trustees v IRC* [1947] AC 447; and *IRC v Baddeley* [1955] AC 572—notwithstanding judicial acknowledgement of the benefits for well-being and morale promoted by recreational activities for adults, because the inclusion of purely social purposes prevented these purposes from being exclusively charitable.

These decisions cast doubt on the status of a number of social trusts that had always been assumed to be charitable, and the Recreational Charities Act 1958 was enacted to restore what was assumed to be the status quo ante in respect of those trusts. This was the thrust of s. 1, with an additional 'social welfare' requirement under s. 1(2). The promotion of amateur sport for its own sake was recognized as charitable by the Charity Commissioners in 2003.

11.5 Legal definition after classifying purposes: the public benefit requirement

In traditional English charity law, in addition to being deemed to have 'charitable character', all charities must also confer a public benefit. The spirit of this has been carried through into the 2006 Act, which points to *continuity* between traditional and new approaches. However, it will also become clear that the new law marks important points of *departure*, suggesting that the public benefit requirement is to have greater prominence still in new charity law, and is intended to promote increasing robustness in the regulation of charitable organizations. In turn, this is believed to be essential for achieving high levels of public confidence in charity, and in the operation of charitable organizations generally. Because, once again, the statutory regime of the 2011 Act (as it consolidates the 2006 Act) can be seen as a project of *continuity* and also *change*, reference is first made to how, traditionally, the public benefit requirement has been manifested in English charity law.

Looking at how public benefit operated in the 'old law' does require looking at each of the four *Pemsel* heads of charitable purpose, but starting with purposes for the advancement of education. From head 2, we then look at how public benefit was accommodated at common law for heads 4, 1, and 3. The test for public benefit for educational charities was very clearly stated, and for this reason it became a benchmark for what is required under the other heads; 'other purposes' under head 4 is considered immediately following head 2 because, as will be explained, this is where the largest concentration of cases can be found.

A two-stage approach to defining 'public benefit'

As has been noted on a few occasions thus far, in addition to having to be capable of being recognized under one of the *Pemsel* heads of charitable purpose, a purpose seeking charitable status also traditionally has had to be a purpose for public benefit. Traditionally, this has required the purpose to have an identifiable public benefit, and to be capable of having a demonstrable effect, whether tangible or intangible, direct or indirect. This flows from the historical significance of recognizing worthy causes as charitable ones. Because of the value of charity for early modern Britain, traditionally, there was a presumption that purposes falling within the first three *Pemsel* heads of charity *would* provide such benefit. However, as it will emerge shortly, this presumption was removed by the Charities Act 2006, as now reflected in the 2011 Act. Although this is a point of clear difference between traditional approaches and new directions envisioned in the Charities Act 2006, the underlying rationale of public benefit is very much one of continuity.

This can be seen in two elements based on tests established in case law, which had to be demonstrated under the old law for public benefit to be satisfied: first, it had to confer to the public a benefit rather than a detriment; and second, it had to benefit a sufficient section of the public. For the first requirement—demonstrating a benefit rather than a detriment—the *National Anti-Vivisection Society* v *IRC* [1948] AC 31 is authority that where a purpose would, on balance, be detrimental to the public, the purposes cannot be charitable. Underpinning this is the rationale that the very reason for treating worthy causes in a special way embodied in charity law is that these are ones for public good. From this, it follows that if there is doubt about whether a purpose does confer a public good, then it cannot be charitable.

In cases in which it was accepted or decided that the purposes were, on balance, beneficial to the public, then the second part of this hurdle had still to be addressed. Thus even where a purpose did fall within one or more of the four *Pemsel* heads and was found to be beneficial to the public (rather than detrimental, on balance), it would not achieve charitable status unless the second public benefit requirement was also satisfied. The purpose also had to benefit a sufficient section of the public. As we will now see, the courts developed different tests for each of the four traditional heads of charitable purpose.

11.5.1 Public benefit and educational charities: the *Oppenheim* personal nexus test

In the case of relief of poverty, even benefiting a small number of people may be regarded as conferring a public benefit, but an altogether different approach was taken elsewhere within *Pemsel*. In relation to education, whilst this was deemed clearly to benefit those in immediate receipt of it, it did not automatically follow that educating a few people constitutes a benefit to the general public. Indeed, given that many of the cases under this head were, in reality, disputes over tax relief, and continue to be so, it would be quite wrong if the education of a privileged few were to be regarded as charitable. At common law under this head, some further additional benefit to the general public or some appreciable sector of it had to subsist, and whilst this was not a requirement for universal access, this had to be reasonably open.

Thus public schools may be charitable as long as they are not operated as profit-making ventures, although their fees may place them beyond the means of the majority. Even scholarships or endowed chairs, which can be enjoyed only by one person at a time, will not present a difficulty in this regard. The problems arise where the purpose is seeking to limit benefit to a group of people so narrow, if not actually so small, that they cannot meaningfully constitute a section of the public. At common law, it could be charitable to provide scholarships that were open to persons following a common profession or calling, or their children and dependants, or people of common nationality, religion, or sex, or the inhabitants of a given area. It is also the case that special provisions for disabled people were also permissible, since they are a section of the public in a meaningful sense.

Explaining the approach taken in trusts for the advancement of education
However, under this head—and all *Pemsel* heads except relief of poverty—it was fatal if the class of potential recipients (however large) was defined in a way that related them to particular individuals or a company. This approach originated in *Re Compton* [1945] Ch 123, in which charitable status was denied to a trust to educate the children of three named families. It is understandable that the courts are reluctant to allow an essentially private arrangement to enjoy charitable privileges, especially tax advantages, but it seems that the principle extends to cases in which the class of potential beneficiaries is defined in terms of a relationship with an employer, even where the employer is a substantial concern. This position was approved in *Oppenheim* v *Tobacco Securities Trust Co. Ltd* [1951] AC 297, with Lord Simonds insisting, first, that the number of possible beneficiaries must not be negligible, and second, that the class must not be defined so as to depend on any relationship to a particular individual or employer:

> Then the question is whether that class of persons can be regarded as such as a 'section of the community' as to satisfy the test of public benefit. The words 'section of the community' have no special sanctity, but they conveniently indicate first, that the possible (I emphasise the word 'possible') beneficiaries must not be numerically negligible, and secondly, that the quality which distinguishes them from other members of the community, so that they form by themselves a section of it, must be a quality which does not depend on their relationship to a particular individual ... A group of persons may be numerous, but, if the nexus between them is their personal relationship to a single *propositus* or to several *propositi*, they are neither the community nor a section of the community for charitable purposes.
>
> (*Oppenheim* v *Tobacco Securities Trust Co. Ltd* [1951] AC 297, *per* Lord Simonds at 306)

In this arrangement, the number of potential beneficiaries was certainly not negligible, with income of the trust fund being directed to be applied:

> ... in providing for ... the education of children of employees or former employees of the British-American Tobacco Co. Ltd ... or any of its subsidiary or allied companies in such manner ... as the acting trustees shall in their absolute discretion ... think fit.

With present employees alone exceeding 110,000, the number of potential beneficiaries was not an issue, and thus it was only the personal nexus rule that was fatal, and this was because they were all connected with the same company. But, as Lord MacDermott pointed out in his dissenting speech, the rule is by no means easy to apply, and produces odd results when the *propositus* (that is, the person immediately concerned) is an employer.

Justifying the approach taken in Oppenheim

Perhaps the subtext for the result in *Oppenheim* was the scope of the trustees' discretion in that case. The benefit to 110,000 or more people may, in fact, have been entirely theoretical. Had the trustees used the funds to pay 15 per cent of fees to those employees who sent their sons to boarding school, only the relatively small number who could afford the other 85 per cent would have benefited. But the *Oppenheim* test may not achieve the desired result in all cases, and perhaps the House of Lords should have focused its findings on how the trustees' discretion was able to limit the number of people who could, in practice, have benefited, rather than the nexus that could be found with the company.

Some loopholes in the personal nexus test are evident in its application in cases such as *Re Koettgen's WT* [1954] Ch 252, and *Caffoor v Income Tax Commissioner* [1961] AC 584, known as so-called 'preference' cases. But in *IRC v Educational Grants Association Ltd* [1967] Ch 123, Pennycuick J found 'considerable difficulty in the *Koettgen* decision' and thought that a preference for a private class might always be fatal, although he did not actually need to decide that. And the *Oppenheim* test does have a certain position, even if this is an inflexible one.

Further requirements of Oppenheim

This test also required that it must be possible to describe the class genuinely as a section of the community, rather than simply a body of private individuals. There are two separate requirements, with one relating to personal nexus and another requiring the class to be capable of being genuinely described as a section of the community, rather than simply a fluctuating body of private individuals. Persons following a common profession or calling, people of common nationality, religion, or sex, or the inhabitants of a town or county can be described as a section of the community. In this respect, special provisions for disabled people are also permissible, since they are a section of the public in a meaningful sense. However, see the distinctions drawn in *Davies v Perpetual Trustee Co. Ltd* [1959] AC 459.

11.5.2 Public benefit under the fourth head

The reason why we need to consider all heads of *Pemsel* in turn to get an overall measure of public benefit at common law is that dicta in *Oppenheim v Tobacco Securities Trust Co. Ltd* [1951] AC 297 suggested that the test of public benefit may vary between the four heads of charity; indeed, 'poor relations' cases were entirely excluded from considerations of the personal nexus test. It is clear that the personal nexus test did apply to the fourth head, but not obviously in the same way as it did under head 2. Here, *IRC v Baddeley* [1955] AC 572 is almost always cited as authority for a more stringent approach to requiring a benefit for a section of the public. The House of Lords held that the persons to be benefited must either be the whole community or the inhabitants of a particular area. If some further restriction is imposed by the trust on who can benefit that has the effect of creating a 'class within a class', then the test for public benefit will not be satisfied.

Viscount Simonds, in *Baddeley*, thought 'that a different degree of public benefit is requisite according to the class in which the charity is said to fall', and that public benefit considerations 'have even greater weight [than in the case of educational trusts] in the case of trusts which by their nominal classification depend for their validity upon general public utility'. This was widely accepted as a position of differing degrees of public benefit depending on into which class the charity could be said to fall (as we shall see when we consider the relief of poverty shortly). And it is said that if a charity falls within the fourth class, it must be for the benefit of the whole community, or at least of all of the inhabitants of a sufficient area.

Baddeley: *a different and additional test*

The *Baddeley* test was regarded as a different, and additional, test from that found under head 2, flowing from the different demands needing to be placed on those purposes only able to achieve charitable status by being purposes beneficial to the community. It is here that demands are most stringent, and any purpose that was able to establish itself as charitable under one of the other *Pemsel* heads would do so for this reason. This was a majority decision, and Lord Reid's dissenting speech harboured quite different views.

The view expressed in this text was always that what constituted a section of the public depended on the purposes of the particular trust, with the courts more likely to strike down arbitrary restrictions that are irrelevant to those purposes, but which simply serve to exclude other sections of the public. This can be seen in *Baddeley* itself, in Lord Simonds' discussion of the rhetorical question, asked in argument: 'Who has ever heard of a bridge to be crossed only by impecunious Methodists?' The limitation merely operated to prevent the purpose from being a public purpose; it could have had no other effect, and a purpose that is not a public purpose cannot be charitable within the fourth head.

Variation within the heads of charity as well as between them?

There is some authority that the test of public benefit can vary even *within* the fourth head itself. In *Re Dunlop* [1984] NI 408 (noted by Norma Dawson [1987] Conv 114), Carswell J took the view that public benefit depended on the nature of 'the advantage which the donor intends to provide for the benefit of all of the public'. In distinguishing *Baddeley* in any case, he was also prepared to distinguish between purposes within the fourth head itself in terms of what is required to satisfy public benefit. And it is also the case that *Baddeley* did not turn on the issue of public benefit, because charitable status failed in any case from its inclusion of purely social purposes.

11.5.3 Public benefit and the relief of poverty

It is unquestioned law that to relieve poverty is to confer a benefit upon the public at large, if only by mitigating the burden of support for the poor, which would otherwise traditionally (and certainly in a pre-welfare-state society) have fallen upon the community. The House of Lords in *Oppenheim* regarded poor relations cases as anomalous and left open the question of whether the personal nexus test applies to them.

The 'poor relations' anomaly stems from the practice of Chancery in the nineteenth century whereby, when faced with trusts expressed to be for poor relations and which would otherwise fail for uncertainty (at a time when the class ascertainability test applied, considered in Chapter 3) or perpetuity, the courts rescued such trusts by holding them charitable. The poor relations cases have been consistently followed, probably explaining why the House of Lords left them alone in *Oppenheim*. The House of Lords considered them directly in *Dingle v Turner* [1972] AC 601 and expressly upheld them. In that case, a trust for 'poor employees of E. Dingle & Co.' was held charitable, when it would have failed under the personal nexus test. The same reasoning must apply to poor relations, and thus this is authority that the personal nexus test does not apply to this head of charity.

A less strict test, but one subject to limitations

Re Scarisbrick [1951] Ch 622 is authority that, to be charitable under this head, it was necessary to show benefit is intended for a genuine class of persons, and not simply for an individual, or group of individuals, who happened to be poor. This was approved by Lord Cross in *Dingle* v *Turner*, and applied in *Re Segelman* [1996] 2 WLR 173. The *Scarisbrick* class of potential recipients was sufficiently wide to be incapable of exhaustive ascertainment ('such relations of my said son and daughters as shall be in needy circumstances'), so the trust was charitable. Once this was satisfied, the public benefit requirements were less stringent than under any other head, and the class to be benefited could be quite small.

11.5.4 Public benefit and the advancement of religion

The dicta in *Oppenheim* suggested that its tests for public benefit applied to all heads of charity except the relief of poverty, and that for religious charities there must also be an element of public contact. Private salvation, however commendable, is not charitable, with this providing further explanation for *Yeap Cheah Neo* v *Ong Cheng Neo* (1875) LR 6 PC 381, because a provision for the performance of ancestor worship could benefit only the family group. In the leading case, *Gilmour* v *Coats* [1949] AC 426, the House of Lords had to consider a gift to a Carmelite priory, housing about twenty cloistered nuns who devoted themselves to intercessory prayer and had no contact at all with the outside world. This was held non-charitable on the grounds that there was no contact with the outside world, and arguments based on Catholic doctrine—that everyone benefited from the intercessory prayers—were rejected because this could not be proved legally; nor could any benefit be found merely in the example of the piety of the women, because it was too vague and intangible. The House of Lords also rejected the argument that, entry being open to all women, the priory should be treated on analogy with an educational institution offering scholarship entry, holding that an educational establishment that required its members to withdraw from the world and leave no record of their studies would not be charitable either.

In *Re Caus* [1934] Ch 162, Catholic masses for the dead were held charitable. Although this case was doubted in *Gilmour* v *Coats*, in principle it seems correct, and *Caus* was applied by Browne-Wilkinson V-C in *Re Hetherington* [1990] Ch 1. Because Catholic masses *are* open to the public at large even when a private function, such as a funerary rite, is incorporated into the celebration, *Caus* is distinguishable from *Gilmour* v *Coats*. In *Re Hetherington*, Browne-Wilkinson V-C was called upon to consider a gift for the saying of masses, which did not exclude the possibility that the masses would be said in private. In practice, however, all or most of the masses would be open to the public. Reviewing the cases, the gift was construed so as to exclude purposes that were non-charitable.

Public and private: distinguishing Gilmour *v* Coats

Neville Estates v *Madden* [1962] Ch 832 shows how mere attendance by the public at a prayer service is sufficient to distinguish *Gilmour* v *Coats*. Here, a trust for the members of the Catford Synagogue was upheld as charitable because it concerned members of a religious group who lived in the world and mixed with their fellow citizens, enabling them thereby to extend their example of religious living to the public at large. Thus religion can be advanced by example, as long as its believers mix in the world in a *physical* sense, with *Neville* as authority that no more is required. While *Re Warre* [1953] 1 WLR 725 suggests differently, *Neville* seems to reflect current favour from the courts and the Charity Commission.

11.6 Purposes that create problems under any head of charitable purpose: disqualification from securing charitable status

Up to now, we have considered that, traditionally, English charity law has demanded that, to achieve charitable status, any purpose must be capable of being recognizable as charitable and it must be for the public benefit. Beyond this, English law has also traditionally demanded one further qualification for purposes seeking charitable status: that there are no so-called 'disqualifying factors' that will prevent a potentially charitable organization from acquiring the legal status of such. This has been alluded to already, particularly in discussion of purposes for the advancement of education and when pointing to the potential difficulties that can arise where a purpose is perceived to have political objectives. Now, we consider how a number of disqualifying factors that can interfere with an organization's ability to acquire charitable status.

11.6.1 Purposes must be exclusively charitable

This is the requirement that a trust must not merely be capable of application to charitable purposes; it must be exclusively so. If it is possible to benefit an object that is not charitable, then the trust will not be exclusively charitable, and as such will fail unless the courts feel able to sever the offending objects from the main part of the otherwise charitable purpose, or to declare that the non-charitable purposes are merely subsidiary. An everyday example of this can be found in the way in which a number of very high-profile UK charities, such as Oxfam and the RSPCA, are able to operate commercial activities, with materials illustrating this to be found on the Online Resource Centre.

The cases here reveal that a great deal has always turned on drafting, and whether terms expressing charitable and non-charitable purposes will be construed conjunctively or disjunctively. For example, if a purpose is described as 'charitable *and* benevolent', it is probable that these will be construed conjunctively: 'benevolent' merely qualifies 'charitable', so only charitable purposes are included. But in *Chichester Diocesan Fund and Board of Finance* v *Simpson* [1944] AC 341, the words 'charitable *or* benevolent' would have permitted the application of all of the funds to benevolent purposes that were not also charitable. The case formed part of the famous *Diplock* litigation concerning the maladministration of the estate of Caleb Diplock, which is considered further in Chapter 17. In *Williams* v *Kershaw* (1835) 5 Cl & F 111, a gift to 'benevolent, charitable and religious' purposes was treated as permitting trustees to select purposes that were benevolent, but not necessarily charitable and religious, with the comma regarded as the word '*or*'.

At common law, with the premise that each case called for independent construction, generally a comma, or the word 'or', would lead to disjunctive interpretation of listed purposes as alternatives, with 'and' being read conjunctively. This generally resulted in 'charitable and … ' succeeding and 'charitable or … ' failing. That this operated generally rather than invariably can be seen in *Attorney-General of the Bahamas* v *Royal Trust Co.* [1986] 3 All ER 423, in which the Privy Council held not charitable a bequest for 'any purposes for and/or connected with the education and welfare of Bahamian children and young people'. This was so on the grounds that education and welfare should be interpreted disjunctively, and that a trust for welfare was not charitable.

In *Simpson*, it was impossible to construe the gift as being confined to charitable purposes, rather than benevolent purposes. But, as we saw in *Re Hetherington* [1990] Ch 1, sometimes it was possible to construe the gift as a whole as being to charitable purposes, because, on construction, excluding non-charitable purposes was possible. This would restrain trustees using trust property for non-charitable purposes: in *Webb* v *O'Doherty*, The Times, 11 February 1991, the officers of a students' union were restrained from making any payments to the National Student Committee to Stop War in the Gulf, or to the Cambridge Committee to Stop War in the Gulf, the purposes of which were not charitable. The union was an educational charity, and the officers were therefore entitled to use its property only for charitable purposes, even though there was nothing in the constitution of the union itself prohibiting such payments.

11.6.2 Purposes that are charitable must not be profit-seeking

Generally speaking, it is incompatible with charitable status actively to seek profit as a primary objective, although fees may be charged and incidental acquisition of profit should not disqualify. In *Scottish Burial Reform and Cremation Society Ltd* v *Glasgow Corporation* [1968] AC 138, the House of Lords held a society charitable for rating purposes (under the fourth *Pemsel* head), the main object of which was the promotion of sanitary methods of disposal of the dead, because the society charged fees, but was not profit-making. This is a further context for discussing the commercial activities of key charities considered in the Online Resource Centre. However, *Re Girls' Public Day School Trust Ltd* [1951] Ch 400 is authority that a purpose that is designed to create profits for a particular individual or individuals cannot be charitable.

11.6.3 Problems arising from political purposes

At common law, a trust could not be charitable under any head if its purposes were, directly or indirectly, political. This ensured at common law that a trust to promote the aims of a particular political party would not be capable of being charitable, and attempts to disguise such objectives as educational trusts generally failed. What is meant by 'political' in this context is wider than what we might consider the meaning of political, and there is a spectrum of activity and intent that can fall within the meaning of 'political', and thus operate to disqualify an otherwise potentially charitable purpose.

Where the objectives involved attempting to bring about a *change in the law*, they could not be charitable, unless change in the law was merely ancillary to the main purpose of the trust. This was one of the reasons for the failure of the National Anti-Vivisection Society to achieve charitable status in *National Anti-Vivisection Society* v *IRC* [1948] AC 31, on the basis that it was for Parliament, not the courts, to decide whether any change in law would be for the public benefit. Lord Simmons also rejected the contention that alteration in the law was merely ancillary to the purposes of the trust, since, in order to abolish vivisection, it would have been necessary to repeal the legislation in place making vivisection lawful.

The activities of organizations such as the RSPCA, which do relate to seeking changes in law, show that this is a matter of degree and that questions of consistency in application can arise. But the reasons for disallowing purposes that are political (beyond being incidental) are found discussed at length in *Southwood* v *Attorney General* [2000] EWCA Civ 204. These centre around the way in which the courts do not consider themselves the appropriate arbiters of whether a change in law is for the public benefit, particularly because there is unlikely to be a complete consensus on matters in relation to which such changes in law are being sought, and in any case these matters are ones rightly pursued through the democratic process.

But older authorities such as *McGovern* v *Attorney-General* [1982] Ch 321 and *National Anti-Vivisection Society* also point to the way in which there is often no absolute consensus that a particular course of action is definitively the right one, and so aligning this with the 'benefit/detriment' test for public benefit is virtually an impossible task, and not one that it is right and proper for the courts to undertake.

It follows from this that any trust the main object of which includes a change in the law of the United Kingdom cannot be charitable, as seen in *Re Bushnell* [1975] 1 WLR 1596, in which money was left to advance awareness of the benefits of socialized medicine and to show that its realization was fully possible only in a socialist state. The testator had died in 1941, before the introduction of the NHS, and one of the grounds upon which the trust was held void was its political bias in favour of socialism; closely related to this was that, in 1941, legislation would have been needed (and was, of course, later enacted) to introduce socialized medicine.

It is also the case that purposes seeking changes in law overseas fall foul of the political disqualification, but with *McGovern* and *Re Strakosch* [1949] Ch 529 pointing to a different reasoning for this. These purposes would fail on the ground that it was not appropriate to be interfering with the affairs of a different nation, and that doing this could actually be highly prejudicial to the interests of the UK in the sphere of international relations. This was applied to Amnesty International's activities in *McGovern*, and even to a trust for the promotion of racial harmony between English and Afrikaans communities in South Africa in *Re Strakosch*. The same position would apply where the aims of a purpose are harmony and peace, if such movements were overtly or covertly to call upon governments to promote specific policies, such as disarmament. One reason sometimes given for denying charitable status to attempts to promote moral objectives is that they necessarily involve a propagandist element biased in favour of only one side of the argument.

Discussion of political issues and campaigning

Whilst there is a spectrum of political aims that are all unacceptable and which will act to disqualify potentially charitable purposes from achieving charitable status, there are also parts of the political spectrum that are legitimate and which will not act as disqualifying factors. This can be seen, for example, in how it was permissible for an educational charity to discuss political issues, and the fact that a political object that is merely incidental will not be fatal. In *Re Koeppler's WT* [1986] Ch 423, a testamentary gift to Wilton Park, the main function of which was to organize educational conferences, was upheld by the Court of Appeal as a gift for charitable purposes, although Wilton Park's objects included the promotion of informed international public opinion, and the promotion of greater cooperation between East and West. Here, Slade LJ distinguished *McGovern*, identifying the existence and significance of political purposes that are incidental. Thus:

> the activities of Wilton Park are not of a party political nature. Nor ... are they designed to procure changes in the laws or governmental policy of this or any other country: even when they touch on political matters, they constitute ... no more than genuine attempts in an objective manner to ascertain and disseminate the truth. In these circumstances I think that no objections to the trust arise on a political score, similar to those which arose in the *McGovern* case.
>
> (*Re Koeppler's WT* [1986] Ch 423, *per* Slade LJ at 437)

Similarly, in *Attorney-General* v *Ross* [1986] 1 WLR 252, Scott J commented that 'there is nothing the matter with an educational charity in the furtherance of its educational purposes encouraging students to develop their political awareness or to acquire knowledge of and to debate and to form views on political issues'. He also observed that there is no reason why a charitable student organization should not affiliate to a non-charitable organization if that enables it to further its own charitable activities for the benefit of students. That is the basis upon which student unions are entitled to affiliate to the National Union of Students, a non-charitable organization. It is, however, essential that the purpose of the affiliation should be to benefit the student body in their capacity as students.

The spectrum of political activity and the difficulty with campaigning

There are limits to the extent to which a charity can go in this direction, and some difficulty has been experienced because, in between political activity, which is fatal to charitable status, and discussion, which is not, there is also campaigning. In making the case in principle for such a distinction in *Webb* v *O'Doherty*, The Times, 11 February 1991, Hoffmann J suggested that 'There is … a clear distinction between the discussion of political matters, or the acquisition of information which may have a political content, and a campaign on a political issue'. However:

> There is no doubt that campaigning, in the sense of seeking to influence public opinion on political matters, is not a charitable activity. It is, of course, something which students are, like the rest of the population, perfectly at liberty to do in their private capacities, but it is not a proper object of the expenditure of charitable money.
>
> (*Webb* v *O'Doherty*, The Times, 11 February 1991, *per* Hoffmann J)

Judicial preference for a conservative approach can be seen in the Court of Appeal's decision in *Southwood* v *Attorney General* [2000] EWCA Civ 204, in which, according to Chadwick LJ at [29]:

> I would have no difficulty in accepting the proposition that it promotes public benefit for the public to be educated in the differing means of securing a state of peace and avoiding a state of war. The difficulty comes at the next stage. There are differing views as to how best to secure peace and avoid war. To give two obvious examples: on the one hand it can be contended that war is best avoided by 'bargaining through strength'; on the other hand it can be argued, with equal passion, that peace is best secured by disarmament—if necessary, by unilateral disarmament. The court is in no position to determine that promotion of the one view rather than the other is for the public benefit.

Alongside this, the Charity Commission takes a more robust approach to encouraging legitimate political activities—crucially, campaigning—than the courts. In response to differing perspectives on what should be permissible, it has acknowledged that some activities fall considerably short of being political purposes, and are actually necessary for achieving the organization's purposes overall. It concedes that *Keoppler*-type distinctions are not always clear-cut. Charity Commission guidance entitled *Speaking Out: Guidance on Campaigning and Political Activity by Charities* (CC9), published in March 2008 (<http://www.charity-commission.gov.uk/Publications/cc9.aspx>), emphasizes the benefits of political advocacy by charities, as well as highlights the difficulties in doing so.

Finally, it is perfectly legitimate for groups to split up their activities among various distinct organizations with their own separate legal structures. This would allow for the situation in which some (but not all) of the group's organizations could engage in political activities, which would allow for charitable status to be claimed in respect of those that did not. This is what Amnesty International tried to do in *McGovern* v *Attorney-General*, by claiming charitable status only for its Prisoners of Conscience Fund. However, this failed, because even the purposes of that subgroup were held to be non-charitable.

Part II **The Charities Acts 2006 and 2011**

As suggested at the outset of this chapter, it will quickly become obvious and apparent from glancing at the texts of the Charities Acts 2006 and 2011 that it is possible for this chapter to provide only a basic outline of how the Acts relate to the legal definition of charity, and the likely relations subsisting between the statutory regime and traditional approaches to defining charity for the purposes of charity law. This proceeds by looking, in turn, at defining 'charitable purposes', and then 'public benefit', and finally at disqualifying factors.

In looking at proposed changes to traditional approaches to the legal definition of charity (and, in due course, the provisions relating to public benefit), attention is, of course, drawn to the relevant sections within the Charities Act 2011, with the text also referencing closely the 2006 Act. Even ahead of the Hodgson Review, it was clear from the way in which the 2006 Act was brought into force—through a series of commencement orders following Royal Assent in November 2006—that its framework was intended to be 'fleshed out' over time. Here, key 'policy' publications from the Charity Commission were to be central to this, in addition to the possible directions from the decision-making powers of the Commission, and the role of the courts and the Tribunal in the light of this.

At this stage, there is one very important element to understanding the statutory definition of charity put in place by the Charities Act 2006. This is the general character of charitable operation has been developed alongside the common law that the statutory regime may embody or from which it may depart. This 'framework' of general character includes matters such as the requirement that, in order to be charitable, a purpose must be exclusively charitable.

11.7 **The 'starting point' for the 2006 Act: the meaning of 'charity'**

The first sections of the Charities Act 2006 attended to what, for the purposes of the proposed new statutory footing for charitable trusts, are meant by the terms 'charity' and 'charitable purpose', and this pattern is now replicated in the Charities Act 2011.

In defining what is meant by 'charity' for the purposes of the law of England and Wales, s. 1(1)(a) provides that 'charity' means an institution that 'is established for charitable purposes only', and by s. 1(1)(b) one that (accordingly) 'falls to be subject to the control of the High Court in the exercise of its jurisdiction with respect to charities'.

What has gone from the 2011 Act that was a key feature of the 2006 Act is the 'conservation' between traditional approaches and future directions in what was s. 1(3) of the 2006 Act. This pointed to the essence of continuity in the legal basis of charity law for the past 400 years, with 'reference in any enactment or document to a charity within the meaning of the Charitable Uses Act 1601 or the preamble to it shall be construed as a reference to a charity as defined by [s. 1 of the 2006 Act].

But the 2011 Act does affirm that the notion of purposes that are exclusively charitable remain at the heart of English charity law. And in replicating the 2006 Act's signals of consolidation and confirmation, and importantly clarification, rather than substantive new direction in law, s. 2's illumination of what is meant by 'charitable purposes' provides, first (by virtue of s. 2(1)), that 'For the purposes of the law of England and Wales, a charitable purpose is a purpose which—(a) falls within section 3(1), and (b) is for the public benefit (see section 4)'.

As a matter of layout, the descriptions of purposes originally located in the same section as the general overview of s. 2(1) now have their own dedicated section, which is s. 3. This does arguably make for greater clarity and accessibility, and this was clearly the intention behind this new dedicated section. Beyond this, the purposes listed in s. 2(2) of the 2006 Act as the statutory list of charitable purposes (which must also be for the public benefit) are now accordingly, under s. 3(1), ones for:

(a) the prevention or relief of poverty;

(b) the advancement of education;

(c) the advancement of religion;

(d) the advancement of health or the saving of lives;

(e) the advancement of citizenship or community development;

(f) the advancement of the arts, culture, heritage or science;

(g) the advancement of amateur sport;

(h) the advancement of human rights, conflict resolution or reconciliation or the promotion of religious or racial harmony or equality and diversity;

(i) the advancement of environmental protection or improvement;

(j) the relief of those in need because of youth, age, ill-health, disability, financial hardship or other disadvantage;

(k) the advancement of animal welfare;

(l) the promotion of the efficiency of the armed forces of the Crown or of the efficiency of the police, fire and rescue services or ambulance services;

(m) any other purposes—

    (i) that are not within paragraphs (a) to (l) but are recognised as charitable purposes by virtue of section 5 (recreational and similar trusts, etc.) or under the old law,

    (ii) that may reasonably be regarded as analogous to, or within the spirit of, any purposes falling within any of paragraphs (a) to (l) or sub-paragraph (i), or

    (iii) that may reasonably be regarded as analogous to, or within the spirit of, any purposes which have been recognised, under the law relating to charities in England and Wales, as falling within sub-paragraph (ii) or this sub-paragraph.

The first three categories of purposes within s. 3(1)(a), (b), and (c) are instantly recognizable from the three of the *Pemsel* heads of charitable purposes, as they were under the

2006 Act, and here, as there, issues of interpretation also highlight differences between the statutory regime and the old law. Here, s. 3(2) explains that:

> (a) in paragraph (c), "religion" includes—
> (i) a religion which involves belief in more than one god, and
> (ii) a religion which does not involve belief in a god, ...

This signals a new direction. It is also notable that the prevention of poverty, as well as its relief, is included, thus suggesting that it will be charitable to seek to prevent poverty and not merely to provide relief for those who fall into it.

It is also so that the 2011 Act reflects the strong consolidation and confirmation of traditional approaches intended in the 2006 Act. The remaining ten heads under s. 3(1) remain (as they were under s. 2(2) of the Charities Act 2006) a mixture of purposes that are recognizable within current understandings of charitable purpose and others that *could* potentially be brought within the scope of the *Pemsel* head 'other purposes beneficial for the community' head, itself built on the spirit and intendment of the 1601 Act. Section 3(2) continues to provide clarification of s. 3(1):

> (c) paragraph (e) [the advancement of health] includes—
> (i) rural or urban regeneration, and
> (ii) the promotion of civic responsibility, volunteering, the voluntary sector or the effectiveness or efficiency of charities,
> (d) in paragraph (g), "sport" means sports or games which promote health by involving physical or mental skill or exertion,
> (e) paragraph (j) [the relief of those in need] includes relief given by the provision of accommodation or care to the persons mentioned in that paragraph, ...

A key difference between the 2006 Act and the 2011 Act in relation to interpretation is how the 'any other purposes' heading (m) is explained. This was part of s. 2's interpretation within the 2006 Act, but what can be brought within the purview of (m) can now be found as subparagraphs of (m) itself. Here, we find replication of what was located in s. 2 as interpretation, which reinforce the connections between the statutory definition of charity and traditional approaches embodied in what is now termed 'old law'.

It was always an open question of whether the 'other purposes' categorization under (m) could achieve anything beyond *Pemsel* head 4, given that whilst a statute may have inherent clarity and perhaps authority beyond the common law, the statutory provision was so strongly premised on the common law. But in terms of accessibility and clarity, the current layout, locating the (m) heading and its interpretation together, would appear to be a positive development.

Elsewhere, new provisions in s. 5 address directly the charitable character of purposes given *ex post* charitable status under the Recreational Charities Act 1958.

11.7.1 Public benefit under the Charities Act 2011

In moving from how the new statutory regime of charity law defines 'charitable purpose', it is now necessary to focus on the insistence that purposes must not simply be of charitable character, but must also be for public benefit. The public benefit requirement was a cornerstone of the traditional legal definition of charity, and thus of the ability of purposes actually to acquire charitable status. This continued within s. 3 of the Charities Act 2006, with these provisions now located within s. 4 of the Charities Act 2011.

We now look at how statutory requirements relating to public benefit show how new law represents an important project of consolidation and clarification, and one that accords considerable respect to existing charity law. According to s. 4(1), a purpose (within s. 3(1)) must be for the public benefit if it is to be considered charitable. As with its predecessor (s. 3(1) of the 2006 Act), this new section does not define what is meant by 'public benefit', but its current meaning can be found explicitly connected with traditional charity law in s. 4(3). At one level, this can be explained in the language of continuity and conservation with traditional law in a way that mirrors the approach taken to the statutory definition of charitable purposes; in this respect, it should not be too difficult to align what are effectively existing charitable purposes with traditional approaches to public benefit. However, there are important questions surrounding what test (for public benefit) might accompany those 'heads' of charitable purpose that are new and are not to be found in traditional law. This is one important respect in which it is not obvious how new law and traditional law might map coherently onto one another, and this is likely to result in much more extensive consideration in the foreseeable future for this text.

For now, the issue is noted in this text and considered a little further in the accompanying Online Resource Centre, but how it actually 'shakes out' as the new law is implemented very much remains to be seen. This is all that can be said with certainty at this point in time, notwithstanding that, in accordance with its statutory duty originally under s. 4 of the 2006 Act, and now located in s. 17), the Charity Commission published in January 2008 guidance on satisfying public benefit in the new regime entitled *Charities and Public Benefit* (<http://www.charitycommission.gov.uk/Library/guidance/publicbenefittext_1.pdf>; the '2008 Guidance'). Again, it remains to be seen what bearing Lord Hodgson's review will have in this regard, but it is also the case, as noted in the previous chapter, that revisions of the 2008 Guidance are already being undertaken, on which more is said shortly (see 'The Charity Commission's 2008 guidance').

Elsewhere in relation to public benefit, it was extremely clear from s. 3 of the Charities Act 2006, and now s. 4 of the Charities Act 2011, that there is a new and radical direction in the sphere of public benefit as it applies to English charity law post-2008—even if this is, at present, a little abstract, even without the revisions being made to the guidance. Here, s. 4 (2) (replicating the 2006 Act) states that there is no longer to be a presumption of public benefit operating in favour of a purpose wishing to secure charitable status. As the Explanatory Notes accompanying the 2006 Act explained, under traditional approaches there lay 'a presumption that purposes for the relief of poverty, the advancement of education, or the advancement of religion ... are for the public benefit'. And in terms of identifying traditional law as that which was not fit for purpose, the Explanatory Notes continued: 'The effect of this presumption is that ... [an] organisation's purpose is presumed charitable unless there is evidence that it is not.' Traditionally, all 'other purposes' charitable under *Pemsel* head 4 had to demonstrate their public benefit, and the effect of the statutory approach under the 2006 Act (and now the 2011) Act is to place all charitable purposes on an equal footing in having to demonstrate their public benefit in order to achieve charitable status.

Section 17 of the Charities Act 2011 follows from the position whereby *all* purposes falling into *all* categories of the new statutory definitional framework have to demonstrate the 'public benefit' dimensions of their purposes. It then falls to the Charity

Commission to issue guidance on demonstrating this. Following the publication of the 2008 Guidance, gleaning some 'hard and fast' detail on how things are likely to work is possible, and this will be considered shortly, along with discussion of the action brought by the Independent Schools Council. Before this, there is now a brief consideration of how the statutory approach to public benefit fits the broader framework of the responsibilities of the Charity Commission in the regulation of the activities and governance of charitable organizations.

The continuing significance of public benefit for the legal definition of charity

The task of determining whether or not a particular purpose is charitable, and thus assessing the merits of a purported public benefit, is vested now in the Charity Commission by the provisions of s. 17 of the 2011 Act. Prior to this, the Prime Minister's 2002 Strategy Unit document entitled *Private Action, Public Benefit: A Review of Charities and the Wider Not-For-Profit Sector* and the government response to it (see Chapter 10) had emphasized the desirability that the Charity Commission should carry out ongoing checks on public character. Government support for this rested on its observation of structural weakness in traditional approaches whereby the only time at which a systematic check is made on a charity's public character is at the point of its registration. The rationale for this reflected opinion that a move to checks that are ongoing could be used to assess any doubts that might arise in respect of the public character of the purpose during a registered charity's operation. Very interestingly, in addition, the government suggested that ongoing checks could be instrumentally used to monitor the 'performance' of certain types of charity, which may accrue benefits for 'underperforming' charitable purposes as they become aware of their position.

What this monitoring proposal does not explicitly point to—but which implication is clearly present in the documentation—is the way in which performance is not being directed towards *under*performance alone, or even in the main. The import appeared instead to be directed towards concerns that might arise from a charity that appears to be *too successful*, and might thereby be deemed to be 'performing' in a manner that is difficult to reconcile with charitable status. An obvious point of reference for this is, of course, the charitable status of independent schools, which became a central reference point for parliamentary debates on the 2006 Act.

The operation of the public benefit requirement under the Charities Act 2006

What can be concluded from this initial overview is that English charity law, as envisioned under the Charities Act 2006 (and now enshrined in the 2011 Act), remains grounded in the concept of public benefit. This is set to continue to be central in securing charitable status under the new regime of charity law, in spite of the extensive and often controversial attention that it attracted at all stages of the 2006 Act's genesis. Although the requirement of public benefit is now enshrined in statute, along with the way in which there will be no presumption of charitable status, what potentially charitable purposes must establish is not being given a clear legal test within the Act. The preferred approach was clearly regarded as being grounded in more generalized notions of public benefit (than those that are specific), and ones that are also highly ambulatory. The role of the Charity Commission in determining this is clear from s. 17, flowing from its role as *regulator* of charitable purposes, through being responsible for their *registration*. Indeed, as well as setting out the mandate for the Charity Commission to issue guidance in order 'to promote awareness and understanding of the operation of the requirement' (amongst the objectives set out in s. 14), to revise guidance where this is appropriate, and to engage in public consultation, under s. 17(5) trustees of a charity 'must have regard to any such guidance when exercising any powers or duties to which the guidance is relevant'.

The Charity Commission's 2008 Guidance

Following the decision of the Upper Tribunal on 14 October 2011 relating to the Charity Commission's guidance on public benefit and fee-charging in relation to educational charities, parts of the 2008 Guidance have been withdrawn. This ruling commenced with an action for judicial review brought by the Independent Schools Council concerning aspects of the 2008 Guidance (centrally, access to benefit under principles 2b and 2c). In a statement in October 2011 and in response to the Tribunal ruling, the Charity Commission announced that the withdrawn 2008 Guidance no longer formed part of its statutory guidance on public benefit to which charity trustees must have regard when carrying out any powers or duties to which the guidance is relevant. It then launched consultation of revision, and draft revised guidance relating to independent schools published on 5 October 2012 has already been criticized as overly long, piecemeal, and unwieldy, and virtually impossible for trustees to follow.

Given the rationale of the Charities Act 2011, it is unlikely that this initial assessment of the draft revised guidance will be welcome, and in any case what happens now remains to be seen. At this point, it seems feasible to provide only an overview of the 2008 Guidance as originally published, and especially aspects of it that remain unaffected by the Tribunal ruling, Full versions are available in PDF and HTML formats, along with a very useful summary of its main thrust, online at <http://www.charitycommission.gov.uk/Charity_requirements_guidance/Charity_Essentials/Public_benefit/default.aspx>

The structure of the 2008 Guidance is essentially as follows.

- The Guidance commences with an introduction explaining the 'public benefit requirement', and the way in which, under the Act, this is a more stringent and robust requirement than previously.
- The Guidance then progresses by linking the points noted in the introduction with the definition of charity under the Act, identifying the way in which the Act sets out 'various descriptions of charitable purposes' representing the 'Meaning of charitable purpose' embodied in s. 2 'and any new charitable purpose that might be recognised in the future'.
- Following this, substantive consideration of public benefit commences in earnest with the observation that there are two key principles of public benefit, each embodying a number of factors that must be considered in all cases.
- The section that follows this illuminates the two principles of public benefit and also provides extensive discussion of the factors that must be considered in relation to them. At this point, the text explains that Principle 1 requires that there must be an identifiable benefit or benefits, and that:
  - by Principle 1a, it must be clear what the benefits are;
  - by Principle 1b, the benefits must be related to the actual 'aims' of the purpose; and
  - by Principle 1c, benefits must be balanced against any detriment or harm.

  Principle 2 requires that the benefit must be to the public or a section of the public, and that:
  - by Principle 2a, the beneficiaries must be appropriate to the aims of the purpose;

- by Principle 2b, where benefit is to a section of the public, the opportunity to benefit must not be unreasonably restricted either by geographical or other restrictions, or by ability to pay fees charged;

- by Principle 2c, people in poverty must not be excluded from the opportunity to benefit; and

- by Principle 2d, any private benefits must be incidental.

- Thereafter, the document considers the 'ongoing' nature of demonstrating public benefit for charities, and relates to the way in which trustees are now under a duty to report on this in their annual reports. Here, guidance given on reporting on a charity's public benefit commences by explaining that the level of detail required in reporting depends on an individual charity's location above or below the so-called 'audit threshold'—that is, the point at which an audit is required, which is if a charity's gross annual income exceeds £500,000, or where income exceeds £100,000 *and* the aggregate value of its assets exceeds £2.8 million. In their reports, trustees must indicate how a charity's aims have been carried out for the public benefit, and also confirm that regard has been had to the Charity Commission's guidance where this is appropriate. In respect of the latter, levels of detailed reporting required will depend on whether the charity is a smaller charity (that is, one that falls below the audit threshold), in which case the requirement is for a brief summary of the charity's main activities in light of the requirement of public benefit, or a larger charity, in which case the reporting requirements are more extensive and trustees are required to provide 'fuller explanation'.

- In the final section, entitled 'Accessing public benefit', the 2008 Guidance explains that, in the case of all applications for registration as charitable organizations, the Charity Commission will assess whether aims are for the public benefit and whether bodies already registered continue to meet the public benefit requirement, which they must do under the new law. It is explained that this is achieved by carrying out generally focused research on the extent to which various types of charity are meeting the requirement, and by working closely with representative professional and umbrella bodies. The Guidance explains that it may also be necessary to carry out detailed individual assessments of particular charities, and, where it is the case that an organization is not meeting the requirement, the Charity Commission will provide clear reasons and an explanation for this, and also advice for trustees on making changes in order to meet the requirements. In this instance, reasonable time will be given for changes to be made, and where there is disagreement with the Charity Commission's assessment, trustees can seek an internal review of a decision made, and will have the right to appeal to the new and independent Charity Tribunal—that is, the First-Tier Tribunal (Charity)—and ultimately to the courts. At this point, the Charity Commission suggests that it is seeking to build constructive relationships and dialogue with those whose activities fall within its regulatory jurisdiction.

It is hoped that, as the statutory regime now contained within the Charities Act 2011 becomes 'bedded in', a closer integration of materials pertaining to the law of charity pre-2006 and approaches post-2006 will be possible. In the meantime, while work on achieving this for the main chapter text is being undertaken, an experimental layout that introduces the statutory regime as 'the law' from the outset and then discusses this alongside traditional approaches can be found on the Online Resource Centre.

Revision Box

1. Ensure that you can identify the three key requirements for achieving charitable status at common law, and that you are able to relate these to the 'special' status of charity and the key advantages of charitable status.
2. Ensure that you can comment on the envisioned relationship between the Charities Act 2006 and the common law relating to the legal definition of charity that it replaced. Would you agree that the 2006 Act was envisioned as a project of 'continuity and change'?
3. Ensure that you can comment on the purpose of the Charities Act 2011 and give examples of how this has changed the appearance of the legal definition of charity as under the 2006 Act.

FURTHER READING

Atkinson (2008) 'Charities and Political Campaigning: The Impact of Risk-Based Regulation Charity Commission' *Liverpool Law Rev* (2008) 29:143–163.

Chesterton (1979) *Charities, Trusts and Social Welfare* (London: Wiedenfeld and Nicholson).

Dawson (1987) 'Old Presbyterian persons: a sufficient section of the public?' Conveyancer 114.

Dunn (2000) 'As "cold as charity"? Poverty, equity and the charitable trust' 20 Legal Studies 222.

Dunn (2008) 'Demanding service or servicing demand? Charities, regulation and the policy process' *Modern Law Review* 71(2) 247.

Dunn (2012) 'Using the wrong policy tools: education, charity, and public benefit' 39 Journal of Law & Society 491.

Iwobi (2009) 'Out with the old, in with the new' 29 Legal Studies 619.

Morris (2000) 'Charities in the contract culture: survival of the largest?' 20 Legal Studies 409.

Rahmatian (2009) 'The continued relevance of the "poor relations" and "poor employees" cases under the Charities Act 2006' 73 Conveyancer 12.

Sloan (2012) 'Public schools for public benefit?' 71 Coventry Law Journal 45.

Warburton (2008) 'Charities and public benefit: from confusion to light?' 10 Charity Law and Practice Review 1.

Waters (2011) 'The advancement of religion in a pluralist society: Part II: abolishing the public benefit element' 17 Trusts & Trustees 729.

 online resource centre   For summaries of a selection of these articles, please visit <http://www.oxfordtextbooks.co.uk/orc/wilson_trusts11e/>

12

··

Cy-près

The Anglo-Norman phrase cy-près (which is sometimes unhyphenated) translates into something like 'as near as possible', and it follows on closely from our study of charity in English law so far. This commenced with a general introduction to charity law, and was followed by a closer look at how 'charity' is defined for the purposes of English law. Both were instrumental in explaining how some 'purposes' and gifts made to them become subject to the special body of trusts law termed 'charity law'. In turn, this is elemental for understanding how the doctrine of cy-près in charity law provides that where property given on trust for charitable purposes cannot be used in the precise manner intended by the donor, the court (and, since about 130 years ago, the Charity Commissioners, and now the Charity Commission) may make a scheme for the application of the property to purposes resembling as closely as possible the donor's original intention. The idea is therefore not to frustrate the intention of the donor (who cannot even be consulted if the gift is testamentary) any more than necessary. The doctrine dates back at least as far as the seventeenth century. It applies only to charities; if private purposes fail, the results are as discussed in Chapter 3 and also Chapters 6 and 7.

12.1 Donors' wishes that cannot be fulfilled: introducing cy-près at common law

A substantial statutory regime now governs the application of cy-près, and there will be much discussion of the Charities Acts 2006 and 2011 as the chapter progresses. But, in contextualizing this, at the heart of traditional applications of cy-près has been what is known in English charity law as 'initial failure' and 'subsequent failure'. Here, 'failure' is a term that has been given to non-fulfilment of the intentions that a donor had in wishing to apply property to charitable purposes. The difference between 'initial' and 'subsequent' failure rests on the point at which fulfilling the donor's terms, as they were specified, cannot be achieved.

So initial failure arises where it is clear from the outset that the donor's intention cannot be fulfilled, such as where the organization that he has singled out for benefit has already ceased to exist, or never actually existed. Subsequent failure, which is much commoner, arises because, at some later time, during the continuance of the trust, it turns out that the purposes cannot be achieved. Cy-près is more easily invoked in the latter case, for once property has been dedicated to charity, there is no possibility of a resulting trust to the donor, which is what will happen if a gift is not found to be charitable, as considered in the previous chapters by reference to *Chichester Diocesan Fund* v *Simpson* [1944] AC 341.

12.1.1 **Cy-près development at common law, and statutory approaches under the Charities Acts 2006 and 2011**

What follows is an examination of the application of cy-près at common law, and how the doctrine's role in charity law has been enhanced by statutory provision. Since the nineteenth century, at common law, when a gift failed from the start, the courts have insisted that, for cy-près to be applied to property, a general or 'paramount' charitable intention must be shown. And, in any case, until 1960 there was scope for applying the doctrine only where the existing trusts had failed by virtue of being impossible to carry out. It is on account of the Charities Act 1960 that the doctrine has been applied more widely. The 1960 Act continued to emphasize a donor's wishes in its extensive referencing of the 'spirit of the gift', particularly in key provisions in s. 13, but a different policy can also be detected within it. Whilst the equitable doctrine espousing 'as close as possible' was very clearly anchored in a donor's presumed intentions regarding his property, this could in some circumstances militate against the efficient operation of charitable enterprises. The 1960 Act was clearly concerned with promoting the efficient running of charities and, notwithstanding its references to 'the spirit of the gift', its application shows that this could occur even at the expense of the donor's intentions.

Following on from the consideration that has been given to the Charities Acts 2006 and 2011 in the previous two chapters, a brief study is now made of the impact that the new legislation has on the operation of cy-près. It is sufficient to say at this point that understanding how the doctrine operates in the modern law requires reference to the Charities Act 1993 and its amendment by the Charities Act 2006 (pursuant to ss. 15–18), and the provisions now found in the Charities Act 2011. But, in essence, the cy-près doctrine will continue to operate in respect of charitable gifts that cannot be applied to the original purposes envisioned by their donor, albeit that there are factors that influence this lying beyond the donor's intentions.

The interactions between the Charities Acts 1993 and 2006 do, of course, provide the opportunity to consider the Charities Act 2006 as a project of continuity and change, in the pursuit of supporting and bolstering charitable activity in the context of demanding enhanced regulation and accountability across the board, with liberalizing the legal regime for small charities straddling both directional considerations. But whilst this chapter touches on these considerations, a much more significant reference point can be found in the rationale of the Charities Act 2011 in providing simplification, accessibility, and clarity in charity law. Indeed, whilst significant development of the law occurred in the implementation of ss 15–18 of the Charities Act 2006 in 2008, this did somewhat convolutedly operate to make insertions into the Charities Act 1993.

Acquiring understanding of law operating in such a way does, of course, present challenges for lawyers who are very familiar with law as it is originally penned, and the rationale and policy of revisions made. Such difficulties are, of course, magnified for others, who must also grapple with what is in force, what is new, and what has changed. Those who are centrally affected are the trustees of charitable organizations, who have to deal with the realities of the legal regime for administering charitable activity 'on the ground'. This would be so in any case, but is particularly notable in that the very first provisions relating to cy-près in the Charities Act 2011 set out a 'duty of trustees in relation to the application of property cy-près'.

This is what commences the provisions relating to cy-près, which are located in Part 6 of the Charities Act 2011. These run from ss 61–75, with this chapter looking at the key provisions that provide an overview of the law relating to applying cy-près in the context of charity. The s. 61 duty sets the tone by providing:

> It is hereby declared that a trust for charitable purposes places a trustee under a duty, where the case permits and requires the property or some part of it to be applied cy-près, to secure its effective use for charity by taking steps to enable it to be so applied.

The whole tenor of the s. 61 duty is very much for trustees to take a proactive approach to using cy-près in order to enhance opportunities for their charitable organizations. This is very significant, and does much to capture why cy-près has been subject to so much statutory enhancement since 1960. This is because, prior to the 1960 enactment, and its modifications by the Acts of 1992 and 1993, and most recently 2006 (prior to the Charities Act 2011), at common law the courts' jurisdiction could apply property cy-près only where what was envisioned by the donor was, or became, impossible or impracticable to carry out. The cases at which we will look show that the courts did, of course, seek to interpret these parameters as widely as possible.

This is consistent with the policy of charity law to encourage any charitable giving at all, and to try to save charitable gifts that might otherwise fail. The legal definition of charity is, of course, elemental in ensuring the former, and it is obvious that cy-près will be very important for securing the latter. But cy-près also bridges the two in as much as heightened perceptions that property dedicated to charity will be well used, even if it cannot be used exactly as foreseen, could be crucial in encouraging charitable giving.

But this rationale was often subtext rather than main text, and even when applying cy-près more widely on account of statutory enhancement, commencing in 1960, reference continued to be made to 'failure' of a trust by the courts themselves and also by the Charity Commission. Unsurprisingly, given its policy of bolstering and supporting charitable activity, the Charities Act 2006 continued to emphasize the essence of utilizing charitable property as effectively as possible in the light of prevailing social and economic conditions.

12.2 Cy-près at common law

As suggested, prior to 1960, at common law, there was scope to apply cy-près to property intended for charitable purposes where carrying out the original purpose was impossible or impracticable, with the language associated with this being centrally that of 'failure' of a gift. The following sections consider this, and the distinction drawn between so-called initial and subsequent failure.

12.2.1 Initial failure and paramount general charitable intention

Here, the application of cy-près turned on whether the intention of the donor was specific or general. If it was to further some specific purpose that cannot be carried out, or to benefit some specific institution no longer in existence, then the gift fails and the property will return to the settlor, or his estate, on a resulting trust, as discussed in Chapter 6. If, however, the intention is a more general one, which might be satisfied by applying the property to a purpose or institution similar to that specified, a cy-près scheme could be ordered. The test, then, is whether a general or 'paramount' charitable intention can be found.

12.2.1.1 Gift to a charity that has never existed at all: operation of cy-près doctrine—general charitable intention

In *Re Rymer* [1895] 1 Ch 19, a gift for a specific seminary that had ceased to exist failed. This is the general position where no paramount (or general) charitable intention can be found. Whether a general charitable intention can be shown is a question of fact. The cases in this section are illustrations of the factors that can be taken into account, but do not lay down general rules.

If the charity specified by the donor has never existed at all, it is usually easier to discover a general charitable intention than where the charity once existed, but has since ceased (as in *Re Rymer*), since only a general intention can be attributed to the donor who fails correctly to specify the beneficiary. For example, in *Re Harwood* [1936] Ch 285, a gift was made to the Peace Society in Belfast, which could not be shown ever to have existed. Farwell J found that there was an intention to benefit societies aimed at promoting peace, and the gift was therefore applied cy-près. A second gift in the will, in favour of the Wisbech Peace Society, which had once existed, but had ceased to do so prior to the testatrix's death, however, was held to have lapsed. Although the case is a good illustration of the operation of the cy-près doctrine, doubt may perhaps be cast on the assumption that the promotion of peace is in fact capable of being charitable.

Finding a general paramount charitable intention: the approach of the courts

In *Re Satterthwaite's WT* [1966] 1 WLR 277, a will listed a number of organizations concerned with animal welfare, which was a haphazard inventory of organizations compiled from the London telephone directory. These organizations were linked by the testatrix's chief concern being to divert her estate to animal charities, because she hated the whole human race. One named institution, the London Animal Hospital, had never existed as a charity, and the Court of Appeal held that it should be cy-près because a general charitable intention could be inferred from the testatrix's known attitude towards the human race, and because all bar one of the other dispositions were made in favour of genuine animal charities.

For Russell LJ, a general intention to benefit animal charities could easily be inferred, whilst Harman LJ expressed 'the gravest doubts'. Perhaps a better explanation aligns this case with *Re Harwood*; Sir Robert Megarry V-C refused to apply what he described as the doctrine of 'charity by association' in *Re Spence's WT* [1979] Ch 483, on the grounds that *Re Satterthwaite* applied only where the body had never existed.

For a paramount general intention to be found, it is also necessary for the other donations to be to charitable organizations of the same type, and a non-charitable body being included among a general list of charities is not evidence of a general charitable intent. In *Re Jenkins's WT* [1966] Ch 249, Buckley J declined to hold that a gift to the British Union for the Abolition of Vivisection (which did exist, but was not charitable) could be taken to be charitable simply by being included in a list of gifts to unquestionably charitable organizations. These cases appear to be extremely fact-dependent and the quite different outcomes that can transpire seem to turn on very little. This, in turn, militates against finding any clear approach that could be regarded as authoritative, and indeed *Re Wilson* [1913] 1 Ch 314 draws attention to the importance of construction in determining the existence or otherwise of a general paramount intention on the part of the donor.

Non-existent body, but no initial failure

Even where the charity specified did not exist, at common law it was possible to save the gift if the institution could be said to continue to exist in some other form. In recent years, many small charities have amalgamated, and it is sometimes possible to regard the new body thus formed as being the same as the old. In *Re Faraker* [1912] 2 Ch 488, for example, a gift to 'Mrs Bailey's charity, Rotherhithe' (which was taken to mean 'Hannah Bayly's Charity') passed to the new charity formed by an amalgamation of Hannah Bayly's Charity with several others.

Gifts that are made to a charitable purpose and not to a charitable body

Another approach taken at common law was to find that the gift was made for the *purpose* of the named charity, rather than for the body itself. If a body is unincorporated, then by definition—following on from the discussion on various available 'forms' for charitable organizations in Chapter 10—the gift cannot be to it, but must be to its purposes; if those purposes can still be fulfilled, the gift would not fail. Since there is no failure, there is no need to show a general charitable intention. But this is, in reality, not an application of cy-près, but rather of finding a substitute trustee to carry out the purposes of the trust.

Where the body is a corporation, however, a gift to it will prima facie lapse if the corporation has ceased to exist, just as a gift to a human individual would lapse if the person concerned had died before the gift was made. The gift may be rescued only on the cy-près principles already outlined—that is, if the court is able to find a general charitable intention going beyond the specific aim of benefiting the named corporate charity. This distinction can be seen at work in *Re Finger's WT* [1972] Ch 286, which concerned gifts to both unincorporated and corporate bodies, with very different results pertaining for organizations that had ceased to exist by the time the testatrix died. Similar principles were also applied in *Re Koeppler's WT* [1986] Ch 423 (considered in Chapter 11), in which Slade LJ construed a gift to a non-existent body as a valid trust for educational purposes.

12.2.1.2 Gifts with conditions attached

Even where the institution to which the donation is made exists, there may be an initial failure if there is a condition in the gift that the donee body finds unacceptable. In *Re Lysaght* [1966] Ch 191, the testatrix left £5,000 to the Royal College of Surgeons (RCS) in order to establish and maintain one or more studentships, but subject to conditions seeking to disqualify Jews and Roman Catholics. The RCS declined to accept the gift on these terms, but it could be saved by finding a general charitable intention on the part of the testatrix to establish medical studentships. The cy-près doctrine operated to delete the condition deemed unnecessary to fulfil the general intention of the gift. A scheme was ordered on the terms of the will as it stood without the condition, and can be seen similarly at work in *Re Woodhams* [1981] 1 WLR 493.

But why *should* gifts like those in *Lysaght* and *Woodhams* fail at all without deletions, given the equitable maxim that 'equity will not let a trust fail for want of a trustee'? Although, in principle, the court should be able to look for an alternative trustee who is prepared to carry out the donor's wishes as they have been specified, cases such as *Lysaght* particularly show that the identity of the trustee can be a 'deal breaker' for gifts. In that case, it was only the RCS that could carry out the testatrix's intentions, and there was no alternative trustee. Both the general principle that a trustee who cannot in good conscience carry out a bequest faithfully as made must 'make way for a trustee who can and will do so' and also the idea that, in some cases, the identity of the trustee is crucial to the settlor's intentions, and without whom these will remain unfulfilled at all, are found in Buckley J's judgment in the case.

12.2.2 Subsequent failure

As suggested, subsequent failure is much more common, and it is here that cy-près had wider application within its traditional parameters of purposes that are impossible or impracticable. Subsequent failure arises when it is unequivocally clear that property has been dedicated to charitable purposes, and so presents none of the difficulties arising in the event of an initial failure. With initial failure, there is a possibility of a resulting trust for the donor, and this will arise where evidence of a paramount general charitable intention can be found. This does not arise in subsequent failure. Where there has been an outright disposition of property in favour of charity and funds cannot be applied to their original envisioned purpose because this is impossible or impracticable, then cy-près will enable them to be applied as close as possible to this.

12.2.2.1 The importance of timing

The importance of timing is shown in *Re Slevin* [1891] 2 Ch 236, in which an orphanage ceased to exist after the date of the donor's death, but before the legacy could be paid over. Because the orphanage had survived its benefactor, by however short a time, the gift was effective in favour of charity and could be applied cy-près. In *Re King* [1923] 1 Ch 243, a surplus remaining after the purpose of setting a stained-glass window in a church was carried out was applied cy-près because it was found that the entire fund (and not only the amount covering the cost of the window) had been dedicated to charity.

The timing of subsequent failure and gifts that are postponed

For questions of timing of a purpose becoming impossible or impracticable, it would not matter that the gift to charity was intended to be postponed until some future date. This is because the relevant date for determining failure was that of the original donation, notwithstanding that the charity at that time obtained only a future interest in the property. Notwithstanding that the interest is a future one, the failure is subsequent rather than initial, as shown in *Re Moon* [1948] 1 All ER 300. The finding that there was an effective gift to charity at that time, and that the failure was subsequent and not initial, was also reached in *Re Wright* [1954] Ch 347, in which the date of the testatrix's death was taken to be crucial in determining the question of whether the gift was practicable.

In *Re Welsh Hospital (Netley) Fund* [1921] 1 Ch 655, a surplus of £9,000 remaining after the winding up of a (charitable) hospital erected at Netley was applied cy-près, but this depended on finding that donors must be taken to have parted with their donations out-and-out to charity (much of the money had been derived from anonymous sources and the issues were essentially those discussed in Chapter 7). There was no suggestion that a cy-près scheme ought to have been automatic on the basis of subsequent failure, but, in *Re Ulverston and District New Hospital Building Trusts* [1956] Ch 622, Jenkins LJ explained *Netley* as a straightforward case of subsequent failure. The earlier case was distinguished because, in *Re Ulverston*, the hospital had never been built and none of the funds ever expended, so the failure was regarded as an initial failure. There being no evidence of general charitable intention and so the fund was not applied cy-près.

12.3 The limitations of 'impossible' and 'impracticable': beyond 'failure' and the alteration of charitable purposes using cy-près

Whilst the common law jurisdiction for applying cy-près served well the needs of purposes that were or had become impossible or impracticable, it had little to offer those that, whilst falling short of this, would experience considerable operating difficulties by virtue of being outmoded or outdated. There was no effective system whereby moribund charities could be modernized and, of course, the cy-près doctrine could not apply if there were no failure.

Even with the courts taking a flexible approach to failure, this provided the limitations of the inherent cy-près jurisdiction. And, indeed, *Re Weir Hospital* [1910] 2 Ch 124 shows the courts asserting these parameters in holding that the Charity Commissioners' approval of a scheme to provide an alternative use for unsuitable premises was ultra vires. Sir Herbert Cozens-Hardy MR's view that the court's primary duty was to give effect to the charitable intentions of the donor, rather than to seek the most beneficial application of the property, was echoed in the findings of Kennedy LJ that neither the court nor the Charity Commissioners were entitled to substitute the intended scheme for one that appeared a preferable direction of the property on the application of 'coldly wise intelligence'.

Re Weir Hospital illustrates that the courts' main concern was not to depart too far from the original wishes of settlors, rather than to promote the efficient administration of charities. However, *Re Robinson* [1923] 2 Ch 332 shows that it *was* permissible under the courts' inherent jurisdiction to eradicate a condition of the trust that, with the passage of time, has become inimical to its main purpose—in this case, a gift of an endowment for an evangelical church requiring a preacher to wear a black gown in the pulpit, which was thought likely to offend the congregation and to reduce attendance.

Similarly, in *Re Dominion Students' Hall Trust* [1947] Ch 183, a colour bar was removed from a trust for the maintenance of a hostel for male students of the overseas dominions of the British Empire, given that the trust's main purpose was to promote community of citizenship among members of the Commonwealth.

These cases sound very much like *Lysaght and Woodhams*, and indeed *Robinson* was applied in *Lysaght*, the key difference being that both of these former cases were ones of initial failure and so required finding a general charitable intention to invoke the cy-près doctrine in the first place. In *Re J. W. Laing Trust* [1984] Ch 143, a term that required trustees to distribute, within ten years of the settlor's death, a fund that, by then, had risen significantly in value (from some £15,000 in 1922, when the trust was set up, to over £24 million in 1982) was struck out. This was because the increase in value had been quite unforeseen when the trust was set up, partly because the settlor had lived much longer than expected (to the age of 98), and because such a distribution would have undermined the support of causes that the settlor wished to benefit.

The offending term was considered 'inexpedient in the very altered circumstances of the charity since that requirement was laid down 60 years ago', but it was not entirely clear whether this expediency test is the same as that being applied in the earlier cases or whether a wider principle is being adopted.

12.3.1 Situations in which no cy-près scheme is required

There were also situations concerning alterations at common law in which no scheme was actually required, such as in *Oldham Borough Council* v *Attorney-General* [1993] Ch 210. This concerned playing fields conveyed to the Council in 1962 for recreational purposes, and which the Council proposed to sell for redevelopment, seeking to provide a new site to be used for exactly the same charitable purposes. The Council expressly disclaimed reliance on the Charities Act 1960, since clearly none of its heads could be applied, and Dillon LJ, giving the only substantive judgment in the Court of Appeal, concluded that the sale of the land would have been approved prior to the Act, since there was no requirement to use *that particular land*. Because the charitable purposes would still be carried out, there was no need for a scheme and the Court was prepared to approve the sale.

12.4 Cy-près and the Charities Act 1960

The Charities Act 1960 gave important statutory authority for the position that scope for the application of cy-près was not confined to failure in terms of impossibility and impracticability. Whilst the courts had arguably been looking at the 'spirit of the gift' for some time prior to this, s. 13 provided an important statement of the legitimacy of such an approach, and even its essence in promoting the proper administration of trusts.

This followed recommendations made by the *Report of the Committee on the Law and Practice Relating to Charitable Trusts* (1952, Cmd 8710; the 'Nathan Committee'), para. 365. In responding to the need to modernize outmoded trusts, which was very limited using the inherent jurisdiction of the courts, s. 13 (5) made this rationale very clear by placing a duty upon trustees to seek the application of property cy-près if and when appropriate circumstances arise. This was the forerunner of the duty now found within s. 61 of the Charities Act 2011.

Then, as now, much of the work of the Charity Commissioners (and now the Commission) consisted in settling and approving schemes of this kind, and with the precise circumstances under which cy-près could be applied, it is clear that it would no longer be necessary to show impossibility or impracticability. For the purposes of s. 13(1), it was sufficient that the original purpose had been fulfilled as far as possible, or could not be carried out according to the directions given and the spirit of the gift, or if there were a surplus left over, or if the purposes had been adequately provided for by other means, or if they become useless or harmful to the community. Cy-près could also apply where the original purposes relate to an area, or class of persons, which has ceased to have any relevance, having regard to the spirit of the gift. There are also provisions for the amalgamation of small charities if that is more efficient.

12.4.1 Illuminating s. 13

Section 13(1) is set out in full on the ground that it formed the basis of provisions of the Charities Act 1993, and then the 2006 Act.

> 13(1) Subject to subsection (2) below, the circumstances in which the original purposes of a charitable gift can be altered to allow the property given or part of it to be applied cy-près shall be as follows:—
>
> (a) where the original purposes, in whole or in part—
>
>   (i) have been as far as may be fulfilled; or
>
>   (ii) cannot be carried out, or not according to the directions given and to the spirit of the gift; or
>
> (b) where the original purposes provide a use for part only of the property available by virtue of the gift; or
>
> (c) where the property available by virtue of the gift and other property applicable for similar purposes can be more effectively used in conjunction, and to that end can suitably, regard being had to the spirit of the gift, be made applicable to common purposes; or

(d) where the original purposes were laid down by reference to an area which then was but has since ceased to be a unit for some other purpose, or by reference to a class of persons or to an area which has for any reason since ceased to be suitable, regard being had to the spirit of the gift, or to be practical in administering the gift; or

(e) where the original purposes, in whole or in part, have, since they were laid down—

(i) been adequately provided for by other means; or

(ii) ceased, as being useless or harmful to the community or for other reasons, to be in law charitable; or

(iii) ceased in any other way to provide a suitable and effective method of using the property available by virtue of the gift, regard being had to the spirit of the gift.

In terms of overviewing the 1960 Act, because of its continuing relevance in 1993 and 2006, s. 13(1)(a)–(e) were generally held to be wider than the pre-1960 definition of failure, and appeared to supersede it. In *Oldham Borough Council* v *Attorney-General* [1993] Ch 210, Dillon LJ took the view that the s. 13 heads were exhaustive, at any rate where alteration of the 'original purposes' were being sought. Broadly, the effect of the section was that an alteration of the 'original purposes' of a charitable gift could be authorized only by a scheme for the cy-près application of the trust property, and that such a scheme can be made only in the circumstances set out in s. 13(1)(a)–(e).

Section 13 defined 'failure'—arguably initial, as well as subsequent, failure—with the section beginning with reference to the 'the original purposes of a charitable gift', which supposes that a charitable gift has taken place. It will not have done so in many cases of initial failure. In that case, the question of whether there has been a failure would continue to be determined on the basis of the pre-1960 law.

In any case, s. 13 (by virtue of s. 13(2)) affected only the definition of when failure occurs for cy-près purposes, and all of the other requirements of the doctrine remained. Thus, for example, it remained necessary to show a paramount charitable intention in the case of an initial failure.

What is clear is that, notwithstanding an emphasis on efficient administration that has persisted thereafter, in interpreting the section, as much effect is given to the intentions of the donor, albeit in understanding these in the light of modern social and economic conditions. For example, in *Re Lepton's Charity* [1972] Ch 276, s. 13(1)(a)(ii) and 13(1)(e)(iii) were invoked in order to increase payment to a church minister from £3 per year to £100 per year. Under the original will of 1715, the testator left land, the profits of which amounted to £5 a year, with a direction to trustees to pay £3 a year to the minister and the residue to the poor of Pudsey.

In 1967, the income from the investments representing the land had increased considerably, and the court felt that, after the change, the relative distribution between the minister and the poor of Pudsey remained as in the spirit of the gift. The main argument in the case was whether s. 13 applied to the trusts in the will as a whole, or to each of the two trusts separately (a trust to pay the £3 a year to the minister, and a separate trust to pay the residue to the poor of Pudsey); only if the spirit of the gift related to the will as a whole could the court alter the relative proportions of each part.

Another case falling within s. 13(1)(e)(iii), but in which the original purposes were neither impractical nor impossible to achieve, was *Varsani* v *Jesani* [1998] 3 All ER 273 (CA). The case concerned a charity, established in 1967 by a declaration of trust, the purpose of which was to promote the faith of a Hindu sect. In 1984, the sect split into two factions, with each side accusing the other of having departed from the true faith. As long as either faction adhered to the true faith, it remained possible to achieve the original purposes, but the effect of the schism was that only one of the factions was making use of the main asset of the charity, a temple in London, to the exclusion of the other faction.

The Court of Appeal, upholding the decision of Carnworth J, felt that the framework within which the faith was practised in 1967 (that is, the original purposes) had ceased to provide a suitable and effective method of enabling the property to be used in accordance with 'the spirit of the gift'; therefore the Court had jurisdiction to order a cy-près scheme. Only the jurisdictional issue was before the Court, and it is not reported what was actually done with the property.

12.4.2 Distinguishing substantive purposes from administrative matters

Section 13 allowed only the original purposes of a charitable gift to be altered, and for this reason it could not be used in *Re J. W. Laing Trust* [1984] Ch 143 to delete a provision relating to distribution that was essentially administrative in nature. Peter Gibson J observed, at 153, that 'it cannot be right that any provision, even if only administrative, made applicable by a donor to his gifts should be treated as a condition and hence part of its purpose'. The same view was taken in *Oldham Borough Council* v *Attorney-General* [1993] Ch 210, in which Dillon LJ considered that the requirement that the actual land given should be used as playing fields was not part of the 'original purposes' within s. 13. In *J. W. Laing*, the condition was struck out under the inherent jurisdiction, whereas in *Oldham* there was no need for a scheme at all, so these are both cases in which the common law applied, but the statute did not.

12.5 Section 13 and the Charities Acts of 1993 and 2006, and beyond

The essence of s. 13 of the Charities Act 1960 was its provision of powers for cy-près to be applied in the five situations set out in the foregoing provisions. This was re-enacted in the Charities Act 1993. The Charities Act 2006 re-enacted some of the 1993 Act, whilst making some amendments to it as far as s. 13 was concerned. Given the rationale for the 2006 Act and its political 'back story', it is not surprising at all that the amendments of law and in policy have the effect that property may be applied cy-près, taking into account not only 'the spirit of the gift', but also the social and economic circumstances prevailing at the time of the proposed alteration of the original purposes. This amendment subsisted by virtue of s. 15(3) of the Charities Act 2006 and was brought into force in March 2008 by the third Commencement Order relating to the Act.

The provisions of s. 13, as amended by the Charities Act 2006 (and centrally s. 14B), are now located in Pt 6 of the Charities Act 2011. The Charities Act 2011, like its predecessors, embodies concerns about the effective administration of charities and seeks to prioritize this in the context of respecting donors' wishes. This latter consideration remains visible in the grounds on which charitable purposes can be altered set out in s. 62, which reference a gift's 'original purposes', and where the significance of the 'spirit of the gift' is acknowledged in subsection (2). And in setting out the 'the appropriate considerations' for applying a cy-près scheme for these purposes, subsection (2) acknowledges the importance of both the social and economic circumstances prevailing that suggest in favour of the alteration of original purposes, and also the donor's wishes embodied in the 'spirit of the gift'. It also acknowledged, perhaps more pointedly than predecessor provisions of s. 14B(3) (inserted by way of s. 18 of the 2006 Act), that these considerations may not necessarily be in harmony with one another.

12.5.1 The Charities Act 2011 and a donor who cannot be identified or who disclaims 'his' property in the context of charitable giving

Part 6 of the Charities Act 2011 also has provision for the application of cy-près in situations in which the donor is unknown or disclaiming. This regime is designed to prevent, in the context of failed charitable purposes, a *West Sussex* (after *Re West Sussex Constabulary's Widows, Children and Benevolent (1930) Fund Trusts* [1971] Ch 1, as considered for non-charitable unincorporated associations in Chapter 7) outcome, whereby those contributors to a fund who could not be identified or could be taken to have made an out-and-out gift would pass to the Crown as *bona vacantia*. The provisions now found in s. 63 of the Charities Act 2011 allow for property given for specific charitable purposes that fail to be applied cy-près by regarding this 'as if given for charitable purposes generally'. The modern ancestry of s. 63 can be found in s. 14 of the Charities Act 1993, which replaced similar provision in the Charities Act 1960 and was designed to rescue property for charity in the event of initial failure, and where a resulting trust to a donor or his estate would ensue on the ground that the property had not been dedicated to charitable purposes. Materials on the Online Resource Centre explain how s. 14 (which was amended by the Charities Act 2006 by virtue of s. 16) was intended to work for donors who could not be identified or who had disclaimed entitlement to 'their' property, and alongside the parallel position of gifts made to unincorporated associations. These materials also explain how the opinion that s. 14 (as it was) acquired a reputation in some quarters as a 'dead letter' of English law, and that it arguably made no difference to the pre-1960 law on account of the fact that its application would be triggered only where property belongs to a donor, which is where Goff J's decision in *West Sussex* is very significant.

12.6 The Charities Act 2011 and assessing the modern law relating to cy-près as law fit for purpose in the twenty-first century

A theme that runs throughout the three chapters of this text considering charity and its legal framework has been to emphasize the Charities Act 2011 as legislation seeking to tidy, simplify, and clarify the law relating to charity rather than as law that alters direction or policy. The Charities Act 2006 was, of course, a key reference point for understanding direction and underlying policy within English charity law, and discussions of the extent to which it embodies 'continuity and change', as suggested, are now closely bound in with the assessment of its fitness for purpose, which have emerged from the Hodgson Review. In looking at the Charities Act 2011 differently—as a statement of simplification and increased accessibility, rather than substantive direction—there is actually much greater scope for doing so in respect of cy-près provisions than was the case in the materials relating to the legal definition of charity.

This is centrally because whilst the Charities Act 2006 provided the first statutory definition of charity, the operation of cy-près has a much longer codified tradition. The statutory framework for cy-près dates back to 1960, and subsequent charities legislation had sought to re-enact this, with some modification and amendment, in 1993 and then 2006. In this regard, much cy-près provision within the Charities Act 2006 sought to insert amendments into the 1993 legislation in a way that made even following this accurately very difficult, let alone discerning policy, and assessing continuity and new direction.

The same is the case for aspects of the 2006 Act detailing the legal status and remit of the Charity Commission, where equally messy insertions were made into the 1993 Act by ss 6 and 7 of the 2006 Act.

In sweeping this complex interaction between charities legislation past and present aside in favour of clear provisions, the Charities Act 2011 does make the law relating to cy-près much more presentable, and capable of being followed and analysed respectively by trustees and charity lawyers—and, as such, it is very welcome indeed.

 Revision Box

1. Ensure that you are able to explain what is meant by 'cy-près' in the context of English charity law in terms of:
   - what the term actually means; and
   - what the facility for cy-près reveals about the significance of the charitable box within English society.
2. Ensure that you can explain how cy-près operated at common law and what has changed about this as a result of charities legislation dating from 1960. In doing so, identify:
   - the continuing significance of the wishes of the donor; and
   - the emphasis given to other considerations in making use of property dedicated to charity.

FURTHER READING

 online resource centre

There is currently no specific reading relating to cy-près at present, and anything that becomes available will be flagged on the ORC accordingly. Please visit <http://www.oxfordtextbooks.co.uk/orc/wilson_trusts11e/>

13

Introduction to trusteeship and an overview of the 'office of trustee'

What is a trustee? The dictionary definition is 'one who is trusted, or to whom something is entrusted; a person in whom confidence is put'. A legal definition is 'one to whom property is entrusted to be administered for the benefit of another'.

(*Spread Trustee Ltd* v *Hutcheson* [2011] UKPC 13, *per* Lord Kerr at 141)

In many ways, this chapter follows on from where we left off in Chapter 5. This is because virtually all of the text up to that point had focused on introducing the 'express private trust' as the paradigm arrangement for conferring the benefits of property, and then explaining what had to be done in order to create a valid express trust of property. At that point, it was noted that the express private trust provides the model for what is known as the 'general law of trusts', but this was not developed any further at that point. This early focus on the existence of express private trusts and their creation was then abruptly brought to a close.

Indeed, Chapter 6 marked the beginning of considering trusts law that is different from the general law of trusts, either because it governs trusts that, although private, are not express, or because it governs trusts that are not private at all. As these latter directions were pursued, the work surrounding the introduction of the express trust and its creation was held in abeyance—until now. Having learned much earlier what happens when an owner of property wants to create a trust of it to benefit others and what is required for him to achieve this, it is now time to learn about the implications of bringing a valid express trust into being. We now look at the consequences of bringing a valid trust into being for each of the 'trust actors' whom we find in the trust arrangement.

Chapter 1 suggested that, once a trust comes into being—that is, once it has been constituted—ownership of property becomes separated, with Chapter 5 explaining that legal title will become vested in the trustee by one of the two constitution mechanisms under *Milroy* v *Lord* [1862] 4 De GF & J 264 and, accompanying this, that equitable title to the property becomes vested in the beneficiary. At this point, the beneficiary acquires not only ownership of the property in equity, but also the capacity to enforce the trust, which, as we learned in Chapter 3, includes the capacity to come to court to force a trustee to carry out the trust.

At this point, as we consider the implications of creating a valid trust, we need to remember that Chapter 1 indicated that. once the trust comes into being. an owner-cum-settlor loses all interest in the property (in this capacity), and that he effectively drops out of the picture because the beneficiary is the only party who can enforce the trust. This is because it is not possible for a settlor to revoke or vary the arrangement once it is created, unless he expressly reserves for himself rights of variation or revocation. So, for considering the implications of a valid trust from the perspective of the actors found in the trust arrangement, the settlor disappears once it comes into being, and we are left with the position of trustee and beneficiary as a measure for what the implications of a valid express trust actually are.

The implications of a valid trust explored through the law relating to trusteeship
The next two chapters consider this through the law relating to trusteeship. Although this appears to focus on trustees rather than beneficiaries, it is the case that exploring what trustees can do and must do—and indeed what they must *not* do—will cast a great deal of light on the position of beneficiaries under the arrangement. This is because the requirements associated with trusteeship are, to a very significant degree, a reflection of the entitlements of a beneficiary. In this regard, we do already have a sense of the kind of role that trusteeship is from the initial introduction to the trust in Chapter 1.

The material in Chapter 1 gave a great deal of introduction to the way in which trusteeship is a highly burdensome office, and one that is characterized by high levels of responsibility and duty, and that this is designed to ensure that the beneficiary is able to enjoy the property as the settlor intended. For example, this is where we discovered that although a trustee holds legal title to (trust) property, this is manifestly different from the type of legal title associated with ownership. This was reiterated when we looked at certainty-of-intention requirements and ones relating to constitution; more generally, material on the certainty of objects provided us with an understanding that trusts are arrangements which trustees actually have to carry out. So we have had a number of glances at the nature of trusteeship, notwithstanding that a comprehensive discussion of this has been held over until now. And at every one of these earlier points, what we have found out about trusteeship has suggested that it is a demanding role and one that carries with it onerous responsibilities.

Up to now, it really has not been clear who might actually act as a trustee and why. Everything up to now has suggested that trusteeship is a very long list of 'down sides'. We will explain the nature of trusteeship and how trusteeship operates in the twenty-first century, and how this might be both similar to and different from the way in which modern trusts law emerged in the nineteenth century. In turn, this actually helps to generate appreciation of the beneficiary's position under the trust arrangement.

It is the case that what trustees must do is very strongly premised on what the beneficiary is entitled to—namely, enjoyment of the property. Here, this introduction to trusteeship builds on our understanding so far to enable us to learn more about who becomes a trustee and why, and what those who become trustees must actually do. As such, these next two chapters, when combined with that considering breach of trust (Chapter 16), are oriented towards two key objectives: first, appreciating the nature of trusteeship and expectations attaching to the 'office of trustee'; and second, appreciating that understanding the nature of the 'office of trustee' can reveal much about the entitlements of a beneficiary under a trust.

13.1 Trusteeship in the twenty-first century: a background and current context

When we were introduced to 'the trust' in Chapter 1, it was suggested that although its origins can be traced to the fifteenth century, it was actually much later that modern trusts started to appear—in the eighteenth century. It was also suggested in Chapter 2 that what we understand as 'modern trusts law' started to be shaped during the nineteenth century. This was on account of the fact that it was then that the trust became popularized.

13.1.1 The emergence of the modern law relating to trusteeship

The modern beginnings of this had started to occur during the eighteenth century, given that it was actually during the seventeenth century that the modern trust appeared (having developed from 'the Use'), but it gathered momentum at this later time because this is when the trust itself became modernized. Chapter 2 explained that this had occurred through the trust's extensive application to family settlements, which were the first modern trusts of real property. By then, it was showing signs of being an extremely useful device for tying up wealth in families (and for reducing exposure to taxation), on principles that had initially appeared in the development of the Use.

As the Use developed into the modern trust, its ability to protect non-legal owners more proactively than simply imposing on the conscience of legal owners who were actually acting unconscionably is why it became such an important way of creating real property rights. And it was recognized that this arrangement would depend upon those who would take responsibility for property to ensure the welfare of others who did not hold legal rights. So as the trust developed from a reactive response to unconscionable conduct, it became common for legal title to be transferred to persons such as clerics and lawyers by owners of property anxious to ensure proactively that the interests of others were protected. This is where legal title to property started to be conveyed to clerics or religious orders 'to the Use' of someone else.

At the time, such persons were seen as pillars of communities, who would enjoy respected positions and status in their communities by virtue of being persons of utmost trust, precisely because they were seen as positions carrying considerable responsibility. Over time, attorneys were brought into this category of persons entrusted with legal title 'to the Use of' another, and both would come to be recognized by equity as positions of utmost loyalty as it developed a special system of governance for what became known as 'fiduciary positions'. But, putting this aside for now, it is from these origins that earliest modern trustees had considerable status in society, which deemed such persons worthy of the considerable responsibility reposed in the trust arrangement.

The significance of the popularization of the trust in the nineteenth century
This is also what would come to make trustees very powerful in the fullness of time, and this is what happened during the nineteenth century when the trust became popularized through the family settlement, which was introduced in Chapters 1 and 2, and about which we will learn more in Chapter 14. These trusts became popular during the eighteenth century, and in the context of the economic transformations that started with industrialization, new classes of person were able to acquire and accumulate property. And, in an increasingly wealthy society, those who were newly wealthy were keen to keep the new-found economic power and opportunity for social advancement that accompanied ownership of property.

Equally, those who historically had a great deal of wealth were keen to safeguard this in new economic climates, being all too aware of the economic and social power attaching to property and its ownership. The trust would be able to assist both of these groups—the newly wealthy and the traditionally wealthy—by being able to limit the use that could be made of property, and thereby tying it into family structures rather than leaving it in the hands of individuals. And as society itself became more wealthy and also more complex, so did its taxation regime; in this climate, it became particularly apparent that the trust was also able to restrict tax liability on dealings with property, as it had done in its earlier form as the Use. It was in this setting that the *law relating to trusts* would emerge on account of the trust's popularization, and in order to achieve both the *facilitation* of trusts and also their *regulation*. The law relating to *trusteeship* was primarily about the latter.

The significance of the popularization of the trust for the development of modern trusts law

The popularization of the trust meant that it became imperative to facilitate the creation of trusts, and so this agenda provided impetus for the modern law of trusts to develop to ensure that those who wished to create trusts were able to do this properly and thus to create arrangements that were effective. This, in turn, set in motion another key agenda, which ensured the development of modern trusts law: the need to regulate the trust, as well as to facilitate it. What was being regulated, as distinct from facilitated, was the separation of ownership of property from its enjoyment, which was the trust's signature feature and key to its popularization. But, from the earliest days of the Use, it was appreciated that giving formal entitlement of ownership to those who were not intended to enjoy the property was risky, as well as beneficial, and that is why many early trustees were clerics and then also attorneys. So it was mainly this regulatory dimension that gave us the modern law relating to trusteeship. This has emerged to fulfil two key functions: to provide a clear position on the entitlement of beneficiaries precisely because they did *not* have ownership of property at law; and also to make very clear statements of responsibility for trustees precisely because they *did* hold legal title to property, but had no entitlement to it.

13.1.2 Focusing on the emergence of the modern law relating to trusteeship

So this is how modern trusts law started to emerge, and we can also now see who might take on trusteeship and why. The earliest days of the Use set the pattern for those who would become trustees when the separation of ownership of property from its enjoyment became popularized. These elements of position and responsibility are central for understanding traditional approaches taken by trusts law to trusteeship. Taking on such responsibility is what people in positions of high status and reposed trust are expected to do, and from this two central themes for studying the modern law of trusteeship become clear: first, that trusteeship is a highly onerous office; and second, that the modern law relating to trusteeship reflects strong adherence both to that put in place during the nineteenth century and, at the same time, to the way in which the office itself is currently changing radically.

As far as the first is concerned, we have already been reminded that the type of legal title held by a trustee in a trust arrangement is legal title that is (effectively) stripped of all benefits of ownership, and that, in this arrangement, the trustee becomes subject to a number of duties that are designed to ensure that the beneficiary will receive all of the enjoyment of the property that the settlor intended. As we unpack this in this chapter and the next, it will become clear just how unattractive trusteeship might appear as we suggest that, as the modern law of trusteeship became formalized, a number of things became clear.

We will learn that the trustee under an express trust falls subject to a number of very onerous duties relating to looking after the assets of the trust and acting in the interests of the beneficiary, and that, traditionally, many of these responsibilities must be carried out by the trustee himself and cannot be delegated to others. We shall also discover that, notwithstanding the onerous nature of expectations of trustees, equity's approach is that there is actually no entitlement to remuneration arising from the office of trustee. We shall learn that there have always been certain ways around the position on remuneration, but that equity takes a more hard-line approach to how trustees are expected to respond to opportunities for personal benefit from their office.

In relation to the second theme, we will then apply all of this to the influences brought to bear on the modern law relating to trusteeship by the origins of the modern law and also recent trends. This requires us to consider the way in which, historically, the role of trustee has been undertaken by those in respected positions, meaning that a large number of trustees have traditionally been family solicitors and also other 'pillars' of the community, such as clerics and persons in 'public office'.

In coming to focus on both of these things, we need to say a little about how the modern law relating to trusteeship emerged and why it did so. This is where we need to understand that, when the law relating to trusteeship started to develop in the nineteenth century, it did so to achieve two key objectives: first, that those who were trustees acted properly rather than improperly when entrusted with legal title to property intended to benefit others; and second, as a result of this, that a clear position emerged on the rights and entitlements of beneficiaries under a trust.

13.1.3 Trusteeship in the twenty-first century

Since the closing years of the twentieth century, there has been a considerable change in the nature of trustees themselves, with the rise of the 'professional trustee'. This is someone different from the traditional trustee, who became one on account of occupying a respected position in society. The professional trustee is someone who actually undertakes providing 'trusts services' as a business, and who will charge often very considerable fees for setting up and administering trusts. Originally, these professional service providers were specialist divisions within financial institutions, such as banks and insurance companies, as well as 'specialist' law firms, but alongside these can be found increasing numbers of (often) sizeable and highly specialized trust service providers, which are commonly called 'trust corporations'. When the term 'trust corporation' is used today by judges, it refers to the way in which those who are professional trustees purvey their services by way of a business. There are legal requirements for qualifying as a trust company and a number are public limited companies; very significantly for this text, they are increasingly being seen in 'trustee litigation', which has traditionally concerned, in particular, family solicitors.

*Issues arising from the changing nature of trusteeship and the emergence
of two key trends*
This has precipitated recognition that the 'rules' governing trusteeship laid down by equity during the nineteenth century might well not be suitable for trustees' activity today. There are two key perspectives on traditional trusts law suggesting quite different things. First, there is suggestion that the law relating to trusteeship developed in the nineteenth century will not provide sufficient protection for beneficiaries to reflect the way in which, increasingly, trustees are likely to be paid professionals for whom providing trusts services is a business, and who ought to be held to high expectations. There is also, second, the view that traditional trusts law is unduly restrictive by not allowing those who are paid professionals enough scope for providing the most efficient services for their clients, which might also mean that trust assets cannot perform to their maximum capability.

From this, the current state of the law appears to be signalling two key trends. The first is greater recognition of the significance of being a professional trustee, both in terms of what is permissible activity and what are considered appropriate levels of liability; the second is a reluctance to depart from some fundamental rules of equity designed to ensure that those who undertake trusteeship do not abuse their positions. These themes remain central as a more detailed look is taken at the way in which the law of trusteeship involves empowering trustees to do certain things and also requiring much of them. This is the focus of the next chapter. This chapter sets the scene for this later development, and also what has been suggested up to now by looking at how trusteeship arises and what its fundamental nature is, and how the 'law relating to trusteeship' can be understood in this light.

General considerations relating to the law of trusteeship

In Chapter 1, it was suggested that a trust can be seen as 'an arrangement whereby a person (a trustee) is made the nominal owner of property to be held or used for the benefit of one or more others'. In this chapter, this very general statement provides a reference point for some of the practical implications of this arrangement, whereby although the trustee does hold legal title to the property, he is not its owner, and he holds legal title solely to ensure that the beneficiary is able to have the benefit of the property without responsibility for it. This is why we will encounter key elements of the considerable body of law that underpins what trustees can do and what constraints are there on their activities, and what will happen if they do not act as they are required to.

Here, much of what trustees can and cannot do, and what will happen if they act outside what is permitted, will be determined by the basis of the trust arrangement itself. There will commonly be some kind of document most commonly referenced as a 'trust instrument', but as a matter of substance rather than form it is the settlor's instructions that will inform how the trust is carried out and what is or is not permitted in pursuit of this.

The general law, and the importance of the settlor's instructions and the 'trust instrument'

In this respect, the 'law relating to trusteeship' that has developed in pursuit of these objectives provides what lawyers call a 'fallback' position. Here, the law adopts an accepted general position for what should happen in any given circumstances, which will be applied where nothing contrary to it is provided in the settlor's instructions. The practical effect of this is that, in most express trusts, what trustees can or cannot do is determined by the terms of the trust. For reasons that will become very significant, the terms of an express trust will also make specific provision for the remuneration of trustees acting under a settlement, and also clauses limiting the liability that they can incur for committing any breaches of trust in carrying out the settlor's instructions.

Although this means that, in many cases, it is the trust that will determine trustees' obligations and empowerments, the general law that we encounter in these materials on trusteeship is very important. This is because, for as long as people set up trusts without taking proper legal advice, provision of a legal fallback position remains of utmost importance. It is also the case that, as a matter of convenience and associated considerations of cost, individual trust arrangements (which are commonly written instruments) can be drafted much more quickly and can be considerably shortened when powers and duties are provided anyway, in the absence of provision to the contrary.

In terms of the nature of the law that we find here, whilst the law relating to trusteeship is traditionally based on case law, increasingly the 'administrative' aspects of trusteeship have become governed by statute. Up until 2000, it was very common for statutory provisions to restate the previous law, or to re-enact earlier statutory provisions either exactly, or only slightly differently, which is why you will notice that some cases that are cited as authority for the interpretation of a particular section of a statute actually pre-date the section currently in force.

It is also the case that, although this idea of a fallback position applies to the Trustee Act 2000, this particular piece of legislation was the product of a longer-standing policy movement, which suggested that the law relating to trusteeship, which remained little altered since its inception during the nineteenth century, was out of step with the current context for trusteeship and was not 'fit for purpose'. More is said about this shortly, but first we need to find out more about the nature of trusteeship.

13.1.4 Some basic considerations of trusteeship

At the end of Chapter 2 and in anticipation of looking at the key requirements of a valid trust, we learned that, when we speak of 'capacity' to create a trust, this refers to the capacity of the settlor. But it was also suggested at that point that we would come back to this question and consider it in relation to who can become a trustee.

Who can be appointed as a trustee?

Much like the capacity of settlor, the capacity to act as a trustee is determined by capacity to hold property at law. This is because, as we know from looking at constitution of trusts and formality arising in the creation of trusts, a trustee will become the new legal owner of trust property once its original owner has settled it. And, in following up the significance of 'trust corporations', a corporation may become a trustee if its constitution so authorizes. For individual human trustees, *Re Vinogradoff* [1935] WN 68 shows that an infant can become a resulting or a constructive trustee, but only of personal property, because, under s. 20 of the Law of Property Act 1925, the express appointment of an infant trustee is void (and s. 36(1) of the Trustee Act 1925 permits the infant's replacement by a person of full age). These restrictions apart, the settlor may appoint trustees as he pleases. Traditionally, certain appointments, such as that of a beneficiary or one of his relatives as trustees, have been regarded as undesirable by the courts, on account of the scope for conflict between the different roles found within the arrangement. The courts have displayed similar caution for those who are solicitors to the trust also being trustees under the arrangement for similar reasons.

These arrangements are very common and they certainly will not be invalid as long as the appointment is properly made. As we know, this will be by virtue of fulfilling formality requirements for transferring trust property from the owner-cum-settlor to the trustee concerned. As it has already been suggested, alongside those traditionally fulfilling the role of trustee, increasingly this is most notably the 'trust corporation'. Traditionally, this has been the executor and trustee company of a large bank, but increasingly there are also dedicated trusts service providers, as well as these 'multifunctional' institutions. The main advantages of appointing a trust corporation are its longevity, financial stability, and expertise, and the fact that it may act alone in circumstances under which two individual trustees would be necessary—but this comes at a cost, and these organizations will commonly charge considerable fees for their services. And in terms of generating the capacity to act as trustee, for a company to be a trust corporation there are qualifications that are contained within the Public Trustee Rules 1912, r. 30, as amended.

What happens if there is no trustee?

We know from Chapter 3 that express trusteeship is voluntary and cannot be forced on anyone, and we also now know that those who are intended to be trustees will commonly be specified when the settlor creates the trust. However, it also happens that sometimes express trust arrangements will not specify individuals, but this will not invalidate the trust, and the equitable principle that 'equity will not allow a trust to fail for want of a trustee' ensures that equity will go to considerable lengths to ensure that there is someone to carry out the mandatory arrangement that comes into being once all validity requirements have been satisfied.

If a trust without trustees arises *inter vivos*, the settlor himself will be the trustee; if it arises by will, the testator's personal representatives will hold the property on trust. Where an instrument creating the trust names someone as having power to appoint trustees, he may use that power to fill the gap. If all else fails, the court will appoint trustees by virtue of s. 40 of the Trustee Act 1925, which can be used in a variety of circumstances, including in the appointment of new trustees once a trust is up and running, should this become necessary (and which can be found considered further on the Online Resource Centre).

Under an express trust arrangement, we know that no one can be compelled to accept office as trustee, but as we learned in Chapter 6 (and developed in Chapters 8 and 9, and will continue in Chapter 17), a person may find trusteeship imposed on him by operation of law in circumstances under which equity imposes a constructive trust or implies a resulting trust. However, once a trustee does accept the undertaking in an express trust arrangement, it is regarded as a once-and-for-all commitment. This office cannot later be renounced, although it is possible for trustees to retire under certain conditions (to which we will come in the next section). This was certainly the position regarding the traditional occupants of trustee office—the clerics and lawyers who were engaged by virtue of being persons of utmost trust—and it is that which can commonly apply to 'trustee corporations', which are capable of indefinite existence.

On this model, it has been par for the course for trustees to die in office, and because of this, with liabilities incurred during a lifetime actually persisting against the estate of a deceased trustee. As the law of trusteeship is configured, any trustee who wishes to disclaim his role for any reason should do so as soon as possible, and preferably by deed. This is because failure to disclaim may lead to a presumption that the proposed trustee has accepted, and acceptance will also be presumed once the trustee has started to act in relation to the property.

How trusteeship can come to an end through retirement and death

The discussion here considers only the position relating to a trustee's retirement and also what happens upon his death, whilst material on the Online Resource Centre considers the circumstances in which a trustee can be forcibly removed from office, with emphasis here on how the court can become involved in who acts as a trustee. At this point, a little more is now said about how a trustee can effectively retire, notwithstanding what has just been said about trusteeship being a once-and-for-all commitment.

There is scope for a trustee to retire in one of several ways. The trust instrument may well provide for this, but more commonly s. 36(1) of the Trustee Act 1925 allows a trustee to find a replacement, and s. 39 allows for retirement without a replacement where that retirement will not leave the trust with fewer than two individual trustees or a trust corporation to act for it.

It is also possible for beneficiaries to consent to a trustee's retirement, and they will be debarred from holding the trustee accountable for any event arising after the date of such consent. This depends on all beneficiaries being *sui iuris* (that is, suffering from no incapacities, such as infancy or mental incapacity) and collectively entitled to the entire trust property, and a beneficiary who consents to a breach of trust has no right of action in respect of that breach (discussed in Chapter 16). The court can also discharge without replacement under its inherent jurisdiction, but only where this will not leave the trust without a trustee. Here, under an order for administration of the trust by the court, the trustee remains in office, but is relieved of responsibility.

So whilst the once-and-for-all nature of trusteeship looks unremitting in theory, in practice the statutory provisions for retirement are almost always sufficient.

In relation to the death of a trustee, the starting point is that where there is more than one trustee, trustees hold their office, and the trust property, jointly. There is a right of survivorship so that, upon the death of a trustee, his office and the trust estate devolve on the survivors. Discussion of the Use, the earliest modern trust, showed how estates were able to pass from generation to generation with few conveyances of legal titles, which was achieved in part by vesting the legal title in a number of 'others' to use jointly, and relying on the right of survivorship on the death of any one of them. Trusts today operate in the same way and for essentially similar reasons, and the equitable rule was codified in s. 18(1) of the Trustee Act 1925, with s. 18(2) making provision for the death of a sole surviving trustee.

13.2 The law relating to trusteeship as seen through the life cycle of an express trust

More is said shortly about the nature of trusteeship and the reasons why it is considered such a burdensome office, and how this can be seen manifested in the law relating to trusteeship. First, we consider how the law relating to trusteeship can be mapped onto three distinct stages in the life cycle of a trust. Here, we look at how legal requirements might be framed around what trustees must do when a trust comes into being, how they must act while the trust is active, and what happens when a trust comes to an end as far as its trustees are concerned.

13.2.1 How trusteeship arises and the appointment of trustees as a trust comes into being

Chapters 3, 4, and 5 considered the creation of a valid trust, which allowed us to glean a considerable amount of understanding about how trusteeship arises. From certainty requirements, we learned that 'equity will not allow a trust to fail for want of a trustee' (of which we have just been reminded), and the work on formalities and constitution, taken together with work on certainty of intention, revealed that express trusteeship must be undertaken voluntarily.

When looking at the constitution requirement and its relationships with formality, we also learned that there are two types of trustee found in an express trust arrangement: the trustee who is chosen specifically for the task in hand; and the owner-cum-settlor who undertakes trusteeship himself. We also learned at that point that the appointment of trustees is the commoner mechanism in the express trust arrangements, and we can now add to this that the intended trustee will normally be clear from the instructions that are given by the settlor, which will commonly be in some form of written instruments, notwithstanding that many trusts can be created very informally.

Initial requirements relating to trust property
This is the normal way in which express trustees are appointed and, in reiterating that trustees become legal owners of trust property, in the creation of an *inter vivos* trust,

they will normally be parties to the deed that creates it, with the effect of vesting in them the trust property. Here, trustees must familiarize themselves with the nature of the property and the terms of the trusts upon which it is held, and ensure that all formalities necessary to vest the property have been complied with.

For *inter vivos* trusts, this will normally be part of the arrangement by which they are appointed (which will usually involve a deed), certainly as far as money and personal chattels are concerned. But, as we learned in Chapter 4 (with this having been signposted earlier), additional requirements are needed to pass title to personal intangible property and real property, with these depending on the nature of the property concerned: for land, this involves satisfying s. 53(1)(b) of the Law of Property Act 1925; requirements surrounding intangible personalty (personal property, not real property) reflect the policy to make dealings with property that is less visible as open and transparent as possible, through requirements of writing, endorsement, or registration.

A self-declaration of trusteeship by the settlor

Where the settlor declares himself sole trustee, there is nothing further required as far as transfer formality is concerned, but trust property that is land must also satisfy s. 53(1)(b) of the Law of Property Act 1925 to be enforceable. In a testamentary trust, in which the same persons are appointed as executors and trustees, executors must vest the property in themselves as trustees, which is notional in the case of most kinds of personalty, but requires a formal assent in the case of land. If other persons are to take over as trustees, the property must be vested in them with whatever formality is required; similarly, when new trustees are appointed to an existing trust, the property must be vested in them so that they hold it jointly with the existing trustees.

Proper vesting of trust property in trustees is vital because the trustees may be held personally liable for any loss arising from failure in this regard, such as missing out on particular investment opportunities through not having the capacity to deal with trust property. A newly appointed trustee must satisfy himself that all is in order and cannot say that it should have been attended to by the other trustees. However, in the case of a newly appointed trustee, some of the formalities of vesting are obviated by s. 40 of the Trustee Act 1925, providing that where he is appointed by deed containing a declaration in appropriate terms, the trust property vests automatically in the new trustee and his co-trustees as joint tenants. But not all property is included within the reach of s. 40, and property that is excluded includes a number of interests and estates in land, flowing from the requirement of writing and/or registration or endorsement in transfers.

Where there is more than one trustee

Trustees appointed to an existing trust (replacing a retiring trustee, for example) must satisfy themselves that the affairs of the trust are in order, and, if not, that steps are taken as soon as possible to put matters right and to recoup any loss. Because carrying out a trust can involve considerable amounts of work, there will often be more than one trustee, which helps to make the task manageable and helps to create efficiencies in trust administration. It also helps to prevent fraud on the part of trustees, because trustees will be able to 'monitor' one another.

However, because *Re Mayo* [1943] is authority that, unless there is express authorization to the contrary, decision-making must be unanimous rather than by way of a 'majority', this suggests that while there are workload and efficiency gains to be made by having more than one trustee, it is also helpful to keep the number small enough to keep to a minimum scope for disagreement. And, returning once more to the workload and efficiency advantages of more than one trustee, it is very significant that the office of trustee is a personal office, which means that the trustee is required to carry out many of the functions of trusteeship himself and that he is allowed to delegate only certain aspects of his role to others.

13.2.2 After creation: expectations in the day-to-day running of the trust

The duty of the trustees in the day-to-day running of the trust is to manage the property so as to preserve the value of the capital and to produce an income for the beneficiaries. Depending on the terms of the trust (with much of this being focused on the trust property itself and what must be done with it), this will require a great deal of management of trust assets by the trustee to achieve this, but it will also require administration, which is why others can become involved.

A trustee who has a portfolio of trust property to manage is likely to want assistance from others who provide ancillary specialist services such as solicitors, accountants, stockbrokers, and estate agents, as he seeks to deal with property to try to maximize assets for the trust. Here, a trustee could probably do at least some of these things himself, but he might nevertheless take the view that it is more efficient for him to concentrate on being a trustee and to engage others to provide supporting services where they are called for. When we come to look at the personal nature of trusteeship, we will see that the law recognizes this and allows trustees to appoint agents to assist them in the proper running of a trust, and thus to delegate to them certain trustee functions. We shall also see that the law also insists that other aspects of their role are carried out by them personally.

It is these two latter considerations that give us insight into how the law relating to trustees has changed much in a few short years in the close of the twentieth century and the dawn of the twenty-first. It also gives us a sense of the extent to which these changes are being driven by the changing nature of trusteeship itself.

Standards expected of trustees in personal performance of the trust

It has already been suggested that the rise of the professional trustee has questioned traditional directions in the law underpinning trusteeship, which has developed to provide support for trustees and protection for beneficiaries, in the context that trustees have traditionally been selected for their utmost trust rather than for their expertise in managing property and its associated administrative demands. This was the case even for family solicitors, and much more convergence of this could be achieved as specialist divisions within law firms and financial institutions started to populate the trust scene.

This marked the arrival of the 'professional trustee', and there are now some commercial enterprises that do nothing other than set up trusts for settlors and administer them. This has precipitated much rethinking of the traditional governance of trusteeship, which underpinned reforms achieved under the Trustee Act 2000, but there is evidence of recognition that the professional trustee had arrived on the scene dating back at least to the 1980s.

Indeed, *Bartlett* v *Barclay's Bank Trust Co. Ltd (No. 1)* [1980] Ch 515 is authority that questions were starting to be asked about whether higher standards should be expected from those who undertake trusteeship as paid professionals, and it is certainly the case that the 'higher standards, enhanced accountability' dimension can be seen in the accommodation in the Trustee Act 2000 of the changing nature of trusteeship. However, another and rather different key theme can be seen in the way in which the Trustee Act 2000 has sought to acknowledge and reflect the changing nature of trusteeship.

The professional trustee and empowerment in carrying out trusteeship

This will become apparent shortly, but what follows now is a brief introduction to the background to the Trustee Act 2000. It has already been suggested that the rise of the professional trustee has been instrumental in emerging views that trusts law dating from the nineteenth century is not obviously fit for purpose. The Trustee Act 2000 is a very significant embodiment of this. This was the result of a policy movement commencing formally in 1997, with the Law Commission's publication of a Consultation Paper *Trustees' Powers and Duties* (CP 146), followed by a report (Law Com. 260) published in 1999, but as Hayton (1990) 106 LQR 87 reveals, the Act was also a reflection of pre-existing dissatisfaction with the law and insistence that much needed to change for it to be fit for purpose in the twenty-first century.

The centrepiece of the Trustee Act 2000

The statutory duty of care applicable to trustees when carrying out their functions under the Act can be seen as the centrepiece of the legislation, but this is not because it recognizes the desirability of a standard of care: equity has always insisted that trustees must carry out their functions prudently. This can be seen from *Speight* v *Gaunt* (1883) 22 ChD 727 (CA), which requires that a trustee acts in a way in which an 'ordinary prudent man of business' would do in his dealings on behalf of the trust. Sir George Jessel MR alludes to the 'ordinary prudent man of business' to state that nothing further is required, but it can also be seen as a statement that nothing less will be sufficient.

However, both of these positions require some further thought on account of the gloss that is placed on the application of *Speight* to trustees by *Re Whiteley* (1886) 33 ChD 347. In the Court of Appeal, Lindley LJ insisted that application of the 'ordinary prudent man of business' test to trustees meant that the standard is what such a person would exhibit in the affairs of 'other people for whom he felt morally bound to provide', given that this would need to be different from him acting in the pursuit of his own affairs. We will discuss the *Speight–Whiteley* approach when we consider investment more extensively in the following chapter, but in this context it shows that the idea of a standard of care for trustees is not of itself new to the Trustee Act 2000.

So it is clear that the idea of a duty of care is not itself new, but what *was* new about the 2000 Act's duty was—as the Law Commission stressed—the creation of a 'uniform duty', with the aim of providing 'certainty and consistency to the standard of competence and behaviour expected of trustees'. This works by applying the same standard of care across each of the functions to which the duty applies. In terms of what the legislation should be, it is clear that the Law Commission envisioned a context of increased professionalism and a diverse business environment within which trusteeship can increasingly be seen to operate.

This is because the statutory duty also provides facility for individual trustees to be judged against the standard exceeding the 'uniform', which is aimed at providing the base-level 'certainty and consistency to the standard of competence and behaviour expected'. This will become clear as we work through s. 1, where it is stated:

1(1) Whenever the duty under this subsection applies to a trustee, he must exercise such care and skill as is reasonable in the circumstances, having regard in particular—

(a) to any special knowledge or experience that he has or holds himself out as having, and

(b) if he acts as trustee in the course of a business or profession, to any special knowledge or experience that it is reasonable to expect of a person acting in the course of that kind of business.

The duty of care applies only in the circumstances listed in Sch. 1, which are the statutory functions of the Act, with exercising the general power of investment (or any other power of investment however conferred) or associated statutory duties being centre stage. We shall come to appreciate how important safeguarding trust assets is in defining the trusteeship—both a trustee's obligations and a beneficiary's entitlements—as we work through the materials, but getting a measure of Sch. 1 generally reveals a range of activities covered by this particular measure of standards in competence and behaviour. By implication, there are activities not covered by this statement of standards, in relation to which standards are drawn from pre-existing legal provisions (rules developed by equity, or statutory provisions that have codified equity's original approaches) and thus are not actionable under the 2000 Act.

Schedule 1 also provides a further reminder of a long-standing approach of English law subsisting as a fallback position in the absence of clear instructions, and the disapplication of the general law where this would contradict specific instructions. This is because Sch. 1, para. 7, provides that 'The duty of care does not apply if or in so far as it appears from the trust instrument that the duty is not meant to apply'.

A different standard for professional trustees?

In situations in which the duty does apply, we can also see an intention in the legislation to hold some trustees in some circumstances to standards that are higher than the 'uniform' baseline expectations. From the background to the Trustee Act 2000 and the wording of the statutory duty of care, we can see an intention in the provisions to hold those who are professional trustees to a standard beyond the basic statutory duty to exercise such care and skill as is reasonable in the circumstances. This is because s. 1 also provides that what amounts to 'reasonable skill and care in the circumstances' will depend on the facts of the case and that, in determining this, specific regard must be given to the factors within s. 1(1)(a) and (b).

The s. 1 criteria give rise to what is often referred to as a combination 'subjective–objective' test. Here, the essence of paragraph (a) is directed towards the trustee concerned, and operates in relation to the qualities that he is representing that he possesses. The trustee's own representations are then pitched alongside and against the objective criteria in paragraph (b), drawn from the standards that can reasonably be expected from a practitioner within the trustee's own business or profession. On this model, it is clear that a higher standard is expected from a specialist professional, and is consistent with Brightman J's suggestion in *Bartlett* v *Barclays Bank Trust Co. Ltd (No. 1)* [1980] Ch 515 that those who are paid professional trustees should be judged against the standards of skill and expertise that they claim to possess.

And by the time the Trustee Act 2000 was being conceived, it was becoming clear that this would be particularly important, given the increasing opportunities for utilizing trust property that were becoming possible on account of new investment opportunities arising from the growing numbers and sophistication of investment products, and an increasing globalization of financial markets. This is also very significant for appreciating why the Trustee Act 2000 can also be seen as reflecting an altogether different set of expectations.

The Trustee Act 2000 and an altogether different direction?

The strength of rationale in favour of enhanced standards for paid professional trustees is clear from the policy movement resulting in the Trustee Act 2000. This reflected a mood that had been gathering strength formally from as early as 1980, which suggested that those who seek actively to distance themselves from persons who were selected as trustees for their esteem and respect 'value', but who lacked expertise and technical knowledge, and then to use this as a justification for providing trusts services by way of a commercial enterprise (and thus to charge considerably for the services provided), should ultimately be held to these representations of skill and expertise.

We know from s. 1 that this has now been actioned through providing a threshold standard for all who perform particular trustee functions, and a higher bar for those representing that they perform these functions with enhanced capabilities. Alongside this, we can also see other aspects of the Trustee Act 2000 reflecting a very different mood, which also started to gather momentum in the last quarter of the twentieth century. This did, of course, reflect increasing acknowledgement of the presence of professional trustees, but it also reflected the changing nature of investment opportunities on account of growing sophistication in financial markets and also their increasing globalization.

The empowerment of trustees in the twenty-first century

From the way in which trusts service providers were increasingly coming from outside traditional 'trusted', but amateur, occupants of this office came calls for those who are professional experts to be given more freedom in carrying out trusts. This is significant because, at the beginning, it was suggested that, as equity developed the law relating to trusteeship, a very significant influence for this was that trustees hold legal title to property to which they are not actually entitled, meaning that trustees must be prevented from acting improperly, but also that they must be compelled to act according to the interests that they are bound to protect. We have already seen through *Re Whiteley*'s gloss on *Speight* v *Gaunt* that a key tenet of this became drawing a distinction between what trustees could do on behalf of themselves and what they were permitted to do on another's behalf, with this being tied in with what was permitted as far as taking risks was concerned, as much as it was about showing prudence and diligence.

With professional trustees came suggestion that whilst this was a sensible approach with trusted, but amateur, trustees, it was inappropriate for professional experts, and moreover that trusts were being deprived of significant benefits through such a restrictive policy. More will be said about this when we look at investment in the next chapter, but these views suggested that trustees (and particularly paid professional ones) should be able to maximize returns for a trust by being empowered to do more things with trust property and to create 'efficiencies' in administration.

The latter point reflects that those who are themselves sizeable market players will be able to secure associated 'administrative' services from lawyers and specialist agents more effectively than those who are not repeat players, but it is with the empowerment to do more with trust property that we can see what appears to be quite a different direction from that which was being sought with the s. 1 duty. If the s. 1 duty is concerned with standard-setting and accountability beyond traditional expectations, then we can see in other parts of the legislation a trend for liberalizing aspects of traditional restrictions on trustees' activities.

This can be seen most clearly in s. 3, which is known as the 'general power of investment' and which has radically altered traditional restrictions on permitted investment opportunities. The traditional position was designed to protect beneficiaries' enjoyment of trust property by limiting risk in investments made with it to those that were listed as approved. The approach taken in s. 3's general power of investment (which does operate subject to the s. 1 duty of care) is that a trustee can make any investment that he would make on his own behalf if the assets were to belong to him absolutely.

Two different directional trends—and an overall measure?

The provisions of ss 1 and 3 of the Trustee Act 2000 are seeking to achieve what appear to be quite different things. On the one hand, s. 1 provides a statutory statement on competence and accountability, making it clear that enhanced expectations apply to paid professionals; on the other, we can see much greater freedom in what trustees can do with trust property provided by s. 3. We can also see how both trends—that for expectation and that for liberalization—have been very much influenced by the professional trust service provider who charges for his business services. In many ways, the Trustee Act 2000 has become consumed by the professional trustee, and much less attention has been paid to how it might impact on those who are more in the traditional mould overall. However, it is also the case that it is hard to get a measure of its effect overall even as far as trustees who are paid professionals are concerned, because enhanced expectations have come with greater empowerment.

This position is complicated still further by the way in which, although the policy of expectations is clear from s. 1, the rise of professional trustees has had one further transformative effect on the law relating to trusteeship—that is, the rising use of trustee exemption clauses (TECs). Discussed further in Chapter 16 (and at length in related materials on the Online Resource Centre), TECs are essentially clauses found in trust instruments, which will limit or even exclude liability that can be incurred by a trustee for breach of trust, which will arise where a trustee's failure to perform the trust as he should causes the trust to experience financial loss.

Holding trustees to higher expectations should increase scope for incurring liability for breach of trust, but as this has happened, so has the use of exclusion clauses increased, which has significant ability to cancel out the intended effects of s. 1. Similarly, greater empowerment in investment opportunities operating subject to the s. 1 duty should increase scope for liability where unwise investments are made, but again the use of TECs has meant that this does not necessarily follow.

13.2.3 **A trust comes to an end: duty in the termination of trusts**

As we know from looking at perpetuity rules in Chapter 3, private trusts can exist only for a limited duration. Sooner or later, a private trust will come to an end and the trustees will be required to distribute the property among the beneficiaries. Needless to say, they must distribute it to those who are properly entitled, and failure in this regard will be a breach for which they may be liable. The onus is heavy, and trustees have been held liable where they made payment on the strength of documents of a beneficiary's entitlement that turn out to be forged, such as the marriage certificate in *Eaves* v *Hickson* (1861) 30 Beav 136. We have also already come across the erroneous belief that a valid charitable bequest was created in the *Diplock* 'exclusively charitable' litigation considered in Chapters 10 and 12 (and again in Chapter 17).

National Trustee Co. of Australia Ltd v *General Finance Co. of Australasia Ltd* [1905] AC 373 suggests that trustees might even be liable where they have acted on legal advice, although this may be a factor that would induce the court to exercise its discretion under s. 61 of the Trustee Act 1925 to exempt the trustees from liability (which is considered in Chapter 16). The problems of wrongful payment are dealt with more fully in Chapter 17, but it may be noted here that trustees may apply to court for directions in doubtful cases or, in the last resort, protect themselves by paying money into court.

Moving away from the trust itself and returning to the nature of trusteeship

After considering the way in which the nature of the law of trusteeship might be shaped by the life cycle of a trust, we now return to look at two key fundamental elements of trusteeship that make the office of trustee distinctive. This is so that we can see how its fundamental nature has affected the law relating to trusteeship, through understanding the personal nature of trusteeship and also the fiduciary nature of trusteeship.

13.3 Understanding the nature of trusteeship from the personal nature of trusteeship and the realities of trust administration

Throughout this book, emphasis is given to the way in which the duty of trustees in the exercise of their discretions is one of a personal nature. Yet although trustees have a hugely onerous job, they will not necessarily be experts in everything that is needed for the safe and profitable running of a trust. Thus it is obviously very important for trustees to be able to employ others to carry out the more specialized aspects of the management of the trust.

Equity has therefore always allowed the employment of agents in effecting specialized administrative functions, the most common examples of which are solicitors, stockbrokers, and accountants. Prior to the enactment of the Trustee Act 1925, two principles had been established by the House of Lords in *Speight* v *Gaunt* (1883) 9 App Cas 1. First, under *Speight* v *Gaunt*, it was permissible to employ an agent where this was reasonably necessary, or in accord with normal business practices. Second, where such an agent was employed, trustees would not be liable for conduct attributable to the agent, as long as proper care was taken in the agent's selection, and the agent was employed within his proper sphere and exercised reasonable general supervision over his work.

In addition to *Speight* being qualified by *Re Whiteley*, the combined effect of these two cases was that it was only ever permissible to delegate administrative aspects of carrying out a trust. Here, the principle in *Speight* distinguished between so-called 'ministerial' and 'fiduciary' functions: delegation could be permitted of the former, but never of the latter. The justification for this was that, when a settlor provides the terms of a trust and appoints trustees accordingly, he is intending them to carry out his instructions personally and is vesting legal title to the property in them for this purpose. In this regard, ability to delegate at all, even ministerial, functions was seen as a concession to this position; hence the requirement of reasonable necessity or 'ordinary course of business'.

13.3.1 Traditional and changing approaches to delegation in the modern law

This distinction was preserved as the law developed and morphed into the Trustee Act 1925, which dispensed with the requirement for delegation being reasonably necessary or in the ordinary course of business. Sections 23 and 30 of the 1925 Act provided for these wider powers of collective delegation by trustees, with the two sections working in tandem (although in a manner that, over time, became widely regarded as confused and difficult to ascertain). Section 23 (now repealed) allowed for the facility of delegation and provided that there would be no responsibility for the default of an agent 'if employed in good faith', while s. 30 relieved the trustees from potential responsibility for the default of an agent by insisting that a trustee was to be 'accountable only for his own acts' and not for those of another unless this occurred through the trustee's 'own wilful default'.

The confusing provisions of the 1925 Act and its preservation of the distinctions made between ministerial and fiduciary functions in the context of delegation were noted in the Law Commission's 1997 Consultation Paper on *Trustees' Powers and Duties* (CP No. 146), with much of this being based on views that the current socio-economic climate rendered personal overseeing of many aspects of running of the trust (and particularly in relation to investment choice and management) impracticable at best and difficult to justify. In its recommendation for 'root and branch' reform, the Law Commission stressed that the essence of professional advice and execution for the efficient administration of trusts and the 'exigencies of business' justified an approach that liberated trustees in their pursuit of the best interests of the trust.

The Trustee Act 2000 breathed completely new life into the position of delegation by throwing out an approach concentrated on specifying circumstances in which a trustee can delegate and putting in its place one that conferred a general power to delegate. It combined this with a prescription of functions that cannot be delegated. The relevant provisions are to be found in s. 11 of the 2000 Act, and the general power can be found in s. 11(1): 'Subject to the provisions of this Part, the trustees of a trust may authorise any person to exercise any or all of their delegable functions as their agent.' What amounts to a 'delegable function' is governed by s. 11(2), which states that it is any function other than:

> (a) any functions relating to whether or in what ways any assets of the trust should be distributed,
>
> (b) any power to decide whether any fees or other payment due to be made out of the trust fund should be made out of the income or capital,
>
> (c) any power to appoint a person to be a trustee of the trust, or
>
> (d) any power conferred by any other enactment or the trust instrument which permits the trustee to delegate any of their functions or to appoint a person to act as a nominee or custodian.

The Trustee Act 2000 adopts the same approach to the liability of trustees as at common law. Here, trustees are obliged to exercise reasonable care in the appointment of agents and also in their supervision, which is achieved through the operation of the s. 1 statutory duty of care.

13.3.2 The personal nature of trusteeship and individual delegation

As far as the entitlement of individual trustees to delegate their functions was concerned, this could be done in respect of all powers including fiduciary powers, under s. 25 of the Trustee Act 1925, as substituted by s. 9 of the Powers of Attorney Act 1971, for up to twelve months. This was clearly designed on the assumption that a trustee would wish to do this only if he were actually absent, such as spending a period of time abroad. These provisions have now been amended by the Trustee Delegation Act 1999, but we do see quite a different policy on delegation in this legislation from that taken in respect of collective delegation under the 2000 Act.

Under the 1999 Act, a delegating trustee must inform any person entitled to appoint trustees and all other trustees of his delegation in writing, to allow them to consider whether he should be replaced. Significantly, here, liability that can be incurred by a delegating trustee by virtue of s. 25(5) is in stark contrast to the position in relation to collective delegation. Those who delegate under this section 'shall be liable for the acts or defaults of the donee (the person to whom delegation is made) in the same manner as if they were acts or defaults of the donor'.

Fuller discussion of the traditional approach and new provisions can be found in more depth on the Online Resource Centre.

13.4 Understanding the nature of trusteeship from the fiduciary nature of trusteeship and the realities of trust administration

From the beginning part of the chapter, we have a clear sense that a number of equity's rules relating to trusteeship *have* been modified over time to give trustees greater scope in delivering benefits for the trust, and more recently to give greater recognition to the rise of the professional trustee in this context. This is particularly the case with powers and duties of trustees, but it has also led to significant reform pertaining to delegation, which is rooted in the personal nature of trusteeship. However, in other respects, there has been unwavering adherence to equity's traditional approach, and this is evident in the way in which equity regards trusteeship as a 'fiduciary office'.

In stressing that equity regards trusteeship as a fiduciary office, we need to be aware that there are other relationships that equity also recognizes as fiduciary. There are some of which we are aware in everyday life, such as that between solicitor and client, and also doctor and patient, and even cleric and parishioner, and equally there are a number of fiduciary relationships that have developed in the context of business dealings, such as that between a director and his company, and an agent and his principal.

In trying to get a sense of where the trustee–beneficiary relationship fits here, there are a number of established recognized fiduciary relationships of which that between trustee and beneficiary is one example, and to a very significant degree this is the relationship that has shaped equity's interest in those known as 'fiduciaries' more generally. It is also the case that equity acknowledges that fiduciary relationships can arise outside established categories of relationship, where this is appropriate in the circumstances. This raises the questions: what does equity regard as a fiduciary relationship and why; and what will the implications of this be? It also raises an even more fundamental question of why equity is interested at all in these relationships.

Equity's development of fiduciary relationships

Equity has developed special rules for relationships that it regards as 'fiduciary', and its interest in these relationships stems from equity's insignia of justice and particularly good conscience. This is the key to equity's recognition of a number of relationships that require a type of governance that is different from any other kind of relationship—personal or business—because of the particular dynamics between the parties. Here, equity recognizes that some relationships are ones in which parties are characteristically of manifestly unequal strength in terms of position and knowledge, and are such that the weaker party is actually in a position of enforced reliance upon the stronger party.

It is for this reason that particular relationships can be described as 'asymmetrical', because, in the absence of proper regulation, they are open to abuse precisely because of this combination of unequal advantage and enforced reliance. This is why eminent US scholar Susan Shapiro (1990) 55 ASR 346 has analysed relationships that can be found classified as 'fiduciary' as ones that are actually 'structurally duplicitous', because they are inherently open to abuse. This is why equity has developed special rules applying to them, which would appear to support such concerns.

The special rules developed by equity show that all fiduciary relationships are regarded as having a particular unique feature that distinguishes them from all others. As Millett LJ explained in *Bristol and West Building Society* v *Mothew* [1998] Ch 1 (CA), at 18:

> A fiduciary is someone who has undertaken to act for or on behalf of another in a particular matter in circumstances which give rise to a relationship of trust or confidence. The distinguishing obligation of a fiduciary is the obligation of loyalty. The principal is entitled to the single-minded loyalty of his fiduciary. This core liability has several facets. A fiduciary must act in good faith; he must not make a profit out of his trust; he must not place himself in a position where his duty and interest may conflict; he may not act for his own benefit or for the benefit of a third person without the informed consent of his principal. This is not intended to be an exhaustive list, but it is sufficient to indicate the nature of fiduciary obligations.

13.4.1 Fiduciary relationships and management of the fundamental obligation of loyalty

This fundamental obligation of loyalty, which is the distinguishing character of fiduciary relationships, is what determines whether equity recognizes a relationship as fiduciary. This has been recently restated in the Court of Appeal in *Sinclair Investments Ltd* v *Versailles Trade Finance Ltd* [2011] EWCA Civ 347. For relationships that equity does recognize as fiduciary, special demands are made on the person who occupies the position of the 'fiduciary'. This is the person who actually owes the obligation of loyalty and is the party (on Shapiro's model) in whose favour the inequalities, or *asymmetries*, of the relationship lie. The person against whom these asymmetries work is known as the 'principal'.

Because this inequality is structural—that is, it is a natural consequence of the relationship between a party who is forced to rely on another who is in a stronger position—equity has seen fit to lay down prescriptive rules, which are commonly known as ones seeking to ensure 'fiduciary integrity'. This is the expectation that the fiduciary always acts impartially in the interests of his principal, on account of the positive duty of loyalty. An application of this general position to the relationship between trustee and beneficiary specifically can be seen in Lord Herschell's judgment in *Bray* v *Ford* [1896] AC 44, at 51–2:

> It is an inflexible rule of equity that a person in a fiduciary position ... is not, unless otherwise expressly provided, entitled to make a profit ... It does not appear to me that this rule is ... founded upon principles of morality. I regard it rather as based on the consideration that, human nature being what it is, there is danger, in such circumstances, of the person holding a fiduciary position being swayed by interest rather than by duty, and thus prejudicing those whom he is bound to protect. It has, therefore, been deemed expedient to lay down this positive rule.

The essence of a fiduciary relationship is that it is one that is governed by equity's special rules; when we look at the trustee–beneficiary relationship specifically, it will become clear that equity's special rules have operated to lay down that trustees are not entitled to be paid for acting in this role, and that trustees must not allow their personal interest to conflict with their duty to carry out the trust wholly and unequivocally in the interest of the beneficiary. At this stage, we need to note that equity's special rules will apply only to relationships that it recognizes as fiduciary.

This is not an issue in established relationships, such as that between trustee and beneficiary, company and company director, and agent and principal, but that equity is prepared to recognize fiduciary relationships that arise in particular circumstances suggests that not all relationships will be recognized as such. This can be illustrated by the considerable body of litigation generated concerning whether fiduciary relationships arise in commercial dealings between parties, in which relationships are ordinarily governed by contract.

The context for much of the litigation in this area—including *Bristol and West BS* v *Mothew*—is that commercial relationships are capable of being fiduciary relationships, but this is not the norm, and commercial dealings are ordinarily characterized by parties acting at arm's length and ultimately in their own interests. That such relationships will not be considered fiduciary is clear from *Re Goldcorp Exchange Ltd* [1995] 1 AC 74, in which the Privy Council refused to recognize the existence of any fiduciary relationship between a company which had sold gold bullion for future delivery and its customers. Lord Mustill observed that 'the essence of a fiduciary relationship is that it creates obligations of a different character from those deriving from the contract itself', and that this was not the case here. But cases like *Mothew*, *Goldcorp*, and also *Halifax Building Society* v *Thomas* [1996] 2 WLR 63 provide a body of authority that, in the absence of this core obligation of loyalty, equity will not recognize a relationship as fiduciary.

As we will see in the material on actions in equity in Chapter 17, much of this litigation today over a century after *Bray* v *Ford* arises because parties who have lost property in commercial dealings wish to demonstrate entitlement to use equity's actions to assist them in recovering it. But in terms of identifying what is at the heart of the positive rule— namely, the obligation of loyalty—we shall find out that, over 150 years before *Bray* v *Ford*, we can see equity's insistence upon this for those who occupy fiduciary positions.

The scope of the duty of loyalty and the practical aspects of fiduciary integrity for trustees

In this study of trusts and trusts law, we are interested at this point in who trustees are and what they must or not do. But, as we come to consider how trusteeship is regarded as a fiduciary office, we do need to recognize that it is one of a number of relationships for which equity has considered it necessary to develop special rules. The result of this is that equity's dedicated branch of 'fiduciary jurisdiction' applies more widely than to trusteeship alone, and this is reflected in the case law that has grown up around this.

Because this body of case law is a statement on how equity manages the duty of loyalty imposed on those who are bound to act wholly and unequivocally in the interests of another, the case law can be seen in more general terms. This means that a number of cases that provide authority for how equity will respond to trustees in the light of the duty of loyalty, and the nature of the liability that can arise here, are not actually cases concerning trustees.

Here, many cases that we regard as authoritative for expectations of trustees are ones that concern company directors, solicitors, executors, and increasingly professionals drawn from commercial dealings. We will find a significant number of company director cases discussed as authorities for trusteeship, so we do also need to understand that the basic duty of loyalty applies across all fiduciary relationships. But precisely how it manifests can vary between different fiduciary positions, because of what is required by the actual 'job description' underpinning it: whilst solicitors and trustees (for example) are both fiduciary offices, the law recognizes that solicitors and trustees also perform vastly different functions. This is particularly significant for our study of trustees, because the law has developed quite a different approach for company directors in recognition that they are intended to be dynamic entrepreneurs operating in the cut and thrust of business.

Applying the duty of loyalty to trusteeship specifically

For trustees, the key manifestation of the duty of loyalty is that, in order to ensure that they are never motivated by anything other than acting in the interests of a beneficiary, trustees are not entitled to make a personal profit from their position *as trustees*. We already know that this stance has even applied to ensure that there is no entitlement to be paid for undertaking trusteeship, and overall this is meant to ensure that a trustee will always be considering the beneficiary as he carries out the trust. In turn, if we relate this back to what Lord Herschell said in *Bray* v *Ford*, we can see that this strict and apparently draconian position is perceived as a positive position, which must be actively set out because the office of trustee is structurally so 'loaded' in favour of a trustee. In other words, in absence of a positive rule, it would be too easy for a beneficiary to lose out in such a situation, because even the most altruistically motivated trustees are only human.

The general principle (which is subject to the exceptions considered in the following section) that trustees (and other fiduciaries) are not entitled to benefit from their fiduciary position does, as suggested, lead to the position that trustees have no automatic right to be remunerated for their service. There are two possible justifications for this position, flowing from the principle of 'no benefit'. First, there is the argument that payment should not be allowed if the prospect of payment affects, or has any possibility of affecting, the manner in which the fiduciary's duties are performed. A fiduciary must act in a manner that is disinterested, and there should be no conflict of interest—or even possibility of conflict of interest—with his duties, which would be created by the prospect of reward. Second, all money and other property acquired by the trustee when acting in his capacity as trustee rightfully belongs to the trust. As we shall see, these two justifications lead to slightly different conclusions, and it is not clear whether the courts have fully adopted the second.

It follows from the general principle that equity has not (subject to exceptions to be set out shortly) permitted trustees to consider themselves entitled to claim remuneration for the performance of their duties. Moreover, it is also clear from case law that, should it transpire that they do obtain a benefit from their trusteeship, they are required to account for it to the trust. Unlike the situations considered in Chapter 17 when we study liability arising from breach of trust, many of the cases that stand as authority for this liability to account are cases in which there has been no loss experienced by the trust and only gain made by the trustee.

While our study of breach of trust will consider how an incompetent trustee is required to make good *losses* that have been experienced by the trust, this chapter is concerned with preventing unauthorized *gains* by the trustee. In this latter situation, the remedy of account is focused on the defendant's gain rather than the claimant's (the trust's) loss. In this respect, a trustee is in a position quite different from that of an ordinary contract breaker, who can generally keep profits that he has gained from the breach, as long as he compensates the other party for his losses.

13.4.2 The duty of loyalty applied to trustees' entitlement to remuneration

However, as we know, increasingly trustees are paid professionals who commonly charge handsomely for their services, and it is difficult to see how trusteeship by way of a business would work if it were not possible to be remunerated for it. But it is also the case that, even traditionally, there have always been a number of ways around this strict general position. The most significant is that remuneration will commonly be fixed by contract between settlor and trustee, as part of the terms of the trust. Where there is one, provision for this will be found in the trust instrument itself, and such an arrangement between trustee and settlor is a legitimate exception to the general principle, because it breaks any possible connection between performance of duties under a trust and personal outcome for the trustee. The logic here is that a trustee will not let remuneration issues incentivize how he carries out the trust because he already knows what the personal outcome for him will be. However, the contract must be one that the company is entitled to make, as was not found to be the case in *Guinness plc* v *Saunders* [1990] 2 AC 663, in which the House of Lords held that the directors were not entitled to keep the £5.2 million that they had 'received'.

Moreover, in the lead-up to the Trustee Act 2000, the Law Commission's 1999 report on *Trustees' Powers and Duties* (Law Com. 260) insisted that the general position of no entitlement was incompatible with the increased professionalization of trusteeship, and it was accordingly recommended that, in the absence of express contrary provision, professional trustees should be entitled to charge as long as the charges are reasonable and do not exceed the amount that trustees would charge in the ordinary course of their business.

This entitlement has now been enacted as s. 28 of the Trustee Act 2000, which provides in s. 28(1) that a trustee is entitled to payment (except to the extent that this is inconsistent with the trust instrument) if:

(a) there is a provision in the trust instrument entitling him to receive payment out of the trust funds in respect of services provided by him to or on behalf of the trust, and

(b) the trustee is a trust corporation or is acting in a professional capacity.

Section 29 provides an entitlement to remuneration for 'certain trustees' where there is no provision elsewhere (that is, in the trust instrument or by any enactment or secondary legislation), where the trustee is a trust corporation (but not a trustee of a charitable trust), or where the trustee is one who acts as a professional trustee. The entitlement that arises is to 'reasonable remuneration out of the trust funds for any services he provides to, or on behalf of, the trust *if each other trustee has agreed in writing that he may be remunerated for the services*' (emphasis added).

However, even prior to the Trustee Act 2000, there were a number of established exceptions to the general position apart from contractual determination, which meant effectively that trustees could be paid for their services, but in theory without disturbing the general traditional position of no entitlement. The key ones are as follows.

- *Entitlement to reimbursement for expenses incurred* This is a long-standing exception to the general position, which is now located in s. 31 of the Trustee Act 2000, and entitles a trustee to reimbursement for expenses from trust funds. However, this is not payment for a trustee's services as such, and is wholly restitutionary.

- *Facility for payment under the court's inherent jurisdiction* The inherent power of the court to award remuneration reflects the courts' willingness to grant remuneration to a trustee in circumstances under which a trustee felt unable to devote his time gratuitously to trust affairs and it was in the beneficiaries' interest that he did so. The authorities and the basis of the jurisdiction were thoroughly reviewed in *Re Duke of Norfolk's ST* [1982] Ch 61, in which the Court of Appeal appeared to have accepted as its justification ensuring the efficient administration of trusts, but also rejected an alternative analysis based on implied contract. This case did also break new ground by extending this rationale to situations in which remuneration provided did not reflect enforced increases of work involved (here, on account of changes to taxation rules), because the Court saw no difference in principle between increasing an already-agreed remuneration and granting remuneration where none was agreed.

- *Facility for payment where a trustee has exceeded his duty* In many cases considered in this chapter, trusts have gained considerably from the zeal of trustees, who have put in a great deal of work well beyond their normal duties or have taken a substantial financial risk. It is arguable that the trust would be unjustly enriched if the trustee were to be required to account for the entirety of his profits, which is why the trustee (or other fiduciary) may (assuming that he has acted in good faith throughout) claim under a common law jurisdiction based on *quantum meruit*, and an equitable jurisdiction to award an allowance that is accepted as working on the same principles.

This can be seen in *Boardman* v *Phipps* [1967] 2 AC 46 (considered at '*Boardman* v *Phipps*: is liability to account a virtual certainty in all profit cases?'), in which although a solicitor as fiduciary to a family trust was not entitled to keep profits received as a result of his position, he was held at first instance to be entitled to an equitable allowance of remuneration, 'on a liberal scale', for his work and skill, and there was no appeal from this aspect of the decision. The Court of Appeal took a similar view in *O'Sullivan* v *Management Agency and Music Ltd* [1985] QB 428, with Dunn LJ observing that 'Although equity looks at the advantage gained by the wrongdoer rather than the loss to the victim, the cases show that in assessing the advantage gained the court will look at the whole situation in the round'.

The basis of the jurisdiction therefore appears to be a discretion in calculating the profit made by the defendant, in cases in which he has benefited the claimant through hard work. *O'Sullivan* extended the law in two respects: first, the Court of Appeal invoked the equitable jurisdiction even though the defendant was not, as he was in *Boardman* v *Phipps*, morally innocent; and second, the remuneration in *O'Sullivan* included even a reasonable profit element (but note that it was not related to the *actual* profits obtained in breach of fiduciary duty, which had to be accounted for).

The basis for the *quantum meruit* claim at common law is that of preventing unjust enrichment, while justification for applying it to trustees can be argued on implied contract reasoning, in which case it is simply a variation on the express contractual provision already considered. In that case, it ought not to be possible for a fiduciary to claim on a *quantum meruit* basis where the express contract would be void. The directors in *Guinness plc* v *Saunders* claimed an alternative *quantum meruit* entitlement, because they had, after all, through their skill brought about a takeover (of Distillers Co.) on favourable terms from which Guinness had undoubtedly benefited. They failed, in Lord Templeman's view, for precisely the same reasons as their claim in contract failed—that is, that the company had no power to authorize payment.

One way of reconciling *Guinness* v *Saunders* (in which Saunders also failed to claim an equitable allowance) with *Boardman* and *O'Sullivan* is that there may have been a conflict of interest. But *Boardman* is not entirely clear that there was not a conflict of interest and certainly raised questions about the existence of conflict—both 'technical' and more tangible—and so perhaps the least unsatisfactory explanation is that it is actually a question of degree of conflict of interest.

It is clear from this material that there are a limited number of circumstances in which trustees and other fiduciaries are entitled to payment. In none of these cases, however, is the amount of remuneration dependent on the manner in which the discretion (if any) of the trustee is exercised. Thus there can be no conflict between the interests of the trust and the personal interests of the trustee. We move on to consider the position in which a trustee (or other fiduciary) in fact gains from his position, and the issue now focuses on whether he is entitled to keep his gain.

13.4.3 Trustees and making profit from the trust

Lord Herschell's famous passage in *Bray* v *Ford* encourages us to think that a trustee should never put himself in a position in which there is any possibility that his duty and interest might conflict, and that because of this he should be required to account for (that is, pay over to the trust) any gains that he makes doing this, whether or not any conflict has actually occurred. This reasoning suggests that it should be immaterial that the trust does not suffer, or even if it gains, from the activities of the trustee, and would also suggest that if no possibility of a conflict arises, then there should be no requirement to account for a personal gain. If we were to use a different premise and say instead that any gains made by a trustee in the course of his duties are the property of the trust, then this would lead to a different outcome. In these circumstances, the trustee should be required to account for profits even if there is no possibility of a conflict of interest. The trustee should have to go further, and show that there is no causal connection between his position and any profit made by him (outside the payment categories outlined at section 13.4.2).

As we work through the cases, it will become clear that the law appears to have adopted this latter stricter position. Indeed, the cases suggest very strongly that, apart from the methods described whereby a trustee (or other fiduciary) becomes entitled to payment, a trustee will rarely, if ever, be allowed to profit from the office of trusteeship. The words 'rarely, if ever' are used deliberately, because although it is not clear beyond doubt, it does appear that trustees are never permitted to profit. And it is clear that whichever of these positions the law has adopted, the law is very strict.

Equity's approach to profit-making and the changing nature of trusteeship
In the course of this analysis, we will also consider whether equity's position is actually too strict, and whether a trust might actually lose out on account of the strong disincentives in place for trustees to go beyond the call of duty in furtherance of those interests that they are bound to protect. This proposition examines competing perspectives that such a position can stifle entrepreneurial conduct on the part of trustees because some of the cases will point directly to this. We will consider this from the viewpoint that this is inevitable if the law insists that a trustee is to exercise truly independent judgement—but perhaps the law accords too high a value to the principle of independence and attaches too little to the encouragement of initiative by trustees.

This discussion will explain that many equitable principles developed in the days when family settlements were the main variety of trust, and initiative was not therefore an especially valued asset in a trustee, and that for some it is inappropriate to apply them in today's 'trustee context'. On the other hand, a strict position provides law that is certain, and makes it clear what trustees may and may not do. And whatever the general principles actually stand for or should do, trustees are able to negotiate terms freely before accepting appointment.

Trying to get a measure of when liability to account will arise (and perhaps when it will not) will be pursued by looking, first, at what is suggested are the clearest cases of where liability arises: situations in which trustees (either directly or by analogy of litigation involving other fiduciaries) have acted in bad faith and liability has arisen. We will then consider cases in which liability has arisen in situations in which there is scope for conflict of personal interest and fiduciary duty, and then situations that suggest that liability will arise even in absence of scope for conflict. This will help us to get a sense of the extent to which the law might be insisting that a trustee must never profit from a trust, and must thus always account to the trust if he does make what are termed 'unauthorized' profits. As we will see when we consider *Boardman* v *Phipps*, profits are regarded as unauthorized when they have been procured without the informed consent of beneficiaries, suggesting that it is possible for beneficiaries to agree to allow this. However, this is uncommon in traditional trustee disputes, and it is clear that nothing less than fully informed consent will suffice. This is one area in which differences as between what is applicable to fiduciaries of different types can be seen, as shown in materials on the Online Resource Centre that discuss the quite different position of corporate fiduciaries extensively.

What follows now is a discussion of how, generally, liability for unauthorized gain becomes 'fixed' to a fiduciary who has breached the duty of loyalty, and when a breach of the duty of loyalty will be found to have arisen.

13.5 Unauthorized profit-making and the nature of liability

The materials in this section have long followed a particular pattern, reflecting that there has, until recently, been relative clarity on the basis of liability incurred once an unauthorized gain has been found and taking a much more open-textured approach to the scope of unauthorized profit-making. The latter continues to occupy much interest, particularly in the normative issues raised by judicial approaches taken, but it is also the case that the former has come very much to the fore recently.

13.5.1 The scope of liability for unauthorized profit-making

Until very recently, it has been possible—and even sensible—to consider the scope of unauthorized profit-making and its relationship with conflict of interest with duty closely together with the nature of liability that is incurred where this arises. This is because the cases show, generally, how the two key ideas run closely together. But recent developments now require us to deal with the two separately at this point in time, and the scope of liability will be dealt with first.

The clearest situation in which liability to account arises is in a case in which the unauthorized gain has arisen from 'wrongdoing' or bad faith on the part of the fiduciary. *Reading* v *Attorney-General* [1951] AC 507 concerned a British Army sergeant who made at least £19,000 illegally by helping smugglers to transport smuggled goods as a result of allowing them to ride in the lorries in his uniform. This profit was confiscated and Reading petitioned unsuccessfully for its return, because, as a fiduciary, he was liable to account for his profits to the Crown. An army sergeant would probably not normally be regarded as a fiduciary, but in this case Reading had used his uniform to deceive the authorities, and this seems to have been the decisive factor. This was followed in *Attorney-General* v *Guardian (No. 2)* [1990] 1 AC 109, the *Spycatcher* case, in which the *Sunday Times* was required to account for the profits that it had received from Peter Wright's deliberate breach of confidence.

Reading was also followed in *Attorney-General for Hong Kong* v *Reid* [1994] 1 AC 324, in which a fiduciary who accepted bribes was required to hold them on constructive trust for the Crown (his employer). *Reid* raises some important issues of scope, because the defendant was liable to account for the unauthorized gain itself and also property purchased with the 'secret commission', which extended to three houses purchased that had substantially increased in value. It is the recent reappraisal of *Reid* that now requires us to consider the nature of liability differently.

The presence of bad faith and the absence of harm?

Returning initially to questions of scope, it is not clear from these 'bad faith' cases that the Crown suffered any loss as a result of the unauthorized gain, and it appears that where there is bad faith, there need not be any harm to the claimant. An interesting example of this can be seen in *Industrial Development Consultants* v *Cooley* [1972] 1 WLR 443, in which the defendant, a managing director for the claimant company, had been negotiating on its behalf a contract with the Eastern Gas Board (EGB). The negotiations failed and it was apparent from the circumstances that the EGB was not at all happy about entering into dealings with Industrial Development Consultants (IDC) under any circumstances. Thus it appeared that, whatever Cooley himself had done, the negotiations between IDC and the EGB would have broken down. This meant that the claimant company IDC had actually suffered no loss from the personal gain that Cooley ultimately achieved for himself after the original negotiations between IDC and the EGB ceased.

After these original negotiations ceased, the EGB began negotiations with the defendant personally, with whom it wanted to work. The end result was that he terminated his contract with the claimant company, obtaining a release on the false representation that he was ill, and contracted with the EGB himself, on terms similar to those originally proposed on behalf of the claimant company. Roskill J held that the defendant was constructive trustee of the benefit of the contract for the benefit of the claimant company. It is noteworthy that the claimant company had lost nothing; in fact, as a result of the case, it gained a 'windfall' resulting from the defendant's breach of duty.

Beyond wrongdoing: conflict-of-interest cases

The wrongdoing cases may be an application of a wider principle that a fiduciary should not put himself into a position in which his duty and interest conflict; after all, a fiduciary accepting bribes or using his position to assist in illegal enterprise is manifestly failing to act with utmost loyalty. A conflict of interest was also assumed to exist in *IDC* v *Cooley*, since the defendant had negotiated for his own benefit in the claimant's time. But conflicts of interest can arise even in the absence of *mala fides*. There are two other clear situations in which a conflict of interest may arise between the trust and the personal interest of the trustee, which the law therefore prevents from arising: first, a trustee may not purchase trust property (or sell property to a trust); and second, he must not set himself up in competition with the trust.

Trustees may not purchase trust property

This rule relating to conflict of interest with duty arises from the way in which, although trustees will routinely sell trust property or make purchases of property for the trust, they will not be permitted either to purchase trust property for themselves or to sell their personal property to the trust. We will see the nature of the problem more clearly as we work through the cases, but essentially this rule exists because it creates obvious scope for conflict on the ground that both selling and purchasing in these circumstances will involve a personal dimension for the trustee that might interfere with his duty of loyalty to the trust.

The issues arising here can be seen from the way in which, in *Holder* v *Holder* [1968] Ch 353, Harman J sought to distinguish what is known as 'self-dealing' from 'fair dealing'. In the former situation, a trustee purchases trust property for himself or sells his property to the trust, and this renders the transaction voidable at the option of the beneficiaries. In the latter situation of 'fair dealing', in which a trustee purchases property from a beneficiary or sells his to one, a transaction is voidable only if the trustee has behaved unfairly. The distinction is not universally accepted, and both are arguably part of a wider principle that a trustee should not profit from his office as trustee.

The rationale for the self-dealing rule is that if a trustee purchases trust property, he can abuse his position and buy at less than the best price obtainable. Similarly, if he sells his own property to the trust, he may be able to demand too high a price. The self-dealing rule is very strict where trustees are concerned, so that there must be no *possibility* of the trustee taking advantage of his position, whether he does so in fact or not. The lengths to which the law goes are shown by *Wright* v *Morgan* [1926] AC 788, in which a trustee who had resigned his trusteeship purchased trust property at a price that had been fixed by independent valuers. One might have thought that not even a possibility of conflict arose here. The arrangements had been made while he was still trustee, however, and the Privy Council held that this sale must be set aside.

It is possible for purchases by trustees to be valid, but only in very exceptional circumstances. It is essential not only that the trustee paid a fair price, as he had in *Wright* v *Morgan*, but also that he took no advantage of his position and made full disclosure of his interest. For example, in *Holder* v *Holder* itself, an executor (Victor) purchased two farms that were part of an estate at a fair price at auction. The Court of Appeal refused to set aside the sale, although, as executor, Victor was acting in a fiduciary capacity. It was clear, however, that Victor had not been active in his role as executor, had indeed purported to renounce it, and had acquired no information as a result of it. He took no part in instructing the valuer who fixed the reserves or in the preparations for the auction. Additionally, the claimant beneficiary had accepted his share of the purchase money in full knowledge of the facts, and so was prevented from taking the action on the grounds of acquiescence.

However, in *Wright* v *Morgan*, both Sachs and Danckwerts LJJ doubted whether the self-dealing rule should apply today where trust property is sold at public auctions, at least in a case in which the sale is arranged by trustees other than the purchasing trustee. However, *Holder* v *Holder* was limited almost to its own unusual facts by Vinelott J in *Re Thompson's Settlement* [1986] Ch 99, a case that concerned the purchase of leases of farms, owned by a trust, by a company the director of which was one of the trustees. Vinelott J explained *Holder* v *Holder* on the narrow ground that the defendant had never acted as executor in a way that could be taken to amount to acceptance of a duty to act in the interests of the beneficiaries under his father's will. He said that the self-dealing rule is an application of the wider principle that a man must not put himself in a position in which duty and interest conflict, or in which his duty to one conflicts with his duty to another. If Vinelott J is right, *Holder* v *Holder* should not be regarded as laying down more than the narrowest of exceptions to the rule, and the same principles apply to sales of property to trusts by trustees.

Trustees must not set themselves up in competition with the trust

The principles that apply here are very similar to the foregoing because the trustee may gain for himself the benefit of any goodwill acquired by the trust, and possibly also useful information. It is not necessary to show that he has actually acquired such benefits, as shown in *Re Thomson* [1930] 1 Ch 203. In this case, an executor was restrained from carrying out a yacht-broking business in competition with the estate. Very interestingly, Clauson J did not think that the outcome would have been different even if the executor had resigned his office, as long as he had contemplated starting a competing business while he was still an executor. There is a logic in this approach, because such contemplation may have affected the manner in which his duties as executor were performed while he was in office. It has been argued that Clauson J's view depends on the specialist nature of the business, but it is difficult to see why this should make any difference. If this is so, then it is so for the law that applies to trustees more specifically, because for corporate fiduciaries there is clearly a much more modified approach to this aspect of conflict of interest and duty.

The scope of the rule against profiting from position: liability to account beyond bad faith or conflict of interest

It is not clear whether these cases are all part of a wider principle that a trustee (or other fiduciary) may not make any profit from his position, but if this is so, then for liability to arise, it should be necessary to establish a causal connection between the profit and the position. If this is so, it paves the way for liability to arise wherever this causal connection can be made, and that it will not be necessary to go further and show either *mala fides* or a conflict of interest. In *Re Macadam* [1946] Ch 73, trustees who used their position to appoint themselves to directorships of a company were held liable to account to the trust for all of the fees that they received as directors. This type of situation can commonly arise in private companies, because eligibility for appointment to directorships can depend on the legal ownership of a minimum number of shares, and indeed trustees may be under a duty to procure their representation on the board if it is necessary in order to safeguard the value of the trust shares.

If liability to account requires only a causal connection between position and profit, then it is significant that not even this was established in *Re Dover Coalfield Extension* [1908] 1 Ch 65, a case similar to *Re Macadam*, but in which a trustee had already become a director before becoming trustee. *Re Gee* [1948] Ch 284 is also similar, because a trustee became a director after refraining from using his vote, which he had by virtue of holding trust shares. He would have been elected anyway, on the basis of the votes of the other shareholders, but he had voted himself; he would even have been elected if he had voted against himself. Harman J held that the remuneration received as director did not have to be accounted for to the trust. In neither of these cases could it be said that the trustees had made any profit by virtue of their position. A closer examination of these cases suggests that they are, in reality, conflict-of-interest cases, since clearly a trustee who stands to gain from his own choice as director cannot advise the trust impartially as to the choice of who to appoint.

A more convincing example that liability will arise upon any causal connection of profit with position can be seen in *Keech v Sandford* (1726) Sel Cas Ch 61, in which the trustee took over the benefit of a lease that had been devised to the trust when that lease expired. Because the lease had expired, this is not a case of dealing in trust property, but the causal connection between position and profit was presumably established, in that he would not have been in a position to take the lease had he not been trustee. The lessor had refused to renew the lease for the trust, on the ground that the beneficiary was an infant, against whom it would be difficult to recover rent. The trustee thereupon took the lease for his personal benefit and profited from it. There cannot have been any actual conflict of interest, because the trust itself could not have benefited, given the views of the lessor, and nor would Lord King LC say that there was any fraud in the case. Yet he held that the trustee had to assign the benefit of the lease to the infant and account for profits received. According to Lord King, the trustee was the one person in the world who could not take the lease for his own benefit, because by so doing he would be profiting from his position. The same principle may apply where a trustee of a lease purchases for himself the freehold reversion, such as in *Protheroe* v *Protheroe* [1968] 1 WLR 519 (CA), but there are also contrary authorities.

A similar principle also appears to be at work in *Regal (Hastings) Ltd* v *Gulliver*, originally reported in [1942] 2 All ER 378 and only in the official reports in [1967] 2 AC 134n—or at least it does at first sight. Regal were considering applying for shares in a subsidiary company, but were unable to afford them, so the directors subscribed themselves and made a profit. The directors would not have been in a position to profit had they not been directors, but arguably there was no conflict of interest, given that Regal was not in a position to subscribe for itself. Yet the directors were held liable to account and, as Lord Russell of Killowen explained at 144:

> The rule of equity which insists on those, who by use of a fiduciary position make a profit, being liable to account for that profit, in no way depends on fraud, or absence of *bona fides*; or upon such questions or considerations as whether the profit would or should otherwise have gone to the plaintiff, or whether the profiteer was under a duty to obtain the source of the profit for the plaintiff, or whether he took a risk or acted as he did for the benefit of the plaintiff, or whether the plaintiff has in fact been damaged or benefited by his action. The liability arises from the mere fact of a profit having, in the stated circumstances, been made.

This is a fairly clear statement that all that needs to be established is the causal connection between position and profit. Arguably, however, there was in fact a conflict of interest, because the directors themselves must have determined that the company could not afford to subscribe for the shares. It would have been difficult for them to advise impartially where they intended to subscribe for themselves and hence obtain a profit.

Boardman *v* Phipps: *is liability to account a virtual certainty in all profit cases?*
Boardman v *Phipps* [1967] 2 AC 46 is authority that liability to account is a virtual certainty in all profit cases, but it is not actually clear on what principle it was decided. Boardman was solicitor to a trust, which owned 8,000 of 30,000 shares in a private textile company with the performance of which Boardman was dissatisfied. The trust had no wish to buy the remaining shares, and in any case was unable to buy them, although it could have applied to court for power to do so.

Boardman decided to purchase them himself, undoubtedly benefiting from information that he had received in his fiduciary capacity (in knowing what price to offer), and did not obtain the consent of all beneficiaries (on which, see further Chapter 14 and especially Chapter 16). The shares later increased in value (partly, perhaps, because of Boardman's management in selling off some of the assets of the newly acquired company), so Boardman made a large profit for himself. And because the trust still had a significant holding in the same company, his activities resulted in a large profit for the trust. There was no claim of bad faith, or any obvious conflict of interest, since the trust did not have the power to purchase the shares itself; in any case, the trust had positively benefited from Boardman's intervention.

By a three–two majority, the House of Lords nevertheless ruled that Boardman held the shares as constructive trustee for the trust, and was therefore liable to account for profits. This is one of the least clear *ratios* in trusts law, because it seems that whilst the majority thought it sufficient that Boardman had profited from the trust, Viscount Dilhorne and Lord Upjohn (dissenting) thought that this was insufficient in the absence of a clear conflict of interest, and took the view that there was no conflict nor even possibility for such.

Unfortunately, the position is muddied because the majority also took the view that there was a (somewhat theoretical) conflict of interest also: the trust might have changed its mind and sought to buy the shares itself, in which case Boardman, as solicitor to the trust, would have had to advise on the application to court. It may be, therefore, that the case does not extend existing principles, except in showing how willing the courts are to find even the most theoretical possibility of a conflict of interest.

A further difficulty with *Boardman* is that, in the Court of Appeal at [1965] Ch 992, Russell LJ had decided the case on an entirely different ground: that all of the information acquired by Boardman in his fiduciary capacity became trust property. Lords Hodson and Guest also seemed to be of this view. Lord Cohen appeared less sure about the trust property point, but was happy to decide the case on causation alone. The property reasoning raises serious difficulties (see, for example, Gareth Jones (1968) 84 LQR 472), especially where information is obtained by somebody who is trustee to several trusts, or where the information is passed on to other, innocent recipients who also profit from it. Partly for these reasons, Viscount Dilhorne, adopting the views of Lindley LJ in *Aas v Benham* [1891] 2 Ch 244, said that information was not the property of the trust, and Lord Upjohn's views were similar. Certainly, the 'information as trust property' reasoning is not part of the *ratio* in the House of Lords.

After Boardman: *is there conclusion and clarification in conflict of interest and duty?*

Although the *ratio* of *Boardman* is not very clear, the weight of authority probably supports the proposition that all that is required is to find a causal connection between the fiduciary's position and the profit obtained. If Boardman would have purchased the shares anyway, even without the information acquired by virtue of his fiduciary position, there would have been no causal connection between the position and the profit, and the case would have been like *Re Gee*. If not, the case is similar to *Re Macadam*, and Boardman was properly held to account.

Although this reasoning suggests that entrepreneurial activity on the part of trustees is undervalued, this reasoning falters rather where Boardman was liberally rewarded on a *quantum meruit* basis for benefiting the trust, on the principles already discussed. What he could not do was to keep any additional profits he made. The law allows private speculators to do so, but takes the view that those who are acting as fiduciaries accept, by taking on fiduciary positions, that their remuneration is limited to the categories described in section 13.4.2, however much they benefit the other party. Although this view may appear harsh, it at least has the merit of ensuring that their discretion will be exercised in an independent manner.

The arguments surrounding the continuing operation of the no-profit rule, as exemplified in *Boardman* (in the context of the unauthorized use of property or opportunities rightfully belonging to the trust), fit essentially into two broad interpretations of the result of the case—namely, its *justifications* and its *implications*. The rule against profiting from a position as fiduciary arises where the justifications in favour of it are strongly outweighed by the opposing position, in which it can be seen to stifle entrepreneurial activity unnecessarily. This might have the result of actually depriving the trust of the benefit of business expertise and acumen from which it might otherwise benefit greatly, as was the case in *Boardman* itself. On this reasoning, the operation of the rule against profit will ensure that the potential (and possibly considerable) benefits for the trust will not be forthcoming in light of the fact that trustees have no incentive to act in a manner that is entrepreneurial, because they are not able to benefit personally from doing so. Indeed, the rule represents an active disincentive for trustees to act in such a way.

The alternative reading of the rule against profiting by virtue of the position of fiduciary is that such a strict 'no profit' rule is required in the interests of certainty and preservation of the principle of fiduciary integrity—or the principle of disinterest that underpins the duty of loyalty.

Entrepreneurialism vs integrity: the same arguments?

The case law in the area of the governance of fiduciary relationships has consistently put at its heart the principle of disinterest. This is promoted as the only position that the law can realistically adopt in order to ensure fiduciary integrity. Indeed, if it were the case that some profits were regarded as being 'authorized' and others not, it would not only become more difficult on a conceptual level to defend the principle of fiduciary integrity, but it would also become impossible to demarcate such distinctions appropriately on a practical level. On such a line of argument (against interference with the principle of fiduciary integrity), this impossible middle way of regarding some profits as authorized whilst others remain unauthorized is also unjustifiable in light of trustees' ability to fix remuneration in advance, so as to avoid 'disappointment' (this was always possible through provision in the trust instrument, even before the enactment of the express power conferred by the Trustee Act 2000).

There are no right answers to the existence of the rule against unauthorized use of trust property, information, and opportunities; what is needed instead are new ways of looking at these two well-worn broad and opposing ideas. Here, materials on the Online Resource Centre discuss perspectives from within English trusts law, which itself promotes the liberalization of trusteeship, and apply these directly to rules relating to profit-making. It balances this with suggesting that this new liberalized context for trusteeship is the very reason why we should take a closer look at the very essence of the fiduciary position.

This draws, of course, on discourses within English law, but also beyond this—and centrally on US scholar Susan Shapiro's work on fiduciaries. This latter perspective draws on two key publications from Shapiro—(1987) 93 AJS 623 and (1990) 55 ASR 346—which can be used to strengthen resolve against profit-making, by providing new theoretical vigour to arguments against further empowering fiduciaries, which already operate in a context in which they benefit from a relationship that is already 'asymmetrical' and actually 'structurally duplicitous'.

Revolutions in trusteeship and the duty of loyalty

Whilst there might be an entreaty to consider the implications of the duty of loyalty in the light of twenty-first-century revolutions in trusteeship and the liberalization of some aspects of trusts law, the cases concerning the fiduciary character of trusteeship do point to a very definite appearance of the law as it stands. These cases suggest that whilst trusteeship and trusts law are becoming transformed in the twenty-first century in some respects, in its governance of trusteeship as a fiduciary office, equity appears to be unwavering in the position that it has adopted clearly since at least 1726 (with *Keech* v *Sandford* pre-dating *Bray* v *Ford* by over 150 years). The essence of *Keech* and *Bray* is seen very clearly in *Mothew*, and was recently restated in *Sinclair*. This is the requirement that trustees must act entirely impartially. As we have seen in these cases, ensuring that they do so is governed by positive rules, and these rules are construed extremely strictly so as to remove as far as possible any inclination that a trustee might have to disregard them.

However, *Sinclair* is also suggesting that perhaps the fiduciary relationship is not as sacrosanct as it might appear from the letter of the no-profit rule. This will now be explored in relation to the implications of its violation.

Unauthorized activity, but no fiduciary relationship

We now move from the scope of the duty of loyalty to the nature of liability for its breach, where we will encounter some very recent unsettledness and actually contention. But, mindful that the 'scope' materials show that liability will arise for unauthorized gains by some mechanism or another, there is an important preliminary point for understanding the nature of liability. This can be illustrated by reference to *Halifax Building Society* v *Thomas* [1996] 2 WLR 63, which also illustrates how fiduciary relationships can arise from the circumstances rather than involving parties in an established fiduciary relationship. Here, it was argued that a fiduciary relationship arose from the defendant mortgagor obtaining a 100 per cent mortgage on the basis of fraudulent misrepresentations. After he defaulted on repayment, the advancing building society argued that Thomas was liable to account for profits made on the property from the explosion of the property market as constructive trustee, given that the profits were the proceeds of fraud. The Court of Appeal held that liability to account for profits and the imposition of a constructive trust were not applicable where there was no fiduciary relationship between the parties. This position can also be seen at work in *Petrotrade Inc* v *Smith* [2000] 1 Lloyd's Rep 486.

13.5.2 The nature of liability for unauthorized profit-making

From these cases, it can be seen that equity will go to some lengths to ensure that any personal benefit from occupying fiduciary positions will not be retained. This is least contentious in cases of wrongdoing and 'clear' conflict of interest in absence of this, and arguably most contentious where there is no obvious conflict. But there is substantial support for liability to account for unauthorized fiduciary gain being cast as widely as possible as a manifestation of the need for positive prohibition because of the inherent vulnerability of the principal and the fragility of human nature, both elucidated by Lord Herschell in *Bray* v *Ford*.

From this, liability incurred is said to transform a fiduciary in receipt of such an unauthorized gain into a constructive trustee, who is not able to retain the benefit, but who holds it on behalf of persons who are properly entitled. In a conventional trust arrangement, this will, of course, be a beneficiary. This position would help to explain even the more contentious aspects of profit-making, such as 'opportunities' deemed rightly to belong to a principal and information 'as trust property' aspects of Boardman, as well as more straightforward ones arising from *Keech* and *Cooley*, and even *Gulliver*.

However, in this context of considering the basis of liability rather than its scope, the most problematic profits made are actually those arising from the most reprehensible conduct, and when looking at *Reading, Spycatcher,* and *Reid,* it was suggested that the Crown had suffered no loss as a result of the illegal conduct committed in each of those cases.

Liability to account for unauthorized gains and the attractions
of constructive trusteeship

Reading was found to be constructive trustee of his illicit gains, and in *Reid* constructive trusteeship was found to extend beyond the secret commission received and actually to property purchased with this. Central to this was the endorsement of the constructive trust in *Reid*, which involved decisive rejection of the contrary approach taken in *Lister & Co.* v *Stubbs* (1890) 45 Ch D 1. *Lister* was authority that liability for a bribe was personal and not proprietary, and thereby that a fiduciary's liability lies in paying over to his principal the value of the secret commission.

Lister explained that this was liability in the species of debt rather than that which incurred constructive trusteeship and, in holding this, the Court of Appeal appeared to attach significance to the bribe not having any antecedence as trust property. This does tie in with what has been said about the payment of secret commissions not exposing a principal to any loss, but this approach also has the implication that liability is limited to paying over the amount of the bribe.

On this reasoning, liability in *Reid* would have been limited to paying over to the Crown the value of the secret commission received by Reid, and would not have extended to liability to account for profits made on the property purchased with this. Thus, in *Reid*, the Privy Council took a very dismissive view of *Lister*, on the ground that the essence of the fiduciary relationship demanded that unauthorized profits are treated by equity as being obtained for the principal, regardless of their origin and antecedence. And *Reid* has since then been regarded as an authoritative statement of English law that liability arises by way of a constructive trust, with all of the implications of a proprietary action in terms of what can be brought within the scope of recovery (the key characteristics of which are considered in Chapter 17*).

A retreat from Reid*? The nature of liability after* Sinclair Investments

Reid can be found applied in a number of cases, including the Court of Appeal decision in *Hurstanger Ltd* v *Wilson* [2007] EWCA Civ 299. However, its supremacy has now been challenged by *Sinclair Trade Finance Ltd Investments Ltd* v *Versailles* [2011] EWCA Civ 347. *Sinclair* concerned the status of proceeds of sale in property dealings embroiled in fraud and sham transacting, and this depended on whether these proceeds were held on constructive trust *for* the original investment company *because* the director had breached his fiduciary duty as such by making a secret profit.

This case thereby reopened the question of whether a secret commission invokes personal liability to 'pay over', or whether it—and any profits generated by it—are held on constructive trust for a principal. In the Court of Appeal, it is Lord Neuberger's judgment that has attracted most attention, with seminal parts including his insistence that there was a line of consistent and reasoned authorities in favour of liability for a secret commission (as distinct from a proprietary interest or opportunity properly belonging to a beneficiary), and that in any case a fiduciary is accountable in equity only for property actually received in violation of the no-profit rule, which can be supplemented with equitable compensation where the principal experiences a 'quantifiable loss'. But, in attacking the very basis of *Reid*, Lord Clarke MR proposed in his judgment at 497:

[I]t seems to me that there is a real case for saying that the decision in *Reid* ... is unsound. In cases where a fiduciary takes for himself an asset which, if he chose to take, he was under a duty to take for the beneficiary, it is easy to see why the asset should be treated as the property of the beneficiary. However, a bribe paid to a fiduciary could not possibly be said to be an asset which the fiduciary was under a duty to take for the beneficiary. There can thus be said to be a fundamental distinction between (i) a fiduciary enriching himself by depriving a claimant of an asset and (ii) a fiduciary enriching himself by doing a wrong to the claimant. Having said that, I can see a real policy reason in its favour (if equitable accounting is not available), but the fact that it may not accord with principle is obviously a good reason for not following it in preference to decisions of this court.

Despite generating criticism that it allows too little incentive to fiduciaries to behave as equity demands they do, this approach can already be seen in a substantial body of case law, including *Cadogan Petroleum plc* v *Tolly* [2011] EWHC 2286, *FHR European Ventures LLP* v *Mankarious* [2011] EWHC 2999, *Horn* v *Commercial Acceptances Ltd* [2011] EWHC 1757 (Ch), and *Page* v *Hewetts Solicitors* [2011] EWHC 2449. However, in the Court of Appeal, *FHR European Ventures* [2013] EWCA Civ 17 noted the continuing controversies and invited the Supreme Court to rule on *Sinclair*'s authority.

Interestingly, the justifications for *Sinclair* do not appear to rest on the proper bounds of fiduciary activity, and emphasis can be found on the manner in which the finding of a trust can disadvantage the position of other claimants in the case of fraud and other wrongdoing. This is an important theme in the significance of trusts and equitable obligations for commercial dealings (alluded to in Chapters 3 and 5, and discussed extensively in Chapter 18), but the upshot of it could well be a liberalization of trusteeship, albeit that this is not obviously intended, in contrast with much of that occurring within the 'general duties' of trusteeship, discussed in this chapter and in Chapter 14. It can also be said to be indirect, by being entirely focused on (liberalizing) the consequences of trusteeship. These wider considerations remain to be explored, but one thing is clear: henceforth, it will be necessary to pay far closer attention to the nature of fiduciary misconduct giving rise to liability for unauthorized gains, and indeed the source and antecedence of the gain, in determining precisely what a principal is entitled to recover following breach of the duty of loyalty by a trustee or other fiduciary.

 Revision Box

1. In looking at the decision in *Boardman* v *Phipps* [1967] 2 AC 46, a case study for considering when liability will arise and when it should, ensure you are able to answer the following questions.
   (a) What is meant by a fiduciary relationship? Explain its key features.
   (b) What does this case suggest for the status of an unauthorized gain or profit in circumstances in which there is no wrongdoing and actual conflict of interest, and even absence of scope for conflict of interest?
   (c) What do the majority and dissenting judgments reveal about the proper scope of fiduciary accountability?
   (d) What arguments can be made both in favour of liberalizing the rules relating to profit-making and in maintaining a hard line against profit-making?
2. In looking at the decisions of *Attorney-General for Hong Kong* v *Reid* [1994] 1 AC 324 and *Sinclair Trade Finance Ltd Investments Ltd* v *Versailles* [2011] EWCA Civ 347, ensure that you are able to answer the following.
   (a) What different approaches can be taken to fixing liability for an unauthorized gain by a fiduciary?
   (b) What are the justifications for each of these approaches, and the merits and limitations associated with them?
   (c) What does *Sinclair* suggest about the future of liability attaching to an unauthorized gain or profit by a fiduciary?

FURTHER READING

Hayton (1990) 'Developing the law of trusts for the twenty-first century' 106 Law Quarterly Review 87.

Jones (1968) 'Unjust enrichment and the fiduciary's duty of loyalty' 84 Law Quarterly Review 472.

Shapiro (1987) 'The social control of impersonal trust' 93 American Journal of Sociology 623.

Shapiro (1990) 'Collaring the crime, not the criminal: reconsidering the concept of white-collar crime' 55 American Sociological Review 346.

This chapter is the first of three providing an extended and thematic study of how trusteeship arises, what the implications of trusteeship are, and what happens when the obligations of trusteeship are not complied with. Therefore it is difficult to isolate reading that overarches a number of these things into one chapter or another, and all pertinent reading will be listed at the end of Chapter 16.

14

···

Powers, discretions, and duties of trustees

The powers and duties at which we will now look follow on directly from the many references that have been made up to now, throughout this text, to trustees 'carrying out' a trust, and from more specific steer for this given in the previous chapter. From the very beginning, in Chapter 1, it was noted that trustees have legal title to property, but that they have nominal ownership of it because what they are required to do is look after it to ensure that those whom the settlor wishes to benefit from it will do so. At an early stage, it was noted that this would require active management of trust property and, by the time we looked at the constitution requirement, it was clear that trustees hold legal title so that they have the capacity to deal with trust property to the benefit of those entitled. When we looked at certainty requirements, we had a slightly different perspective on this, in as much as we learned that trustees need to be able to identify beneficiaries so that they can be located and property given to them. In the previous chapter, we learned that the law relating to trusteeship aims to ensure that trustees act properly when carrying out the trust and with only the interests of the beneficiary influencing their conduct. We also discovered then that they would be held to certain standards in carrying out the trust, and in turn it was intimated that this was very important because, in order to equip a trustee to use trust property to benefit others, his office carried with it a number of powers.

In this chapter, we learn more about what these powers actually are, and we will also learn about the way in which equity has tried to countervail these powers with constraints in the form of duties that accompany their exercise. This will, in time, anticipate the way in which any failure of a trustee to do what he is required to, and any commission of an unauthorized act by him, will amount to a breach of trust (which we consider in Chapter 16).

In this chapter, we encounter both powers and duties, and so it might be wise to think back to what we learned about the nature of powers in Chapter 2, and then in relation to certainty of objects in Chapter 3. This is because similar distinction exists between the duties of the trustee's office, on the one hand, and his powers and discretions arising from it, on the other. Trustees have discretion as to whether or not they will exercise a power and if, after proper consideration, they decide in good faith not to exercise it, then the beneficiaries have no ground for complaint. This is not the position with duties, because generally (although this becomes significant when we consider trustees' liability) where there is a duty to act in a particular way, this is not discretionary, and the statutory duty of care under s. 1 of the Trustee Act 2000 will apply to all of the duties that are specified as subject to it in Sch. 1 to the Act.

In view of the different types of situation in which trusts come into being, it is only to be expected that powers and duties will vary according to the character of the trust—for example, whether the trustees are required to accumulate or distribute the income and so on. However, it will be seen that some kinds of power are, in principle, widely available to trustees. Most of these are now statutory in nature and they are chiefly concerned with facilitating the management of the trust. For example, there will be much attention given to the trustees' obligation to invest the funds of the trust according to powers of investment conferred on them by the trust instrument or the Trustee Act 2000. They must also ensure the proper payment of tax and, at some stage, they may well have to consider matters such as the sale of trust property or making provision for infant beneficiaries. Accounts of trust business must be kept and copies supplied to the beneficiaries; in this vein, it is usual and desirable for trustees to meet in order to transact trust business, and records of such meetings must be minuted in a diary or minute book.

The duties of trustees will vary considerably, and some duties will frequently be modified by the trust instrument itself. Others, such as the duty to make proper distribution of trust property, are inherent in the nature of any trust, although even here the trust instrument may limit the personal liability of the trustees in the event of breach of trust. There are also certain fundamental duties that are fiduciary in character—namely, the duty of loyalty, carrying with it the duty not to profit from the trust—and which will apply to all trustees. Other common duties will include the safe keeping of trust property, the proper custody of documents of title, investments, etc. It will also become clear later that trustees have certain duties towards the beneficiaries. These include the duty to inform them of their rights and provide information regarding the affairs of the trust, and the duty to distribute the property in accordance with entitlements to it. They must also consider the need to maintain fairness between the beneficiaries.

Before starting to look at the powers that are given to trustees to equip them to carry out the trust in accordance with the settlor's instructions, and duties that are imposed to ensure that they do so properly, reference to the settlor and his instructions does actually provide a very important introduction to this general discussion. This is because most of these general powers and duties will, in practice, be modified (limited or enhanced) or excluded by the express terms of a particular trust in question. This is very significant because most express trusts today are created by deed of settlement or will, will be prepared with expert legal advice, and will generally seek to give the trustee the widest powers possible. This is often because 'tax saving' is a very important motivating force for creating trusts, and so a settlement will want to equip a trustee with as much scope to achieve maximum gains for the trust property; so the general law has much more application to older and less professionally oriented trusts. It is also the case that trustees themselves will be able to influence the scope of their powers and particularly the limitations of their duties, as we will discover when we consider trustee exemption clauses (TECs) in Chapter 16.

It will be apparent that the administration of all but the simplest of trusts calls for a considerable degree of business competence, and nowadays most trusts of any size will have a professional trustee, such as a bank or trust corporation, to act for them. The professional may act either as a sole trustee or in conjunction with one or more individuals. This sort of mixture can be useful in family settlements, combining the expertise of the professional with the more intimate knowledge of family circumstances supplied by the private trustee. However, it should also be noted here that the powers and duties described in this chapter apply to express trusts, under which trusteeship has been voluntarily undertaken, and increasingly by paid professionals who no longer simply freely accept trusteeship, but actively seek it as a business activity.

This point is made to clarify the different position of constructive trustees, who have trusteeship imposed on them by equity. The scope of their empowerment, and particularly the extent of their duties, is unclear. It is difficult to determine the extent to which the statutory duty of care applies to them, with it being very difficult to reason this from the vast number of very disparate circumstances in which constructive trusteeship arises. One view of this is that this militates against the application of the duty of care on account of the fact that, at the most extreme end of the constructive trust's operation, a person can become such a trustee without knowing it and remains ignorant until the matter is determined by the court. In the absence of definitive guidance, it must also be noted that an argument in favour of the duty applying to a constructive trustee can be made from the way in which the legislation expresses the duty of care applying to trustees exercising the powers prescribed 'however conferred'.

We shall now take a look at some key duties that arise for trustees in carrying out a trust, before moving on to how they are empowered to do them. We will then look at investment as a case study for how power and duty interact specifically.

14.1 An overview of trustees' duties

In many respects, we can see the duties that arise for trustees as countervailing forces for the empowerment that they have in order to work for the good of the trust. We have already considered fiduciary duties, which set out the core obligation of loyalty for trustees, and it has already been suggested that this is an example of a duty that cannot be modified in any way, shape, or form. We need to bear this in mind, of course, but the focus of this chapter is duties that arise in the everyday running of a trust. There are a number of possible starting points for this, including duties that arise in relation to how trustees must act in relation to the beneficiaries when carrying out a trust.

14.1.1 General duties focused on beneficiaries themselves

This is very significant for framing our ideas on what trustees are compelled to do, because although a beneficiary is entitled to enforce the trust, and indeed is the only one in a position to do so, it will become apparent that this does not translate directly into exerting control over what is happening, or even having to be informed about what is happening. This is because a trustee's instructions come from the settlor who created the trust in the first place. As we know from Chapter 1, one of the reasons for creating a trust is that it gives an owner of property control not only over who benefits from this, but also over how this is achieved. This means that it is the settlor's instructions that a trustee is duty bound to carry out, and there is no principle in support of beneficiary control over how the trust is carried out. This is a position of principle in as much as it respects the settlor's wishes, but it is also pragmatic, because a trustee who is compelled to carry out the trust might become hopelessly handicapped in fulfilling this overriding duty towards the trust as a whole if beneficiaries were to have much steer. Thus the court will never compel the trustees to act under orders from the beneficiaries where a power or discretion has been entrusted to the trustees alone. This will hold as long as the trust continues, although if the beneficiaries collectively wish to do so, they can bring the trust to an end and resettle the property on any terms that they wish, under the *Saunders* v *Vautier* doctrine (after *Saunders* v *Vautier* (1841) 10 LJ Ch 354, which is considered further in Chapter 15).

In this regard, *Tempest* v *Lord Camoys* (1882) 21 Ch D 571 shows that, whilst a trust is operational, the court will not interfere with a trustee's bona fide decision making. But whilst trustees have no obligation even to consult with the beneficiaries as to how a power or discretion should be exercised (apart from under the Trusts of Land and Appointment of Trustees Act 1996, as a result of which trustees are under a statutory duty to consult beneficiaries in possession and to give effect to their wishes so far as is consistent with the general intentions of the trust), they will in practice do so.

The courts' mindfulness in protecting trustees from zealous beneficiaries extends this general position to trustees' obligations to discourse reasons for decision making, with *Re Beloved Wilkes's Charity* (1851) 3 Mac & G 440 as authority that trustees are not compelled to give reasons for exercising powers or discretions that are conferred to them. It was held that, in the absence of evidence that the trustees had exercised their discretion unfairly or dishonestly, the court would not interfere. This will present problems for a beneficiary wishing to challenge a decision made by trustees, because if trustees are not required to give reasons for their decisions, it will generally be impossible to know whether they have exercised their discretions in a proper manner. This does not instinctively feel compatible with equity's recognition that trusteeship is a powerful office, and one in which custodians of trust property must act properly.

Where trustees do declare their reasons

In what has to be a huge disincentive for trustees to disclose the reasons behind their actions, where they choose to do so, the court may consider their adequacy. In *Klug v Klug* [1918] 2 Ch 67, a trustee whose daughter was a beneficiary refused to consider the exercise of a power of appointment in her favour, and from the correspondence it appeared that her reason was annoyance that the daughter had married without her consent. Neville J held that the trustee had not exercised her discretion at all, and that it was the duty of the court to interfere. Where the trustees take steps to keep the basis of their decisions private, however, there appears to be little that a beneficiary can do if the decision is not obviously unreasonable or fraudulent.

Beneficiary access to matters of 'trust business'

This leads to the question of whether the beneficiaries are entitled to have access to any written records of how the trustees have conducted the trust business. It is usual practice for trustees to keep a trust diary or minute book in which they record decisions affecting the trust, but there is no requirement that the reasons for trustees' decisions should be recorded. Traditionally, however, beneficiaries have been entitled to access to documents connected with the trust, known as 'trust documents', and indeed have been considered to have a proprietary interest in such documents. If those documents were to disclose the reasons for a decision, this would seem to offer the beneficiaries a way around the difficulty that trustees will not be compelled to disclose reasons. In *Re Londonderry's Settlement* [1965] Ch 918, the Court of Appeal effectively closed this door. A beneficiary who was dissatisfied with the sums appointed to her by trustees pressed them to disclose various documents connected with the settlement, and the trustees sought directions from the Court. The Court of Appeal considered that 'trust documents' had not previously been defined with any degree of clarity, and concluded that all documents held by trustees *qua* trustees are prima facie trust documents, but that documents containing confidential matters about which a beneficiary is not entitled to know should not be disclosed, either (in the view of Harman J) because they are protected by analogy with the rule that trustees need not disclose reasons, or (according to Salmon LJ) because a document that a beneficiary is not entitled to see cannot be a trust document.

From this, it would appear that a beneficiary is forced to bring a hostile action, which is fraught with difficulties not least because it will hinge on a beneficiary having substantial evidence of misconduct. It is not obligatory, or even usual, to have trust accounts subjected to an audit, but this may be done at the absolute discretion of the trustees, who may employ an independent accountant and charge the costs to the trust fund. By s. 22(4) of the Trustee Act 1925, an audit is not to be carried out more frequently than once every three years, unless the nature of the property or other special difficulties so require. Any trustee or beneficiary may apply for an investigation and audit of the trust accounts by virtue of s. 13 of the Public Trustee Act 1906. A copy of the auditor's report is supplied to the applicant and to each trustee.

Although it is clear that beneficiaries do have the right to see such trust documents, it is not entirely clear that this arises in the way in which it is traditionally explained in *Re Londonderry* on the basis that these are 'trust property' and thus entitled to be distributed through access being made available. This is on account of the decision in *Schmidt* v *Rosewood Trust* [2003] UKPC 26. This decision suggests that a beneficiary's right to these documents arose from the court's inherent jurisdiction to ensure that the trust was properly administered, and so access is actually governed by the court's discretion to refuse or grant this as the circumstances are appropriate. This appears to be supported by the decision in *Breakspear* v *Ackland* [2008] Ch 220, which is authority that the courts will refuse access to matters that are regarded as confidential, and a trustee has declined access and even refused to give reasons for this. Given that the courts' inherent jurisdiction, as explained in *Schmidt*, is concerned with the proper supervision and performance of trusts, it is not clear where this leaves beneficiaries who suspect that something is amiss, which is why they have sought access to records of 'trusts business' in the first instance. But it does also reinforce the point that trustees are required—and indeed duty-bound—to carry out the trust properly, and that in some instances zealous beneficiaries might be able to undermine this by burdening trustees with their requests to be informed.

14.1.2 Judicial control over trustees' discretions: the rule in *Re Hastings-Bass*

Notwithstanding the approaches to trustees' decision making above, the rule in *Re Hastings-Bass* [1975] Ch 25 operates to ensure that where a trustee has not exercised a power or has exercised a power inappropriately, this can be overturned by the courts. This will have the effect that the power will be considered to have been exercised in the former situation and its exercise will be considered void in the latter. As seen in *Mettoy Pensions Trustees* v *Evans* [1990] 1 WLR 1587, the rule in *Re Hastings-Bass* has traditionally been applied in situations in which it is found that the trustee would have acted differently had he taken into account factors that should have been taken into consideration, or had he not taken into consideration factors that should not have been considered.

Where this rule is invoked, this will have the effect that the course of action that should have been taken is deemed to have been taken, as seen applied in *Abacus Trust Co. (Isle of Man)* v *NSPCC* [2001] STC 1344, with *Abacus Trust Co. (Isle of Man)* v *Barr* [2003] ChD 409 and *Sieff* v *Fox* [2005] 3 All ER 693 considering what must be present for it to be invoked. Fundamentally, *Barr* requires for there actually to be a breach of trust, and that a trustee's decision will not be declared invalid merely on account of ignorance or mistake on the part of the trustee, which does not amount to a breach, however unforeseen or unpalatable the consequences of this mistake or incomplete information might be. More is said about breach of trust in Chapter 16, but once the rule has been invoked, *Sieff* suggested that, in most situations, the appropriate question was one of whether a trustee *would* actually have decided differently, but could extend to situations in which he *could* have acted differently.

Much of this concern with the relevant question of 'would' or 'could' appeared to be related to the position of pension trusts, which are, as we know from Chapter 7, 'special arrangements' under which beneficiaries provide consideration for rights enjoyed under a settlement, rather than being in the position of 'windfall' recipients of another's generosity.

A number of decisions in addition to those above demonstrated this to be a very much 'live' response to trustee decision making including *Gallaher* v *Gallaher* [2004] EWHC 42, *Burrell* v *Burrell* [2005] EWHC 245, *Betafence* v *Veys* [2006] EWHC 999 (Ch), [2006] All ER (D) 91, and *Donaldson* v *Smith* [2007] WTLR 421, prior to *Pitt* v *Holt; Futter* v *Futter* [2011] EWCA Civ 197. In *Pitt*, the Court of Appeal re-examined the scope and application of the rule in *Hastings-Bass*. At the time of writing, this case had been granted permission to appeal to the Supreme Court, but the outcome of the Court of Appeal case was to put strict limits on the rule in *Hastings-Bass*, and in future it will be much more difficult for trustees to succeed in applying to the Court to set aside actions that later turn out to have unforeseen and adverse consequences.

14.1.3 The duty to act even-handedly as between beneficiaries

So there is considerable variation in what beneficiaries are entitled to know about how trustees carry out the trust and in the documentation that they are permitted to access, but there is no question that a trustee is duty-bound to act even-handedly as between beneficiaries. This has two dimensions to it: even-handedness between beneficiaries per se; and even-handedness between different types of beneficiary under a trust arrangement. The general requirement that trustees act in an even-handed way to all those entitled under a trust flows from the way in which, as we studied certainty-of-objects requirements, we saw that trustees are fiduciaries who are expected to carry out the trust in a rational manner that is based on a sound understanding of the terms of the trust and the class of objects under it. This means that it is not open to trustees to show favouritism to any particular beneficiary on account of his own 'quirks', and that exercising of powers and discretions must be consistent with holding fiduciary office even if, as we have discovered, it may not be straightforward for a beneficiary to raise a complaint because the court will not ordinarily force trustees to explain their actions or produce evidence for them (apart from trust accounts). There are also considerations that flow from the way in which Chapter 1 suggested that settling property on trust enables property to be used not only to benefit a number of people, but also to benefit them successively.

The duty to act even-handedly where there are different types of beneficiary
Nothing further was said about using property to provide so-called 'successive benefits' in Chapter 1, but now we need to understand that creating successive benefits from property means that there are not only different beneficiaries that a trustee must consider in order to act even-handedly, but also different types of beneficiary to consider. In explaining what we might mean by 'benefits of property that are successive', as the term suggests, these are benefits from property—or interests in trust property—that will take effect after one another. This will work whereby one type of benefit or 'interest' will come into being as another comes to an end. This creation of a successive interest became known as making a 'settlement', which is from where we get the term. There is also more terminology that we need to understand, which flows from the way in which, as we discovered in Chapter 2, the first modern trusts were trusts of land; this is where we see first the creation of successive interests in property. This meant that what became subject to these settlements (successive interests) were benefits from (or interests in) property that was land.

This is very significant for the titles given to beneficiaries in a scheme in which there are successive interests, which can be explained by reference to a typical arrangement within such settlements. Here, property will be settled on trust for one (type of and possibly numerical) beneficiary, and then for others (and a different type of beneficiary) upon the death of the former. Such an arrangement will typically be expressed as 'for the benefit of A for life, then to B for life, and then to C and D equally'. And because this arrangement was developed around land, the person who is 'A for life' is known as a 'life tenant' under a settlement, while those who receive the property following A's death are known as 'remaindermen', which is language that will be familiar from studying the law of real property. This is the typical traditional arrangement, but successive interests can be created in any type of property and for any 'chunk' of time, provided that the arrangement does not infringe perpetuity requirements. However these are configured, the existence of successive interests in property does raise special considerations for how a trustee fulfils his duty to act even-handedly towards all beneficiaries.

Tensions arising in the duty to act even-handedly

We will come back to the decision in *Nestlé* v *National Westminster Bank* [1993] 1 WLR 1260 when looking at the significance of investment of trust assets, but for present purposes it introduces the duty to act even-handedly amongst beneficiaries and the more fundamental point that not all beneficiaries will have the same interests in (even the same) trust property. In prefacing this with the wide discretion that trustees have in relation to investment (which is discussed shortly), *Nestlé* insists that a trustee 'must act fairly in making investment decisions which may have different consequences for differing classes of beneficiaries'. Even the quite different reading of 'the so-called duty to act impartially' emerging from *Edge* v *Pensions Ombudsman* [2000] Ch 602—that this is actually nothing more complex than requiring trustees to exercise discretion properly—leaves no doubt that there will commonly be different 'beneficiary interests' for a trustee to balance.

How a trustee achieves this will introduce us to further terminology, which is used to classify different beneficiary types in arrangements with successive interests, and in anticipation of this we need to understand the scope of the duty to act in an even-handed way towards beneficiaries. This requires a trustee not only to have regard to the beneficiary whose interest is 'live' at any given time, but he must also consider those who will come to benefit in the fullness of time—another life tenant, if there is one, and then those who will receive the property absolutely eventually. So how does a trustee consider prospectively the interests of those with more distant benefits and who are not entitled to the property as yet in relation to someone whose interest currently exists? We get a clue as to how this is achieved from learning what these different beneficiary types are termed in addition to 'life tenants' and 'remaindermen'. The way in which these beneficiary types are also termed, respectively, 'income beneficiaries' and 'capital beneficiaries' also helps us to understand what issues arise for a trustee in fulfilling his duty to be even-handed as amongst all beneficiaries.

Essentially, those who are life tenants are known as 'income beneficiaries' because they are entitled to the income benefits generated by the management of trust property. We will look closely at investment shortly, whereupon it will become clear that a trustee is duty-bound to safeguard trust assets, and then he is empowered to do this to try to maximize what can be 'earned' on trust assets. In this context, an income beneficiary is entitled to income that arises from a trustee's duty to safeguard trust assets and which is earned on trust property. Precisely how income is generated will depend on what type of property is subject to the trust (either because that is what has been given by a settlor, or because a trustee has exercised his power to acquire more suitable property for the trust, on which more is said shortly). In Chapter 2, it was suggested that trust property is commonly shares; in this case, income will be dividends earned on the shareholding rather than the shares themselves, and where the trust property is one of a number of financial instruments, then what is earned by way of income will be interest. Perhaps the easiest way in which to understand this is to use the example of trust property that is land: in this situation, rent that is generated on the property will be income, whilst the property itself—a house or a flat, or even commercial property—is the capital asset.

Giving the example of the way in which land can be both a source of income and a capital asset does lead neatly to the way in which, in managing trust property, a trustee is required to select property or ways of dealing with it that will generate sufficient income for a life tenant, and also be capable of delivering capital benefits to the remainderman. If this is not a challenge enough in itself, it is also the case that the investment strategies required for each of them are not always compatible. This is because an income beneficiary will be keen for investment to make maximum yield over a shorter term and will be less concerned about longer-term considerations, whilst the remainderman has the opposite interest. The trustee must manage both by taking certain steps to ensure that a fair balance is maintained between the capital and income of the trust. This is to ensure that capital is preserved for those entitled in the future, while at the same time allowing a reasonable income to those currently entitled. The rules relating to apportionment arise from this principle, and although it is nowadays usual practice to exclude their operation where possible, they are by no means without relevance, particularly in their application to accretions to the trust fund. It has been said that, in special circumstances, the court itself may direct an apportionment (*Re Kleinwort's Settlement* [1951] Ch 860), but this does not appear to have been done in practice. It is also the case that the Law Commission has recently looked at this matter, and so having some background on traditional rules is useful for understanding current debate and policy.

Apportionment and Howe v Earl of Dartmouth

Some types of property are inherently unsuited to being held for successive interests. A wasting asset, which will soon be used up, provides no benefit to the remainderman, whilst one on which interest may not accrue for many years (such as a reversionary interest in land) will provide no present income for the life tenant. Settlors might not fully appreciate this when generously deciding to give the benefits of property to others on trust, or that the 'investment value' of a particular type of property might dramatically change in different market conditions. In these circumstances—however they might arise—the obvious course of action for a trustee who must achieve fairness as between the beneficiaries is often to sell the property, and to invest the proceeds in something more suited to providing an income for the life tenant and an addition to capital for the benefit of the remainderman. There will not be any difficulties here if the trust instrument directs a trustee to do this. Here, *Howe* v *Earl of Dartmouth* (1802) 7 Ves Jr 137 compels trustees to sell in other circumstances, even if there is no express direction, in some testamentary trusts of personal property (but not land), and where there is no contrary intention expressed in the will.

Where a duty to convert (that is, to sell) arises under this principle, the normal date at which the property should be converted is one year from the death of the testator— that is, at the end of the 'executors' year' allowed for the administration of the estate to be carried out. If there is power to postpone the sale and conversion, however, this cannot apply, and the valuation for the purposes of apportionment is taken to be the date of the death. It will usually not be possible to convert and reinvest on either of these specific dates, so some principle is needed for apportioning the income from the asset until actual conversion. This is unnecessary if there is a clear intention that the tenant for life should have the actual income, or if the property is realty (and so not subject to the rule in *Howe* v *Earl of Dartmouth*) and no contrary intention appears, in which event the life tenant will receive the actual income. This is because otherwise complex actuarial calculations are required, which turn on the precise nature of the property.

For property that produces no present income, such as a reversionary interest, the principles deriving from the decision in *Re Earl of Chesterfield's Trusts* (1883) 24 Ch D 643 apply, and apportionment between capital and income is calculated by a formula. In effect, an assumption is made of 4 per cent interest, compounded annually. Suppose that the property produces £1,000 at sale. The capital element will be the amount which if invested at 4 per cent compound interest would have produced £1,000: this will be less than £1,000, and the income will be the rest. Where the asset produces income, the life tenant is entitled to 4 per cent of its value as interest, and if extra income is actually produced, it accrues to capital. There is also a formula, based on an assumption of 4 per cent compound interest, for apportioning the payments of liabilities out of the fund (such as funeral expenses, and settling debts of the testator) to capital and income. This formula derives from *Allhusen* v *Whittell* (1887) LR 4 Eq 295. It seems likely that none of these formulae could easily be applied without employing the services of an accountant, to the obvious detriment of the fund, which is one reason why they are in fact frequently ignored.

Income and capital, apportionment, and law reform
Other difficulties are that the value of specific proportions and percentages does not transfer well over different periods of time, especially in climates of economic instability. This gives trustees real difficulty in determining whether to go with what is set out or to try to calculate a more realistic value. The law here is dominated by a number of equitable principles developed through case law, which, as the Law Commission's report on *Capital and Income in Trusts: Classification and Apportionment* (Law Com. 315) noted in 2009, reflect the presumed intention of a settlor or testator who creates successive interests in property that life tenants and remaindermen should enjoy the benefits of the trust equally. As a lone statutory provision, there is also s. 2 of the Apportionment Act 1870, which provides that income beneficiaries are entitled only to the proportion of income that is deemed to have accrued during the period of entitlement. However, a number of the equitable rules are disapplied from modern trusts and there has long been talk of replacing these with a statutory duty of a more general nature. This would be to hold a fair balance between beneficiaries, with express power to trustees to convert capital to income and vice versa, and a duty to have overall regard to the investments of the trust. The effect of this, if enacted, would be to simplify the actuarial calculations required in these situations.

In 2004, the Law Commission published its Consultation Paper on *Capital and Income in Trusts: Classification and Apportionment* (CP No. 175). It was described by the Law Commission as a project to reform the complicated rules governing:

(1) classification of trust receipts and outgoings as 'capital' or 'income'; and

(2) the requirement that trustees apportion capital and income in order to keep a fair balance between different beneficiaries.

And in connecting this directly with the foregoing equitable rules, the Law Commission noted in its 2009 report that whilst all of the traditional rules are 'theoretically logical and sensible developments of the classification rules and the duty to balance', they are commonly excluded from express trusts because they require complex calculations relating (usually) to relatively—or even very—small sums.

The remit of the consultation, in this respect, has arisen from the reappraisal of trusteeship that arose from the Trustee Act 2000. This text has already made many references to this far-reaching modernization of the office of trustee, which did, of course, include provisions relating to investment of trust assets. However, the Law Commission noted in its 2004 Consultation Paper that at the time when the (then) Trustee Bill was heading towards becoming law, concerns were expressed as to whether the Act would 'tackle the difficulties caused in the management of trust estates by the distinction which trust law draws between income and capital' (para. 1.5).

In the Consultation Paper, the Law Commission identified the principal issues arising from its consideration of how income and capital are classified in trusts law as follows. First, in relation to private trusts, these would be an appraisal of the rules that govern trusts receipts as income or capital, and consideration of the statutory and equitable rules that require conversion of the original trust property or apportionment between the capital and income accounts. Thereafter, the Law Commission intended to consider the impact of these rules on charities.

Following the project's suspension in 2007 on account of the cohabitation project, the Law Commission's report was published in 2009, in which the Law Commission reiterated that it regarded the remit of this project as being:

> ... to examine the complicated rules governing the treatment of trust receipts and outgoings as capital or income and the extent to which trustees who have to distinguish between income and capital should be able to invest on a 'total return' basis, with reference particularly to trusts for interests in succession and to charitable trusts with permanent endowment.

The recommendations of the report can be found summarized on the Online Resource Centre, where there is also discussion of the Trusts (Capital and Income) Act 2013, which received Royal Assent on 31 January 2013.

14.2 Powers and discretions arising from trusteeship

There is a considerable variety of powers and discretions that equity has conferred (and which, over time, statute has enshrined) designed to allow a trustee scope for providing benefit for those entitled to trust property. There are those that relate to general matters associated with an active trust and also ones directed at more specific aspects of this.

14.2.1 Powers arising that relate to general matters in trusts administration

In this regard, power to sell some or all of the trust property is usually given by the trust instrument, either expressly or by implication, and even in the absence of such power trustees will often be permitted to sell by statute, or as a last resort by order of the court.

Because this has applied to property that is land traditionally, we have had to learn about trusts arising from the Settled Land Act 1925 and also statutory trusts for sale. However, in the former case, this is such a rare occurrence that it is hardly a mainstream consideration anymore, and statutory trusts for sale (which contained a duty to sell, with an implied power to postpone) have now been replaced by ones under the Trusts of Land and Appointment of Trustees Act 1996, which gives trustees wide powers of sale, but (unlike the predecessor trust for sale) not duties to sell. In relation to personal property, the Trustee Act 1925 contained a number of provisions for the sale, which authorize sale of trust property by trustees (including its s. 16) in situations in which no such power was expressly or impliedly given in the trust instrument itself. However, under the new regime, there is no statutory power of sale except in the case of trusts of land, and the Trustee Act 2000 does not include any provision authorizing the sale of (personal) property except for the purposes of varying investment.

In dealings with trust property, and closely connected with the sale of trust property and the acquisition of property to enhance a trust's performance, it would be of little value to be able to sell trust property unless the purchaser were able to obtain a valid receipt for the transaction. Thus s. 14 of the Trustee Act 1925 gives a power, notwithstanding anything to the contrary in the trust instrument, to issue an effective receipt. The receipt of such a receipt in writing from a trustee operates to exonerate the purchaser from any obligation to ensure that the trustees apply the money received in accordance with the trust. This is very important from the perspective of the purchaser, because his awareness that the property he has purchased is the subject of a trust might otherwise be taken to ensure that he holds it as constructive trustee under the equitable notice doctrine.

Trustees are also empowered, and indeed expected, to acquire trust property where this is appropriate; the power to acquire land is conferred by provisions within Pt III of the Trustee Act 2000. These new powers are extensive, and apply to the purchase of leasehold and freehold land. By the provision of s. 8, such purchases can be made for the purposes of investment, for occupation by a beneficiary, or for any other purpose. By the provisions of s. 8(3), the trustee is given all of the powers of an absolute owner, and this is a significant specific power because the purchase of land, other than loans that are secured on land, is an exception to the general power of investment (see 'The general power of investment: s. 3'), which allows a trustee to make any investment as he could do if he were absolutely entitled to the property. The trustee is subject to the duty of care in s. 1 in the exercise of these powers. And, in this vein, s. 34 of the Trustee Act 2000 gives trustees wide powers to insure trust property, which reflect that predecessor provisions under s. 19 of the Trustee Act 1925 were regarded as being very restrictive by limiting this power to insuring against loss or damage by fire, but not against other very important insurable risks. This very limited power stemmed from the fact that 1925 pre-dated many forms of insurance that are available to (and increasingly regarded as being indispensable within) commercial dealings. The exercise of this power is now subject to the statutory duty of care.

We have already seen that, in carrying out the trust, trustees may wish to have the assistance of others, and we have already learned (in Chapter 13) that there are a number of 'delegable functions' under s. 11 of the Trustee Act 2000 that can be collectively delegated by the trustees to others. This is part of the new regime for the appointment of agents, custodians, and nominees under Pt IV of the Act. Here, we can find wide powers for the holding of trust property by custodians and nominees. Perhaps most important under this head is the new statutory duty in Sch. 1, para. 3, under which trustees must labour in the appointment of agents, custodians, and nominees, while s. 22 places upon trustees the duty to review the activities of this category of delegatee. Over and above compliance with these duties for the appointment and review of such persons, by the provision of s. 23 of the Trustee Act 2000, trustees incur no liability for any default committed by agents, custodians, or nominees so appointed. Trustees are themselves subject to the statutory duty of care in validly delegating to others.

The power to compound liabilities arises from the way in which, as the legal owner of the property, a trustee has the right to maintain an action with regard to the trust property. Where the claim itself is a legal claim, it will be the case that it is only the trustee as legal owner who can sue. This is very important, particularly where debts are owed to the trust. Notwithstanding this, litigation is still a risky business, perhaps especially so in the pursuit of debts owed, in which instance it is far from clear that there will be recovery of what is owed and there is expense entailed in the debts pursuit. To this end, s. 15 of the Trustee Act 1925 gives discretion to trustees in their dealings with persons who are in contention with the trust (commonly because they owe the trust money), and effectively allows trustees to weigh up litigation risk. When exercising this power under s. 15 of the Trustee Act 1925 (or any corresponding power, however conferred), trustees are subject to the statutory duty of care as provided by s. 1 of the Trustee Act 2000.

14.2.2 Powers arising from more specific aspects of an active trust

The powers of maintenance and advancement arise from the way in which trustees are able to use trust property for the benefit of those who are not yet entitled to benefit from any income or capital. This situation will arise for infants who will become entitled, but are not so yet, but who will require financial support during their minority. Here, we find statutory powers conferred by the Trustee Act 1925, relating to what we term 'maintenance' and also 'advancement', and the court also has inherent jurisdiction in this regard.

The statutory power of *maintenance* under s. 31 of the Trustee Act 1925 can arise only where the beneficiary is entitled to receive intermediate income under the trust. This will be the case either where his interest is vested or where it is a contingent interest that carries the intermediate income. If there are prior interests (that is, others are entitled to the benefit of the property prior to him) or if the beneficiary's interest is as a member of a class of discretionary beneficiaries, the power will not be available at all. Where income is available and the trustees have the discretion as to whether to maintain the beneficiary, s. 31 provides guidance on such matters as the age of the infant, the requirements that he may have, and the general circumstances of his case. Subject to contrary intention in the trust instrument, the power to maintain ceases when the infant obtains majority. This is the 'contingency'. Even if his interest is still contingent, the trustees must pay the whole of the income to him until he obtains a vested interest or dies.

The power of *advancement* permits trustees to pay capital sums to, or on behalf of, a beneficiary some time before he is entitled to claim the fund. The power may be given by the trust instrument or, subject to a contrary intention, s. 32 of the Trustee Act 1925 may be invoked. The statutory power allows trustees at any time to pay or to apply capital money for the 'advancement or benefit' of any person entitled to that capital or a share thereof. Subject to that limitation, the powers are wide and apply whether the interest is vested or contingent, or whether it is in possession, in remainder, or in reversion. Up to one half of the beneficiary's share may be advanced. The trustees' discretion whether to exercise their power of advancement is absolute, so long as it is for the 'advancement or benefit' of the beneficiary. The ambit of the power is very wide, and it is popular in schemes that are designed as tax-saving devices. In this context, it can be seen as a device operating for schemes that are designed to avoid tax on capital transfers, which is itself an instrument for circumventing the avoidance of estate duty (by ensuring that gifts were made more than seven years before death), and was designed to tax family capital at least once per generation.

The key case here is that of *Pilkington* v *IRC* [1964] AC 612, which arose from a proposed advancement of part of a contingent share of Penelope Pilkington, who was an infant beneficiary, under the terms of a fund established by her uncle so long as she attained majority (of 21 years). The House of Lords held that the trustees' wish to advance to Penelope a sum of £7,600, which was to be settled on other trusts for her, was a proper course of action, and it did not matter that the very purpose of the advancement was resettlement and that the very purpose of this resettlement was avoiding duty payable on death—in other words, tax avoidance.

But, in *Re Pauling's ST* [1964] Ch 303, the Court of Appeal stressed that trustees must be satisfied that the advancement is for the benefit of the advance, and, further, that where advancement is for a particular purpose, trustees must ask themselves whether the beneficiary is likely actually to carry this out. From this, no payment should be made where a beneficiary is left to do as he pleases, but *Pauling* left open the question of whether the trustees can recover money that the beneficiary requests for a particular purpose and then applies to something quite different.

14.3 Trustees, and powers and duties arising in investment of trust property

It has already been suggested that the study of investment can be regarded as a meeting point for trustees' powers and duties. In turn, this is because, in many ways, investment is a meeting point for everything that we have learned about express private trusts up to now. We can see that managing the trust property is integral to why the trust has developed to allow ownership of property to be separated from its enjoyment, and why it is necessary to give legal title to trustees and to create 'validity' requirements that ensure that this will happen.

The very *raison d'être* of creating trusts is to provide benefits of property, whether this is to provide genuine enjoyment of property for another in ways in which are akin to a gift, or whether this is more strategic, with 'wealth preservation' and tax avoidance in mind. Enabling trust property to achieve this is why trustees are regarded as custodians of trust property, and has been a central reason why, historically, it has been permissible for trustees to delegate only administrative or ministerial functions to others, because looking after trust property has been regarded as something that the settlor intended those whom he has selected as trustees to carry out. Investment has traditionally been regarded as the paradigm illustration of the office of trustee as a personal office, and the duty to safeguard trust assets is a core element of the law relating to trustees' duties. This has implications for the commencement of trusteeship and a trustee's conduct while the trust is active. And, in pointing to a cycle of the significance of investment for a trust, as we shall discover in Chapter 16, the perceived failures of trustees in this regard can be seen in how many 'investment cases' have influenced the law relating to breach of trust.

We already know that, when a trust commences, trustees must acquaint themselves with the terms of the trust and the state of the property that they are to hold, and that, as part of this, they must ensure that funds are appropriately invested, and that all securities and chattels are in proper custody, and all steps must be taken to secure any property that is outstanding. In *Re Brogden* (1888) 38 Ch D 546, trustees were held liable where they refrained from suing to enforce a covenant to pay £10,000 into the settlement, notwithstanding that their motivation was reluctance to endanger the family business, which formed a significant part of the covenanter's estate. But equally, in *Ward* v *Ward* (1843) 2 HL Cas 777, trustees were not liable for failure to sue a beneficiary who might have been ruined by the action, along with his family, who were also beneficiaries. However, *Ward* is regarded as an extreme case; in *Re Brogden*, the Court of Appeal found that the only excuse for the trustees' failure to sue was that the action was considered to be fruitless. This was not an appropriate reason for failing to enforce payments due to the trust. Subsequently, s. 15 of the Trustee Act 1925 came to the aid of trustees in weighing up litigation risks, and now, subject to the statutory duty of care under the Trustee Act 2000, trustees in the exercise of their powers are able to compound liabilities and allow time for the payment of debts and will not incur liability.

14.3.1 Empowerment *and duty* arising in the protection of trust assets through investment

Once assets have been 'collected' in this manner in this initial phase by the trustees, they must then be protected for the longer term, which requires the trustee to make decisions on how to invest trust property properly. In this regard, two central principles can be seen to operate: first, trustees have a general duty to act fairly as between the beneficiaries; and second, the trustees must make investments that are appropriate. We already know that the operation of the former principle requires that, in making his selection of investments, the trustee must be mindful of those for whom the property must provide an income and also those who have ultimate entitlement to the property. These materials will allude to this on occasions, but will focus mainly on the duty to make appropriate investments, and how trustees are empowered to do this.

The duty to make appropriate investments
In respect of this, the enactment of the Trustee Act 2000 signals the arrival of a new approach to investment that is radically different from the traditional caution of the law relating to investment by trustees in contrast with normal investment culture and practice. The law will provide the fallback position whereby it will apply in the absence of express powers of investment conferred in the trust instrument. It is very common for professionally drafted trusts to contain such express powers, but it could well be that the enactment of a general power to invest by the Trustee Act 2000 might also reduce the need for such express provisions.

14.3.2 Definitions of 'appropriate investment' past and present: contextualizing the Trustee Act 2000

The policy of the law until the changes introduced in the 2000 Act was that of restriction and the need for caution. We can see this in a very generalized way through the interaction of *Speight* v *Gaunt* [1883] 9 App Cas 1 and *Re Whiteley* [1886] 33 ChD 347, where *Re Whiteley* was intended to serve as a reminder that, in a trust arrangement, a trustee is not dealing with his own property, but rather with property belonging to those whose interests he is bound to protect. In the context of investment, this would require the same prudence as if the trustee were investing his own property, but it would also prevent him from undertaking the same level of risk as if he were investing his own property. We have already had advanced notification of how the Trustee Act 2000 might have liberalized this position, but the 'risk containment' idea of *Whiteley* is very plain in the policy of the Trustee Act 2000's predecessor, the Trustee Investment Act 1961.

The general policy of the 1961 Act was that, in their selection of investments that would be appropriate for a particular trust, trustees were required to choose from a limited pool. Availability within this pool was itself limited to investments that were seen as safe and low risk. This took the form of an 'approved list' of investments that were designed to be profitable whilst being safe, and the significance of this approved list could be seen from the fact that deviation from this amounted to a breach of trust by the trustees. This approach was one of the most criticized aspects of trusts law that were not fit for purpose in the Law Commission's enquiries from 1997 and 1999, which gave rise to the Trustee Act 2000. In its 1997 Consultation Paper on *Trustees' Powers and Duties* (CP No. 146), the Law Commission described the approach of the 1961 Act as 'over cautious and restrictive', and it even suggested that the regime placed huge and unnecessary burdens upon trustees, and that there was evidence of serious underperformance by some trusts on account of its lack of congruence with the tremendous opportunities offered in the diversified investment market of the late twentieth century. The Law Commission suggested that, instead, trustees should have the same power as individuals in the making of investments, and that making this subject to a duty of care would compel regard to the need for diversification and suitability. There would be a further safety check built into such a differently focused regime from requiring trustees to seek proper professional advice in such matters.

14.3.3 The Trustee Act 2000: responding to calls for a more liberalized approach

In response to the criticism of investment regimes contained within the Trustee Act 1925 and the Trustee Investment Act 1961, s. 3 of the Trustee Act 2000 provides trustees with new wide statutory powers. Here, the opening part of the section is a very important statement of recognition of the significance of investment for trusts, and the intention to sweep away much of what is outmoded and to replace it with a more appropriate and facilitative legal framework governing investment.

The general power of investment: s. 3
Section 3(1) states that: 'Subject to the provisions of this Part, a trustee may make any kind of investment that he could make if he were absolutely entitled to the assets of the trust.'

While the remainder of the discussion of the new legal regime now in place will focus on the limitations of trustees' powers of investment, as well as their scope, this statement of intent should remain foremost a matter of context. Indeed, s. 3(2) defines this statement of intent as the 'general power of investment'. Significantly, unlike in the provisions of the Trustee Investment Act 1961, there is no requirement under the new legislation that there should be any division of the trust fund, but the general power of investment is subject to the 'safeguards' prescribed by ss. 4 and 5. These safeguards essentially refer to the duty of trustees to have regard to the 'standard investment criteria', and the obtaining and consideration of proper advice.

Section 4 and the standard investment criteria
Neither the idea of 'standard investment criteria' nor their precise composition within the Trustee Act 2000 can be regarded as new, and they have in essence been re-enacted

from the Trustee Investment Act 1961. According to the provisions of s. 4(1), trustees must have regard to the standard investment criteria when exercising any power of investment, whether this is part of the general power of investment conferred by the 2000 legislation or is from a different source (for example, the trust instrument itself, when the power is an express one provided rather than a general one available to all trustees). Indeed, in this respect, the general power of investment operates subject to restrictions or exclusions on such activity, which are contained within the instrument that has created the trust. Under s. 4(2), trustees must take into account the standard investment criteria when exercising *any* investment powers. And, as part of this process, they should, from time to time, review whether or not investments made should in any way be varied from their original composition. Again, this need to review is defined in terms of reference to the standard investment criteria, and provides the benchmark against which such an assessment must be made.

The standard investment criteria: a twin set of objectives

The standard investment criteria are composed of two measures of the appropriateness of any given investment, and this is reflected within the legislation:

- the *suitability* to the needs of the particular trust of the type of investment that is being considered is enshrined in s. 4(3)(a); and
- the need for *diversification* in so far as this is appropriate to the needs of the individual trust is signposted within the provisions of s. 4(3)(b).

The requirement that the type of investment chosen should be suitable for the nature of the trust requires that the trustee should look at the type of investment that he wishes to make to judge its appropriateness for the needs of the particular trust, and to assess its suitability. The needs of individual trusts will, of course, vary considerably, and accordingly so will the factors that will influence questions arising in the assessment of suitability. But it is clear from authorities such as *Cowan* v *Scargill* [1985] Ch 270 that the calculus of suitability cannot include trustees' personal views on ethics or politics when considering the most favourable financial returns. Indeed, it is clear from *Buttle* v *Saunders* [1950] 2 All ER 193, which pre-dates this, that if maximizing the trust's assets requires acting improperly (although not illegally), then trustees are duty-bound to do this—in that case, by 'gazumping' a purchaser of the property in favour of another higher offer.

The requirement of diversity is of essence in 'portfolio theorization' of investment, which takes as its standard of risk assessment the risk level of the *entire portfolio* and not of *individual investments* within it. It is this global consideration of assessing risks taken in investments that articulates that trustees must ensure that investments are appropriately spread, and thus that risk is evened out. It would be surprising if the duty to ensure diversification were not applicable to the exercise of all powers of investment (and not simply the s. 3 general power), and indeed it is so applicable to all powers of investment. Whilst this is a duty that cannot be excluded or restricted, and notwithstanding its general policy of promoting the spirit of a portfolio approach in all exercising of investment power, by the provisions of s. 4(3)(b) the duty to ensure diversification applies (only) 'in so far as is appropriate to the circumstances of the trust'. Thus whilst the import of diversification is within the legislation without dispute, its provisions recognize that there are nevertheless limitations on its appropriateness (for example, on grounds of size of the trust and its assets).

Section 5 and the duty to take advice in the exercise of the power of investment

Given the investment opportunities available in the context of financial markets, which are increasingly saturated with 'investment products' and operating in an increasingly globalized context, for all but the most expert professional trustees managing investment opportunities will be the most demanding aspect of their office. This is, of course, pursued through exercising significant powers and labouring under increasing 'duty' scrutiny. Some assistance is provided 'at source' for market participants by so-called 'conduct of business' rules, which are at the heart of the United Kingdom's regulatory regime for financial markets. Although this is itself highly dynamic, key reference points in this context can be found focused on requiring a seller of regulated products to be mindful of the level of expertise of the client, as well as to act in a client's best interest, to obtain the best execution, and to communicate in a manner that is clear, fair, and not misleading.

Also very significantly, under s. 5(1), before exercising power of investment (irrespective of its source), the trustee must (subject to the exception provided in s. 5(3)) obtain and consider proper advice. This proper advice refers to the way in which the power of investment (from whatever source) should be exercised, with regard to the standard investment criteria. By the provisions of s. 5(2), when a review is being made of the suitability of investments (by reference to the standard investment criteria and in furtherance of s. 4(2) of the 2000 Act), the trustee must obtain and consider proper advice as to the way in which the investments should be varied. This requirement marks a considerable point of departure from the 1961 legislation under which the duty to seek and consider advice was much narrower, while s. 5(3) seeks to deal with the situation in which the trustee is himself an experienced financial adviser, by providing that 'a trustee need not obtain such advice if he reasonably concludes that in all of the circumstances it is unnecessary or inappropriate so to do'.

The question of what amounts to 'proper advice' is provided for in the Act's definition in s. 5(4) as 'the advice of a person who is reasonably believed by the trustee to be qualified to give it by his ability in and practical experience of financial and other matters relating to the proposed investment'. This definition has been lifted from the provisions of the 2000 Act's predecessor, the Trustee Investment Act 1961.

14.3.4 Empowerment and concomitant duty: the combined effects of ss. 3 and 1

We have suggested that the Law Commission saw the liberalization of investment behaviour by trustees as being coupled with requiring them to take professional advice, and also being subject to a duty of care. Adoption of this latter policy can be seen from the way in which the s. 3 general power is one of those that is specified as operating subject to the s. 1 statutory duty of care by virtue of Sch. 1. Here, the threshold standard of competence requires fulfilment of ss. 4 and 5 for all trustees, and in this regard we can see that this liberalization of the law might make things more complicated for certain trustees who do not have a great deal of 'market savvy'. Such a trustee may well have liked the restrictions of the 1961 regime, which limited him to making a selection from a prescribed list, taking comfort from the fact that equity has never required trustees to 'play the market' aggressively, and has espoused the view that trustees are not guarantors of performance and can be held responsible only for failing to act prudently.

The new liberalized approach under s. 3 is, of course, subject to the s. 1 duty of care. Amongst service providers who called for reform—to lift restrictions on 'maximizing' a trust's possibilities—will have been many who are not only subject to the s. 1 threshold standard in principle, but also are theoretically held to higher standards. As we discovered when we considered the s. 1 duty itself, these are additional factors shaping what is expected from an individual trustee in the light of general expectations of everyone occupying this role, and which are designed to reflect particular skills and expertise of which the individual trustee has made representations. However, at that point it was also noted that, notwithstanding the intended import of differentiating on the basis of skill and representation, it might be difficult to see whether the duty would actually influence liability that can be incurred by trustees in default of reaching the required standard. This is because it was suggested that those to whom this would most likely make a difference in principle were actually those most likely to insist on limiting liability by way of a trustee exclusion clause in practice. This is considered further in Chapter 16, where we will find out just how significant 'bad' investment choices are in precipitating actions for breach of trust.

When we looked at the s. 1 statutory duty, we also learned that although it seeks to create a universal standard, it is not actually a universal duty, and will not apply to arrangements to which there is evidence that it was not intended to apply. In short, the effect of Sch. 1, para. 7, is that operation of the duty can be excluded by the trust instrument. In these circumstances, a trustee's performance will be judged against equity's standards of prudence as applied to investment specifically (see especially *Nestlé* v *National Westminster Bank plc* [1993] 1 WLR 1260), bearing in mind that again it is open to trustees to use trustee exemption clauses.

 Revision Box

1. Joining the materials from this chapter with the previous chapter's introduction to trusteeship, ensure that you can answer the following.
   (a) In what way can the duties of a trustee under an express arrangement be seen as a measure of a beneficiary's entitlements under it?
   (b) How can the duties of a trustee be explained in reference to the 'life cycle' of an active trust?
   (c) What issues arise where there are a number of beneficiaries under a settlement?
   (d) How do rules relating to the administration of an active trust seek to balance the entitlements of a beneficiary with equipping the trustee actually to carry out the trust?
2. Ensure that you understand the nature of trusteeship in the twenty-first century by reference to:
   – growing dissatisfaction with the legal framework for trusteeship dating from the latter years of the twentieth century;
   – the rise of the 'professional trustee'; and
   – the way in which the Trustee Act 2000 can be seen to embody two key trends— that is, increased liberalization and also accountability—and how these aims can conflict.

FURTHER READING

This chapter is the second of three providing an extended and thematic study of how trusteeship arises, what the implications of trusteeship are, and what happens when the obligations of trusteeship are not complied with. Therefore it is difficult to isolate reading that overarches a number of these things into one chapter or another, and all pertinent reading will be listed at the end of Chapter 16.

15

Variation of trusts

As a general rule, as we have seen throughout this book, trustees are bound to carry out the settlor's wishes, and any deviation from the terms of the trust will amount to a breach of trust. Nonetheless, circumstances may arise in which an extension of the trustees' powers, or even a substantial alteration in the beneficial interests of the trust, would be desirable in the interests of efficient administration or for the sake of preserving the value of the beneficiaries' entitlements.

15.1 Some basic considerations around variation explained

The main reason for wishing to vary trusts is to reduce liability to taxation, and that is what this chapter is really about. Yet although it has become apparent that equity permits trustees to have discretion in many aspects of performing the trust, it has also become apparent that equity does not generally allow them to recast its terms. Until recent statutory reforms, therefore, the inherent powers of the court to vary have been extremely limited, especially where tax planning is the motive.

There are nevertheless circumstances other than those provided for by statute under which variation is possible.

Express powers to vary
Obviously, the trust instrument itself may have been drafted so as to confer upon the trustees powers far wider than those contemplated by the general law. Modern trust instruments generally contrive to allow the trustees considerable discretionary powers, and not uncommonly provide for variation of the beneficial interests themselves, by means of suitably drafted powers of appointment. The terms of such powers must, of course, be strictly observed, but it is often possible through careful drafting to obviate the need for recourse to more complex variation procedures. Reliance upon express powers contained in the trust instrument, needless to say, creates no exception to the duty not to deviate from the terms of the trust, for such powers are themselves among the terms of the trust.

Saunders *v* Vautier: *variation with the collective consent of the beneficiaries*
In the absence of express powers, it may be possible to effect a variation in the trust by taking advantage of the rule in *Saunders v Vautier* (1841) 10 LJ Ch 354. Collectively, the beneficiaries, as long as they are all adult, *sui iuris*, and between them entitled to the entirety of the trust property, can bring the trust to an end and resettle the property on any terms they wish. Thus, in a simple settlement of property upon a life interest for X with remainder for Y, X and Y may agree to end the trust and divide the capital between them immediately. More complex settlements may require more sophisticated

measures, involving perhaps the actuarial valuation of future entitlements and possibly the need for insurance against any risk of loss, but the principles are basically the same.

The beneficiaries can also collectively consent to any act by the trustees that has the effect of varying the terms of the trust, without going through the process of dissolving and resettling the property, which may involve a number of separate conveyances, all attracting stamp duty.

It is very important, however, to appreciate the limits of the *Saunders* v *Vautier* doctrine. First, it depends on the beneficiaries all being collectively entitled. Thus donees under a power cannot use it, and although beneficiaries under a discretionary trust usually can, they will not be able to unless the entire class of objects is ascertainable.

Second, it turns upon all of the beneficiaries being able to consent to dissolve the trust, or to what would otherwise be a breach of trust by the trustees. If some of the beneficiaries are infants, or if the settlement creates any interests in favour of persons who are not yet born or ascertained, variation of the trust upon this basis will not be possible. This is a serious limitation when dealing with family settlements of the usual type, which almost invariably give interests to non *sui iuris* persons. As will appear in section 15.4, this is the difficulty tackled by the Variation of Trusts Act 1958.

Third, unless the trustees also agree, the beneficiaries cannot vary an existing trust and keep it on foot, instead of dissolving it and resettling the property. This can be seen in *Re Brockbank* [1948] Ch 206, which gives a general flavour of the issues, although the law underpinning it has now changed. According to Vaisey J at 209:

> It seems to me that the beneficiaries must choose between two alternatives: either they must keep the trusts of the will on foot, in which case those trusts must continue to be executed by trustees ... not ... arbitrarily selected by themselves; or they must, by mutual agreement, extinguish and put an end to the trusts.

Walton J expressed similar views in *Stephenson* v *Barclays Bank Trust Co. Ltd* [1975] 1 WLR 88. One of the reasons he gave was that otherwise the beneficiaries could force upon the trustees duties quite different from those that they had originally accepted. This reasoning would seem to survive the Trusts of Land and Appointment of Trustees Act 1996.

15.2 The limited inherent jurisdiction of courts to vary trusts

The problem arises in relation to persons unable to give consent—especially children and unborn persons. As will be explained in section 15.4, the Variation of Trusts Act 1958 confers upon the court a discretion to give its approval to a proposed variation on behalf of such persons if the court is satisfied that such a variation would be for their benefit. Before considering the effect of that Act and other statutory provisions, however, it is necessary to outline the extent to which the courts have traditionally been willing to permit a variation of trust under their inherent jurisdiction, where not all beneficiaries are adult and *sui iuris*.

It has long been recognized that the court may, in the case of necessity, permit the trustees to take measures not authorized by the trust instrument. In *Chapman* v *Chapman*

[1954] AC 429, the House of Lords indicated that this inherent jurisdiction is narrow, encompassing for the most part only emergency and salvage. Originally, this seems to have been confined to cases in which some act of salvage was urgently required, such as the mortgage of an infant's property in order to raise money for vital repairs. Gradually, it was widened to cover other contingencies not foreseen and provided for by the settlor, but the House of Lords reaffirmed in *Chapman* v *Chapman*, unanimously approving the formulation of Romer LJ in *Re New* [1901] 2 Ch 534, that some element of emergency still needs to be shown.

Chapman v *Chapman* applies only to variations in the *beneficial interests* as such. There is a wider inherent jurisdiction regarding the administration of the trust fund. For example, as seen in Chapter 13, in *Re Duke of Norfolk's ST* [1982] Ch 61, the court authorized payment of remuneration to a trustee under its inherent jurisdiction.

The courts may also approve compromises of disputes regarding the beneficial entitlements on behalf of infant or future beneficiaries. Arguably, this is not a matter of genuine variation of the trust, since by definition its terms are not clear; hence the dispute. The courts, however, showed a willingness to extend the term 'compromise' to cover situations in which no real dispute had arisen, and approval was sometimes granted to what were, in reality, mere variations worked out between the beneficiaries. This broad conception of the inherent jurisdiction was firmly disapproved by the House of Lords in *Chapman* v *Chapman*, and held to be confined to instances in which a genuine element of dispute exists.

Thus, in *Re Powell-Cotton's Resettlement* [1956] 1 All ER 60, the Court of Appeal decided that there were no disputed rights where an investment clause was ambiguous and it would have been advantageous to the beneficiaries to replace it with a new clause. In *Mason* v *Farbrother* [1983] 2 All ER 1078, genuine points of difference were found to have arisen where two contending interpretations of an investment clause had widely different implications for the permitted range of investments. The court, however, was reluctant to approve the substitution of a new clause under its inherent jurisdiction, preferring to rely upon s. 57 of the Trustee Act 1925. In *Allen* v *Distillers Co. (Biochemicals) Ltd* [1974] QB 384, the court was asked to approve a settlement of the claims of the child victims of the drug thalidomide, and the question arose as to whether the court could postpone the vesting of capital in the children to an age greater than 18. Eveleigh J, on the basis of the rule in *Saunders* v *Vautier*, held that there was no inherent jurisdiction to order such a postponement, but found it to be authorized by the terms of the settlement itself.

Clearly, therefore, the inherent equitable jurisdiction is of limited value to those whose main motive for variation is to reduce liability for taxation.

15.3 Statutory powers to vary trusts apart from the Variation of Trusts Act 1958

The Matrimonial Causes Act 1973, as amended

The narrowness of the court's inherent jurisdiction to give approval to variations in the terms of trust is offset by several statutory provisions. A particularly useful and important addition to the jurisdiction was made by the Matrimonial Causes Act 1973, which, by ss. 24 and 25, gives a wide power to make orders affecting the property of parties to matrimonial proceedings, so as to avoid the unfairness that sometimes arose where the property of a married couple, in particular the matrimonial home, came under the rules governing resulting trusts (see Chapter 8). The court may order provision for either spouse to be made by payments in cash, by transfers of property, or by the creation of a settlement for the benefit of a spouse and children.

More important in the context of variation, s. 24(1)(c) and (d) allow for variation of an pre- or postnuptial settlement, including settlements made by will or codicil, and also permit the making of an order extinguishing or reducing the interest of either of the spouses under such a settlement. The term 'settlement' has been widely interpreted to include any provision (other than outright gifts) made for the benefit of the parties to a marriage, whether by themselves or by a third party, and the acquisition of a matrimonial home has been held to be a settlement (*Ulrich* v *Ulrich* [1968] 1 WLR 180). Further, the court has the power to vary or discharge any order for a settlement or variation under s. 24(1) made on or after a decree of judicial separation if the separation order is rescinded or the marriage subsequently dissolved.

The Mental Health Act 1983, as amended

The power given by s. 96(1)(d) of the Mental Health Act 1983 to the Court of Protection to make a settlement of a patient's property also allows the judge to vary the settlement as he thinks fit if it transpires that some material fact was not disclosed when the settlement was made, or if substantial changes in circumstances arise.

The Trustee Act 1925

The foregoing provisions are designed to meet rather special situations; more general powers may be made available to trustees by virtue of provisions contained in the Trustee Act 1925 and the Settled Land Act 1925. Section 57(1) of the Trustee Act 1925, in effect, widens the inherent jurisdiction with regard to 'emergency' by making the jurisdiction available in any case in which it is 'expedient':

> (1) Where in the management or administration of any property vested in trustees, any sale, lease, mortgage, surrender, release or other disposition, or any purchase, investment, acquisition, expenditure, or other transaction, is in the opinion of the court expedient, but the same cannot be effected by reason of the absence of any power for that purpose vested in the trustees by the trust instrument, if any, or by law, the court may by order confer upon the trustees, either generally or in any particular instance, the necessary power for the purpose, on such terms, and subject to such provisions and conditions, if any, as the court may think fit and may direct in what manner any money authorised to be expended, and the costs of any transaction, are to be paid or borne as between capital and income.

The section operates as though its provisions were to be read into every settlement, but it is clearly limited to matters falling within the management or administration of the trust property, and does not permit the alteration of beneficial interests under the trust.

Applications under the section are usually heard in chambers and so are not generally reported, but the few reported cases show that it has been used to authorize a sale of settled chattels, to partition or sell land where necessary consents had been refused, to purchase a residence for the tenant for life, and to sell prematurely a reversionary interest.

Settlements of land do not fall within s. 57(1) of the Trustee Act 1925, but they may be varied by recourse to s. 64(1) of the Settled Land Act 1925, which allows the court to make an order authorizing the tenant for life to effect any transaction affecting or concerning the settled land, or any part of it, if the court is of the opinion that the transaction would be for the benefit of the settled land, or any part of it, or of the persons interested under the settlement. The transaction must be one that could have been effected by an absolute owner. The section is not confined to cases of management or administration alone, although it includes such purposes and allows alteration of the beneficial interests with a view to reducing tax liability. In the days of estate duty, the especial vulnerability of the strict settlement to onerous charges might be mitigated by rearrangement of the beneficial interests under this section.

This section was invoked by Morritt J in *Hambro* v *Duke of Marlborough* [1994] Ch 158, to allow the eleventh Duke of Marlborough (as tenant for life) to execute a conveyance, the effect of which was to disinherit the Marquis of Blandford, who (the trustees had concluded) displayed unbusinesslike habits and lack of responsibility.

The Settled Land and Trustee Acts (Court's General Powers) Act 1943, as amended by the Emergency Laws (Miscellaneous Provisions) Act 1953, permanently extends the court's jurisdiction to authorize the expense of any action taken in the management of settled land or land held on trust for sale in the context of ss. 57 and 64 to be treated as a capital outgoing where the action is beneficial and the income insufficient to bear the expense.

The inherent jurisdiction to make provision for infants is somewhat extended by s. 53 of the Trustee Act 1925, which allows the court to authorize dealings with the infant's property with a view to application of the capital or income for the infant's maintenance, education, or benefit. 'Benefit' has been interpreted to cover dealings having the effect of reducing estate duty for the benefit of the infant: *Re Meux* [1958] Ch 154.

In *Re Meux*, the proceeds of sale of property were to be resettled upon the infant, and so could be regarded as an 'application' for the infant's benefit. However, in *Re Hayworth's Contingent Reversionary Interest* [1956] Ch 364, a proposal to sell an infant's contingent reversionary interest to the life tenant for cash, thus ending the trusts, was thought not to be for the benefit of the infant. Other types of dealing approved under the section have included the barring of entails to exclude remote beneficiaries (*Re Gower's Settlement* [1934] Ch 365) or to simplify a proposed application to the court for approval of a further variation under the Variation of Trusts Act 1958 (*Re Bristol's Settled Estates* [1965] 1 WLR 469).

15.4 **The Variation of Trusts Act 1958**

The decision of the House of Lords in *Chapman* v *Chapman* [1954] AC 429 curtailed, as explained, the broad approach previously developed by the courts in the exercise of the inherent jurisdiction to approve compromises or 'disputes', and the Law Reform Committee was asked to consider the question of the court's powers to sanction variations, which resulted in the report entitled *Court's Power to Sanction Variation of Trusts* (Cmnd 310, 1957). The Variation of Trusts Act 1958 was based on these recommendations and provides a new statutory jurisdiction independent of the Trustee Act 1925 or the Settled Land Act 1925.

Under s. 1(1) of the 1958 Act, the court has discretion to approve, on behalf of the following categories of person, any arrangement varying or revoking all or any of the trusts, or enlarging the trustees' powers of management and administration over the property subject to the trusts. The categories are as follows:

(a) infants or people who are mentally incapacitated; or

(b) people who have a mere expectation of benefiting under the trusts, but those with interests, whether vested or contingent, should consent on their own behalf (see further section 15.4.1); or

(c) any person unborn; or

(d) any person with a discretionary interest under a protective trust.

Proposals to vary the beneficial interests under a trust may be approved, provided (except in the case of persons falling under s. 1(1)(d)) that the court is satisfied that such variation will be for the benefit of the persons on behalf of whom approval is given. In deciding whether to approve a proposed settlement, the court will consider the arrangement as a whole, since it is the arrangement that has to be approved and not only those aspects of it that happen to affect a person on whose behalf the court is being asked to consent.

15.4.1 Use of the 1958 Act

Where an extension of the trustee's powers of management is sought, the jurisdiction of the Act is invoked in preference to s. 57 of the Trustee Act 1925 wherever possible. The courts have shown themselves willing to approve the insertion of powers of advancement or a period of accumulation, or to terminate an accumulation, among other matters.

As far as investment is concerned, in *Trustees of the British Museum* v *Attorney-General* [1984] 1 WLR 418, Sir Robert Megarry V-C took the view that the powers conferred by the (then in force) Trustee Investments Act 1961 were becoming outdated, and that the effects of inflation and the character of the trust may amount to special circumstances in which it would be proper to give approval under the 1958 Act. The decision was based on the changes of investment pattern—including the movement from fixed-interest investments to investments in equities and property—that had occurred between 1961 and 1983.

The reasoning is by no means of universal application, however, and indeed Sir Robert Megarry V-C's judgment is in quite restricted terms. At the time of the case, investing in equities was relatively risk-free, and there had been a more or less continuous bull market for some eight years. That is not the case today. Sir Robert Megarry V-C also said, at 425:

> The size of the fund in question may be very material. A fund that is very large may well justify a latitude of investment that would be denied to a more modest fund; for the spread of investments possible for a larger fund may justify the greater risks that wider powers will permit to be taken.

The main application of the Variation of Trusts Act 1958 has been to vary the beneficial interests for tax-saving purposes, and this has been assumed to be its natural sphere of operation. Some would argue that those who cannot give a valid consent to schemes that would be for their benefit, such as infants and the unborn, should not be deprived of the advantages that their consensual counterparts could obtain on *Saunders* v *Vautier* principles; nor should their incapacity prevent the opportunity of gain to the trust as a whole.

Persons on whose behalf the court may give its approval

The way in which the statute works is to allow the court to give consent on behalf of beneficiaries who are not *sui iuris*, but the principles underlying the rule in *Saunders* v *Vautier* were preserved by the Act in as much as the court will not provide a consent that ought properly to be sought from an ascertainable adult, *sui iuris* beneficiary. Hence the limits placed on s. 1(1)(b).

The difficulty with s. 1(1)(b) arises in relation to interests that are very remote, such as interests in default of appointment or in the event of a failure of the trust. The subsection allows the court to consent on behalf of:

> (b) any person (whether ascertained or not) who may become entitled, directly or indirectly, to an interest under the trusts as being at a future date or on the happening of a future event a person of any specified description or a member of any specified class of persons, so however that this paragraph shall not include any person who would be of that description, or a member of that class, as the case may be, if the said date had fallen or the said event had happened at the date of the application to the court, ...

It is the words after 'so however' that cause the problem, since those persons have to consent on their own behalf; the court cannot consent for them. There is no problem over, for example, potential future spouses, since they clearly have a mere expectation of succeeding. They clearly come within the first part of s. 1(1)(b) and the court can consent on their behalf. But if somebody is named in the instrument as having a contingent interest, however unlikely that contingency is to arise, the court cannot consent on his behalf. He must consent himself to any variation.

The scope and limitation of the 1958 Act

This can seriously limit the scope of the 1958 Act. For example, in *Re Suffert's Settlement* [1961] Ch 1, the court could not consent on behalf of a cousin who benefited only if Miss Suffert died without issue, and even then subject to a general testamentary power of appointment. Other examples are *Re Moncrieff's ST* [1962] 1 WLR 1344 and *Knocker v Youle* [1986] 1 WLR 934. In the latter case, the court could not consent on behalf of sisters who would benefit only in the event of failure or determination of the trust, and Warner J felt constrained to adopt a fairly literal interpretation of the Act.

The application should be made by a beneficiary, preferably by the person currently receiving the income, but the settlor may also apply and, as a last resort, the trustees may apply, but only if no one else will apply and the variation is in the interests of the beneficiaries. Otherwise, it is undesirable for trustees to apply, because their position as applicants may conflict with their duty to guard the interests of the beneficiaries impartially. The settlor, if living, and all of the beneficiaries, including minors, should be made parties, special attention being paid to ensure proper representation for minors and the unborn.

What is 'benefit'?

The general scheme of the 1958 Act is to give a wide discretion to the courts, but the one limit on the discretion is that, except for persons within s. 1(1)(d), the court may not approve a variation unless it is satisfied that such variation will be for the benefit of those persons on behalf of whom approval for the variation is given. Stamp J took the view in *Re Cohen's ST* [1965] 1 WLR 1229 that the benefit must be to those persons considered as individuals and not merely as members of a class.

The benefit requirement does not extend expressly to a variation proposed on behalf of a beneficiary under a discretionary protective trust (s. 1(1)(d)), but the court has an unfettered discretion as to the exercise of its powers under the Act and, in *Re Steed's WT* [1960] Ch 407, the Court of Appeal refused its consent in such a case, in which it thought that no benefit was shown (see further under 'Assessing financial benefit: long-term considerations vs short-term considerations').

Nature of benefit

It is not possible to state categorically what the court will regard as benefit, except that it will adopt the test of what a reasonable *sui iuris* adult beneficiary would have done in the circumstances.

Financial benefit is clearly included, and most tax-saving schemes will satisfy the requirement, since such saving preserves the total quantum of property available for distribution among the beneficiaries.

Assessing financial benefit: long-term considerations vs short-term considerations

In assessing financial benefit, the court may have to balance short-term against long-term factors, and take account of the character of the persons on whose behalf approval is sought. In *Re Towler's ST* [1964] Ch 158, Wilberforce J was prepared to postpone the vesting of capital to which a beneficiary was soon to become entitled upon evidence that she was likely to deal with it imprudently. In *Re Steed's WT* [1960] Ch 407, the proposed scheme was for the elimination of the protective element in a trust relating to land. The principal beneficiary, who was a life tenant (but not *sui iuris* because of the protective element), wanted a variation such that the trustees held the property on trust for herself absolutely. Clearly, this was in theory to her financial advantage, but evidence suggested that advantage would in fact be taken of the life tenant's good nature by the very persons against whose importuning the settlor had meant to protect her, and the Court of Appeal refused its consent (considered further at 'The relevance of the settlor's wishes').

Although it will be rare for the court to look beyond the financial advantages contained in the proposed arrangement, the unfettered discretion given by the Act to the courts can lead them to refuse a variation where there is a clear financial benefit. In *Re Weston's Settlements* [1969] 1 Ch 223, the Court of Appeal refused to approve a scheme that would have removed the trusts to a tax haven (Jersey), where the family had moved three months previously, on the ground that the moral and social benefits of an English upbringing were not outweighed by the tax savings to be enjoyed by the infant beneficiaries. Harman LJ said that 'this is an essay in tax avoidance naked and unashamed', and Lord Denning MR noted, at 245, that:

> There are many things in life more worthwhile than money. One of these things is to be brought up in this our England, which is still 'the envy of less happier lands'. I do not believe it is for the benefit of children to be uprooted from England and transported to another country simply to avoid tax ... Many a child has been ruined by being given too much. The avoidance of tax may be lawful, but it is not yet a virtue.

Re Weston is perhaps atypical, and the court will not always refuse approval to the removal of a trust from the jurisdiction. It will depend on the circumstances. In *Re Windeatt's WT* [1969] 1 WLR 692, a similar scheme was approved by Pennycuick J, but in that case the family had already been in Jersey for nineteen years and the children had been born there; there was no question of uprooting them. Similarly, in *Re Seale's Marriage Settlement* [1961] Ch 574, Buckley J approved a scheme removing the trusts to Canada, to which country again the family had moved many years previously, with no thought of tax avoidance, and had brought up the children as Canadians.

In reality, the use of the 1958 Act to export trusts is quite common, but *Re Weston* shows that all circumstances will be taken into account and that the existence of a clear financial benefit will not necessarily be conclusive.

Another possibility, included for the sake of completeness, is that some beneficiaries will benefit at the expense of others. An example is *Re Remnant's ST* [1970] Ch 560, in which Pennycuick J approved the deletion of a forfeiture clause in respect of children who became Roman Catholics. Some of the children were Protestant and others Roman Catholic, but the court approved the deletion of the clause on policy grounds (as being liable to cause serious dissension within the family), although this was clearly to the disadvantage of the Protestant children. The settlor's intentions were also not considered conclusive; indeed, they were overridden.

The courts may go further and approve schemes where there is a positive disadvantage in material terms. In *Re CL* [1969] 1 Ch 587, the Court of Protection held that there was a benefit to an elderly mental patient in giving up, in return for no consideration, her life interests for the benefit of adopted daughters. This was, in effect, giving approval to a straightforward gift by the beneficiary, from which in strictly material terms she could not possibly benefit. The lady's needs were otherwise amply provided for, however, and the court, in approving the arrangement, took the view that it was acting as she herself would have done, had she been able to appreciate her family responsibilities.

These cases should not be regarded as typical, however. Assuming that a proposed arrangement is otherwise unobjectionable, it will be rare for the court to look beyond the financial advantages contained therein.

The extent of court's discretion

The only constraint on the court's discretion under the Act is the requirement that it must be satisfied of a benefit, except in the case of persons under s. 1(1)(d). However, even if it is clear that the court has *jurisdiction* to consent to a variation, it has an unfettered discretion to exercise its powers under the Act '*if it thinks fit*'. Thus, whereas the court cannot approve a variation except where the Act so provides, it has an unlimited discretion to refuse its approval where it is given jurisdiction under the Act.

It follows that, even where a benefit is clearly shown for the persons on whose behalf approval is sought, the court is not required to approve. For persons under s. 1(1)(d), it is not even required that a benefit be shown, yet the court, in its discretion, refused to approve a variation in *Re Steed's WT* [1960] Ch 407.

The relevance of the settlor's wishes

In *Re Steed's WT* [1960] Ch 407, the Court of Appeal was undoubtedly influenced by the views of the settlor, who in his will had clearly expressed his concern about the welfare of the beneficiary under the protective trust, for whom approval was sought. Yet although the settlor's views can be relevant, they are rarely paramount: they were overridden in *Re Remnant's ST* [1970] Ch 560, and it was the settlor who applied for the variation in *Re Weston's Settlements* [1969] 1 Ch 223. Moreover, the Court of Appeal held, in *Goulding* v *James* [1997] 2 All ER 239, that they have no relevance at all unless they relate to someone on whose behalf the court's approval is required. In *Goulding* v *James*, the proposed variation (which was clearly for the benefit of the testatrix's unborn great-grandchildren, for whom approval was sought) would have frustrated her desire to restrict the ability of two adult, *sui iuris* beneficiaries to touch the capital of the estate. Since the court's approval was not required for the adult beneficiaries, however, who were able to consent for themselves, the settlor's views were entirely irrelevant.

What are the risks involved?

Sometimes, a proposed arrangement may involve some element of risk to the beneficiary for whom the court is asked to consent. An element of risk will not prevent the court from approving the arrangement if the risk is one that an adult beneficiary would be prepared to take. Such a test was applied by Danckwerts J in *Re Cohen's WT* [1959] 1 WLR 865.

In *Re Robinson's ST* [1976] 1 WLR 806, the fund was held on trust for the claimant for her life, with remainders over to her children, one of whom was under the age of 21 (the age of majority at the time). The claimant was aged 55 and expected to live for many years. The variation proposed was to divide up the fund, giving the claimant an immediate capital share of 52 per cent (the actuarial capitalized value of her share), and the children dividing the balance in equal shares. The children who got their share immediately and those who were over the age of 21 consented to the variation; the court was asked to approve variation on behalf of Nicola (who was aged 17).

Before the introduction of capital transfer tax (CTT) in 1975, division of the fund in this way, by giving the children their interests immediately rather than on the death of the life tenant, was almost certain to reduce liability to estate duty, because at that time there was no liability to estate duty on any advance made more than seven years before the death of the life tenant. The same is true today under inheritance tax. However, for a short period following the Finance Act 1975, which introduced capital transfer tax, all *inter vivos* gifts were also taxable, albeit that liability was lower as long as the transfer was made more than three years before the death of the life tenant.

At the time of *Re Robinson's ST*, therefore, the division would not necessarily have favoured Nicola. The transfer would have been taxed immediately, so that the value of the fund would be reduced. On the other hand, Nicola would get her share immediately and would not have to wait for the death of her mother. Whether this would be to her benefit or not would depend entirely on how long her mother was likely to live. If she were to die immediately, Nicola's share would be less than she would have received under the unvaried trust, since tax would have been paid on it. It was calculated, however, that, given the mother's life expectancy, the deficiency would be made up in income on her share between the date of the variation and her mother's death.

Templeman J took the view that the court should require evidence that the minor would at least not be materially worse off as a result of the variation. He adopted as the test whether an adult beneficiary would have been prepared to take the risk: a 'broad' view might be taken, but not a 'galloping, gambling view'. The arrangement was approved, subject to a policy of insurance to protect the minor's interests, but Templeman J did not require the entirety of the possible loss to be covered, the view being taken that the saving in premium on a lesser cover was worth the small risk.

Re Robinson's ST can be illustrated as in Figure 15.1.

		Mrs Robinson	Children
Before proposed variation	Capital	Life interest on 100%	Remainder on all, but subject to CTT
	Income	Income on all until death	Income on all, but only after Mrs R's death
After proposed variation	Capital	52% immediately	48% immediately, perhaps with lower CTT
	Income	Immediate income on 52%	Immediate income on 48%

Figure 15.1 *Re Robinson's ST* [1976] 1 WLR 806.

A different type of case was *Re Holt's Settlement* [1969] 1 Ch 100. The trust provided for a life interest of personal property for Mrs Wilson, and then to her children at the age of 21 in equal shares. The variation proposed was that Mrs Wilson should surrender the income of one half of her life interest to the fund, but another effect of the proposed variation was to postpone the vesting of the children's interests until they reached the age of 30. The court was asked to approve the variation on behalf of Mrs Wilson's three children, who were aged 10, 7, and 6.

The surrender of the income (the real purpose of which was to reduce Mrs Wilson's liability to surtax) was also clearly to the advantage of the children, since the value of the trust property would be increased. However, the postponement to the age of 30 (on the grounds that it would be undesirable for Mrs Wilson's children to receive a large income from the age of 21) was clearly to their disadvantage. Megarry J approved the variation on the same test adopted in *Re Robinson*.

Benefit must be to individuals, not only to the class as a whole

In *Re Cohen's ST* [1965] 1 WLR 1229, Stamp J held that, in considering questions of benefit under the 1958 Act, the court was being asked to consent on behalf of beneficiaries who were not *sui iuris* considered as individuals, and not merely as members of a class. It follows that if only one member of the class can be envisaged who cannot possibly benefit from the proposed variation, even if the class as a whole will benefit, the court will refuse its consent.

In *Re Cohen's ST*, the variation sought, with a view to saving estate duty, was to substitute for the death of the life tenant (who was an elderly lady) a specified date (30 June 1973) for the vesting of her grandchildren's interests. It was very unlikely that the life tenant would survive beyond 30 June 1973, although, of course, it was a theoretical possibility. Consent was sought on behalf of infant and unborn beneficiaries.

There was no problem regarding the infant beneficiaries, although even here an element of risk was involved. They all stood to gain from the tax advantages of the proposed variation. If, however, the life tenant were to die before 30 June 1973, any infant grandchild who died between her death and the specified date would inevitably lose out (the grandchild would have taken under the unvaried, but not under the varied, settlement). Also, the share of all of the infant beneficiaries would be reduced if further grandchildren were to be born between her death and the specified date. On balance, however, these risks would be worth taking, given the likely saving in estate duty (the principles applicable being those considered in the previous section).

Risks to beneficiaries and unborn grandchildren

The difficulty in *Re Cohen's ST* concerned unborn grandchildren. Although it was unlikely, it was theoretically possible that the life tenant would live beyond the specified date. Had she done so, it was also theoretically possible for an unborn grandchild to be born after 30 June 1973, but before the life tenant's death. Any such grandchild would take under the unvaried settlement, but not under the proposed variation, and therefore could not possibly benefit from the variation. Of course, the chances of *both* of these events occurring were very low, and it may well be thought that the class of unborn grandchildren, as a whole, might be prepared to take the risk of the life tenant living beyond the specified date, and having further grandchildren before she died. Weighed against the tax advantages of the proposed variation, it might be thought that any reasonable unborn grandchild would be prepared to take this risk.

Stamp J held that it is not permissible to consider only the position of the class as a whole. If any individual grandchild were born after the specified date, but before the life tenant's death, then, under the proposed variation, he or she would lose his or her entire interest. That individual would clearly not consent, since he or she would have no conceivable benefit. Since it was therefore possible to envisage unborn persons who could not possibly benefit, this was fatal to the proposed variation, and Stamp J refused his consent. It was not enough that the proposed variation would benefit the class as a whole if it were possible to envisage *a single individual* who could not possibly benefit.

The argument that any unborn individual would have a greater chance of being born before 30 June 1973, because (since the life tenant was unlikely to live that long) more time would probably be available in which to be born, was also rejected on the ground that the court would not ascribe chances to a disembodied spirit. Stamp J observed, at 1233:

> Now it is of course perfectly true that as a result of this variation there would be a greater chance of there being some person or persons now unborn becoming beneficially interested in the trust fund [by being born], but to say that some particular unborn person will, immediately on the variation taking effect, have a better chance of being born within the qualifying period or a better chance of satisfying the necessary conditions seems to me to involve an excursion into metaphysics, on which I am unwilling to embark. Such a proposition seems to me to involve the logical conclusion that the court must regard one whose body may come into the existence in the future as having nevertheless such a present imaginary existence as to enable the court to ascribe to him a present chance of coming into existence at some specific time or during some specified period. My mind recoils at the idea of the unborn having prior to his birth such an identity as to enable the court to ascribe to him any such chance, or to enable one to say that he can more or less easily satisfy a condition of coming into existence during some particular period.

Only once birth (albeit in the future) had occurred could chances of benefit be ascribed to any individual.

Re Cohen's ST was distinguished in *Re Holt's Settlement* [1969] 1 Ch 100. In this case, the settlement was in essence that Mrs Wilson gave up part of her income from the fund (so increasing the size of the fund), but that vesting of the children's interest in possession would be postponed. If a child was born the year after the variation, and his or her mother died very soon afterwards, that child could not possibly benefit. The benefit from Mrs Wilson surrendering part of her income under the trust would be minimal if Mrs Wilson were to die soon after the birth, whereas the postponement would operate entirely to the newborn's disadvantage. *Re Cohen's ST* was distinguished, however, because in this case two possibilities had to manifest: first, the unborn person had to be born next year; and second, that child having been born (and thus having become a legal entity), his or her mother had to die shortly afterwards. The first chance could be disregarded on *Cohen* principles, but not the second. Both were independently unlikely possibilities, so approval for the scheme was given. Even once the theoretical unborn child had been born, he or she would still have been well advised to agree to the variation, and accept the slight risk of his or her mother dying shortly afterwards.

It follows that the reasoning in *Cohen* applies only when the date of *vesting in interest* (in other words, the date on closing the class) is altered, and does not apply merely to alterations in *vesting in possession* (on which more can be found on the Online Resource Centre).

It might be objected that two independent chances also had to occur in *Cohen* before an unborn beneficiary was certain to lose: first, the hypothetical beneficiary had to be born after 30 June 1973; and second, the life tenant had to live beyond the date of the beneficiary's birth. However, no unborn beneficiary born after 30 June 1973 could possibly gain from the variation, and he or she might lose, so there could be no advantage in the hypothetical beneficiary consenting to the variation. In this regard, the proposed variation in *Re Cohen's ST* differed from that in *Re Holt's Settlement*, in which the hypothetical beneficiary had a good chance of benefiting from the variation.

15.5 Variation or resettlement? And the juristic basis for variation

According to Megarry J in *Re Ball's Settlement* [1968] 1 WLR 899, the courts will not approve a proposal for a total resettlement that alters completely the substratum of the trust. This is a question of substance, not form.

In *Re Holmden's ST* [1968] AC 685, Lord Reid took the view that a variation under the 1958 Act must be regarded as one made by the beneficiaries themselves, rather than by the court, with the court acting merely on behalf of those beneficiaries who are unable to give their own consent and approval. His view did not form part of the *ratio* of the case, nor was it explicitly shared by his brethren, but it was accepted as being good law by the Court of Appeal in *Goulding* v *James* [1997] 2 All ER 239, probably as part of the *ratio*, since it followed that the adult *sui iuris* beneficiaries could consent to the variation for themselves, and that any reservations the settlor might have had were irrelevant. Since, however, as we have seen, even where all beneficiaries are *sui iuris* and consenting, they may not be able to vary the trusts in all circumstances, it must follow that the jurisdiction under the Act takes the form of a *Saunders* v *Vautier* revocation, followed by a resettlement (this presumably requires the consent of the trustees, since the resettlement cannot be forced on them against their will).

On this view of the matter, however, it arguably follows that the adult beneficiaries at least ought to give their consents in writing so as to comply with s. 53(1)(c) of the Law of Property Act 1925. In fact, however, variations are seldom in writing. In *Re Viscount Hambleden's WT* [1960] 1 WLR 82, it had been stated that the court's approval was effective for all purposes to vary the trusts, and this has been relied upon in countless subsequent instances. The problem was posed directly in *Re Holt's Settlement* (see 'Risks to beneficiaries and unborn grandchildren'), in which Megarry J—aware that thousands of variations may have been acted upon without writing conforming with s. 53(1)(c)—accepted, although without enthusiasm, two grounds put forward by counsel in favour of the view that no writing was necessary. First, it might be said that, in conferring express power upon the court to make an order, Parliament had impliedly created an exception to s. 53. Second, and alternatively, the arrangement might be regarded as one in which the beneficial interests passed to their respective purchasers upon the making of the agreement, that agreement itself being specifically enforceable. The original interests under the (unvaried) trusts would thus be held, from the moment of the agreement, upon constructive trusts identical to the new (varied) trusts and, as constructive trusts, would be exempt from writing under s. 53(2). Whether or not these reasons are regarded as adequate, the assumption that no writing is required has continued to prevail.

The point was also important in *Re Holt's Settlement* because the order of the court took effect after 15 July 1964, whereas the original trust had been set up in 1959, and Megarry J thought that the provisions of the Perpetuities and Accumulations Act 1964 (on which, see the Online Resource Centre) could apply. If all that the court had done had been to provide consent, then the perpetuity period would have been that applicable to a 1959 instrument (that is, the common law period).

Revision Box

1. From reading the materials on the variation of express trusts, ensure that you can answer the following questions.
   (a) What is meant by 'variation' of a settlement?
   (b) What issues arise in decisions to vary trusts and what, if any, policy considerations arise as a result?
   (c) In what circumstances will a variation of an original settlement be sought?
   (d) What are the key provisions that allow for the variation of trusts?

FURTHER READING

Riddall (1987) 'Does it or doesn't it? Contingent interests and the Variation of Trusts Act 1958' 51 Conveyancer 144.

online
resource
centre

For a summary of this article, please visit <http://www.oxfordtextbooks.co.uk/orc/wilson_trusts11e/>

16

Breach of trust

This chapter follows the consideration given to the nature of trusteeship, considered in Chapter 13, and the nature of duties that arise from this, examined in some detail in Chapter 14. In terms of 'locating' breach of trust within this text's overall coverage of trusteeship, generally speaking, any failure to comply with the duties laid upon the trustee will amount to breach of trust. This is so whether the duties arise from the trust instrument itself, where there is one, or whether they arise from obligations imposed by equity. Such failure may take the form of some positive action, such as investing in unauthorized securities, or an omission, such as neglecting to have the trust property placed in the name of the trustee. Even a merely technical act of maladministration may result in liability if, in fact, it causes a loss to the trust estate.

16.1 A question of liability: what is breach of trust?

This can be illustrated by reference to *Armitage* v *Nurse* [1998] Ch 241, in which, according to Millett LJ, at 251:

> Breaches of trust are of many different kinds. A breach of trust may be deliberate or inadvertent; it may consist of an actual misappropriation or misapplication of the trust property or merely of an investment or other dealing which is outside the trustees' powers; it may consist of a failure to carry out a positive obligation of the trustees or merely of a want of skill and care on their part in the management of the trust property; it may be injurious to the interests of the beneficiaries or be actually to their benefit.

In addition, at least in the case of an express trust, it does not matter how the trust was created (although the duties imposed on constructive trustees, as we have seen, may be less). Volunteer beneficiaries are entitled to have their interests protected to the same extent as those who have given consideration, and it is of no relevance either that the trust was created voluntarily by the same person who, in his capacity as trustee, is now charged with breach of trust. In other words, a settlor-trustee is liable to the same extent as any other trustee.

16.1.1 The basis of liability

The basis of a trustee's liability is compensation to the beneficiaries for whatever loss may have resulted from the breach, or, if an unauthorized profit has been made, the restoration to the beneficiaries of property rightfully belonging to the trust. The objective is not to punish the trustee, so his personal fault is immaterial once a breach is established. Of course, fault, in an objective sense, may be relevant to the question as to whether there has in fact been a breach, there being, as we have seen, a general standard of care based on normal business practice.

In many of the cases considered in other chapters, the trust had generally not suffered a large loss, and the remedy sought against the defendant was actually account of profits. In most of the cases considered in this chapter, the remedy sought is compensation for breach. In *Target Holdings Ltd* v *Redferns* [1995] 3 WLR 352, the House of Lords held that this is governed by principles similar to damages at common law. The claimant company, Target Holdings Ltd, was persuaded to advance approximately £1.5 million on a mortgage, on the assumption that the selling price of the property was to be £2 million. In fact, the property was sold for £775,000. The defendant solicitors acted for both vendor and purchaser. They had taken the money advanced, and paid it over to the purchaser and associated companies before the purchase and mortgage were executed, and in this respect (because they had paid the money away before being authorized to release it) were clearly in breach of trust with the claimant.

The purchasers later became insolvent and the claimant sold the property, but for only £500,000 (so that it had lost around £1 million), and sued the defendants for breach of trust. The defendants argued that the claimant had suffered no loss, because the defendants had obtained for the claimant exactly the mortgages to which it was entitled. The claimant would have suffered exactly the same loss, whether or not the defendants had paid out the money in breach of trust. The House of Lords held, in principle, in favour of the defendants: that a trustee who committed a breach of trust was not liable to compensate the beneficiary for losses that the beneficiary would, in any event, have suffered if there had been no such breach. The defendants would therefore not be liable on the assumed facts that the transaction would have gone through anyway, even in the absence of Target's advance. If the assumed facts were wrong and Target's advance was necessary for the transaction to go through at all, then Target would be entitled to be compensated for the entire loss that it had suffered, since in that event, but for the breach of trust, nothing would have been paid over.

There are no degrees of breach, however. Liability can attach to a trustee who has acted honestly in the beneficiaries' interests, just as it can to a trustee who has acted fraudulently for his own ends. Further, since the standard of care is objective (that is, it is measured against the level of competence of a notional reasonable man, rather than that of the particular trustee), liability can attach to a trustee who lacks the knowledge or skills to avoid the breach and is doing his incompetent best, if that best is not up to the objective standard required. Protection of the beneficiaries, and not the nature of the wrongdoing, is the crucial element.

The court may, however, take into account degrees of culpability in exercising its discretion to grant relief from liability, or in fixing the amount of interest that the trustee may be liable to pay on the sum lost to the trust estate, both of which are considered shortly.

What is not a breach of trust: distinguishing breach of fiduciary duty from breach of trust

When we look at what is said about breach of trust in *Armitage* v *Nurse*, we need to be aware that breach of trust is often considered closely alongside what is termed 'breach of a fiduciary duty', and we need to be able to understand that they are different. In this chapter, we are concerned with breach of trust; from *Armitage* v *Nurse*, it is clear that the scope of breach of trust is considered to be acts and omissions that define what a trustee must do—either from general law or according to the trust's terms—and which will make him liable *for* breach of trust if he does not do as required. Breach of fiduciary duty is different, because it is not of itself a wrongful unlawful act; instead, it refers to the situation in which a prima facie lawful act becomes a wrongful act because of the fiduciary obligation of loyalty that is imposed by equity, which disallows a trustee's duty to the trust and his interest to conflict.

Where a trustee makes investments that are imprudent, or which are not permitted by the terms of the trust, he has committed a breach of the duties that are imposed on him to ensure the proper administration of the trust. We can get a measure of this from looking back at the proper administration of trusts (initially in Chapter 13, and then Chapter 14), and liability for breach of trust will arise where a trustee fails to do what is required and the trust suffers a loss as a result of this. Where a trustee commits a breach of a fiduciary duty, we refer to situations in which he has breached the duty of loyalty that underpins all fiduciary relationships. So in setting himself up in competition with the trust, as long as he continues to administer the trust properly, a trustee will not commit a breach of trust. But even a trustee who does this properly will breach equity's special rules for fiduciaries by breaching the duty of loyalty. Where he does commit what we now know is a breach of fiduciary duty, we know from Chapter 13 that he can be restrained from the offending conduct and he must account for any unauthorized profit made.

This explains why equity treats wrongful dealings with trust property *by* a trustee (such as misappropriating it, or distributing it to persons not entitled to it) as a breach of trust, which must be compensated, whilst treating conduct that would not ordinarily be wrongful were it not for him placing himself in a position of conflict *as breach of* the fiduciary duty of loyalty.

16.1.2 **The personal nature of a trustee's liability**

A trustee is liable personally for his own breach of trust, and not vicariously for breaches committed by fellow trustees. In *Re Lucking's WT* [1968] 1 WLR 866, Lucking had committed a breach of trust in entrusting large sums of money to a manager without adequately supervising him. His fellow trustee, Block, was not liable for Lucking's breach of trust, but was entitled to rely on what Lucking had told him about the company's affairs, unless he had a positive reason to disbelieve him.

However, a trustee who passively permits a breach to occur may thereby put himself in breach of his own duties because, although trustees are not required to police each other's conduct, they are expected, as we have seen, to be active in the administration of the trust. Thus a trustee who leaves funds under the control of a fellow trustee without enquiry, or who fails to take steps to obtain redress if he discovers a breach, will be in dereliction of his own duty to the beneficiaries.

The personal nature of trusteeship can be appreciated through examining case law under the 1925 Act. By virtue of s. 30, 'A trustee ... shall be answerable and accountable only for his own acts, receipts, neglects, or defaults, and not those of any other trustee ... nor for any other loss, unless the same happens through his own wilful default'. In *Re Vickery* [1931] 1 Ch 572, Maugham J assumed that s. 30 had altered the law, at least in relation to liability for agents, for he interpreted the phrase 'wilful default' as meaning 'a consciousness of negligence or breach of duty, or recklessness in the performance of duty'. If this meaning is applied in relation to co-trustees, the section clearly confers extra protection.

Apart from *Re Vickery*, it is generally accepted that s. 30 did not alter the previous law: the section does not alter the principle that a trustee remains liable for his own acts, upon which the liability in the section is based. Under the previous law, liability was incurred where a trustee handed over money without securing its proper application, or permitted a fellow trustee to recover money without enquiring what he did with it, or refrained from taking steps to obtain redress for a breach of which he was aware. It has yet to be decided whether, in these circumstances also, it will be necessary to prove that a passive trustee was guilty of 'wilful default', as defined in *Re Vickery*, but we would suggest that this is unlikely. This position must now be seen in light of the repeal of s. 30(1) by the 2000 Act: the current position appears to be that a trustee now labours under the requirement to establish that he acted properly.

A trustee will not, upon accepting office, become liable for breaches committed prior to his appointment. His first steps on taking office, however, should be to examine the documents and accounts of the trust; if he discovers that a breach has occurred, he should take action against the former trustee to recover the loss. Failure to do so may itself amount to a breach for which he will be liable, save perhaps in the rare case in which he can show that action would have been futile (because there would then be no causal relationship between the breach and the loss).

A trustee cannot escape liability for his own breach of trust by retiring from office: even after his retirement, he remains liable for breaches committed while he was in office, and his estate remains liable after his death. He will not be liable for breaches committed after the date of his retirement, unless it can be shown that he retired in order to facilitate a breach of trust (*Head* v *Gould* [1898] 2 Ch 250).

16.1.3 Liability as between trustees

The liability of trustees is said to be 'joint and several', which means that if two or more trustees are liable, a beneficiary may choose to sue some or all of them, or perhaps only one, and recoup the entire loss from those against whom he chooses to proceed. Similarly, he may levy execution against any one of them for the whole amount.

As between themselves, however, the trustees were, until 1978, regarded by equity as being equally liable, so that a trustee who was compelled to pay more than his fair share of the loss could in turn enforce a contribution from the others. In enforcing equal contribution, equity disregarded any differing degrees of involvement in the breach. Thus, in *Bahin* v *Hughes* (1886) 31 ChD 390, a passive trustee was liable to the same extent as an active one.

There were exceptions to the principle of equal contribution, which were unaffected by the 1978 legislation (considered in the next section), as follows.

(a) *Where there has been fraud* A fraudulent trustee is solely liable and can claim no contribution from the honest trustees.

(b) *Where a trustee has got money into his hands and made use of it* In this instance, the trustee will be liable to indemnify a co-trustee, who is obliged to replace the funds.

(c) *Where one trustee was a solicitor and the rest relied on his judgement* (Re Partington *(1887) 57 LT 654)* The mere fact that a trustee happens also to be a solicitor will not make him liable to indemnify the other trustees, for it is necessary also that the others rely on his judgement. Thus he will not be liable if it is shown that the other trustees were active participators in the breach, and did not participate merely in consequence of the advice and control of the solicitor (*Head* v *Gould* [1898] 2 Ch 250).

(d) *Where a trustee is also a beneficiary* In this case, he will be required to indemnify his co-trustees to the extent of his beneficial interest, and not merely to the extent that he has personally received some benefit from the breach (*Chillingworth* v *Chambers* [1896] 1 Ch 685). Only after that interest is exhausted will further liability be shared equally. The principle seems to be that a beneficiary may not claim any share of the trust estate until he has discharged his liabilities towards it.

16.1.3.1 Departing from the principle of equal responsibility

The equitable position has been affected by the Civil Liability (Contribution) Act 1978. Under this Act, any person liable in respect of damage suffered by another person, including damage arising from breach of trust, may recover a contribution from any other person in respect of the same damage. By s. 2(1), the amount of the contribution is 'such as may be found by the court to be just and equitable having regard to the extent of that person's responsibility for the damage in question'—and may, by virtue of s. 2(2), amount to a total indemnity. The Act therefore gives the court a discretion (but not a mandatory duty) to depart from the rule of equal distribution and to have regard to degrees of fault.

The Act does not apply to the limited number of exceptions to the general equitable principle described in the last section, and may indeed not affect the equitable position at all, since it is left to the court to determine what is 'just and equitable'. One other situation is clearly unaffected by the 1978 Act: if all of the trustees were involved in a fraud, equity would not allow those who paid the damages to claim any contribution from the rest, on the ground that a claimant could not base a claim upon his own wrongdoing. The 1978 Act makes no special provision for such a case, but while the court is theoretically free to exercise its discretion in allocating liability to contribute, it is inconceivable that a fraudulent trustee would be allowed to sue.

Where some, but not all, of the trustees are excused from liability under s. 61 of the Trustee Act 1925, it would seem to follow that those who are not excused can claim no contribution from them. Under the 1978 Act, the excused trustees would seem not to be persons who are liable in respect of any damage, so presumably the court cannot direct them to contribute.

16.1.4 **Trustees and criminal liability**

In the course of a breach of trust, criminal offences may be committed, but breach of trust is not of itself a criminal offence. There used to be a difficulty about theft, because the trustee, as legal owner of the trust property, could not be guilty of stealing it, and a special offence of 'conversion by a trustee' had to be created in order to make him punishable. However, by virtue of the provisions of the Theft Act 1968, a trustee may be guilty of ordinary theft. This is possible through the statutory definition of theft found in ss. 1(1) and 5(2) of the 1968 Act. Section 1(1) provides that 'A person is guilty of theft if he dishonestly appropriates property belonging to another with the intention of permanently depriving the other of it'.

The significance of s. 5(2) rests on the 'problem' that the trustee is actually the legal owner of trust property. Section 5(2) contains provisions for the meaning of property 'belonging to another' for the purposes of the s. 1(1) definition. By virtue of s. 5(2), 'property belonging to another' includes property held on trust so that:

> ... where property is subject to a trust, the person to whom it belongs shall be regarded as including any person having a right to enforce the trust, and an intention to defeat the trust shall be regarded accordingly as an intention to deprive of that property any person having that right.

This chapter is primarily a consideration of how breach of trust arises and the key dimensions of how the personal remedies against a trustee who has committed a breach of trust will operate. Previous editions reflected this position, and, accordingly, attention paid to trustees' criminal liability was brief and confined to the foregoing references to ss. 1(1) and 5(2) of the Theft Act 1968, to draw attention to the way in which a trustee who misappropriates trust funds can also be guilty of theft and thus incur criminal liability. Although it was always deemed necessary to point to the way in which, according to the criminal law, a legal owner of property can nevertheless be guilty of its theft, this was also deemed sufficient.

There was always scope for considering the way in which the criminal law dimension formed part of a 'bigger picture' of questions of trustee liability and accountability for the property that is entrusted to him for the beneficiaries. In this vein, it may well be the case that the threat of *criminal* liability serves important functions in deterring misappropriations of trust property, because of the *stigma* that is believed by many to attach to exposure to criminal culpability. However, at this point, it is now necessary to give criminal liability arising from the office of trustee much fuller consideration on account of the Fraud Act 2006.

Notwithstanding, this chapter remains a consideration of the consequences in equity that attach to a trustee's breach of his duties; this progresses from looking at what amounts to a breach, and how this becomes a 'measure' of the liability that can be incurred upon being found in breach. To preserve this emphasis, at this point only very brief reference is made to indicate that trustees *can* incur criminal liability in addition to that arising in equity. The more extensive consideration of the criminal consequences of trusteeship that is necessary in light of this recent change to English criminal law will close this chapter on breach of trust.

16.1.5 Bankruptcy of a defaulting trustee

If a trustee who is liable for a breach becomes bankrupt, the claim in respect of the breach is provable in his bankruptcy. His duties towards the trust are not affected by his bankruptcy, so the odd situation arises whereby he has a duty (as trustee) to prove in his own bankruptcy (as debtor to the trust). If he fails to do this, he commits a further breach of trust, which is not affected by any subsequent discharge from bankruptcy, and he will be liable to the trust for the resulting loss (that is, the dividend that he would have received in the bankruptcy).

16.2 Qualifications and defences to liability

English law's position on trustee liability is that, where there is a breach of a duty, this gives rise to breach of trust. The numerous ways in which breach of trust can arise have been explained, with illustrative reference made to Millett LJ's judgment in *Armitage* v *Nurse*. In terms of what 'breach of trust' means, within the spectrum of its possible manifestations is that a trustee is liable to account, to the beneficiary, for losses experienced by the trust and its assets. This is the position in principle, and it is—like liability across legal regimes—liability that operates within certain limitations. In trusts law, these limits are defined in reference to the defences that a trustee accused of breach of trust may be able to invoke.

16.2.1 Consent or participation by beneficiaries

A beneficiary who consents to or participates in a breach of trust will not usually be able to succeed in a claim against the trustees, even if he has obtained no personal benefit from the breach. The consent or participation of one beneficiary will not, of course, prevent those who did not consent from claiming, and if it is uncertain which beneficiaries have consented, the court may order an inquiry. No particular form of consent is required.

To be effective, consent must be that of an adult who is *sui iuris* and not acting under an undue influence that prevents him from making an independent judgement. In *Re Pauling's ST* [1964] Ch 303, trustees of a marriage settlement had made a series of advances in breach of trust because the trustees did not ensure that the moneys advanced were used for their proper purpose. A wide range of defences was argued, both before Wilberforce J and in the Court of Appeal, but on this issue several of the payments that went to benefit the parents were presumed to have been the result of undue influence over the children. Whether undue influence has been exercised is a question of fact, depending on circumstances. The trustees will not be liable if it cannot be shown that they knew, or ought to have known, that the beneficiary was acting under such influence.

In *Re Pauling's ST* itself, the Court of Appeal held that, where a presumption of undue influence existed, as between a parent and child who was still subject to parental influence (albeit a child who had reached her majority), an advance to the child that was given to her parents could not be retained by the parent unless it was clear that:

(a) the gift was the spontaneous act of the child; and

(b) the child knew what her rights were.

It was also desirable that the child had obtained independent and, if possible, professional advice.

In this regard, the courts treat with suspicion gifts from children to their parents, whereas the reverse is true of gifts the other way round (see, for example, the presumption of advancement in Chapter 6).

16.2.1.1 Acquiescence and the requirement of 'consent'

Consent involves more than mere awareness of what the trustees are proposing to do; otherwise, trustees could protect themselves by simply telling the beneficiaries beforehand. In *Re Pauling's ST* [1962] 1 WLR 86, Wilberforce J explained, at 108, that:

> [T]he court has to consider all the circumstances in which the concurrence of the *cestui que trust* was given with a view to seeing whether it is fair and equitable that, having given his concurrence, he should afterwards turn round and sue the trustees.

He went on to say that it is not necessary that the beneficiary should know that what he is concurring in is a breach of trust, provided that he fully understands in what he is concurring. Nor is it necessary that he should personally benefit from the breach. This statement of the law was neither approved nor disapproved by the Court of Appeal in *Re Pauling's ST* [1964] Ch 303 itself, but was approved by the Court of Appeal in *Holder* v *Holder* [1968] Ch 353, in which a beneficiary was held unable to set aside a sale after affirming it and accepting part of the purchase money.

16.2.2 Release or acquiescence by beneficiaries

A beneficiary will also be unable to succeed in his claim if, on becoming aware of the breach, he acquiesced in the breach or released the trustee from liability arising therefrom. A partial defence succeeded on the basis of the acquiescence doctrine in *Re Pauling's ST* [1964] Ch 303.

Release suggests some active waiver by the beneficiary of his rights. A waiver requires a positive act that is intended to be irrevocable. It is like making a gift and, as with gifts, no consideration need move from the donee (in this case, the trustee). As with consent, there need not be any particular formalities and release may even be inferred from conduct.

If a release cannot be shown, it may still be possible to show that the beneficiary acquiesced in the breach. It is usually accepted that the acquiescence doctrine is based on an implied contract, whereby the beneficiary is taken to have agreed not to rely on his rights. The evidence required for this intention to be inferred is less than in the case of release, and the doctrine is often applied where a beneficiary has done nothing to pursue his claim.

Delay in making the claim is not, in itself, evidence of acquiescence, but where the length of time between the breach and the claim is very great, slight additional evidence will suffice. As in the case of consent, the release or acquiescence must be that of an adult who is *sui iuris*.

Undue influence or lack of full knowledge will prevent the trustee from relying on these defences, the test being as in the consent doctrine (see section 16.2.1).

16.2.3 Impounding a beneficiary's interest

The court has an inherent power to impound the interest of a beneficiary, thus providing the trustee with an indemnity to the extent that the beneficiary's interest will suffice to replace the loss to the trust.

The power can arise where a beneficiary has merely consented to the breach, but only if some benefit to him can be proved, and then only to the extent of that benefit. If the beneficiary has gone further and actually requested or instigated a breach, the power can be exercised whether or not he has received a personal benefit from the breach.

Needless to say, the trustee has to show that the beneficiary acted in full knowledge of the facts, but it is not necessary to show that he knew that the acts he was instigating or consenting to amounted to a breach.

There is also a statutory discretion to impound. Section 62(1) of the Trustee Act 1925 (replacing an earlier enactment) provides that:

> Where a trustee commits a breach of trust at the instigation or request or with the consent in writing of a beneficiary, the court may, if it thinks fit, make such order as to the court seems just, for impounding all or any part of the interest of the beneficiary in the trust estate by way of indemnity to the trustee or persons claiming through him.

The courts seem to have treated this largely as a consolidating section, rather than as extending their powers, except that Wilberforce J in *Re Pauling's ST (No. 2)* [1963] Ch 576 thought that it gave an additional right, among other things, to deal with a married, female beneficiary. This additional right is no longer necessary, because of changes in legislation on family property, and that part of the section was repealed in 1949.

The effect of the court making an order impounding a beneficiary's interest is that the beneficiary is not only debarred from pursuing his own claim against the trustee, but also liable to replace the losses suffered by the other beneficiaries, to the extent ordered by the court, and perhaps up to the full value of his own interest. To this extent, the trustee is protected at the beneficiary's expense.

The discretion is a judicial discretion, and although the section appears to extend the inherent power of the court by giving a discretion to impound a beneficiary's interest regardless of whether he obtained a benefit, it has received a restrictive interpretation. It seems that the court will make an impounding order in any case in which it would have done so before the Act—generally speaking, in any case in which the beneficiary has actively induced the breach (for which it has never been necessary to show benefit).

16.2.3.1 Requirement of full awareness by beneficiary

It must, of course, be shown that the beneficiary was fully aware of what was being done. In *Re Somerset* [1894] 1 Ch 231, a beneficiary had urged the trustees to invest in a mortgage of a particular property, but had left them to decide how much money they were prepared to invest. Lindley MR said, at 265:

> In order to bring a case within this section the *cestui que trust* must instigate, or request, or consent in writing to some act or omission which is itself a breach of trust, and not to some act or omission which only becomes a breach of trust by reason of want of care on the part of the trustees.

The words 'in writing' have been held to apply only to consent, and not to instigation or request (*Griffith* v *Hughes* [1892] 3 Ch 105). So a request or instigation need only be oral.

The power to impound will not be lost on an assignment of the beneficial interest; nor is it lost when the court replaces the trustees in consequence of the breach. In *Re Pauling's ST* [1962] 1 WLR 86, the trustees resisted removal because they were claiming an indemnity out of the interests of the parents. Wilberforce J held that they were entitled to such indemnity and that this would be unaffected by their replacement. They were therefore unable to use this as a ground for continuing in office (see *Re Pauling's ST (No. 2)* [1963] Ch 576).

Apart from statute, it is the practice, where trustees have under an honest mistake overpaid a beneficiary, for the court to make allowance for the mistake in order to allow the trustee to recoup as far as possible (*Re Musgrave* [1916] 2 Ch 416). An overpaid beneficiary is not compelled to return the excess, but further payment may be withheld until the accounts are adjusted.

If a payment is made by mistake to someone who is not entitled, the trustee may recover on an action for money had and received if the mistake was one of fact, but not if it was a mistake of law (*Re Diplock* [1947] Ch 716). It is also certain that the error must be corrected where trustee-beneficiaries overpay themselves.

16.2.4 **Trustee liability and the lapse of time**

Lapse of time may protect a trustee in one of two ways. By the Limitation Act 1980, limits are set upon the time within which certain actions for recovery may be brought, while in cases not covered by statutory limitation, a defendant may rely on the doctrine of laches.

16.2.4.1 Limitation Act 1980

By s. 21(3) of the Limitation Act 1980, any action by a beneficiary to recover trust property or in respect of any breach of trust (other than situations covered by the self-dealing and fair-dealing rules) must be brought within six years of the date on which the right of action accrued.

A right of action in respect of future interests is not treated as having accrued until the interest falls into possession: this was also part of the *ratio* in *Re Pauling's ST* [1964] Ch 303 (discussed in this chapter).

Under s. 21(1), no period of limitation applies where the action is in respect of any fraud to which the trustee was a party, or privy, or where (in summary) it is sought to recover from the trustee trust property still in his possession or the proceeds of sale of such property. Protection is also lost where the trustee converts trust property to his own use. Conversion to the trustee's own use, however, implies application in his own favour, so that if the funds have been used to maintain an infant beneficiary, or dissipated by a fellow trustee, the protection of limitation remains available.

Where fraud is the issue, this must be fraud by the trustee himself. In *Thorne* v *Heard* [1894] 1 Ch 599, a trustee was protected, by a section (in similar terms) of an earlier Act, where he had left trust funds with a solicitor who had embezzled them, the trustee himself being no more than negligent. Where the trustee is in possession of trust property or its proceeds, however, no dishonesty need be shown. Fraud for these purposes is wider than common law fraud or deceit, but nevertheless requires unconscionable conduct on the part of the trustee, something in the nature of a deliberate cover-up. In *Bartlett* v *Barclays Bank Trust Co. Ltd (No. 1)* [1980] Ch 515, the bank was held able to rely on what is now s. 21(1) of the 1980 Act in respect of income lost outside the limitation period, since, being unaware that it was acting in breach of trust, it could not be guilty of fraud for these purposes.

Section 22 prescribes a limitation period of twelve years for actions in respect of any claim to the personal estate of a deceased person. It is often hard to determine at what point executors have completed the administration of an estate and become trustees, but it is thought that the twelve-year period will apply, although for all other purposes the executors would be regarded as trustees.

Claimants 'under disability' are permitted an extended period in which to bring an action by s. 28; by s. 32, where fraud, concealment, or mistake is alleged, time runs only from the point when the claimant discovers the fraud or mistake, or could with reasonable diligence have discovered it.

It should be noted that a person other than a bona fide purchaser for value without notice who receives property from a trustee also falls within these rules.

16.2.4.2 The equitable doctrine of laches

Where no statutory limitation period applies, the defendant may rely on the equitable doctrine of laches—that is, he may show that it would be unjust to allow the claimant to pursue his claim in view of the time that has elapsed since it accrued. The court has a discretion to allow or refuse the defence, and mere delay may suffice, but, where

possible, the courts have preferred to regard delay as furnishing evidence of acquiescence by the claimant.

16.2.5 Trustee Act 1925, s. 61

The Trustee Act 1925, s. 61, gives the court a wide discretion to excuse honest and
reasonable trustees from liability for breach of trust. It applies also to executors. The
section provides:

> If it appears to the court that a trustee ... is or may be personally liable for any breach of
> trust, whether the transaction alleged to be a breach of trust occurred before or after the
> commencement of this Act, but has acted honestly and reasonably, and ought fairly to
> be excused for the breach of trust and for omitting to obtain the directions of the court
> in the matter in which he committed such breach, then the court may relieve him either
> wholly or partly from personal liability for the same.

Dishonesty will obviously disqualify a trustee from obtaining relief, but a trustee is
also required to act 'reasonably'. The standard applied appears to be the same as that
for breach of trust itself—that of the prudent man of business in relation to his own
affairs—and the bank failed on this test in *Bartlett* v *Barclays Bank Trust Co. Ltd (No. 1)*
[1980] Ch 515. Failure to obtain directions might be thought to fall below this standard,
but the section implies that relief may nonetheless be granted.

Unauthorized investments appear to be the most common circumstances in which
applications are made, and it may not be easy to show that this sort of risk-taking meets
with the standard of the prudent business person. Reasonable conduct may be more easily
shown where the breach consists in some error made in the course of a complex administration. Professional trustees may claim the protection of the section, but the courts have
been less ready to excuse failure where a high standard of expertise is professed by the
trustee: see, again, *Bartlett* v *Barclays Bank Trust Co. Ltd (No. 1)* [1980] Ch 515.

It may be that even if the trustee is shown to have acted honestly and reasonably, the
question of whether he ought fairly to be excused will be separately considered.

16.3 Trustee exemption clauses

Traditionally, the only coverage given in this textbook to exemption clauses was the
observation that '[t]here is no reason why an appropriately drafted exemption clause
in the trust instrument should not protect a trustee who would otherwise be liable for
breach of trust'. This was accompanied only by a reference to *Armitage* v *Nurse* [1998] Ch
241 as authority for this position.

The essence of the trustee exemption clause (TEC) is much like it sounds. Like exemption clauses found in contract law, the TEC is a mechanism to restrict or exclude liability that may otherwise be incurred in the course of trusteeship. The context for such
clauses is the occurrence of breach of trust, which flows from the duties to which trustees are subject in their administration of the trust, or from the trust instrument, or
duties imposed by law; it is any failure to comply with these duties that will amount to
a breach of trust. And, as was made clear earlier, there are no 'degrees' of breach of trust:
a breach can be innocent, as well as fraudulent, and the law does not even distinguish

flagrant incompetence from incompetence arising from misfortune. It is even the case that liability for breach of trust is not confined to situations that have detrimentally affected the trust: liability will arise equally where the breach has actually brought beneficial consequences for the trust. In short, all incidences of breach of trust leave the trustee open to incur liability for it.

This scope of breach of trust should therefore explain trustees' attempts to limit or exclude the liability that it is possible for them to incur; even trustees who are competent and bona fide might, with very good reason, elect to try to protect themselves in such a manner. This also serves as a reminder of the very close relationship between performance of the trust and its breach—itself a further illustration of the very close interrelationship between all of these chapters on trusteeship and the way in which the essence of trusteeship is actually very difficult to 'parcel' into more discrete aspects for study. Indeed, just as TECs can be seen as a mechanism to protect trustees against breach of trust, they can also be seen as a measure of trustees' duties. This latter analysis emphasizes them as devices to 'manage' expectations of trustees in the performance of their duties. In light of this 'dual perspective', this consideration of TECs would therefore be equally at home in Chapter 14 as it is in the present one, and passing reference was indeed made to these mechanisms in that chapter.

16.3.1 Trustee exemption clauses: common law and pressure for reform

Traditional coverage of TECs was so brief that, whilst *Armitage* v *Nurse* [1998] Ch 241 was cited as the leading case for their validity in English law, there was no actual quotation of the key passages of the judgment of Millett LJ. However, materials on the Online Resource Centre that consider TECs show how coverage became far more extensive post-2002 on account of the reactions generated by *Armitage*, characterized by concern that what was permissible at common law gave far too much facilitation to trustees to avoid the consequences of breach of trust. The Online Resource Centre materials also discuss how any study of the modern law relating to TECs includes explaining what is meant by 'duty modification' clauses, and also 'extended powers' or 'authorization' clauses.

This discussion is grounded in work undertaken by the Law Commission, which resulted in the adoption of a different approach, designed to rebalance the respective needs of trustees, and also settlors and particularly beneficiaries. The full narrative is located within the Online Resource Centre materials, and it is only possible to give coverage to key aspects of the journey from *Armitage* to current approaches. So what precisely did *Armitage* permit, and what is the approach now? Under *Armitage*, the common law allowed considerable scope for trustees to limit liability for committing a breach of trust, or even to escape this altogether. Indeed, in accepting that liability for breach could be excluded for conduct that fell short of amounting to 'actual fraud', Millett LJ conceded, at 242, that:

> the view is widely held that these clauses have gone too far, and that trustees who charge for their services and who, as professional men, would not dream of excluding liability for ordinary professional negligence should not be able to rely on a trustee exemption clause excluding liability for gross negligence.

After *Armitage*, a flurry of cases followed, initially with *Bogg* v *Raper* (1998–99) 1 ITELR 267, *Wight* v *Olswang (No. 2)* (1999–2000) 2 ITELR 689, and *Walker* v *Stones* [2001] QB

902. And whilst the Law Commission's work was well under way, *Armitage* was followed in *Barraclough* v *Mell* [2005] EWHC 3387 (Ch) and, in the context of a pension settlement, in *Baker* v *J. E. Clark & Co. (Transport) UK Ltd* [2006] EWCA Civ 464.

In 2002, the Law Commission published its Consultation Paper on *Trustee Exemption Clauses* (CP No. 161). This was an extremely interesting and highly readable document, which provided an excellent point of reference for much of the coverage on trusteeship in this text in earlier chapters. In this more general sense, it provides an excellent opportunity to review understanding of many of the core issues, as well as an opportunity to examine them more critically. In July 2006, the Law Commission published its consequent report of the same name (Law Com. 301, Cm. 6874). In looking at the range of issues, in both documents, spanning traditional and evolving understanding of trusts and their creation, and the economics of trust formation—in terms of how economically viable the creation of a trust is, in the light of how costly it is to be administered by trust service providers—in the initial consultation, the Law Commission explained, at para. 1.5, that the central problem for its inquiries was that:

> English law does not at present provide a readily available means for beneficiaries to claim that a trustee exemption clause should not be invoked by a trustee and, as a result, trustees have considerable scope to protect themselves from liability for breach of trust. The question arises whether reliance on trustee exemption clauses is seriously endangering the interests of those whom the trust relationship is directed to promote.

In setting out a typical pattern for exemption clauses following *Armitage*, where trustees sought routinely to exclude liability 'for any loss or damage which may happen to the Trust fund … at any time or from any cause whatsoever', unless such loss or damage was caused by 'actual fraud', the Law Commission lamented that there could be no doubt that such clauses are valid and that they would be interpreted in a way by which liability for losses caused to the trust arising from negligence, and even from gross negligence, can validly be excluded. This meant that English law had adopted a position whereby a trustee could protect himself (in the words of presiding Millett LJ in *Armitage* itself) 'no matter how indolent, imprudent, lacking in diligence, negligent or wilful he might have been, so long as he has not acted dishonestly'.

Striking the best balance

From this, the Law Commission was forced to conclude that the protection of beneficiaries under English law was 'weaker than in the past'. And whilst the Law Commission accepted that there was no possibility of absolute protection of beneficiaries, it also insisted that the very weak protection afforded by *Armitage* had to be reconciled with the position that beneficiary protection is 'one of the prime concerns of trust law'.

16.3.2 The 2002 Consultation Paper and the 2006 report: core concerns and key recommendations

At the heart of the Law Commission's work in 2002 was independent work commissioned from Dr Alison Dunn. This provided the core around which the Law Commission could consider the fundamental considerations of a trust, together with changing patterns of trust formation—centrally, the growing presence of trust formation in commercial dealings, and the increasing importance of pension scheme trusts—and the economics of trust service provision in this context. This is set out in extensive detail on the Online Resource Centre.

The Online Resource Centre materials also consider the Law Commission's initial recommendations following the close of the consultation in 2003, and examine them alongside those emerging from the 2006 report, published in light of responses received to the consultation. From this, a general picture emerged that the presence of TECs was inevitable, but that common law provided far too much scope for trustees to avoid liability for breach of trust and that, often, settlors commonly had little or no awareness that such mechanisms were being deployed.

Striking a new balance and a new approach to regulation

In its 2006 report, the Law Commission reiterated that serious concerns continue to pertain to the use of exemption clauses; this is because they are able—at their most extreme—actually to exclude liability, and this also renders them capable of undermining attempts that may be made to regulate them. But it sought to balance this with its assertion that '[s]uch clauses are often included in trust instruments for perfectly good and practical reasons not motivated by an intention to avoid liability for breach of trust'. In so doing, the Law Commission conceded that it had been 'unable to frame legislative regulation in a way which would effectively distinguish between these two types of use, other than by creating a complicated system with even greater potential adverse impact'. Thus, in the report, the Law Commission shifted its focus to an alternative strategy, which reflected a core set of issues on which it did remain convinced following the consultation, but which would be pursued through a system of 'rule of practice' rather than legislation.

The Law Commission suggested that such a rule of practice would be the most 'appropriate and effective means of influencing and informing trustees so as to secure the proper disclosure of exemption clauses', because '[r]egulated persons would be required to adhere to defined good practice'. Such a scheme would not suffer the same defects that could undermine one based in statute because '[c]ompliance with the rule would be a matter of professional conduct for the trustee'. Being in breach of good practice in this manner will not invalidate the clause or affect a trustee's reliance upon it, but it will 'render the trustee open to professional disciplinary measures'. In turn, this amounted to a 'proportionate response' to any failure by a trustee to ensure adequate settlor awareness of any exemption provisions within the trust instrument.

The report thus recommended, at para. 1.2.2, the following rule of practice in arrangements that are not between commercial parties or pensions trusts (or ones that are charitable):

> Any paid trustee who causes a settlor to include a clause in a trust instrument which has the effect of excluding or limiting liability for negligence must before the creation of the trust take such steps as are reasonable to ensure that the settlor is aware of the meaning and effect of the clause.

The Online Resource Centre materials pay considerable attention to how and why the Law Commission concluded that negligence was the appropriate benchmark for limiting or excluding liability, why the rule would be focused on 'paid trustees', and also why certain types of trust would not be subject to the rule of practice. But in focusing here on those who would fall subject to it, the Law Commission noted in the report that, from its communication with regulatory and professional bodies, a large number, including the Law Society and the Institute of Chartered Accountants in England and Wales, set to work quickly on designing regulation to this effect; government was also urged to 'promote the recommended rule of practice as widely as possible across the trust industry', and regulatory authorities were encouraged to adopt 'a version of the rule appropriate to the particular circumstances of their membership, and to enforce such regulation in accordance with their existing codes of conduct'.

A much more critical and actually normative discussion of the Law Commission's work can be found on the Online Resource Centre. This explores all of the stages of the Law Commission's involvement in some depth, and it also asks whether the Law Commission was correct to conclude that the presence of TECs is inevitable in English law and considers some of the merits and disbenefits of a 'self-regulation' approach, drawing on interdisciplinary perspectives from history, criminology, regulation, and professions and professionalism. In focusing on the current position, following the publication of the report, the Law Commission's website reiterated that the trust service industry should adopt a non-statutory rule of practice, and that this should be enforced by the regulatory and professional bodies that govern and influence trustees and the drafters of trusts.

It also documented that several professional bodies are working towards introducing regulations for their members that are intended to be binding, and which embody that the use of clauses in trust instruments which have the effect of limiting or excluding liability for negligence must be disclosed and explained, with paid trustees taking reasonable steps to ensure that settlors understand the meaning and effect of such clauses before including them in trust instruments. There was also the recommendation that those who actually draft trusts also be subject to the rule.

16.3.3 Adoption of the rule of practice and the approach of the courts

The Law Commission also noted that its approach has been 'welcomed by the Better Regulation Executive', with affirmation from the latter that '[w]ith complex and important issues such as trustee exemption clauses it is all too easy to play it safe and legislate', and that it was good to see that 'the Law Commission has listened to people on all sides of the debate and developed a proportionate risk-based approach to the issue'.

This optimism was certainly in place in September 2010, when the government accepted the Law Commission's recommendations. In a statement, then Under Secretary of State for Justice Jonathan Djanogly confirmed that the government would be promoting further uptake by writing directly to the relevant regulatory and professional bodies to urge them to adopt the Law Commission's recommended approach.

Indeed, this position has very recently provided the basis for the Privy Council decision, in *Spread Trustee Ltd* v *Hutcheson* [2011] UKPC 13, in which (as summarized by Lord Mance)—in accordance with the codes of conduct or regulatory and professional bodies, under which any *paid* trustee including a clause exempting from any type of negligence must, before creation of the trust, take reasonable steps to ensure the settlor's awareness of its meaning and effect—the argument was raised that any provision exempting from liability for gross negligence should be regarded as invalid as a matter of law, whether the trustee be professional or not, paid or not.

This case was on appeal from the Guernsey Court of Appeal. In Guernsey, the regulation of exemption clauses is statutory, and there, on account of original statutory provision and amendments to it, exemption clauses will not relieve trustees from liability for fraud, wilful misconduct, or gross negligence. There is much that is revealing for the position of English law within this three–two majority judgment, and much of the thrust of the majority judgments was directed at applying the Guernsey statute to the clause in question.

But, more generally, an interesting starting point is Lady Hale's dissenting discussion of the benchmark of negligence. With reference to the Trust Law Committee's 1999 Consultation Paper on *Trustee Exemption Clauses*, she recounts the commentary upon the Court's reluctance to distinguish between ordinary and gross negligence, notwithstanding that 'there is a long and respectable line of authority ... dealing with the concept of gross negligence in the common law and distinguishing it from ordinary negligence'.

Lady Hale's view was very much that, whilst the duties and liabilities of active trustees are said to be of infinite variety, central to the notion of trusteeship was 'the reposing of reliance on a responsible person or agency to manage property in a manner that will benefit those who are the beneficiaries of the trust'. From the dissenting judgment of Lord Kerr, we have an even more powerful reminder of the *raison d'être* of restricting the scope that trustees have for excluding liability for breach of trust and, within this, strong endorsement that negligence is the most appropriate benchmark for this:

> If ... the placing of reliance on a responsible person to manage property so as to promote the interests of the beneficiaries of a trust is central to the concept of trusteeship, denying trustees the opportunity to avoid liability for their gross negligence seems to be to be entirely in keeping with that essential aim.
>
> (*Spread Trustee Ltd* v *Hutcheson* [2011] UKPC 13, *per* Lord Kerr at 1413)

16.4 Personal remedies against trustees

The materials here concern the issues arising when a breach of trust *has* occurred and when a financial remedy is sought on the ground that losses have been incurred as a result of this.

16.4.1 Measure of liability

The measure of liability is the actual loss to the trust estate that arises, directly or indirectly, from the breach, usually with interest. Where an unauthorized profit has been made, the trustees must account for this profit, but this will be the limit of their liability. It should also be noted that the trustees are liable only for losses that arise causally from a breach of trust. They are not required to act as insurers for the beneficiaries, and any losses that arise despite the exercise of due diligence on the part of the trustees must be borne by the trust estate.

Subject to these limitations, assuming that the claimant can establish a causal connection between the breach and the loss, there are no rules governing remoteness of damage such as apply in tort or contract. Inquiries as to what a reasonable trustee ought to have foreseen or contemplated are not relevant in this context. This may not matter as much as in, for example, a tort action, because the spectre of virtually unlimited liability—such as could occur in a negligence action, for example, if a cigarette end negligently thrown away were to cause a large ship to explode—is unlikely to arise. The value of the trust property, and profits from its use, provide a natural limit to liability without the need for additional remoteness rules, but trustees could find themselves in difficulties where, for example, the property unexpectedly increases in value. Nor, incidentally, can a trustee set off against the amount that he is obliged to restore to the trust funds the tax that would have been payable on that amount had he not lost it through his breach (*Re Bell's Indenture* [1980] 1 WLR 1216).

Further, a trustee cannot set off a profit made in one transaction against a loss made in another. The reason is that any profits made out of the trust property belong to the beneficiaries, so the trustees have no claim against those profits to lessen their own liability for loss caused by a breach. A frequently quoted authority is the old case of *Dimes* v *Scott* (1828) 4 Russ 195.

If the profit and loss can be seen to be part of the same transaction, however, the principle of *Dimes* v *Scott* will not apply. In *Bartlett* v *Barclays Bank Trust Co. Ltd (No. 1)* [1980] Ch 515, loss had resulted from a disastrous development, but another development had produced a profit. While acknowledging the general rule, Brightman J allowed that gain to be set off against the loss, remarking that it would be unjust to deprive the bank of an element of salvage in the disaster. The explanation was that the loss and gain arose from the same policy of speculation in the *Bartlett* case, and that, where gains and losses arise in a single dealing or course of dealing, the trustees will be liable only to the extent that a net loss results.

16.4.2 Investments

Many of the cases concern losses arising from improper use by the trustees of their powers of investment, and some specific points should be noted, as follows.

(1) If trustees make an unauthorized investment, they will be liable for any loss that is incurred when that investment is realized. There are, however, qualifications to this principle, as follows.

    (i) If the beneficiaries are all *sui iuris* and collectively entitled to the entire trust property, they may adopt the unauthorized investment as part of the trust property. It is not clear whether, if they do this, they may nonetheless call upon the trustees to make good any loss that arises from that investment: *Re Lake* [1903] 1 KB 439 seems to suggest that they may, but this result appears contrary to principle. If the beneficiaries do not unanimously agree to adopt the investment, the trustee's duty is to sell it and to make good any loss.

    (ii) The trustee is alternatively entitled to take over the investment for himself, subject to refunding the trust estate, the beneficiaries having a lien on the investment until the refund is made.

    (iii) If an unauthorized investment brings in a greater income than an authorized one would have done, and this income has already been paid over to a beneficiary, the trustees cannot, it seems, require him to repay the excess above what he should have received, or to set off this excess against future income.

    (iv) In *Nestlé* v *National Westminster Bank plc* [1993] 1 WLR 1260, Staughton LJ observed that trustees will not be liable if, although they applied the wrong criteria in their choice of investments, their decision is nonetheless justifiable on objective grounds, making it difficult to show loss to the trust.

(2) Where unauthorized investments are improperly retained, the measure of liability is the difference between the present value of the investment and the price that it would have raised if sold at the proper time. In *Fry* v *Fry* (1859) 28 LJ Ch 591, for example, the trustees were liable for the difference between the offer of £900 and the sum eventually obtained.

(3) If the trustees are directed by the trust instrument to make a specific investment, and either they make no investment at all or they invest the fund in something else, their liability is to supply the same amount of the specific investment as they could have acquired with the trust funds had they purchased it at the proper time. Account will be taken, however, of any payments that the trustees would have had to make regarding the investment if they had acquired it at the correct time.

Where the trustees are given a choice of investments, but make no investment at all, they will be liable to replace only any deficit in the trust fund, with interest. This is simply because it cannot be assumed that any particular investment would have been chosen by the trustees if they had acted properly, and it is therefore impossible to base their liability on the value of any particular investment.

(4) A trustee who uses trust money in his own business will be liable to hold any profit that he makes as a constructive trustee for the beneficiaries, or to account for the money with interest, whichever happens to be the greater. If he mixes trust money with his own, the beneficiaries may demand the return of the trust money with interest, or else claim a share in the profits proportionate to the amount of the trust money employed in the venture. Any loss must, of course, be borne by the trustee, and where he has become insolvent, the beneficiaries may have a proprietary claim for the return of the trust fund, in preference to his creditors (see Chapter 17).

16.4.3 Interest

Normally, a trustee will be required to replace a loss with interest. Traditionally, the rate of interest was 4 per cent, which was in line with the rate produced on old-style trustee securities, but this is now recognized as unrealistic, and the proper rate at present appears to be that allowed from time to time on the court's short-term investment account established under s. 6(1) of the Administration of Justice Act 1965 (*Bartlett* v *Barclays Bank Trust Co. Ltd (No. 1)* [1980] Ch 515).

A trustee may be liable for a higher rate, at the discretion of the court. If he has actually received more than the standard rate, he will be liable for what he has actually received. Similarly, if it can be shown that he ought to have received more than he did, he will be liable for what he should have received, for example where proper investment producing a higher rate has been wrongfully terminated. Traditionally, if the trustee was guilty of fraud or other active misconduct, the rate was raised from 4 per cent to 5 per cent, on the presumption that this represented what he had actually received. On the same presumption, compound interest may nowadays be charged, and it seems that this will be a matter of course if the trustee was under a duty to accumulate. Despite the frequent reiteration that higher rates are charged merely as reflecting the actual gain made by the defaulting trustee and not by way of penalty, the extent of the trustee's misconduct may be a relevant factor in the court's exercise of its discretion (see *Wallersteiner* v *Moir (No. 2)* [1975] QB 373).

16.5 Trustees and criminal liability: examining the implications of the Fraud Act 2006

16.5.1 The significance of the criminal law and its limitations

It has been noted that the criminal law may be a very important mechanism for protecting trust property and promoting compliance with lawful behaviour on the part of trustees. However, this notwithstanding, it is also the case that the function of criminal law is different from civil wrongs such as breach of trust (along with commission of a tort or breach of contract) because in today's society it represents the state's concern to protect citizens from harm by making some harms liable to criminal punishment. Thus, for a beneficiary, the criminalization of misappropriations of trust property might have a deterrent effect, and could help to assuage anger against a trustee who has misappropriated property, but unlike remedies found in the civil law, the criminal law does not engage in financial recompense to victims. This is highly significant because, in the context of misappropriation of trust funds, a beneficiary is most likely to be concerned with restoration of the trust property.

16.5.1.1 Fiduciary conduct and the limitations of the Theft Act provisions

Another factor that can severely limit the use of criminal law in the context of trustees' conduct is that it is clear, from the commencement of this chapter, that not all breaches will involve misappropriations of property by a trustee. This is very important because the legal definition of 'theft' hinges on 'appropriation' of property belonging to another. So while some trustees might simply misappropriate trust property, Chapter 13 pointed to numerous examples of trustees' behaviour that, in different ways, illustrated trustees profiting from their fiduciary positions that did not involve this. There was reference, for example, to trustees' 'interested' transactions with the trust's business or its property, and of course to unauthorized profit-making. All of these examples pointed to equity adopting a very strict approach to making trustees accountable where they have in any way compromised their fiduciary responsibilities and, under recently enacted provisions of the Fraud Act 2006, these activities have the potential to become criminal offences alongside actual misappropriation of trust property. Fuller discussion of the new provisions, their likely reach into fiduciary activity, and the possible implications can be found on the Online Resource Centre.

 Revision Box

1. In joining these materials on breach of trust together with the study of trusteeship in Chapters 13 and 14, ensure that you can answer the following questions.
    (a) What is meant by breach of trust and how is a breach of trust committed?
    (b) How does breach of trust differ from breach of a fiduciary duty?
    (c) What are the remedial consequences of breach of trust compared with breach of duties at common law arising from breach of contract or commission of a tort?
    (d) What defences are available to a trustee acting in breach?
2. From reading the chapter materials and any Online Resource Centre materials, ensure that you understand the significance of trustee exemption clauses (TECs) by considering:
    – what is meant by TECs;

→

> – what issues arise in the use of TECs; and
> – what the implications for trusts law might be in the growing use of these mechanisms for restricting/excluding liability for breach of trust.

FURTHER READING

Chambers (2005) 'The consequences of breach of fiduciary duty' 16 King's College Law Journal 186.

Dal Pont (2001) 'Wilful default revisited: liability for a co-trustee's defaults' 65 Conveyancer 376.

Edelman (2013) 'Two fundamental questions for the law of trusts' 129 Law Quarterly Review 66.

Hayton (1990) 'Developing the law of trusts for the twenty-first century' 106 Law Quarterly Review 87.

Hayton (1999) 'English fiduciary standards and trust law' 32 Vanderbilt Journal of Transnational Law 555.

Hicks (2001) 'The Trustee Act 2000 and the modern meaning of "investment"' 15 Trust Law International 203.

Jones (1968) 'Unjust enrichment and the fiduciary's duty of loyalty' 84 Law Quarterly Review 472.

Lee (2009) 'Rethinking the content of the fiduciary obligation' 73 Conveyancer 23.

Lowry (1994) *Regal (Hastings)* fifty years on: breaking the bonds of the ancien régime' 45 Northern Ireland Legal Quarterly 1.

McGrath (2012) 'Constructive trusts: an analysis of *Sinclair* v *Versailles*' 4 Lloyd's Maritime and Commercial Law Quarterly 517.

Mitchell (2008) 'Dishonest assistance, knowing receipt, and the law of limitation' 72 Conveyancer 226.

Nolan (2009) 'Controlling fiduciary power' 68 Cambridge Law Journal 293.

Sealy (1962) 'Fiduciary relationships' 20 Cambridge Law Journal 69.

Seneviratne (1999) *The Legal Profession: Regulation and the Consumer* (London: Sweet & Maxwell).

Shapiro (1987) 'The social control of interpersonal trust' 93 American Journal of Sociology 623.

Shapiro (1990) 'Collaring the crime, not the criminal: reconsidering the concept of a white-collar crime' 55 American Sociological Review 346.

 online resource centre   For summaries of a selection of these articles, please visit <http://www.oxfordtextbooks. co.uk/orc/wilson_trusts11e/>

17

Remedies associated with missing trust property: actions in equity and the basis for liability

This chapter follows on directly from the previous one looking at breach of trust, because it is entirely about what a beneficiary under a trust can do where there has been a breach of trust that has resulted in trust property going missing. Its length and its focus are premised on the way in which, in these circumstances, the liability of a trustee to pay compensation for a breach of trust is likely to have limited value. The reasons for this will be explained in due course, when it will also be explained why the responses developed by equity to address the limitations of a trustee's liability to provide equitable compensation for a breach of trust have become popular with other claimants who have lost property, but who are not beneficiaries under a trust. In this regard, we will need to understand how accommodating equity has been in making those actions that it developed for a beneficiary under a trust more generally available, and how equity has actually facilitated this.

Ahead of any of this, we do need to be sure that we understand how equity works, with a view to appreciating the nature of the different actions that it has developed to assist an owner of missing property, which were designed specifically with trust property in mind. It is important that we appreciate the significance of the common law and its own development as something that has influenced equity's development, and not simply in a general sense of understanding how these two jurisdictions work differently. This is because this area of law requires us to look at how equity facilitates the recovery of property alongside the actions for achieving this that are available at law. This flows from the general introduction that we had to equity's emergence and the development of its own distinctive remedies in Chapter 1.

In Chapter 1, it was suggested that equity's origins are best understood by looking at those of the common law, which sought to put in place a system of law that was based on a series of rights and entitlements, and responsibilities and duties, relating to a number of 'interests' that an individual might be concerned to safeguard. We can see this in relation to an individual's personal safety and that of his property, and the agreements that he reaches with others. These are rights that law was prepared to recognize as universal and applying to everyone, and ones that in due course became supported by a number of remedies developed in order to enforce the universal position. When these rights were breached by others, law would provide a remedy for the wronged party, which was a recourse arising as of right and which would, in turn, provide a certain, albeit inflexible, outcome. At that point, it was suggested that equity developed so as to be able to deliver a 'gloss' on common law entitlements enforced through its remedies, by delivering different outcomes in respect of individual cases and individual defendants where the circumstances called for this. This is how equity became a personal jurisdiction, which ultimately became embodied in the maxim that 'equity acts *in personam*'. It was also noted that these different outcomes arose from equity's discretion, which meant that a claimant had no entitlement to seek equity, and was required to 'do equity' in order to seek it and to come to it with 'clean hands'.

The maxim that 'equity acts *in personam*' continues to govern much of equity's operation today, and provides the basis for a number of equity's most common and readily recognizable remedies, including injunctions, specific performance, and rescission. We shall find out that it also provides the basis for the more specialized remedies developed by equity about which we do not know much yet. This includes a trustee's liability to provide equitable compensation for a breach of trust, which we encountered in the previous chapter. More will be said about this shortly, but for now we need only to be aware that this is an action that is available for one party to pursue—the beneficiary—and he can do so only against a specific person—the trustee who has acted in breach. We will also encounter other personal actions shortly, along with much more explanation of what makes a personal action so-called and what other types of action we can find alongside this.

This point does signpost for us that equity does not only act *in personam*, to which we have already had an introduction in Chapter 1, where it was explained that equity has actually developed rights in property that are 'hard-nosed' property rights for a beneficiary under a trust, which do not depend on discretion or what is 'fair, just or reasonable'. This becomes very significant for us when we learn about how equity assists with the loss of property.

17.1 An introduction to equity's actions concerning lost property

This chapter on equity's actions for missing trust property follows on quite directly from the previous chapter on breach of trust, which itself had close connections with the material relating to trusteeship in Chapters 13 and 14. Its more general links with chapters on trusteeship arise on account of the fact that we study the law relating to trusteeship as a reflection of the rights and entitlements of a beneficiary who owns trust property in equity. In this regard, we know from looking at *Armitage v Nurse* [1998] Ch 421 in the previous chapter that a breach of trust can arise from a range of acts and omissions on the part of a trustee. Here, *Armitage* is very significant for this chapter from the way in which Millett LJ identifies specifically amongst those inactions or actions that can amount to a breach of trust 'actual misappropriation or misapplication of the trust property'. This *does* happen, and this chapter considers what a beneficiary can do in this situation and why the normal action for breach of trust—one for equitable compensation—is of limited value in situations in which trust property actually disappears.

In Chapter 1, we learned that a beneficiary's equitable title to trust property can, in any case, be lost where this property comes into the hands of (that is, is sold to) a bona fide purchaser for value without notice, and lots of other things *can* happen to trust property: it can be misappropriated or stolen by a trustee, who might keep the property; if this is money, it might be placed in his bank account; or he might invest it, or just dissipate it. This property might also be passed onto someone else, who may or may not be a bona fide purchaser: here, someone other than the trustee will actually have the 'trust property' and the trustee will have proceeds from its wrongful sale. So there are a number of problems potentially facing a beneficiary where property has been applied in breach of trust, in terms of what happens to the property and who comes into possession of it. And because this is 'hot property', a great deal *can* happen to it and, in reality, *does* happen to it.

To reflect this, there are a variety of actions that may be open to a beneficiary. We already know about the personal action against the offending trustee of 'equitable compensation' for losses incurred to the trust by parting with trust property in breach of trust. But there are also mechanisms that can assist a beneficiary in these circumstances, including ones that are focused on actually recovering the property. But this will raise issues about what has actually happened to the trust property. This means determining which actions are *actually* available to a beneficiary in the particular circumstances, and what will be the best one(s), depends on what has actually happened to the property. Establishing this is central to what can be 'recovered' by a beneficiary and from whom. Here, it is vital for the beneficiary to be aware of the full range of possible actions, together with the full range of potential defendants. The significance of this last point is that there may be others (other than the original trustee acting in breach) who can incur liability for having some involvement in the breach or its aftermath.

17.2 Preliminary considerations for understanding equity's actions for missing property

Before any of this can take place, three very important matters will help us to put together a picture of what potential actions are available to a beneficiary where trust property has been misappropriated or misapplied, and for generating an appreciation of their nature and requirements, and also the strength and limitations of each. There is also one final consideration that explains why cases that we will encounter show us that it is not only a beneficiary under a trust who might wish to use these actions that equity developed with a beneficiary in mind. This was noted a little earlier, and we need to understand why equity might want to make its 'beneficiary actions' available to others and how it might achieve this. This requires us to understand these actions as actions developed for a beneficiary in the first instance, which leads us straight into the three important matters that help to clarify what we need to be aware of when considering the nature of equity's beneficiary actions.

The nature of a beneficiary's 'equitable title' under a trust

A beneficiary owns trust property 'in equity' or has 'equitable title'; while legal title binds the world, equitable title binds everyone except a 'bona fide purchaser [of the property] for value and without notice [of the trust]'. As an example of an equitable right that is a 'right *in rem*', this gives the beneficiary proprietary interest in trust property itself, and not only as an action against a particular person. This explains how a beneficiary can potentially have access to personal and proprietary actions when trust property has been dealt with in breach of trust.

Classifying beneficiary actions as 'personal' and 'proprietary'

We know that equity has developed numerous remedies, and we now know that this includes some specific ones that have been designed especially to assist a beneficiary where trust property is missing because a trustee has committed a breach of trust. The development of a range of actions for a beneficiary in this situation—some personal, some proprietary—reflects equity's recognition that much can happen to property wrongfully parted from those rightfully entitled to it. Proprietary remedies—which have been developed by the common law, as well as equity—attach to the property *itself*, allowing the property's recovery *by* those who are entitled to it *from* whoever has hold of it. This acknowledges the reality that, when property is taken from its owner, it is unlikely to remain in the same hands, and even in the same form. Generally, proprietary approaches have several attractions for a beneficiary whose property has been taken from him through a breach of trust: a proprietary action will allow 'specific recovery' of a specific asset by its rightful owner; it will confer protection for an owner where there is an insolvency; and potentially it can facilitate a 'recovery' by an owner that reflects increases to its value whilst it has been missing.

The last of these is quite a specialist consideration of equity's scope and so will be considered in some detail later on, but in terms of understanding equity's more general approach to missing property, more can be said on the significance of specific recovery of an asset, and also how a beneficiary can be protected in the event of an insolvency and why this might be important. Taking the former first, although a proprietary action makes specific recovery of a particular asset possible in principle, given all that can happen to property, in reality what will be recovered in most cases is the representative 'cash value' of the property. So for most cases (particularly ones involving personal property), the value of a proprietary claim lies in the entitlement that it confers for full value of the property (with the scope also to recover increases in value), and often there will be substitution of the original property for something else—usually something that has been purchased with the proceeds of an unauthorized sale of property.

A beneficiary's ownership of trust property in equity is what will protect his position where the person who (wrongfully) holds it becomes insolvent. This is because this is a type of ownership—a right *in rem*—and so this means that whoever acquires the property (other than a bona fide purchaser) does not own it. Where a person becomes bankrupt or a business insolvent (that is, is unable to pay his debts), his property is taken from him and given to either a trustee in bankruptcy or a company liquidator for the purpose of satisfying as many of the debts as possible. This means that any property to which a bankrupt holds title (this can be a trustee, or someone else who has acquired the 'hot' trust property) could be at risk of being taken away and used for these purposes. This is what would happen if the beneficiary were not to continue to own the property in equity. But because a beneficiary does own the property in equity, it cannot be used as if it were owned by the bankrupt, so the beneficiary can claim this as his and does not have to 'join the queue' with others who are making claims against a debtor's property. The possibility of bankruptcy and multiple claims is also important for understanding why a trustee's personal liability to provide equitable compensation is of a much more limited value. This is a personal action that the beneficiary has against a trustee acting in breach, and so its success will depend on the trustee actually having personal assets to satisfy the claim, and he could also have a number of other creditors.

However, notwithstanding the advantages of proprietary remedies, the availability of a suite of different actions that are personal and proprietary reflects that a lot can happen to missing property. Property that has been taken wrongfully from an owner can be destroyed, or can be lost by being transferred to an unknown person—which means that trying to identify the missing property or its substitute is not feasible. Here, an action against a particular person for having received the property might appear to be all that is possible, but, as you will discover for one action, it is even possible to incur liability without ever receiving hot property.

The significance of trust property being 'misappropriated or misapplied'
In focusing on how a beneficiary can recover trust property dealt with improperly and in breach of trust, we know that a breach can be committed innocently by a trustee as much as by a trustee acting fraudulently. The term 'misapplication' reflects that whilst

a lot of situations will involve a trustee actually misappropriating (and indeed stealing) trust property for his own purposes, actions for a beneficiary will also result from different situations. We encountered *Re Diplock's Estate* [1948] Ch 465 in studying the legal definition of charity, and this shows that trustees (and those whose actions are treated as if they were a breach of trust, as explained shortly) who are honest and diligent are capable of 'misapplying' trust property if they distribute it otherwise than is permitted. Here, situations that do not involve attempts to misappropriate trust property and are not consciously seeking to use trust property improperly are still regarded as 'wrongdoing' for the purposes of establishing breach of trust, and the liability that can be incurred. This is because, where trust property goes missing as a result of this, they are situations in which a beneficiary who is *rightfully* entitled to the property will want to recover it.

The availability of beneficiary actions for persons who are not beneficiaries

For all of these reasons, equity saw fit to develop a number of special actions that are designed to help a beneficiary in situations in which trust property goes missing. These are designed for him to be able to assert his claim to his property where this is possible, and to be able to have recourse in a number of ways where this is no longer possible because the property cannot be found, has been destroyed, or has fallen into the hands of the only person who can possibly trump a beneficiary's claim—that is, a bona fide purchaser. In due course, it will become apparent just what significant scope this gives a beneficiary on account of all of the different scenarios that can potentially be catered for by equity's actions. This is particularly so with the equitable proprietary 'tracing claim', which has become very popular with claimants who are not beneficiaries under trusts, but who wish to be able to use what equity has developed for beneficiaries when their property goes missing. It is not only beneficiaries whose property goes missing from wrongful dealings with property, and whilst the common law has also developed actions for those who are legal owners of property facing these very difficulties, because equity works differently from the common law, equity's actions have traditionally been perceived as being more accommodating than what is available at common law.

For this reason, those who are not beneficiaries under a trust have been keen to try to claim entitlement to use equity's actions. We know from Chapter 1 and the introduction to this chapter that, generally, equity's remedies are not available as of right, and so it will become clear that, traditionally, equity has made its beneficiary actions available to others in some circumstances and that this has been underpinned by 'requirements' that will be automatically satisfied by a beneficiary, but which will need to be demonstrated by others. As we work through the material, it will become clear that some can establish these as easily as beneficiaries, because equity's responses to trusteeship are actually part of its much more extensive jurisdiction of fiduciary conduct, with the executors in *Re Diplock* illustrating this for us. But it will also become clear that other claimants will have to establish their entitlement to use equity's actions much more actively.

And in terms of how equity achieves this as a matter of jurisdiction, we need to think back to the distinctive facets in modern equitable jurisdiction that we first encountered in Chapter 1. Those materials introduced us to the way in which, substantively, equity's jurisdiction could be considered as being 'exclusive', with the creation of new rights that the common law would not offer, and 'concurrent', where equity's distinctive remedies sit alongside and supplement the common law's actions. In this vein, we can regard the availability of equity's actions for recovering property to persons other than beneficiaries under a trust as possible on account of concurrent jurisdiction. We shall consider this further when we come to look at equity's tracing rules.

17.3 Equity's responses to missing trust property: developing an overview of beneficiary actions

The main focus of this picture of beneficiary actions is the proprietary tracing action, which has been developed by equity and is the action that every claimant who has lost property wants to use on account of its combination of the general advantages of proprietary actions with equity's flexible approach. There are also personal actions, with the essential difference between an action being personal or proprietary being that the latter amounts to an assertion of ownership over trust property (or property treated to all intents and purposes as if it were trust property), whoever might have this, including an innocent party who has no idea what has happened. We then move on to consider the liabilities of third parties who may no longer be in possession of the property, or where that property is no longer identifiable. Because this liability will not attach to the property itself, it is regarded as personal liability.

Throughout, there will be considerable emphasis placed on the huge complexities and uncertainties that explain why this is a very difficult area of law—an area that has, until very recently, been very unsettled and uncertain. This is not only on account of pressure brought to bear by those other than beneficiaries who are seeking to use equity's actions for property that they have lost, but also because a number of very different principles have influenced 'conversations' on how the law should be developing. In this vein, there will also be reference to key recent developments, both as part of the general discussion and also as a specific focal point. This will ensure that, at the very least, we can get a sense of the complex issues raised by the actions that are potentially available and a measure of what their current requirements appear to be, and how particular actions relate to others that are available.

What follows now is an overview of the key actions available, with a view to appreciating their nature and their requirements, and also the strength and limitations of each, bearing in mind that making a clear statement of current law is difficult. This is a time of significant change, with numerous traditional principles and requirements currently being reassessed, along with distinctions traditionally drawn between different actions. Our consideration of all of this will start by looking at the proprietary action traditionally known as 'tracing'. This is a good place to start, because this is the action that every claimant who has lost property wants to be able to bring; whether or not he can do so depends on the circumstances, but this is the most attractive claim, in principle, for someone who has lost property.

17.4 Proprietary actions traditionally known as 'tracing'

Tracing is a term of art that has traditionally been applied to actions or remedies that have provided a claimant with a means of 'following' property belonging to him into the hands of others. The reason why tracing is such a significant action and the most desirable action for those who have lost property is that it is a proprietary action. As we know, all proprietary actions are premised on a claimant being able to assert a claim over property subject to the action, and this means that the claimant is permitted to treat specific property or (as we will see) a proportion of it as his property. Traditionally, these elements have all added up to a claimant being able to follow that which he should have because it is his into the hands of others who should not have it, and to recover it for himself on that basis.

Although some of the traditional terminology associated with tracing has been challenged recently—particularly in the landmark case of *Foskett* v *McKeown* [2000] 3 All ER 97—it remains essentially about seeing or finding property belonging to the claimant in the hands of others, and enabling the claimant to recover it for himself. A further tradition in the study of tracing is that there have always been two distinct routes by which property belonging to a claimant can be followed into the hands of others, because both the common law and equity have developed tracing rules designed to assist owners who have lost their property. Here, we will see how there has been a traditional division of tracing rules into those that are available at common law and those available in equity. As part of this, we will also learn that dicta in the House of Lords' decision in *Foskett* v *McKeown* has challenged this.

So that we can get a feel for tracing without having to reflect on new challenges to traditional ideas as yet, it is much more straightforward to get a basic grasp of things by exploring tracing through the distinct tracing rules that have developed at common law and in equity. But before even this, we need to understand why tracing is the claimant's action of choice. This is so because tracing attaches to (following, at least traditionally) the property, and because of this it is an action that can be pursued against anyone. For those able to take advantage of common law rules, this literally means everyone, because ownership at law is a universal right that binds (and is thus good against) the world, on account of the maxim *nemo dat quod non habet*. For those entitled to trace in equity, this action can be used against everyone except a bona fide purchaser. This wide 'net' of persons from whom an owner can recover *his* property includes those who are innocent, as well as those who have the property knowing that its provenance is not proper. This is very significant, because some actions can be pursued only where there is some fault on the part of the person being pursued. So this explains why tracing is the action of choice for a claimant, but it does not explain why we are looking at tracing rules at common law.

Why look at common law tracing at all?

Given that we know that it is only those who hold legal rights who are able to use actions at law, it is not obvious why we need to look at tracing rules developed at common law at all for our focus on a beneficiary under a trust. The obvious reason for this is that a beneficiary does not hold rights that law will recognize and thus enforce, and so it would not be possible for a beneficiary to use law's tracing rules. In addition, we have already been told that rules that equity has developed for a beneficiary on account of such persons not being able to use actions at law are very popular amongst persons who have lost property, but who are not beneficiaries. This last point suggests that there are some serious shortcomings with tracing rules at law, which is true; before finding out what these are, we shall see how they might arise, because we do know that legal actions are known to be certain and also inflexible.

One reason why it is important to have an awareness of tracing rules developed at common law is that while this is not a feasible action for a beneficiary himself, it can be used on his behalf by a trustee; this will not be appropriate in all circumstances, but it might be in some. More generally, there are advantages to getting a feel for tracing rules at common law as well as in equity, in that this does help to clarify understanding of what a beneficiary can or cannot do and why. This is also helpful for appreciating why claimants who are not beneficiaries might wish to utilize what equity has developed for beneficiaries. Furthermore, common law tracing is theoretically simpler and works in more straightforward ways than that in equity, and so provides effective 'building blocks' for understanding equity's approaches, which, although more flexible, are also more complicated mechanically.

So tracing at common law is a much easier way into appreciating the central concepts of a claimant being able to identify a specific asset as his asset, and the ability to trace the asset by following it into the hands of another. And their first factor in common is that both types of tracing start with an owner whose property is wrongly taken from him and who is seeking to have it restored to him. In a proprietary tracing action, the claimant is seeking the return of the actual property itself, or its equivalent substitute, and this is premised on being able to *establish* that a specific asset (or a proportion of it) *belongs to him*.

In addition, it will become apparent that tracing rules developed at common law and in equity have always shared similarities as well as differences, and we will also learn that recent trends are suggesting that the differences between them are becoming less pronounced. Indeed, we shall consider judicial calls for there to be one universal set of tracing rules that would be available to all owners of property, be they owners at law or in equity, and so this is a further reason why we need to have a good grasp of common law tracing rules, as well as ones in equity.

Part I **Tracing at common law**

When reference is made to property that 'belongs' to a claimant, with a beneficiary under a trust, 'ownership' of an asset will always be ownership in equity. But property gets separated from its rightful owners in all kinds of circumstances and can 'go missing' from outright owners, who will be just as concerned to recover it. To trace or follow an asset at common law, a claimant must be its legal owner. The common law will recognize only 'universal' legal rights and entitlements at law, and this is indicative of what tracing at common law actually requires, and what it is capable of achieving. This, and the way in which legal title to property is not easily 'lost' by its owner, reveals key strengths of common law tracing as an option for an owner of property that has been stolen, who is seeking to recover it by tracing it into the hands of another. However, it has also been at the heart of its traditional weaknesses in this area.

Where we refer to property not being 'easily lost' by its owner, what we mean is that legal title to property is not easily lost even when property goes missing from its owner. This is because the operation of the *nemo dat* rule means that a thief cannot pass on title to property even where stolen property is passed on from one person to another, as it tends to be; in these circumstances, an owner of property can recover it from the person who now has it, who may or may not know that it is stolen. We will consider how a legal owner does this shortly, but first we need to make what might seem an obvious point, but may not always be so: although the *nemo dat* rule makes it difficult for a legal owner of property to lose title to it, there are exceptions to the rule which have developed. These are beyond the scope of our considerations here, except that we need to be aware that this can happen and that, if it does, the original owner cannot use common law tracing rules, because he no longer owns the property at law. So an owner can use common law tracing rules when he loses property in circumstances under which he retains legal title to it.

Once we have established that an owner of property has lost only the property itself and not title to it, where an owner can trace his property into another's hands, he can make a claim for 'specific delivery'—namely, its return or recovery. This works where the claimant 'finds' property to which he holds legal title in the hands of another and can assert his claim to it. This is illustrated by the case of *Taylor* v *Plumer* (1815) 3 M & S 562, which also establishes that an owner can claim as his any property that is a substitute for that originally taken from him.

Sir Thomas Plumer instructed his stockbroker to purchase some bonds and provided money for this purchase. The stockbroker purchased different investments and bullion with Plumer's funds, and attempted to abscond with these. He was caught and Plumer seized the property; upon the stockbroker's bankruptcy, his assignees then brought an action to recover this from Sir Thomas, but failed. The investments and bullion were held to be Sir Thomas's own property. In effect, Plumer's money was traced into the investments and bullion, for, according to Lord Ellenborough, 'the product of or substitute for the original thing still follows the nature of the thing itself, as long as it can be ascertained as such'.

17.5 The significance of the common law tracing claim and its scope

Where the property concerned is personal property rather than real property, although historically the court has discretion to order specific delivery (return) of the property, there is no absolute right to the return of the actual property itself. This means that the significance of the proprietary tracing claim is that it entitles the claimant to the full value of the property, in preference to the claims of the defendant's other creditors. And, in terms of its scope, as *Taylor* v *Plumer* suggests, the common law evolved not simply to allow recovery of a specific asset that a claimant can identify as 'his', but also to allow a claimant to be able to recover *substitute* property when the original property has been sold, and there are proceeds of sale, or new property purchased with the proceeds of sale. Here, the claimant's right to trace the property continues as long as it remains possible to show that what the defendant holds is simply a substitute for the original property belonging to the claimant. In *Re Diplock's Estate* [1948] Ch 465, Lord Greene MR explained this as the claimant ratifying (or adopting) the wrongful sale of his property and purchase of different property, to enable him to claim the substitute property as its legal owner. Authority for this can be found in *Taylor* v *Plumer* itself, with a more interesting exposition of substitution coming from property that is money being paid into a bank account considered in *Re Diplock*. Here, provided that the money is not mixed with any other funds, Lord Greene MR suggested, at 519, that there was no reason why the common law would not allow the substitution of the money into the cause of action, and vice versa, because:

> If it is possible to identify a principal's money with an asset purchased exclusively by means of it, we see no reason for drawing a distinction between a chose in action such as a banker's debt to his customer and any other asset. If the principal can ratify the acquisition of the one, we see no reason for supposing that he cannot ratify the acquisition of the other.

We can see this principle at work in *Banque Belge pour L'Etranger* v *Hambrouck* [1921] 1 KB 321, prior to *Re Diplock*, and this passage within *Diplock* was subsequently approved by

Millett J in *Agip (Africa) Ltd* v *Jackson* [1990] 1 Ch 265, but he thought that it was limited to following an asset into a changed form in the same hands. This suggests that this can be applied only to following the same asset from one recipient to another, and that the common law would not necessarily allow free tracing of causes of action from one person to another. So these authorities suggest that substitutions of property can be in different forms of property for the purposes of being followed by a legal owner seeking its recovery, but that complications can arise where the new property changes hands as well as form.

17.6 The limits of tracing at common law and the 'money had and received' claim

This proprietary tracing claim depends on the claimant being able to trace or follow his actual property, or its product or substitute (under *Taylor* v *Plumer*), into the defendant's hands. Difficulties arise with currency where title passes to the recipient upon receipt: the *nemo dat* rule does not apply here, because title passes on receipt and the obligation is to pay the 'bearer on demand'. The cause-of-action cases of *Hambrouck* and *Diplock*, among others, do not cause these difficulties, because whilst there may appear to be no substitute asset, actually there is one on account of the form of the money. In this case, what is being passed from one person to another is not currency, and so the problems created by transfer of ownership on receipt of it do not apply here. Where there is instead an amount of money being represented by a cheque or other negotiable instrument, and this is paid into a bank account, it is transformed into a cause of action that an original owner can trace. This is clear in the House of Lords' decision in *Lipkin Gorman* v *Karpnale Ltd* [1991] 2 AC 548, which provides authority for what normally happens where what an original owner has lost is currency. Title to currency is passed upon receipt, and so in situations in which there is no cause of action that an owner can trace, the law has developed a different approach to make sure that those who are wrongfully parted from their money do not lose out. Here, the law imposes on the recipient of money stolen from the claimant an obligation to reimburse the claimant with an equivalent sum. The leading authority for this is *Lipkin Gorman*. From this, we can see that this is a personal action, which appears to arise from the defendant having been unjustly enriched at the expense of the claimant, which is a so-called 'restitutionary' claim.

The action for money had and received: its workings, scope, and limitations
The workings for the 'money had and received' claim will be explained shortly, and arose from the way in which this case concerned the use of stolen money for gambling purposes by a solicitor. The solicitor, Cass, was a partner at Lipkin Gorman and was a regular client of the respondent casino. Cass was cashing cheques as an authorized signatory to fund his gambling habits, and he stole a large sum of money from the firm's clients' account, which he took to the respondent's Playboy Club and gambled away. The appellants successfully claimed the club's winnings from Cass's gambling.

Although liability arises on receipt of property, the restitutionary claim can be defeated in circumstances under which the recipient has not been unjustly enriched. This is because receiving stolen money in return for full consideration is not to be unjustly enriched (at the claimant's expense) at all. This means that a defendant must argue that he has not been unjustly enriched by showing that he has provided consideration. This was argued unsuccessfully in *Lipkin Gorman* itself, in which the 'consideration' alleged to have been provided related to an unenforceable contract. Indeed, those involving gaming and wagering were rendered null and void by virtue of s. 18 of the Gaming Act 1845, and so gambling contracts are not, in law, contracts for consideration.

A defence to liability to make restitution?

However, it is still possible for a defendant who has provided no consideration to escape the obligation to make restitution in full by showing that he has 'changed his position'. The change-of-position defence was successfully argued in *Lipkin Gorman* alongside the unsuccessful attempt to show that consideration had been provided. This can be invoked where the defendant has altered his position in good faith, so that it would be inequitable to require him to make restitution in full. In *Lipkin Gorman*, this limited what the claimant firm was able to recover from the casino, with paying out money as winnings to Cass constituting a change of position by the club, which general position has recently been restated in *Haugesund Kommune v DEPFA ACS Bank* [2011] 1 All ER 190, with Pill LJ's insistence that it is 'founded on a principle of justice designed to protect the defendant from a claim to restitution in respect of a benefit received by him in circumstances in which it would be inequitable to pursue that claim or to pursue it in full'.

It has been applied in *Bank Tejarat v Hong Kong and Shanghai Banking Corporation (Ci) Ltd and Hong Kong and Shanghai Bank Trustee (Jersey) Ltd* [1995] 1 Lloyd's Rep 239, in which the defendant was able to show that it had changed its position, having paid money away, in good faith, before the claimant claimed the money, on the basis that it had been subject to a fraudulent transaction.

It is not yet clear whether the change-of-position defence applies only to money had and received, or to any of the restitutionary claims considered in this and the following section, but there is some suggestion that it applies in tracing claims in equity. However, as *Campden Hill Ltd v Chakrani* [2005] EWHC 911 (Ch) suggests, this is controversial. It is also not clear what happens when money is paid to a second recipient, but Millett (1991) 107 LQR 71 argues that, because the action is personal and not proprietary, what happens to the money after it has been received by the first recipient is irrelevant.

But, more generally, the defence is regarded as evolving and not being 'fixed in stone'; according to Pill LJ in *Haugesund*, its development up to now has been on a case-by-case basis and this pattern can be expected to continue.

17.7 The traditional limitations of tracing at common law

As we work through these materials, and especially when we come to look at equity's tracing rules, it will become apparent just how few successful common law tracing claims can be found in the case law. The requirement for the common law tracing claim is that it is possible for the claimant to show that what the defendant holds is either the claimant's actual property or a substitute for the property that originally belonged to the claimant. This works in *Taylor v Plumer* situations, in which it is clear that the property held by the defendant has been purchased with proceeds of the unauthorized sale of the claimant's property (which the claimant then ratifies). We know this also works where the claimant's money (other than currency, for which we will discover special rules have had to be developed) or proceeds of an authorized sale are placed in a bank account that substitution with a cause of action is something that is traceable. So this is how the common law rules have evolved to give owners of property scope to recover it in a variety of situations, accepting that property wrongfully taken from its owner will often change hands, as well as form.

However, despite this apparent scope, it is actually very difficult for the claimant to establish that what a defendant holds is his actual property or its substitute, and the most significant problem here is how the common law reacts where money has been placed in a bank account. On *Diplock* principles, as illustrated by *Hambrouck*, this will not cause problems where a bank account contains only money once belonging to the claimant, or the proceeds of a sale of his property, but, as a number of cases testify, if a bank account contains any money from any other source, then the common law will not recognize this as property over which the claimant can assert his ownership and his entitlement to its return. This is because although so-called 'mixed funds' will contain the claimant's property, it is no longer identifiable as *his* property, because it is mixed with property that does not belong to him.

Agip (Africa) v *Jackson* [1992] 1 Ch 265 shows how this limitation operates in relation to money that comes into contact with other sources, in this case following payment orders fraudulently altered by the company's chief accountant. The claimant sued the fraudulent recipient at common law for the full amount received by it; had this succeeded, it would have been irrelevant that the recipient had disposed of all but US$45,000 of the money. But because the money had 'travelled' through the New York clearing bank system, it could not be traced through it, and the Court of Appeal upheld Millett J's finding that, at this point, the money had clearly became mixed with other money.

It is also the case that mixed funds, which will also disallow tracing at common law, can also be mixed goods, such as we have already encountered in the certainty cases (such as *Re Wait* [1927] 1 Ch 606 and *Re London Wine* [1986] PCC 121), and *Clayton's Case* (1816) 1 Mer 572, to which we will come when considering equity's tracing rules. This inability to recognize a claimant's assertion of ownership where his property has become mixed with that of others is the common law's biggest limitation as far as the proprietary tracing claim is concerned. This gives us an insight into why equity's rules are so attractive to claimants and it has already been noted that equity has extended the availability of this 'action' originally conceived for beneficiaries under a trust to others who are not. However, while successful common law tracing claims are rare, they are not unheard of, and one did succeed in *Lipkin Gorman* in relation to money held by the casino that could be proven to have come from the firm's client account, which could be followed, with enthusiasm for this approach also to be found in *Foskett* v *McKeown* [2000] 3 All ER 97. Furthermore, the decision in *FC Jones & Sons* v *Jones* [1996] 3 WLR 703 suggests greater flexibility in common law tracing, and indeed that it is becoming more like tracing in equity. But this is not easy to understand in the light of the common law's traditional refusal to trace into mixed funds, and so does require some thought, and will be considered again as part of examining 'new trends in tracing' following a look at traditional approaches of tracing in equity.

17.8 **Tracing in equity**

The starting point for understanding tracing in equity is, like common law tracing rules, an owner of property who has wrongfully been separated from it. In this case, we already know that, as equity originally conceived 'tracing in equity', the wronged owner is a beneficiary under a trust. And in this context tracing has the same significance as it did for common law tracing rules, and has traditionally been associated with a rightful owner of property following this into the hands of someone who is not entitled to have it, and then asserting his claim to it and demanding its return to him.

We do know that a beneficiary owns trust property in equity rather than law: as we know from as far back as Chapter 1, legal title is held by trustees under a trust arrangement, and a beneficiary's ownership of trust property is possible on the basis that equity was able and prepared to evolve 'hard-nosed property rights', which are not determined on discretion or fairness and justice. We also know that the reason why a beneficiary will be in the position of losing his property is because those who hold title to it at law have committed a breach of trust by either stealing it or by somehow using it in a way that is contrary to the terms of the trust or general law, which has resulted in it becoming lost from its rightful owner. So we can see how beneficial owners of property might become separated from it, but this does not by itself explain why equity developed the facility for tracing. Before looking at what equity has developed, we need to understand more about why equity has developed a proprietary remedy regarded traditionally as allowing beneficiaries to follow trust property or its substitute into the hands of others.

The requirements and scope of tracing at common law tell us that, even where there is an outright owner, in which case legal rights are very strong and not easily lost, property does still fall into the 'wrong' hands. So now consider the scope for improper dealings with property in a trust setting: although what is being held is nominal legal title, held only to further the interests of beneficiaries, a trustee *is* the apparent owner of property. There is no protection from common law here, because law does not recognize a beneficiary's position. As far as equity is concerned, through formality requirements in the creation of trusts and a number of 'trusteeship' rules, we can see that equity has always been mindful that holding legal title as trustee can encourage misconduct rather than propriety. Given what can happen to trust property when it is misappropriated or misapplied, perhaps it is not surprising that equity has developed the proprietary remedy of tracing. But it is not necessarily obvious either, especially given that we already know about other beneficiary actions concerning the improper use of trust property. This is clear from the way in which we encountered liability to account for unauthorized profits and a trustee's liability to provide equitable compensation whenever a breach of trust is committed in Chapters 13 and 16, respectively.

Tracing rules for lost property and other 'wrongdoing' with trust property

The first thing to note is that, in developing tracing rules for the recovery of 'missing' trust property through enabling a beneficiary to follow property belonging to him into the hands of another, equity has taken quite a different approach from situations in which a trustee has made an unauthorized profit. An unauthorized 'profit from position' does not amount to misappropriating trust property, and instead arises from a trustee's personal interests conflicting with his duty to the trust; equity responds by imposing a constructive trust over this profit in furtherance of a trustee's liability (to account for his unconscionable conduct). Where property *is* misappropriated by a trustee, *Foskett* v *McKeown* [2000] 3 All ER 97 is authority that this *can* give rise to a proprietary action for recovery of assets, but this is liability arising from the process of tracing, rather than creating a constructive trust. This is explained by

Lord Millett as what a beneficiary is and is not entitled to where property actually goes missing:

> It does not entitle him to priority over the trustee's general creditors unless he can trace the trust property into its product and establish a proprietary interest in the proceeds. If the beneficiary is unable to trace the trust property into its proceeds, he still has a personal claim against the trustee, but his claim will be unsecured.
>
> (*Foskett* v *McKeown* [2000] 3 All ER 97, *per* Lord Millett at 109)

It will become clear that this distinction drawn between a proprietary action for the recovery of assets and unauthorized profit-making reflects that equity's approach to tracing missing property is to impose a 'charge' or lien *over it* rather than to impose liability to account *for it*. And, in turn, both are different from a trustee's liability to provide equitable compensation following a breach of trust, because this is a personal action, which is subject to all of the limitations of personal actions, which are only as good as those who are defendants to them, in terms of what assets this particular defendant has and who else might be owed money by him.

So what is equity's approach to tracing? Traditional approaches have hinged on three requirements to be met by a claimant. Although these are stringent, for those entitled to trace in equity there is much more flexibility than there is for those tracing a claim at common law.

Tracing in equity: two key cases, three requirements, and equity's concurrent jurisdiction

This is where we now find out what equity's tracing rules are for the recovery of lost property. We shall come to understand why equity's approach is regarded as more flexible than that at common law, but first we need to understand more about its requirements and availability. This is where we need to have a sense of how equity fits in with changing ideas on tracing, which were alluded to earlier, and getting a measure of this requires us to consider that this has been a highly dynamic area of law. This is also one that has been rather unsettled in the past decade or so, on account of its being influenced by a number of different ideas on how competing claims to property should be resolved. The issues here are more straightforward where a claim is as between a rightful owner of property and another who is responsible for parting him from his property, but, as we will see, things can get very difficult where the rightful owner of property is only one of the innocent parties who has become involved in the wrongdoing of others. To start with, the key cases *Westdeutsche Landesbank* v *Islington LBC* [1996] AC 669 and *Foskett* v *McKeown* [2000] 2 WLR 1299 help to set out some of these considerations, even though the reasons why these cases (and particularly *Foskett* v *McKeown*) are so significant will become clear only as we progress.

Westdeutsche Landesbank v *Islington LBC* arose from the way in which this particular London local authority sought to manage its finances. It concerned particularly borrowing arrangements that it made by entering into a 'rate swap' agreement with the Westdeutsche Landesbank, which resulted in Islington receiving advances of several million pounds from the bank. These arrangements were then declared to be *ultra vires* for local authorities, and so the bank sought to recover its money. The issue arising in the case was whether the bank could recover so-called 'compound' interest. The bank was particularly keen to do this, because this would give it a much better return on the amount advanced to Islington: this arrangement means that, when interest is added to the principal sum advanced from that moment on, the interest that has been added *also itself* earns interest, and is said to be *compounding* interest. It was found by the House of Lords that compound interest was not recoverable by the bank in the circumstances, because the local authority was not a trustee of the money advanced, and nor was the local authority otherwise in a fiduciary relationship with the bank in respect of the money.

Foskett v *McKeown* concerned contracts made by a group of purchasers for plots of land for holiday homes in Portugal. The financial arrangement for this was that money paid by the purchasers was to be held on trust until the development had been completed; the trustee was Timothy Murphy. The development was never completed and the money collected from the purchasers was dissipated. At one point, Murphy effected a life insurance policy, the beneficiaries under which were Murphy's wife and his three children. The premiums, which cost £10,000 a year, had been paid with a mixture of Murphy's own money and £20,440 that had been misappropriated by Murphy from the purchasers. Five years later, Murphy committed suicide, and the insurance policy paid out £1 million. In a dispute between Murphy's children (beneficiaries under the life policy) and the purchasers, the life policy beneficiaries argued that what the purchasers could recover from the fund was limited to return of the £20,440. The purchasers argued that their entitlement was to 40 per cent of the proceeds of the policy (which represented a share proportionate to the value of the premiums that were paid with the misappropriated trust money). A majority in the House of Lords found in favour of the purchaser claimants.

17.9 Rules relating to equitable tracing: two key cases casting light on three key requirements

These cases are very significant for this discussion of tracing in equity in terms of what it can achieve and what is required of a claimant in order to be permitted to use equity's mechanisms. From these cases, we already get a sense that equity can achieve a great deal and that those who are entitled to use its tracing rules can be treated generously, and it has already been suggested that equity's tracing rules are popular amongst claimants. This is where we have to start to think about requirements because not everyone will be able to use equity's rules where their property is missing.

As far as equity is concerned, we know that these rules were developed to provide beneficiaries under a trust with protection as a reflection of what could happen to property that is ostensibly owned by others (namely, trustees), and where it is possible for these people successfully to represent to others that this property is theirs to deal with as outright owner. Where this involves dealing with a bona fide purchaser, this will destroy a beneficiary's ownership of the property in equity. So equity has always been mindful that much can happen with trust property that should not, and its tracing rules embody these concerns. So as far as satisfying equity's requirements to use its tracing rules, it will not be an issue for a beneficiary to demonstrate entitlement, although, as we will discover, for any tracing action in equity the property must not be destroyed and it must remain the beneficiary's (and not become a bona fide purchaser's). But there are other 'requirements' that must be met, which demonstrate that it is not only a beneficiary under a trust who wishes to use equity's tracing rules to recover his property.

So why would anyone other than a beneficiary wish to use equity's tracing? From what has been suggested throughout about equity's workings and its recognition of the trust, we can see that equity created tracing rules for those who lose property and who cannot use tracing at common law. However, we also now know that tracing at common law is subject to the very significant restriction that, once lost property becomes mixed with other property, law will not allow a claimant to assert that this is his property. Equity does not work in this way, and this is why claimants who are, in principle, entitled to trace at law will commonly wish to be able to use equity's rules, because law can assist them only if their property remains uncontaminated by anything else. Given the circumstances in which owners are forcibly parted from their property, it is almost always going to be the case that it does become mixed up with other property. For law, traditionally this has been fatal; for equity, it has never been a problem. This is centrally because of equity's charge or lien mechanism, but before we explain this further, we need to understand how equity extends its tracing rules to those who are not beneficiaries under a trust.

17.9.1 Extending the reach of equity's tracing action beyond a beneficiary

There are two elements to understanding this extended reach: the first is how, jurisdictionally, equity can enable others in this way; and the second is how this jurisdictional enabling is manifested in requirements to be met in order to use equity's actions. As we shall see, there are requirements that mean that even a beneficiary cannot use equity's tracing rules, but equally there are others that a beneficiary never has to satisfy because these rules were originally developed with him in mind.

Taking the first, the jurisdictional basis for recognizing a claimant who is not a beneficiary under a trust, the simplest position stems from the way in which, although the trustee–beneficiary relationship is the paradigm fiduciary relationship, there are a number of others, and in this context there are other non-trustee fiduciaries who deal with property belonging to others in circumstances under which it can (and indeed does) go missing. In this category, we find solicitors, executors, and company directors, among others, who are within equity's established categories of fiduciary relationships, and also others such as financial services professionals, who are brought under the rubric of 'fiduciary' by satisfying the 'duty of loyalty' criteria set out in *Bristol and West Building Society* v *Mothew* [1998] Ch 1. In relation to these persons, equity will treat their wrongful conduct, which has resulted in the claimant's property being missing, as if it were a breach of trust. This is one respect in which equitable tracing rules become available where the wrong committed was not done so by a trustee, but equity will also allow its 'beneficiary actions' to be used more generally where the claimant has been a victim of fraud.

We can now start to put these building blocks together through examining the requirements that must be satisfied for a claimant to use equity's tracing rules to find his property in the hands of another and to assert his claim to it. These will be set out initially, as follows, and then the detailed requirements and also the significance of each one will be considered in turn.

(1) There must be an initial fiduciary relationship.

(2) The claimant must own an equitable proprietary interest.

(3) The right to trace must not have been lost.

Taking each one in turn, we can learn more about how these rules were developed with beneficiaries in mind, and start to appreciate how entitlement of others to use them has been developed and what limitations have always applied to these rules—even for the paradigm claimant, a beneficiary.

(1) There must be an initial fiduciary relationship
As far as a beneficiary under a trust is concerned, this is not a requirement that really applies to him because, under a trust arrangement, there will always be a fiduciary relationship on the basis that trusteeship is a paradigm fiduciary office. We also know that, where wrongdoing committed by a fiduciary other than a trustee involves loss of property (belonging to those in relationships of enforced reliance with such persons), equity will treat the wrong as if it were a breach of trust, and this is straightforward because there will always be an initial fiduciary relationship in these circumstances.

In Chapter 14, we learned that this jurisdictional reach extended to persons such as company directors, who are within the established category of fiduciary relationships, but we also referenced *Bristol and West BS* v *Mothew* [1998] Ch 1, which is authority that fiduciary relationships can arise from the circumstances. And the way in which property becomes lost through the actions of a number of persons to whom it is entrusted is a central reason for the amount of litigation around the 'fiduciary relationship/ commercial professional relationship' issue. This was seen illustrated by *Re Goldcorp* [1995] 1 AC 74 and *Halifax* v *Thomas* [1996] Ch 217, among others, and it is significant here because one of the consequences of being able to show the existence of a fiduciary relationship is that this will allow a claimant to trace in equity. Here, *Chase Manhattan Bank NA* v *Israel British Bank* [1981] Ch 105 suggests that, where property goes missing outside the relationships that equity's special system of fiduciary governance emerged specifically to protect, this is not a difficult requirement to satisfy. This was reinforced in *Shalson* v *Russo* [2003] EWHC 1637 (Ch), suggesting that, although it must be appropriate for a fiduciary relationship to arise, a flexible view of this is taken—especially where the claimant has been a victim of theft or fraud.

Everything up to now has suggested that satisfying the fiduciary relationship requirement is not difficult in practice, even for someone who is not a beneficiary under a trust, but it is also the case that the requirement itself has been heavily criticized. This can be seen in *El Ajou* v *Dollar Land Holdings plc* [1993] 3 All ER 717, and it does appear that the requirement itself might well have arisen as a historical accident. This view proposes that the pedigree of the fiduciary relationship requirement began with *Re Hallett's Estate* (1890) 13 ChD 696, and the extension of *Hallett's Estate* principles for tracing into mixed funds by *Sinclair* v *Brougham* [1914] AC 398. The latter case was highly complex and its *ratio* extremely difficult to follow; it was overruled in *Westdeutsche LB* v *Islington LBC* [1996] AC 669.

It has long been thought that *Re Diplock's Estate* [1948] Ch 465 was authority for an 'initial fiduciary relationship' requirement, and this appears to have arisen from the way in which *Sinclair* was interpreted in *Re Diplock's Estate*. In *Re Diplock*, this was interpreted as authority that an initial fiduciary relationship was required. Nevertheless, the traditional view—that this is a requirement—was affirmed by the House of Lords in *Westdeutsche*. Although a number of authorities point to the way in which a fiduciary relationship can arise on account of the presence of theft or fraud, the House of Lords also criticized the requirement again in 2000, in *Foskett* v *McKeown*. This means that future directions remain unclear. Most recently, at first instance, it was held in *Campden Hill Ltd* v *Chakrani* [2005] EWHC 911 (Ch) that *Foskett* v *McKeown* had *not* decided that it was no longer necessary to identify a fiduciary relationship as a precondition to tracing in equity, and this itself followed the approach taken in *Shalson* v *Russo* [2003] EWHC 1637 (Ch).

(2) The claimant must own an equitable proprietary interest

Once again, this is an example of what is almost a non-requirement for a beneficiary under a trust, in as much as it is one that is satisfied automatically. Indeed, one of the first things that we learned about a beneficiary under a trust is that he is owner of the trust property in equity, and that this has arisen from equity's development of hard-nosed property rights for those who do not have rights to property at common law. This will not be a problem for either the recovery of missing 'company property' following wrongdoing by a director, or the recovery of the contents of a solicitor's client deposit account, or from the maladministration by *Diplock* executors. But the class of claimant who is seeking to establish a fiduciary relationship arising from facts presents a more interesting position regarding proprietary interest. As we know, seeking entitlement to trace in equity is a strong force in much of the 'fiduciary/professional commercial relationships' cases, and in these circumstances equitable proprietary interests can arise for a number of other claimants, such as those who are unpaid sellers (as some of the *Aluminium Industrie Vaassen BV* v *Romalpa Aluminium Ltd* [1976] 1 WLR 676 cases illustrate), and even victims of theft and fraud (as illustrated by *Shalson* v *Russo* [2003] EWHC 1637 (Ch)).

(3) The right to trace must not have been lost

We will already have a sense of the perceived value of tracing in equity from the lengths to which claimants who are not beneficiaries, or those within traditional categories of relationships of utmost loyalty or enforced reliance, are prepared to go in order to establish entitlement to use equity's rules. The reasons for this will become clear shortly, but the requirement that the right to trace has not been lost is perhaps particularly interesting for us at this stage for two reasons. First, unlike the others, it is a requirement that *does* apply to a beneficiary in as much as it can materially affect his entitlement to trace. This means that any claimant who has satisfied the first two requirements (actively or automatically) can lose the right to trace, which is closely related to the second reason why this is such an interesting requirement—that is, that it forces us to confront not only the value of the equitable tracing claim, but also its limitations.

The right to trace can be lost in a variety of circumstances, with the first two being connected, respectively, with the continuing existence of the property itself and also the claimant's entitlement to it. The other situation in which the right to trace can be lost is perhaps the most interesting, because this can still happen even if both the property and the claimant's entitlement to it continue to exist. In this last situation, the right to trace can be lost in circumstances under which it is considered inequitable to allow tracing. Each of these is now explained in more detail.

As we learned when we first encountered the significance of a proprietary claim, this is a claim that attaches to the property itself, which means that an owner of property can focus on recovering the property regardless of who has it. However, because this is an action that attaches to property itself, it can persist only as long as the lost property still exists, and so a proprietary action will always be lost where the property is destroyed (such as by water damage or fire) or where the processes of manufacturing mean that it is no longer identifiable as the claimant's property. This position seems also to apply to bank accounts that are overdrawn, with *Ultraframe* v *Fielding* [2005] EWHC 1638 (Ch) and *Re BA Peters plc, Atkinson* v *Moriarty* [2008] EWCA Civ 1604 as authority that no tracing into an overdrawn bank account can occur (notwithstanding contrary dicta in the Court of Appeal in *Foskett* v *McKeown* [1998] 2 WLR 298 (CA)). In circumstances in which the property does still exist, and has not been destroyed, a claimant will lose his entitlement to trace where the property ceases to belong to him; for those who hold equitable interests in property, this will happen where the property is acquired by someone who is a bona fide purchaser. This can be seen in many older cases and was reaffirmed by the House of Lords in *Foskett* v *McKeown* [2000] 3 All ER 97.

For these reasons, that it can become inequitable to trace property is perhaps the most interesting requirement of equitable tracing and limitation of it. This is because the property does still exist and so does the claimant's entitlement to it. So why would equity insist that the right to trace is lost in circumstances under which the claim remains a possibility in principle, but where allowing it would be inequitable? The situations in which this will arise are all reasoned from the way in which tracing in equity works by declaration of a charge on the property and because allowing tracing in these circumstances would be inequitable. How this can be explained is best presented through the facts of *Re Diplock* [1948] Ch 465, as affirmed in *Ministry of Health* v *Simpson* [1951] AC 251.

This case concerned the will of Caleb Diplock, which gave the residue (that is, the amount left from a person's property after 'specific' bequests have been made) of his property 'to such charitable institutions or other charitable or benevolent object or objects in England' as his executors should, in their absolute discretion, select. The executors believed that this created a valid charitable trust, and accordingly distributed £203,000 among 139 different charities. Diplock's next-of-kin successfully challenged the trust's validity, because, on a matter of construction, the gift would not satisfy the requirement of being exclusively charitable. Diplock's next-of-kin were able to recover money from the various charities, and being able successfully to use a proprietary claim against some of the charities conferred the advantage that it allowed the next-of-kin to claim interest. However, this was a very important case for considering the limits of a proprietary equitable tracing claim, given that the recipients of the property were unaware that it was misapplied to them and, in some cases, had used it for their own purposes, believing it to be a valid gift to them.

In these situations, it was considered inequitable to allow the next-of-kin to make a tracing claim in respect of property that had been used to make *improvements to land*, as seen in *Re Diplock* [1951] AC 251, with suggestion also that it would be inequitable to declare a charge on the property where this has been used for the *payment of debts*. So the right to trace was not lost by the fact that the volunteer charities were innocent recipients of an executor's wrongdoing—because successful tracing claims were brought against some of them; what made the difference was that tracing was considered inequitable where these innocent charities had then used the property in question in ways that either could not be reversed or were not easily reversible. As we will find out, the next-of-kin were entitled to recover their property even here, but this was on a different basis and led to a more limited recovery than would have been possible through a tracing claim.

There is also some authority that the right to trace can be lost where the defendant has changed his position in good faith, with *Boscawen* v *Bajwa* [1996] 1 WLR 328 suggesting that, where the defendant acts in reliance of receiving the misapplied property, the (restitutionary) change-of-position defence from *Lipkin Gorman* should also be available in a tracing action. But *Campden Hill* v *Chakrani* [2005] EWHC 911 (Ch) shows this to be controversial, and it is unclear to what extent a change of position affects the right to trace in equity.

Having considered the requirements for bringing a tracing claim using equity's rules, it is now time to learn what these actually are and what they can achieve.

17.9.2 **The scope of what is possible by tracing in equity**

Traditionally, tracing in equity has been more flexible and able to achieve more than tracing at common law. Like the common law, equity allows the owner of property (here, the owner of the equitable proprietary interest, as explained) to trace property (or its representative value) itself directly or through direct or 'clean' substitutions of one item or type of property for the original one misapplied, and this is the easiest situation in which a wronged (equitable) owner will find himself. But when things get difficult because the misapplied property has become mixed with other property not belonging to the claimant, the common law has struggled, whilst equity has been very flexible. This is known as a 'mixed fund' of wrongfully applied trust property or the proceeds of its sale, and usually concerns money in bank accounts, although you will also see that it can apply to goods as well. This idea of equity's assistance to a beneficiary where there is a mixed fund is centrally what we will consider before looking at new trends in tracing. This starts with considering how tracing in equity in these circumstances might actually work.

How it works by following a 'charge' over property into the hands of others
Although this is central to the discussion that follows, the basic idea of a charge over missing trust property is not very easy to grasp. We do get some explanation in *Re Hallett's Estate* (1890) 13 Ch D 696, but it is more likely to come to life when we look at the key cases. According to Sir George Jessel in *Hallett* at 709, and anchoring this to the situation in which what is being traced is property that has been purchased using trust money, in such situations:

> ... the beneficial owner has the right to elect either to take the property purchased ... or ... he is entitled at his election either to take the property, or to have a charge on the property for the amount of the trust money.

As indicated, in the most straightforward cases the original trust property may still exist unaltered; in these circumstances, equity—like the common law—will allow a beneficiary to follow this into the hands of another, whether the original trustee himself, or someone else to whom the property has been passed on, but who is not entitled to take free of the claimant's equitable interest (to be considered shortly). This is the case for both the actual property, or substitute property, up to which point we see equity providing for beneficial owners what the common law developed for legal owners; in these circumstances, equity allows recovery of the actual property itself, or what is known as a 'clean substitute', because this is a straightforward swap of the original property for something else. A clean substitute is what pertains where there has been no contamination of the property being claimed with property belonging to anyone else. However, as we discovered when we looked at common law tracing rules, where property is wrongfully taken from its owners, it is more likely that this, or its substitute, or the proceeds of an unauthorized sale of either, will become contaminated with money from other sources, as happened in *Re Diplock* [1948] Ch 465. This is where's equity's charge mechanism comes into its own and makes possible that which has never been so at common law.

Equity's key traditional advantages: tracing into mixed funds
As we will discover, the 'charge' mechanism works by way of a claimant in equity asserting a charge over the property or a proportion of it, and this forms the basis of his claim.

For an owner of property who is seeking to claim what is clearly his actual property or an identifiable substitute for it, common law tracing is a relatively straightforward and uncomplicated course of action. As *Taylor* v *Plumer* (1815) 3 M & S 562 suggested, common law tracing has evolved to allow return of the property actually stolen or its equivalent substitute. We have also seen that the common law has had to develop different rules for currency, and the position is more complicated where the property or its proceeds are placed in a bank account.

An important distinction between tracing in equity and at common law can be seen in the application of *Re Hallett's Estate* (1890) 13 ChD 696, which is authority that it has always been possible to trace money into mixed accounts when tracing in equity, while not being able to do this has been seen as the biggest limitation of the common law's rules. Here, the idea of a charge over the property is central both to the ability to trace into mixed bank accounts and the clear scope for recovering increases in value of the property.

Both propositions are best explained through the key facts of *Re Hallett's Estate*. Hallett, who was a solicitor, was a trustee of his own marriage settlement. Hallett paid some of the money from that trust into his own bank account, into which he also paid money entrusted to him for investment purposes by one of his clients. Hallett made various payments into and out of the account, which, at his death, contained sufficient funds to meet the claims of the trust and his client, but not those of his personal creditors as well. It was argued (using the rule in *Clayton's Case* considered at section 17.9.3) that payments out of the fund had been made with trust money and that *what remained was Hallett's own money*; a finding in favour of this would have meant that funds were available to satisfy Hallett's personal creditors. It was held that the trustee's own money had been dissipated first, because a trustee cannot assert that he has (wrongfully) dissipated trust money when he clearly had the right to spend his own.

The starting point for understanding what is happening here is the earlier suggestion that determining the most suitable remedy will depend on working out what has happened to the property. The wrongdoer might have passed it on to another, but could well have misappropriated it for his own purposes, and so retained it, and where he would be very likely to place it in a bank account. Here, a claimant will be seeking to trace property into the bank account concerned. Where a trustee (or other wrongdoer) has placed this in an existing bank account that contains other money, he has 'mixed' trust property with other money, and *Hallett's Estate* is authority that equity allows tracing property into accounts containing mixed funds. Precisely how and what a beneficiary can recover will depend on how funds are mixed, which can reflect a number of possibilities.

Using a trust example, we see that mixtures can occur as follows:

(1) money rightfully belonging to the trustee, as well as the beneficiary;
(2) money rightfully belonging to the trustee, the beneficiary, and other innocent parties; or
(3) money belonging to the beneficiary and other innocent parties, but not the trustee.

All of these are situations that can arise from a wrongdoing trustee, but it is not always the case that mixing is done by this person. In this regard, the first scenario is dealt with effectively using *Hallett*, where equity regards the trustee as spending his own money first, with the result that the beneficiary can trace against any balance remaining; so is the second, up to the point that it concerns a wrongdoer's property. Problematic issues arise in the last two in which the beneficiary is one innocent claimant amongst others, with the third scenario arising where it is actually an innocent volunteer who mixes the property rather than the trustee. This happens where the innocent volunteer adds wrongfully applied trust funds to his own moneys, not realizing that what he has received is wrongfully applied trust money and that this is property to which he is not entitled.

Scenarios (2) and (3) illustrate that where the mixed fund is a mixture of the beneficiaries' property and that of other innocent parties, a different approach is required to determine that which belongs to the beneficiary; we also need to understand how equity facilitates tracing at all in these situations. But even before we consider how other innocent claims can complicate things, it is clear that applying *Hallett* has not always been straightforward.

While Sir George Jessel's judgment indicates that the beneficiary has a choice in terms of 'taking the property' or 'enjoying a charge over' substitute property or proceeds of sale of the original property, it is not always this simple. This is because *Hallett* also suggested that where property purchased was genuinely 'mixed property' because it had been purchased with a trustee's money as well as trust property, this no longer gave entitlement to claim the property itself, because it could not truly be said to be the beneficiary's property. In these circumstances, *Hallett* suggested that the beneficiary's entitlement was limited 'to a charge over the property purchased for the amount of trust money laid out in the purchase'. But this has been rebuked in *Foskett* v *McKeown* [2000] 3 All ER 97, in which Lord Millett suggested, at 131, that the basic rule is that:

> Where a trustee wrongfully uses trust money to provide part of the cost of acquiring an asset, the beneficiary is entitled *at his option* either to claim a proportionate share of the asset or to enforce a lien upon it to secure his personal claim against the trustee for the amount of the misapplied money. It does not matter whether the trustee mixed the trust money with his own in a single fund before using it to acquire the asset, or made separate payments (whether simultaneously or sequentially) out of the differently owned funds to acquire a single asset.

(Emphasis original)

Applying Re Hallett's Estate: *difficulties presented where there is more than one innocent claimant*

For the most part, these rules need to be understood in the context that what is being claimed against is a depleted fund, which is unlikely to be sufficient to satisfy losses experienced by all of the parties. This is particularly problematic where there is more than one innocent party. Obviously, we are concerned with the position of the beneficiary, but other innocents who might be caught up in claims to a mixed fund include a trustee's creditors or clients. The same difficulty—that of competing innocent claims—will also arise where the person mixing the money, including the wrongfully applied trust property, is innocent, such as the situation in *Re Diplock* [1948] Ch 465. These situations raise issues about how to permit recovery amongst equally innocent claimants, given that although a mixed fund *can* give rise to a profitable investment, it is more likely to be a fund insufficient to satisfy all potential claims.

17.9.3 A mixed fund that is insufficient to satisfy all claims to it

Having introduced the likelihood that, in these situations, the claims made against a mixed fund are likely to outstrip the assets available to satisfy them, it is also likely that many mixed funds will contain money belonging to the wronged beneficiary, the wrongdoing trustee, and also other innocent claimants. And while the justifications for preventing trustees from keeping the fruits of wrongdoing through mechanisms such as *Re Hallett's Estate* are clear, often the beneficiary will not be the only innocent claimant. These situations raise issues about how to permit recovery amongst equally innocent claimants, given that although a mixed fund can give rise to a profitable investment, it is more likely to be a fund insufficient to satisfy all potential claims against it.

Traditionally, the approach taken in these situations has been the application of the rule in *Clayton's Case* (1816) 1 Mer 572. Here, on a principle of 'first in, first out', the first payment into a mixed account is considered to be 'appropriated' to satisfy the earliest debt, and it was applied in the Court of Appeal in *Re Diplock*. This approach has been criticized for being very unfair on early 'contributors' to a mixed fund, and to a significant extent this is because the rule in *Clayton's Case* was developed around dealings with goods rather than funds of money. In these circumstances, where purchases and sales of goods are being made all of the time, it is easy to see how goods—and particularly perishable ones—which are purchased at an earlier time are not assumed to be ones that are 'left' at a later date. So the approach taken to mixed funds of money was a later development of *Clayton*, in order to provide a clear resolution to the difficulties created by situations in which claims against a mixed fund far outstrip what it is capable of satisfying, which is what commonly happens, even if it is not seen as a resolution that is very fair and it will always operate against the claims of earlier contributors to mixed funds.

This is why *Clayton* has been extensively criticized, and policy discourses have shown a long-standing preference for the approach of dividing an insufficient fund rateably amongst all of its contributors—that is, in proportion with their actual contributions and this is known as *pari passu* (meaning 'on an equal footing'). This was identified as the mechanism of choice for insolvency law by the 1982 *Report of the Review Committee on Insolvency Law and Practice* (Cmnd 8558; the 'Cork Report'). However, judicial reluctance to depart from *Clayton* can be seen in the Court of Appeal's decision in *Barlow Clowes International Ltd* v *Vaughan* [1992] 4 All ER 22, which insisted that *Clayton's Case* normally applied because the Court was bound to regard it as authoritative on account of the *ratio* of *Re Diplock*. However grudging this might appear, it did suggest that *Clayton* was a presumption and that alternative approaches could be pursued where there was evidence that they should be, as was actually done in *Barlow Clowes* itself, which did appear to be consistent with *Re Diplock*. This suggested that there was scope for the presumption of *Clayton* to be departed from without too much difficulty and, as Leggatt LJ suggested, 'During the 175 years since the rule in *Clayton's Case* was devised, neither its acclaim nor its application has been universal'. Even Woolf LJ's insistence that the rule was 'settled law' was unenthusiastic, claiming that this was (only) so 'short of [intervention from] the House of Lords'. In *Foskett* v *McKeown*, the House of Lords responded, and the case is strong authority in favour of *pari passu*, with more recent signs of departure from the traditional approach evident in *Russell-Cooke Trust Co* v *Prentis* [2003] 2 All ER 478 and *Commerzbank AG* v *IMB Morgan plc* [2004] EWHC 2771. For an alternative to *Clayton* and also *pari passu*, see Lowrie and Todd [1997] Denning LJ 43, on the North American rolling charge mechanism.

17.9.4 The position of innocent claims where the fund has been invested profitably

In the vast majority of cases, applying the rule in *Re Hallett* will reflect the difficulty that there are likely to be a number of competing claims to a mixed fund, and not only that of a beneficiary, and that in reality it is likely that there will not be enough to satisfy losses experienced by all of the parties. However, it might also be the case that mixed money has been used to purchase assets (usually investments) which have actually performed very well. Here, *Re Oatway* [1903] 2 Ch 356 is authority that the operation of *Re Hallett* does not prevent a beneficiary from enjoying a charge (or lien) over any property purchased from the mixed account. There had been some doubt about this in *Re Hallett*, and *Sinclair* v *Brougham* suggested that this was not possible and that the beneficiary's remedy was limited to a charge on the property for the amount of trust money expended in its purchase. This is a surprising result, given the strict rule against profits by trustees, and some doubt was cast on this in *Re Tilley's WT* [1967] Ch 1179, albeit that this was *obiter* and a decision at first instance.

In *Re Tilley*, a sole trustee who was also a life tenant had mixed a small amount of trust money in her own bank account before embarking on a series of property speculations, which were so successful that, on her death, her estate was worth £94,000. The beneficiaries entitled in remainder claimed a share of this wealth in the proportion that the trust money in the account bore to the balance of the account at that time. Ungoed-Thomas J held them entitled only to the return of the trust money with interest. This decision was based on a finding of fact that Ms Tilley had not invested the trust money in property, but had merely used it to reduce her overdraft. However, Ungeod-Thomas J suggested that, in different circumstances, where a trustee has in fact laid out trust money towards a purchase, the beneficiaries would then be entitled to the property and any profit to the extent that it had been paid for with trust money. The position was clarified in the House of Lords in *Foskett* v *McKeown*, albeit that the Court of Appeal took a different view, as considered in the next sections. The basic rule can be seen in Lord Millett's judgment in the same passage as that set out in the previous section:

> Where a trustee wrongfully uses trust money to provide part of the cost of acquiring an asset, the beneficiary is entitled *at his option* either to claim a proportionate share of the asset or to enforce a lien upon it to secure his personal claim against the trustee for the amount of the misapplied money. It does not matter whether the trustee mixed the trust money with his own in a single fund before using it to acquire the asset, or made separate payments (whether simultaneously or sequentially) out of the differently owned funds to acquire a single asset.
>
> (*Foskett* v *McKeown* [2000] 3 All ER 97, *per* Lord Millett at 131, emphasis original)

17.10 Current understanding of the rules of tracing

Up to now, much of the discussion of the House of Lords' decision in *Foskett* v *McKeown* in 2000 has focused on the majority decision, which is itself best understood from what had happened in the Court of Appeal in 1998. In this earlier decision, which was also a majority ruling, the purchaser beneficiaries were held only to be entitled to a charge on the proceeds to secure their restitutionary claim for the value of their money that was used for the payment of the life policy premiums. However, in May 2000, the House of Lords ruled that, as beneficiaries under a trust, they were entitled to trace in equity into the policy proceeds, and to do so in proportion to their contributions to the premium payments. Indeed, it was held that the beneficiaries' claim was simply an assertion of an equitable proprietary interest arising from the mixing of the value of the premiums with the value of the policy, which was analogous with the mixing of moneys in a bank account. It thus followed that the beneficiaries were entitled to a pro rata share of the policy moneys. This becomes very significant for considering how many findings of the majority in *Foskett* can be seen as a commentary on the changing nature of the tracing claim. However, this also requires us to consider the views of the minority, who concurred with the Court of Appeal.

17.11 The changing nature of tracing, and the significance of *Foskett* in the Court of Appeal and the House of Lords

As we will discover shortly, for the majority, this outcome was seen as a vindication of the beneficiaries' proprietary interest in the fund and their entitlement to a pro rata share. The dissenting view, of Lords Hope and Steyn, was that such a misapplication of trust moneys (to pay for insurance policy premiums) did not entitle the purchaser beneficiaries (not to be confused with the named beneficiaries under the deceased man's life policy) to a pro rata share in the property. It was suggested instead that this situation was more akin to use by a trustee of moneys held on trust for maintenance of his own property (thus invoking the principle that a trustee cannot profit from his own breach of trust) rather than mixing money in bank accounts. This was discussed at length in the Court of Appeal by Sir Richard Scott V-C, the essence of whose reasoning was that it followed that, unless it could be demonstrated that he obtained a profit as a result of the expenditure, a trustee's liability to repay extended only to the money misapplied, thus invoking *Re Tilley's WT* principles. This entitled the purchasers to no more than the return of their contributions plus interest.

We shall come to consider the significance of proprietary entitlement shortly, but first we find some very interesting views on the nature of tracing itself being expressed by the majority in the House of Lords, and particularly Lord Millett. This is where we need to go back to the earlier suggestion that tracing has traditionally been regarded as a proprietary remedy, which would permit the beneficiary to proceed against a particular asset in the defendant's hands. However, *Boscawen* v *Bajwa* [1995] 1 WLR 328 and *Foskett* v *McKeown* show growing judicial consensus that tracing is better viewed as an exercise in 'identification' rather than following. This can also be seen in academic writings, such as those of Peter Birks, including (1993) LMCLQ 218. In both cases, Lord Millett devoted considerable time to a discussion of the nature of tracing; accordingly, in a tracing claim, 'the claimant claims the new asset because it was acquired in whole or in part with the original asset. What he traces, therefore, is not the physical asset itself but the value inherent in it'. This meant that, according to his Lordship at 128:

> Tracing is thus neither a claim nor a remedy. It is merely the process by which a claimant demonstrates what has happened to his property, identifies its proceeds and the persons who handled or received them, and justifies his claim that the proceeds can properly be regarded as representing his property. Tracing is also distinct from claiming. It identifies the traceable proceeds of the claimant's property. It enables the claimant to substitute the traceable proceeds for the original asset as the subject matter of his claim. But it does not affect or establish his claim. That will depend on a number of factors including the nature of his interest in the original asset. He will normally be able to maintain the same claim to the substituted asset as he could have maintained to the original asset.

This rationale was followed closely in *Ultraframe (UK) Ltd* v *Fielding* [2005] EWHC 1638 (Ch). On this reasoning, having successfully traced property, a claimant may be entitled to assert a legal proprietary right or an equitable proprietary right, depending on the nature of his interest in the original property. This view of tracing makes the distinction between equitable and common law tracing much less significant than has traditionally been the case, and possibly even redundant, according to Lord Millett in *Foskett* v *McKeown*, at 128:

> There is thus no sense in maintaining different rules for tracing at law and in equity. One set of tracing rules is enough … There is certainly no logical justification for allowing any distinction between them to produce capricious results in cases of mixed substitutions by insisting on the existence of a fiduciary relationship as a pre-condition for applying equity's tracing rules.

And in terms of explaining the difference between tracing and following in pursuit of his mission to equate tracing with 'identifying' property, Lord Millett suggested, at 127, that:

> These are both exercises in locating assets which are or may be taken to represent an asset belonging to the plaintiffs and to which they assert ownership. The processes of tracing and following are, however, distinct. Following is the process of following the same asset as it moves from hand to hand. Tracing is a process of identifying a new asset as a substitute for the old. Where one asset is exchanged for another, a claimant can elect whether to follow the original asset into the hands of a new owner or to trace its value into the new asset in the hands of the same owner.

So we have a definite sense of traditional ideas—that tracing is all about a claimant following property that he owns into the hands of someone who should not have it and seeking its return—falling out of favour. We can also glean from this that tracing is better considered a process for identifying property, over which a proprietary claim can then be asserted. But getting a sense of what all of this actually means, or might mean, is not altogether straightforward. This is partly because a number of these ideas have been developed little, if at all, since *Foskett*, given that in so far as they might have been given further thought judicially, this has been through a number of decisions at first instance. So what can we make of reasoning that a claimant identifies his property and then asserts a (legal or equitable) proprietary entitlement to it, which is achieved through the process of tracing, because tracing is better regarded as a process rather than a remedy?

At this point, it is necessary, and indeed possible, to have only some idea of what is happening. And in trying to understand what all of this might amount to, there is a clear rationale, and the first thing that we do need to appreciate is that, in many ways, these issues set out in *Foskett* and developed a little subsequently are at the tail end of a much bigger movement in this sphere. This is one that has now subsided considerably, but was the way in which the mid-to-late 1990s and the early 2000s was a period of time during which the whole area of recovering missing property was embroiled in a much bigger debate over what the *mechanisms* for recovering missing property *should be seeking to achieve* and what their *legal basis* should be.

What should proprietary entitlement amount to (and for whom)?
This time of very significant debate was a battleground between principles of *proprietary entitlement* and *restitution*, which can be seen reflected in the differences in approach

between the Court of Appeal and the House of Lords in *Foskett*. To explain these terms a little, 'proprietary entitlement' is where we find legal rules that are seeking to preserve the entitlement of owners of property in circumstances of a defendant's bankruptcy, and also to ensure that an owner of property is able to achieve the full benefit of the property, including any increases in value; 'restitution' is concerned with protecting different interests, and seeks to prevent the unjust enrichment of one party at the expense of another. One can see how both of these different approaches could potentially apply in situations in which an owner of property is forcibly separated from it, and another who is not entitled to it actually has it. In the case of proprietary entitlement, conferring protection from the insolvency of the person in whose hands the property lies, and also the facility of recovering increases in value, is extremely valuable for a claimant. Restitution looks at things differently and considers the position of those who receive property in these circumstances, as well as those who have lost it.

This debate was settled in the House of Lords in *Foskett* in favour of proprietary entitlement, but there had been a great deal of pro-restitution force beforehand, as was clear from the commentary generated by the decision in *Westdeutsche* and as was evident in the Court of Appeal's decision in *Foskett*. In this context, the House of Lords' decision in *Foskett* was very much reasserting proprietary entitlement, but it also went further, by setting out the stall for what 'proprietary entitlement' should mean and to what it should amount. Much of this flows from the way in which *Foskett* illustrates a strong movement towards making tracing a more universal mechanism, evident from suggestion that there really should not be separate regimes for 'owners' with different proprietary interests in property. In turn, it is possible for us to consider what universal tracing rules might look like. In the course of doing so, we can check our understanding of traditional tracing rules at common law and in equity by thinking about how a universal set of tracing rules might adopt the good aspects of both, and work to exclude the disadvantages of each.

What might a universal set of tracing rules look like?

So, if we try to visualize a universal set of tracing rules premised on proprietary entitlement, what might these rules look like? Here, we need to think about how this should take on the flexibility of equity and also the simplicity of the common law. The former can be seen in equity's very accommodating approach to 'mixed substitutions', its approaches to competing innocent claims, and also its facility for allowing recovery for increases in value. In terms of joining this with the simplicity of the common law, we would focus on the much more elementary requirements of using tracing at common law, which means that all that is required is that the claimant owns the property. Obviously, in a universal approach, this would be better expressed as requirement of a proprietary interest in property—be this legal ownership or ownership of property in equity—but this would dispense with the fiduciary relationship requirement, which many find very hard to justify. We can see criticism in *Foskett* of the way in which it appears to have arisen as a result of historical accident and, from the cases, we can see that there is commonly little 'issue' about whether it has been satisfied. But there is also post-*Foskett* authority suggesting that it is still a requirement. So the creation of a universal set of tracing rules would be an opportunity to consider whether this requirement should remain.

In these circumstances, the combined strengths of the common law with those of equity would be available to everyone (universally) who has a proprietary interest in the missing property, and would not distinguish or discriminate between what type of interest is held, be it legal or equitable. Because there is so much more development actually needed to make more sense of this, this is all that is being said at this point in time—except, that is, to note the rationale for this movement, which it was suggested does exist: that anyone who has had their property taken from them wrongfully should be able to seek its recovery and that, in facilitating this, the law should seek to treat all those in this unfortunate position *equally*.

Part II Personal actions arising from breach of trust

Where trust property is missing following a breach committed by a trustee, we know from Chapter 16 that, following breach of trust, the trustee is liable to provide 'equitable compensation'. This is a personal action, remembering also that the personal nature of a trustee's liability means that trustees are liable only for their own breaches and not vicariously for breaches of others. The materials in this second part of the chapter do continue to be concerned with the recovery of property wrongly applied in breach of trust, but focus differently on the personal actions that are available and why they might be important. In this respect, and in introducing the significance of personal actions for missing property, a trustee's personal liability to compensate for the breach of trust will be measured by the losses that have been caused to the trust by his maladministration.

It was suggested earlier that unless the claimant (we are mainly concerned with a beneficiary here) can establish the right to trace the property (belonging to him in equity and wrongly applied by a trustee) and establish a proprietary interest in property that can be 'identified', *Foskett* v *McKeown* is authority that the beneficiary's claim against the trustee acting in breach of trust is a personal one; in Chapter 16 on breach of trust, it was explained that this was distinguishable from the liability incurred by a trustee for an unauthorized profit, which is imposition of a constructive trust. It is important to remember this, because constructive trusts *are* to be found in assisting a beneficiary's recovery of trust property, but not used against the trustee acting in breach. Instead, where constructive trusts are found, they are used for 'fixing' liability for the property applied in breach of trust upon those who are otherwise unconnected with the trust, and who are known as 'strangers' to a trust.

The parameters of 'stranger' liability arising from breach of trust

So how and why can persons other than a trustee acting in breach ever incur liability for wrongful applications of trust property? This is because where there is a breach of trust (or a wrong regarded as equivalent to it) and property goes missing as a result of this, others can also become involved in this. We can see how others can become involved in property becoming missing from understanding that there are two types of stranger liability in which liability arises by way of constructive trust. Here, we find liability that arises for actually receiving trust property (or that which belongs to another who is using equity's actions), which acknowledges that misapplied trust property is often very quickly passed on to other persons, and in which case a tracing action cannot be used unless this person actually retains the property. This type of recipient liability does not require retention of the property and liability is said to be 'complete' on receipt of the property. Liability can also arise for assisting a trustee's breach of trust. This arises for those who have actually participated in the original breach committed by the trustee (or conduct that is regarded as equivalent with it), and this other person may even have instigated it. Although, in this type of 'accessory liability', such a person never actually receives any property, it is treated as a form of constructive trusteeship.

In addition, there are potentially strangers who can incur liability following a breach of trust, but who do not do so by way of a constructive trust. This situation arises where those who receive wrongfully used trust property (or property of non-beneficiary claimants who can use equity's actions) *are* strangers to a trust, and they do receive it, but they do so innocently. This means that they receive the property without knowing that the person dealing with it is not entitled to do so, or is doing so improperly (such as the executors in *Re Diplock*). Such recipients *are* liable because they are not bona fide purchasers able to take the property free of the trust, but, unlike other recipients of wrongfully used property, they have not acted reprehensibly. Such persons are known as 'innocent volunteers' and *Westdeutche* [1996] AC 699 (HL) is authority that whilst it is appropriate for liability for innocent volunteers to arise, it is not appropriate for this to be by imposition of a constructive trust. The reasons for this can be understood from the way in which Chapter 6 analysed constructive trusteeship as a response to unconscionable conduct by those who hold legal title to property, and this is clearly not the case for an innocent volunteer recipient.

We will come to look at how liability for strangers who are innocent volunteers is configured in due course, but first we will look at liability for strangers who are not innocent.

17.12 Liability for persons who *are* 'strangers', but who *are not* 'innocent'

As this heading suggests, these issues are explored first in relation to the liability that can be occurred by others who are in some way involved when a trustee commits a breach of trust. Traditionally, the liability of strangers to a trust in this category has been divided into two categories, called 'knowing assistance' and 'knowing receipt', with the latter often including reference to dealing to become 'knowing receipt and dealing', as evident in *Barnes* v *Addy* (1874) 9 Ch App 244. But, more recently, there has been a changing focus of terminology of and even the fundamental basis for liability, which requires us to look closely at both types of liability.

At the outset, as a general observation, both are regarded as forms of constructive trusteeship, even though an assistant 'accessory' to a breach of trust never actually receives (trust) property. This means that a beneficiary only ever has a personal action against an accessory because trust property does not actually pass into his hands, but with the extent of this liability recently considered in *Fiona Trust & Holding Corporation* v *Privalov* [2010] EWHC 3199. This is unless the accessory has also received property that he might or might not still have, in which case the claimant potentially has a wider range of possible remedies.

Liability for those who 'know': common ancestry and what is currently required
What both these forms of liability have in common is awareness that a breach of trust has been committed. This raises questions of *what* precisely must be known, or *how much* must be known, for liability to arise. The traditional 'starting point' is *Baden Delvaux* [1983] BCLC 325 (more recently reported at [1992] 4 All ER 16), identifying five categories of knowledge (the 'five degrees of *Baden Delvaux* knowledge'), as follows:

(i)   actual knowledge;

(ii) wilfully shutting one's eyes to the obvious;

(iii) wilfully and recklessly failing to make such inquiries as an honest and reasonable person would make;

(iv) knowledge of circumstances that would indicate the facts to an honest and reasonable person; and

(v) knowledge of circumstances that would put an honest and reasonable person on inquiry.

Current approaches to both species of stranger liability will now follow, but first you should ensure that you understand two things: first, that both share this common ancestry classification of so-called *Baden Delvaux* knowledge; and second, that current approaches have been much influenced by the difficulties that have traditionally arisen from mapping *Baden Delvaux* classifications onto the involvement of strangers in breaches of trust, or situations that are treated as if they were so. Traditional applications of *Baden Delvaux* have led to a very confused and inconsistent body of case law, especially in respect of knowing receipt, where the receipt of property in fast-moving commercial transactions has presented particular difficulties for establishing what the threshold for liability should be. We can also see some disagreement within these cases even as to what type of action was actually at issue, and it is common to find cases critiquing earlier authorities as 'not truly a case concerning' knowing receipt or knowing assistance.

The way in which these issues are set out in cases tells us how the courts have struggled with what is required as far as each of these species of 'knowing' liability is concerned. For liability that has traditionally been termed 'knowing assistance', a number of key cases—notably, *Belmont Finance Corporation* v *Williams Furniture Ltd (No. 1)* [1979] Ch 250—have indicated a relatively strict requirement for 'actual knowledge', which has appeared to embrace *Baden Delvaux* categories (i), (ii), and (iii). Others, including *Agip (Africa) Ltd* v *Jackson* [1991] 3 WLR 116 (CA), have suggested a different approach, whereby a defendant can be found liable by virtue of having either 'actual knowledge' or 'constructive knowledge', ensuring that any of the *Baden Delvaux* categories are capable of giving rise to such liability. The position for knowing receipt has been even less clear, with much of this on account of the issues arising with receipt of property in commercial transactions. Some authorities have suggested that constructive knowledge or constructive notice will suffice: respectively, *Belmont Finance Corporation Ltd* v *Williams Furniture Ltd (No. 2)* [1980] 1 All ER 393 and *Agip (Africa) Ltd* v *Jackson* [1990] Ch 265. Others have suggested that this is not sufficient, but without being very clear on the point, with several cases, including *Eagle Trust plc* v *SBC Securities Ltd* [1993] 1 WLR 484 and *Polly Peck International plc* v *Nadir (No. 2)* [1992] 4 All ER 769, emphasizing the particularly problematic aspects of this within commercial dealings.

The modern law relating to both types of stranger liability are now considered, commencing with knowing assistance, on account of the fact that much has changed here, including the actual basis for liability to arise.

It has been explained that this is always a personal action and—like the trustee actually committing the breach—an accessory is jointly and severally liable for any loss that the beneficiary suffers as a result of the breach of trust. Like the 'express' trustee, a constructive trustee accessory will incur liability to account to the trust for any profit that he has made as a result of being involved in the breach (see, for example, *Ultraframe* v *Fielding* [2005] EWHC 1638 (Ch)). This is the liability that can be incurred, its basis and mechanism, and what follows is a look at how liability can arise and who will be liable, and in what circumstances.

17.13 The modern law on liability for being an accessory to a trustee's breach of trust: movement away from knowing assistance and towards 'accessory liability'

The traditional terminology for this liability was 'knowing assistance', with *Baden Delvaux* providing insight into what had to be known by someone in order to render him a knowing assistant of a breach of trust. This entire approach was swept aside in *Royal Brunei Airlines* v *Tan* [1995]] 3 WLR 64, in which the Privy Council suggested that a more appropriate term for this liability is 'accessory to a trustee's breach of trust'. This rethinking was clearly influenced by the difficulties generally experienced in finding a 'correct' *Baden Delvaux* standard, given the differences of approach evident in the case law, but there was also a much more specific difficulty with the law as traditionally framed. As the judgments in *Tan* make clear, case law governed by knowing assistance principles had resulted in too much focus on whether the trustee whose original breach was being assisted was honest or otherwise, because it was traditionally thought that this type of liability could be incurred only by an assistant where the original breach was itself fraudulent. *Royal Brunei Airlines* v *Tan* stated unequivocally that, in the case of accessory liability, there is no requirement for a dishonest or fraudulent breach of trust by the trustee, and to take a different position meant that a very fraudulent accessory could escape liability simply because the trustee himself was innocent. In other words, the term 'accessory liability' was intended to focus liability on the conduct of the accessory, rather than the circumstances of the breach itself.

17.13.1 Developments since *Royal Brunei Airlines* v *Tan*: *Twinsectra Ltd* v *Yardley*

As part of its refocusing of 'assistance' liability upon the accessory rather than the original trustee, *Royal Brunei Airlines* v *Tan* suggested that, rather than being premised on knowledge (the *Baden Delvaux* approach), accessory liability is more appropriately focused on the honesty or otherwise of the accessory, and the speech of Lord Nicholls discussed this extensively. The basic approach in *Tan* was followed by the majority in the House of Lords' decision in *Twinsectra Ltd* v *Yardley* [2002] 2 WLR 802, and thus the phrase 'dishonest assistance' is now widely employed (alongside that of accessory liability). It is also the case that *Twinsectra* considered the degree of dishonesty that is required in order for liability for dishonest assistance to arise.

The case involved two solicitors and a loan transaction, and raised questions as to the status of the loan transaction and whether it was subject to a (*Quistclose*) trust or otherwise. The existence or otherwise of a *Quistclose* trust (after *Barclays Bank Ltd* v *Quistclose Investments Ltd* [1970] AC 567, discussed in Chapter 18) hinged on whether or not the (second) solicitor, Sims, held the loan subject to a trust (arising from its mandated application towards a purpose specified by the lender, through his instructions), and the question of accessorial liability involved the other (first) solicitor, Leach. This followed the way in which the loan was, in the event, not applied in accordance with the lender's instructions, and then was not repaid. Twinsectra sued three parties: the two solicitors and the client, Yardley. Sims was sued because his release of the money to the client amounted to breach of trust. The money was released to the client through Leach, and it was alleged that Leach's failure to take any steps to ensure the correct application of the money amounted to dishonest assistance of a breach of trust; this occurred when Leach paid out the money in contravention of the lender's instructions, acting on Yardley's behalf.

In respect of liability as an accessory, it was found at first instance that the first solicitor had not been dishonest, although he had deliberately shut his eyes to the implications of the undertaking. The Court of Appeal reversed this finding and gave judgment against Leach for the proportion of the loan that had not been applied in the acquisition of property. The House of Lords' consideration arose following an appeal by Leach as to whether or not he had assisted in the breach of trust that had been committed by Sims (the Court of Appeal finding that the loan was subject to a trust was upheld on *Quistclose* principles) and could incur personal liability on account of doing so.

In considering what meaning might appropriately be given to the term 'dishonesty' in this context, it was held that, for an accessory to be liable:

(1) he had to have acted dishonestly by the ordinary standards of reasonable and honest people; *and*

(2) he had to have himself been aware that, by those standards, he was acting dishonestly.

This looked a combination objective–subjective test.

So, in focusing attention on dishonesty in this way, as Lord Hutton understood the law, a completely subjective approach—the 'Robin Hood' test (whereby a person is only regarded as dishonest if he transgresses his own standard of honesty, even if that standard is contrary to that of reasonable and honest people)—is not accepted in the courts. The difference between an objective test and one that combines objective–subjective criteria was explained as follows: the former will involve the court determining that the defendant's conduct is dishonest as judged against the 'ordinary standards of reasonable and honest people, even if he does not realise this', while the latter makes reference to the defendant *himself* within a broad setting of objectivity. This latter combination test rests on whether the defendant's conduct was dishonest by the ordinary standards of reasonable and honest people, and that he *himself* realized that, by those standards, his conduct was dishonest.

The majority in *Twinsectra* appeared to prefer the combination test, with Lord Millett dissenting in favour of an objective test, believing this to be what Lord Nicholls had intended in *Tan*. But the majority approach clearly attached much significance to Lord Nicholls's judgment. In explaining how the law determines dishonesty, we can see clearly the significance of an objective approach: '[I]n the context of the accessory liability principle acting dishonestly, or with lack of probity, which is synonymous, means simply not acting as an honest person would in the circumstances. This is an objective standard.' However, Lord Nicholls continued, at 391:

> Ultimately, in most cases, an honest person should have little difficulty in knowing whether a proposed transaction, or his participation in it, would offend the normally accepted standards of honest conduct. Likewise, when called upon to decide whether a person was acting honestly, a court will look at all the circumstances known to the third party at the time. The court will also have regard to personal attributes of the third party, such as his experience and intelligence, and the reason why he acted as he did.

Lord Hoffmann's concurrence with Lord Hutton was manifested in his view that dishonesty requires a dishonest state of mind, which amounts to 'consciousness that one is transgressing ordinary standards of honest behaviour', and that wrongful conduct of this species requires more than mere 'knowledge of the facts'. Lord Millett's view was that liability as an accessory to a breach of trust does not depend upon dishonesty in the normal sense of that expression. It is sufficient that the defendant knew all of the facts, which made it wrongful for him to participate in the way in which he did. Indeed, His Lordship contended that the only subjective elements allowed by *Tan* were the defendant's experience, his intelligence, and actual state of knowledge, and there was no requirement that he must have realized that he was acting dishonestly.

Lord Millett's preferred test, set out at 135, was an objective one, in which liability was not dependent upon the defendant's appreciation that he was acting dishonestly, or even his detailed knowledge about the details of the trust and its breach:

> It is sufficient that he knows that the money is not at the free disposal of the principal. In some circumstances it may not even be necessary that his knowledge should extend this far. It may be sufficient that he knows that he is assisting in a dishonest scheme.

Lord Hoffmann's view of Lord Millett's judgment was that it was not open for the House to concur with a view other than that 'consciousness that one is transgressing ordinary standards of honest behaviour' was required for conduct to be wrongful and capable of incurring liability.

And, in speaking for the majority, Lord Hutton concluded that the test for accessory liability was substantially the same as the test in criminal law for dishonesty, as laid down in *R v Ghosh* [1982] QB 1053. This became a source of much criticism, which was generated by *Twinsectra*, because it was suggested that it was inappropriate to import tests for criminal liability into determinations of civil liability. This was evident in Lord Millett's dissent. More generally, it appeared difficult to square with the spirit and intendment of *Royal Brunei Airlines v Tan*, which sought to liberalize accessory liability by transferring focus away from the trustee (and whether his initial breach of trust was dishonest or not) and placing it firmly upon the accessory himself. In this vein, it was asked whether the very welcome decision in *Tan* would be able to achieve its full potential in the sphere of accessory liability in the wake of *Twinsectra*. Predictably, following *Twinsectra*, suggestions were made in some quarters that the position it appeared to adopt—in what had to be present for accessory liability to be incurred—was too 'pro-defendant' (see Ryan (2006) 70 Conv 188).

17.13.2 **Developments since *Twinsectra Ltd* v *Yardley* and the current state of play**

Almost as quickly as the *Twinsectra* test started to attract academic scrutiny, an objective approach was being asserted in the courts in *Dubai Aluminium v Salaam* [2002] 3 WLR 1913 and *Tayeb v HSBC Bank plc* [2004] 4 All ER 1024, and the issue was considered comprehensively again in *Barlow Clowes International Ltd (in liquidation) v Eurotrust International Ltd* [2006] 1 All ER 333. The background for this case can be gleaned from earlier references to *Barlow Clowes v Vaughan* in this chapter, and from its discussion in Lowrie and Todd [1997] Denning LJ 43, which explain how, during the 1980s, a fraudulent scheme that purported to offer high returns on UK gilt-edged securities ('gilts') was run by Clowes and operated through a company called Barlow Clowes International. Thereafter, it was into Isle of Man-based bank accounts maintained by Eurotrust International that investors' funds were paid during 1987. The three defendants in this action were Eurotrust International itself and also two principal directors; in the High

Court of the Isle of Man, Barlow Clowes International claimed that the two defendants and, through them, Eurotrust International had dishonestly assisted Clowes and an associate in misappropriating investors' funds.

The High Court found all three defendants liable for dishonest assistance, and all three appealed, whereupon the appeals of the first and third defendant (the company and one principal director, respectively) were dismissed. However, the appeal of the second defendant—Henwood—was allowed, on the ground that it was not supported by evidence. It was at this point that Barlow Clowes International appealed to the Privy Council.

Originally, in the High Court of the Isle of Man, it had been found that Henwood could incur liability for dishonestly assisting the misappropriation of sums paid into bank accounts during 1987. The Court found that he strongly suspected that the funds passing through his hands were funds received by Barlow Clowes International from members of the public who believed that they were investing in gilts. From this, it was found that no honest person could have assisted the subsequent disposal of the assets to Clowes and his associate, and that his decision not to make enquiries amounted to a conscious strategy to avoid running the risk that he would encounter the truth. In the Privy Council, counsel for Henwood argued that, on *Twinsectra* principles, the High Court's findings in respect of Henwood did not satisfy the *Royal Brunei Airlines* test (also sometimes referenced as the '*Tan* test' or the '*Tan* approach') for dishonesty as this appeared in light of *Twinsectra*.

The Privy Council was unanimous in its rejection of the defendant's argument, and upheld the original findings in respect of Henwood. This precipitated the Judicial Committee's reflections on the majority approach in *Twinsectra*, which had been relied upon by the defendant's counsel. Especially significant in light of the nature of these reflections, this Judicial Committee included Lords Nicholls (author of the *Tan* approach) and Hoffmann (part of the majority in *Twinsectra*). The Privy Council's judgment was delivered by Lord Hoffmann, who sought to clarify the position of dishonesty under *Tan* in light of the apparent effect of *Twinsectra*. His Lordship particularly sought to clarify that, in *Twinsectra* in 2002, the House of Lords did not seek to alter or refine the *Tan* test, but he accepted that there might have been an element of ambiguity left by *Twinsectra* concerning what was actually required for liability to arise.

However, Lord Hoffmann suggested that this was much less so than had been suggested in some subsequent commentary. This was because *Twinsectra* had not put emphasis on what the defendant's views on generally acceptable standards of conduct might be; instead, for liability to arise, what was required was that the defendant's knowledge of the transaction had to be such as to render his participation contrary to normally acceptable standards of honest conduct and thereby transgressory. There was no requirement that he should have had reflections about what those normally acceptable standards were. For a useful commentary on how this decision emphasizing consciousness of transgression as 'the better interpretation of the *Royal Brunei* test' and also the way in which Lord Hoffmann's allusion to 'an element of ambiguity' is rather an understatement in what appeared to be rather a significant retreat from *Twinsectra*, see Ryan (2006) 70 Conv 188.

17.13.3 The *Twinsectra* test after *Barlow Clowes*: the significance of *Abou-Rahmah*

In this very informative article, Ryan suggests that while there is a very attractive simplicity in Lord Nicholls's *Royal Brunei Airlines* proposition that '[i]n most situations there is little difficulty in identifying how an honest person would behave', a consideration of both *Twinsectra* and *Barlow Clowes* provided a salutary reminder of the 'formidable difficulties' confronting judges, who must *apply* the test. In turn, more recent case law provides a salutary reminder of the way in which it can very quickly become apparent that decisions that appear to clarify the law do not, in fact, do so. Just a short time after *Barlow Clowes*, the Court of Appeal considered this again in *Abou-Rahmah* v *Kadir Abacha* [2006] EWCA Civ 1492. And while two Lord Justices of Appeal (Rix and Pill LJJ) both took the view that the case could be determined without engaging with the controversies left open by *Barlow Clowes'* implications for *Twinsectra*, Arden LJ enthusiastically engaged with this first opportunity for an appellate court to consider *Barlow Clowes*. Arden LJ considered that *Barlow Clowes* should be followed, but she also ensured that the controversies continued by suggesting that this did not depart from, or amount to, a refusal to follow the *Twinsectra* approach. Instead, *Barlow Clowes* provided guidance as to the proper interpretation to be placed on it as a matter of English law, showing how 'the *Royal Brunei* case and the *Twinsectra* case can be read together to form a consistent corpus of law'.

Arden LJ's reading of the cases was that the widely held interpretation that *Twinsectra Ltd* v *Yardley* required both an objective and subjective test was a wrong interpretation, with the accurate position being clarified in *Barlow Clowes*. According to Arden LJ, it was not a requirement of the standard of dishonesty that the defendant should be conscious of his wrongdoing; instead, the test was 'predominantly objective', but with subjective aspects. On this reasoning, the position was that taken by Lord Nicholls in *Royal Brunei Airlines* v *Tan*, with an assessment (of dishonesty) being made on the basis of what the defendant actually knew at the time (thus accounting for the *subjective* elements) rather than what a reasonable person would have known or appreciated. On the facts, it was found that although a bank manager had a general suspicion that two individuals might possibly be involved in money laundering, he did not have any particular suspicions about the two transactions that were being litigated. This meant that the judge at first instance was correct in finding that this did not amount to dishonesty.

Abou-Rahmah received important endorsement in *Starglade Properties Ltd* v *Nash* [2010] EWHC 148 (Ch) and, in the intervening period, *AG Zambia* v *Meer Care and Desai* [2007] EWHC 952 provided important support for a test that was objective, but in which determining a breach would involve 'a subjective assessment of the person in question in the light of what he knew at the time as distinct from what a reasonable person would have known or appreciated'.

On the facts of *Starglade* (which can be found set out in the Online Resource Centre), it was found that the defendant's conduct was not dishonest for the purposes of liability for dishonest assistance, because, in the absence of specific advice knowledge, his conduct was not conduct that would have transgressed generally accepted standards of commercial behaviour by a person in his position, even if he had had greater commercial experience. More generally, in finding this, Strauss J also confirmed a number of qualities attaching to dishonesty for the purpose of establishing liability for dishonest assistance, which were set out by the Court of Appeal in *Abou-Rahmah*, and it did appear from *Starglade* that *Abou-Rahmah* provided an up-to-date statement of the law. The case appeared to suggest that *Abou-Rahmah* might be the 'last word' on the standard required for accessory liability, without actually being clear about whether it affirmed *Abou-Rahmah*'s proposition that *Tan*, *Twinsectra*, and *Barlow Clowes* provide a 'consistent corpus of law', and that the 'retreat from *Twinsectra*' is something that has been invented by commentators.

However, the Court of Appeal, at [2010] EWCA Civ 1314, then ruled that whilst the correct standard was to apply the ordinary standard of honest behaviour to the facts of the case, Strauss J had been wrong to rule that, where a body of opinion might regard the conduct as honest, dishonesty could not be found. Indeed, differing views on dishonesty would not militate against a finding of dishonesty, and such determinations are for the court to make and then apply to the facts of the case. In *Starglade* itself, the deliberate removal of the assets of an insolvent company in order to defeat the legitimate claims of creditors was not considered in accordance with the ordinary standards of honest commercial behaviour, and contemporaneously *Aerostar Maintenance International Ltd* v *Wilson* [2010] EWHC 2032 (Ch) had suggested that dishonesty meant 'not acting as an honest person would in the circumstances' and for the most part was to be equated with 'conscious impropriety'.

Starglade has now been applied in *Halliwells LLP* v *Nes Solicitors* [2011] EWHC 947 (QB), in which the defendant was found to have transgressed the 'ordinary standards of normal commercial behaviour', and in *Secretary of State for Justice* v *Topland Group plc* [2011] EWHC 983 (QB), in which it was found to be the court that determined whether the conduct was 'commercially unacceptable'.

17.14 The modern law on liability for being a knowing recipient of property belonging to another

The application of court-determined dishonesty is likely to continue to generate litigation interest, and it will be interesting to observe how this will be approached where there are competing views on dishonest or honest conduct from which to choose. But, in terms of its basic premise, the law on dishonest assistance appears to be relatively well settled. In this vein, *Starglade* also provides a neat segue for the following material, which moves on to discussing the other type of personal liability that can be incurred by a 'knowing' stranger. This is because it illustrates for us the way in which a number of cases will actually be multiple-action cases in which defendants are alleged to be accessories to a breach of trust and *also* knowing recipients of wrongfully applied property. In some ways, this is not surprising, given that these actions are designed to be part of a package of responses seeking to assist those who are wrongfully separated from property belonging to them; in this respect, in *Starglade*, there was also a claim for knowing receipt of trust property. However, generally, this is also a contributing factor for the difficulties that have traditionally subsisted in mapping these actions onto *Baden Delvaux* knowledge, and even distinguishing them from one another. This is how we get decisions suggesting that a particular authority is not truly a decision on one or another of these actions, and did instead concern the other. Unfortunately, this has been particularly the case with liability known as 'knowing receipt'.

Finding acceptable parameters for this type of liability has always been particularly problematic in cases in which property is exchanged in commercial transactions, where it passes from hand to hand at great speed, as well as very frequently, and so there is very little time to investigate its provenance. This is why 'notice' requirements for application of the bona fide purchaser have become much attenuated in this context, and this has made mapping *Baden Delvaux* knowledge onto these types of situation difficult for the purposes of liability for knowing receipt.

Indeed, the commercial context is also very significant for understanding why there is a significant body of law relating to whether or not there has even been a 'receipt' of property for the purposes of determining liability for its knowing receipt before we even consider what might amount to 'knowing'. Here, key cases are *Agip (Africa) Ltd* v *Jackson* [1990] Ch 265 (see especially per Millett J at 286), *El Ajou* v *Dollar Land Holdings* [1994] 2 All ER 685, *Charter plc* v *City Index Ltd* [2007] 1 WLR 26, and *Uzinterimpex JSC* v *Standard Bank plc* 2008] EWCA Civ 819.

As part of this, *El Ajou* also lists the ingredients of this offence, at 700, which requires:

> ... first, a disposal of his assets in breach of fiduciary duty; secondly, the beneficial receipt by the defendant of assets which are traceable as representing the assets of the plaintiff; and thirdly, knowledge on the part of the defendant that the assets he received are traceable to a breach of fiduciary duty.

The materials now focus on the third element, in terms of *what* must be known for there to be knowledge. But unfortunately, unlike the case of accessory liability, there has not been a clear defining moment (a '*Tan* moment', for want of a better phrase) for this species of liability.

The modern law, without a 'Tan *moment', but with a key case?*
It was never very clear what categories of *Baden Delvaux* knowledge were required for knowing receipt, with the earlier materials suggesting that there was actually considerable disagreement in the case law. However, whilst the position of knowing receipt in the modern law has always been far less clear and far less certain than dishonest assistance, the interest generated *has* clustered around one 'key' case: the Court of Appeal decision in *BCCI (Overseas) Ltd* v *Akindele* [2000] 3 WLR 1423. Indeed, in *Akindele*, Nourse LJ suggested, in reaction to *Tan* (albeit that this was before *Twinsectra*, among others) that, given that there was a settled test of dishonesty for knowing assistance, the same position should be established for 'knowledge' in the case of knowing receipt.

Akindele was in turn anchored to the approach adopted in *Re Montagu's ST* [1987] Ch 264, which was described as a seminal judgment and is authority for the 'want of probity' approach. Here, a defendant who was not dishonest could incur liability as a knowing recipient, and thus dishonesty was not a requirement; instead, what was required was for the 'recipient's state of knowledge' to be such as 'to make it unconscionable for him to retain the benefit of the receipt'.

Akindele *as a defining moment? Issues unclarified and subsequent developments*
This approach was considered by the Court of Appeal to be capable of avoiding difficulties of definition and allocation of liability, which caused problems in earlier categorizations and especially the inconsistencies arising from applying *Baden Delvaux* (which, it was noted in *Akindele*, was in any case a knowing assistance case). The difficulty with *Akindele*, and especially with its own references to *Tan* as a defining moment (for dishonest assistance), was that it did not actually clarify what the differences between dishonesty and unconscionability might amount to.

There was some clarification provided by the Court of Appeal in *Criterion Properties plc* v *Stratford UK Properties LLC* [2003] 1 WLR 2108, stating that the question of unconscionability could not simply be answered by reference to whether or not there was knowledge of the circumstances giving rise to the breach of duty, and thereby favouring a flexible approach to it. Yet when that case was heard by the House of Lords, it was decided that neither it, nor *Akindele*, were truly concerned with knowing receipt, and *Crown Dilmun* v *Sutton* [2004] EWHC 52 (Ch) is critical of the looseness of the conscionability approach.

However, the Court of Appeal in *City Index Ltd* v *Gawler* [2007] EWCA Civ 1382 accepted that *Akindele* 'represents the present law'. This was so albeit that the uncertainties generated by *Akindele* did not appear to have been resolved by it, or indeed by *Charter plc* v *City Index Ltd* [2008] 2 WLR 950, which insisted that 'liability for 'knowing receipt' depends on the defendant having sufficient knowledge of the circumstances to make it 'unconscionable' for him to retain the benefit'. Subsequently, *Independent Trustee Services Ltd* v *GP Noble Trustees Ltd* [2010] EWHC 1653 (Ch) and *Law Society of England and Wales* v *Habitable Concepts Ltd* [2010] EWHC 1449 (Ch) have applied *Akindele*. And then, in what gives us a strong sense of déjà vu, not to mention also circularity, the Court of Appeal, in *MCP Pension Trustees Ltd* v *AON Pension Trustees Ltd* [2010] EWCA Civ 377, [2011] 1 All ER (Comm) 228, strongly endorsed *Montagu* on the significance of 'forgetting' in making determinations of 'want of probity'.

Knowing receipt, 'Tan *moments', and the significance of* Twinsectra

Considering what the effect of current case law might be is not easy, but it does raise the question of whether a '*Tan* moment' has ever been considered for liability for knowing receipt. We can see that liability, once known as knowing assistance, has been completely reconfigured and we also know that, in many respects, liability for knowing receipt has been more problematic than this. This is where we turn to one of the key cases in that '*Tan*' trajectory for dishonest assistance to consider its thoughts on knowing receipt. *Twinsectra* v *Yardley* is, of course, best known for opening up the 'dishonesty controversy' in relation to accessory liability or dishonest assistance, but it is also a source for appreciating differing views on what should be required for liability for knowing receipt to arise. In *Twinsectra*, Lord Millett suggested (*obiter*) in favour of liability which is receipt-based, and this means that it is established when (trust) property is received and it is not premised on showing fault on the part of the recipient (here, manifested in knowledge). Lord Millett continued by stressing that this meant that the cause of action in this case was restitutionary, which we know is a case based on preventing an unjust enrichment, and this has already been shown by reference to the common law action for money had and received.

If this approach were adopted, it would mean that the beneficiary's action for what has traditionally been known as knowing receipt would be restitutionary (that the recipient has been unjustly enriched at the beneficiary's expense—and so presumably subject to a change of position defence?), rather than by way of the imposition of a constructive trust. Adopting such a view might even cast doubt on the differences that are traditionally regarded as having subsisted between principles of unjust enrichment and constructive trusts. However, *Westdeutsche Landesbank* v *Islington LBC* [1996] AC 669 is authority that a difference between them is regarded as appropriate (pursued through reference to liability incurred by innocent volunteers, where imposition of a constructive trust was considered to be inappropriate), and in *Akindele* itself Nourse LJ was not convinced that 'strict liability coupled with a change of position defence would be preferable to fault-based liability' in many cases.

In coming full circle and ending this discussion where we started, we can see the decision in *Starglade* v *Nash* at first instance (the Court of Appeal did not touch its observations in this regard) reaffirming the traditional view of fault-based liability based on knowledge and without needing to show dishonesty. In finding that the defendant was liable as a knowing recipient (having found that he was not liable as an accessory), Strauss J also affirmed the continuing significance of *Akindele*—namely, that liability for knowing receipt would arise in circumstances under which the recipient's state of knowledge made it unconscionable for him to retain the benefit of the receipt of the property. This is, of course, the approach developed in *Akindele* from the want-of-probity approach taken in *Re Montagu's ST*. This suggests that, in *City Index Ltd* v *Gawler* [2007] EWCA Civ 1382, the Court of Appeal was correct to conclude that *Akindele* 'represents the present law', but *Starglade* also confirms that the uncertainties generated by what actually will operate to render receipt of property unconscionable had not been clarified.

17.15 The personal action in equity against 'innocent volunteers'

This action stems from the way in which, in cases where it is theoretically possible to bring a proprietary tracing claim in equity, it is deemed inequitable to do so. In these circumstances, a claimant will not be able to vindicate his proprietary entitlement in this way on account of two key factors: the first is that the defendant is a volunteer who received the property innocently and without knowing of the owner's proprietary entitlement; the second is that this recipient has actually then used this property for purposes that are neither reversible nor can easily be reversed. We saw this being applied in *Re Diplock*, in which we learned that the recipients could not take the property free of the owner's entitlement because they were not bona fide purchasers. Here, this particular action can be seen as recognition that the owner who lost the property remains entitled to it, because his title has not been lost to another.

Equally, this 'personal action in equity' is acknowledgement that, because of the circumstances, an owner's rights will not be fully vindicated. Essentially, this action is seeking to strike a balance between competing claims between two innocent parties who are both victims of a trustee's breach of trust (albeit that this can arise without dishonesty on the part of the trustee, as was the case in *Diplock* itself). This action recognizes that volunteers should not take free of a beneficiary's interests, and also acknowledges the position of an innocent recipient who has actually acted on this property being 'his' in ways that cannot be undone. The action seeks to achieve this by not being as extensive in scope as other beneficiary actions, and quite clearly it is intended to be different in scope from the action that a beneficiary would have in personal actions against a knowing stranger. Most significantly, it is different from what is recoverable through tracing, where increases in value are recoverable even from innocent volunteers, on account that it is only ever a bona fide purchaser against whom a tracing action cannot be brought.

The difference between a tracing action against an innocent volunteer and the personal action is that the property has actually been applied irreversibly by this recipient. In these latter circumstances, what can be recovered is limited to the principal sum that was misapplied, and the action may be available only in the administration of estates, as suggested in *Re Montagu* [1987] Ch 264. Even if it applies more generally to volunteers (which is the view of some), it can be used only once all remedies against wrongdoers have been exhausted. However, as suggested earlier, it would appear that, to qualify for this extent of liability and to escape the full consequences of a tracing claim, something more than a change of position (established in *Lipkin Gorman* v *Karpanale* [1991] 3 WLR 10) is required to be shown by the volunteer recipient, and that nothing short of irreversible use of the misapplied property will enable a volunteer recipient to have to repay this limited recompense to the rightful owner of the property.

17.16 Personal actions, proprietary entitlement, and restitution: a postscript

Given the context that where trust property 'goes missing', it will often end up in the 'wrong hands', much of considering the actions available to a beneficiary concerns how a person who *receives* the property can be liable to the beneficiary. Property wrongfully received in this way may either be retained by the recipient, or passed onto another, and from the mid-1990s onwards questions of liability became dominated by considerable disagreement as to whether the basis for the beneficiary's recovery of (wrongfully applied trust) property should be restitutionary (and thus based on 'unjust enrichment principles'), or based on proprietary entitlement. By way of reiteration:

- where liability is restitutionary, it is said that liability arises because the recipient is unjustly enriched at the rightful owner's expense (in this case, the rightful owner is the beneficiary); and

- where liability is based on proprietary entitlement, it is said to arise because the recipient of wrongfully applied property has interfered with the owner's (the beneficiary's) property rights attaching to the property.

Most recently, *Foskett* v *McKeown* is authority for a triumph of proprietary entitlement principles in tracing cases. This is a central development on the ground that applying these different approaches can lead to very different outcomes in terms of what can be recovered by the beneficiary, and the way in which these can be seen as representing different degrees of fairness and appropriateness from the perspective of a liable recipient, and also an owner wrongfully parted from his property. Here, the favour shown by the courts for principles of proprietary entitlement does, in many ways, mark a full circle back to where this text commenced: the importance of property—and particularly the *ownership* of property in English law.

A very good analysis of the triumph of proprietary entitlement in the context of tracing can be found in Tang Hang Wu (2001) 25 Melbourne U L Rev 295, but it is also the case that these issues of the basis of liability can be seen in recent developments in the personal remedies that attach to the receipt of trust property, and particularly considerations of whether equity's remedy for knowing receipt should evolve to be more like the common law action for money had and received, which is very effective. Indeed, in *Abou-Rahmah* v *Kadir Abacha* [2006] 1 All ER, Rix LJ suggested that the courts (still) consider that this area of law is 'in flux or at any rate subject to a process of analytical change'.

In assessing whether the law should develop in such a way, it *is* the case that the precise scope of the change-of-position defence in the common law action is unclear. However, some clarity is evident from subsequent decisions in *Niru Battery Manufacturing Co* v *Milestone Trading Ltd* [2004] 2 WLR 1415, *Barros Mattos Junior* v *MacDaniels Ltd* [2005] 1 WLR 247, and *Abou-Rahmah* v *Kadir Abacha*, clustering around the change-of-position defence. In *Niru Battery*, it was held that, in order to defeat the defence of change of position, it did not have to be shown that the recipient had been dishonest; rather, what needed to be shown was that he had not acted in good faith. A person who had, or thought that he had, good reason to believe that a payment had been made to him by mistake failed to act in good faith if he paid the money away without making enquiries of the payer. It was held, in *Barros Mattos Junior,* that an innocent recipient of stolen money could not rely upon the defence of change of position where the circumstances in which this arose were considered to be wrongful. This meant that, in the case, the defendants were not able to rely on foreign exchange transactions that were illegal under Nigerian law, and accordingly the defence failed. In *Abou-Rahmah* v *Kadir Abacha*, attention was drawn to the significance of whether the conduct was considered to be 'commercially acceptable', but it was also considered (by the majority) that a general suspicion of involvement in a money-laundering scheme was not sufficient, and that there must have been particular suspicions about the two payments in question.

In terms of the significance of this for the effectiveness of common law, it has been argued (see Martin (1998) 62 Conv 13) that equity, too, should provide a personal action based on the same principles. Furthermore, it is clear, from *Kleinwort Benson Ltd* v *Lincoln City Council* [1998] 3 WLR 1095, that the scope of restitutionary actions has also now been extended to cover situations in which money is paid over under a mistake of law, as well as to those in which money is paid over under a mistake of fact, where it has traditionally been recognized.

 Revision Box

1. Ensure that you understand and can answer the following.
   (a) Why, following a breach of trust, may pursuing an action for equitable compensation not be satisfactory for a beneficiary?
   (b) Why it is necessary to have a suite of actions that are both proprietary and personal, and which are also available against a range of defendants?
   (c) Why is a proprietary action a claimant's action of choice?
2. In relation to equity's tracing action, ensure that you can explain the following.
   (a) Why do so many non-beneficiary claimants wish to use equity's tracing rules and what is the jurisdictional basis of this?
   (b) What are the requirements for tracing in equity?
   (c) What is meant by a 'unitary system of tracing' and to what degree does English law currently embody this?
3. In relation to equity's personal actions, consider the following.
   (a) What is meant by 'strangers' to a trust and why is it said that there are two types of stranger?
   (b) How does the type of stranger appear to influence the nature of liability?
   (c) Summarize the current law relating to dishonest assistance.
   (d) Summarize the current law relating to knowing receipt.
   (e) Summarize the key features of the personal *Diplock* action.

FURTHER READING

Andrews (2003) 'The redundancy of dishonest assistance' 67 Conveyancer 399.

Birks (1992) 'Mixing and tracing' 45 Current Legal Problems 69.

Birks (1993) 'Persistent problems in misdirected money: a quintet' Lloyd's Maritime and Commercial Law Quarterly 218.

Conaglen (2011) 'Difficulties with tracing backwards' 127 Law Quarterly Review 432.

Hayton (2012) 'The extent of equitable remedies: Privy Council versus Court of Appeal' 33 Competition Law 161.

Lowrie and Todd (1997) 'In defence of the North American rolling charge' Denning LJ 43.

Martin (1998) 'Recipient liability after *Westdeutsche*' 62 Conveyancer 13.

Millett (1991) 'Tracing the proceeds of fraud' 107 Law Quarterly Review 71.

Millett (1998) 'Restitution and constructive trusts' in Cornish (ed.) *Restitution Past, Present and Future: Essays in Honour of Gareth Jones* (Oxford: Hart Publishing).

Mitchell (2008) 'Dishonest assistance, knowing receipt, and the law of limitation' 72 Conveyancer 226.

Panesar (2012) 'Equitable tracing: Part 2: A change in English law' 134 Trusts and Estates Law & Tax Journal 23.

Pawlowski (2011) 'Tracing into improvements, debts and overdrawn accounts' 17 Trusts & Trustees 411.

Pearce and Shearman (2012) 'The pursuit of proprietary remedies for fiduciary duty' Denning Law Journal 191.

Ryan (2006) *'Royal Brunei* dishonesty: clarity at last' 70 Conveyancer 188.

Ryan (2007) *'Royal Brunei* dishonesty: a clear welcome for *Barlow Clowes*' 71 Conveyancer 168.

Sheehan (2010) 'Property in a Fund, Tracing and Unjust Enrichment' 4 Journal of Equity 225.

Shine (2012) 'Dishonesty in civil commercial claims: a state of mind or a course of conduct?' 1 Journal of Business Law 29.

Stevens (2001) 'Vindicating the proprietary nature of tracing' 65 Conveyancer 94.

Thompson (2002) 'Criminal law and property law: an unhappy combination' 66 Conveyancer 387.

Wu (2001) *'Foskett* v *McKeown*: hard-nosed property rights or unjust enrichment?' 25 University of Melbourne Law Review 295.

 For summaries of a selection of these articles, please visit <http://www.oxfordtextbooks.co.uk/orc/wilson_trusts11e/>

18

Trusts arising in commercial dealings

The creation of a dedicated study of trusts in commercial dealings has been an idea that has taken shape over the past few years. As new cases arise and new editions of the text are prepared, it has become ever more apparent that cases involving trusts principles that have been created, and honed and developed, by equity over several centuries are increasingly ones concerning commercial dealings. These are dealings involving the exchange of goods and services between parties who ordinarily deal 'at arm's length' in relationships that are governed by contract. There are now a large number of cases showing that parties who are litigating as a result of their commercial interactions are increasingly arguing the applicability of rules and principles developed by equity in order to protect beneficiaries under a trust to their rather different circumstances. We have seen a number of examples of this throughout this text, and to this extent, while there is some new commercial material for this edition, there are many other examples that have been a mainstay of earlier editions showing that this trend for seeking to use trusts principles in litigation for matters arising from commercial dealings is not of itself new.

This dedicated chapter now brings together material that has previously been distributed across its different parts, according to the substantive area of trusts law to which it could be seen to be related. Here, it draws together material that does have connections of origin and context, but which connections had not been noted before now. And, as the chapter was originally conceived, this was intended as a celebration of the diversity of use that can be made of trusts in contemporary society. Focusing on trusts that are not anomalous by virtue of being recognized by equity as charitable, this chapter was always intended to anchor this celebration of twenty-first-century diversity with the flexibility and adaptability of a device that equity started to develop more than 500 years ago.

So this was always going to be a location for noting that commercial dealings can be found in current litigation concerning validity requirements of express trusts, access to equity's beneficiary actions for assisting an owner whose property has become 'lost', and the significance of implied trusts in contemporary society. To this extent, this chapter has remained faithful to its original intended direction. However, as the materials have been collated and thought has been given to their analysis, it has become clear that, yes, trusts are becoming more commonly found in commercial dealings, but this seems to be signalling developments of a more significant nature. This increasing prominence of commercial dealings in analysing traditional trust principles is suggesting that this new context for trust principles might actually be becoming a new paradigm for trusts law, and its future evolution and development.

18.1 Introducing trusts arising in commercial dealings

What this means is that the nature of where trusts are being found in litigation involving commercial dealings might actually have the scope to alter significantly the nature of trusts law. It has been suggested at various points in this text since Chapter 1 that the first modern trusts appeared in the eighteenth century, and also that the trust became popularized during this time and into the nineteenth century. This was precipitated by the 'family settlement' trust, which was the first truly modern trust. This heightened focus on the trust arose because it was able to achieve restrictions on the free disposal of property by those who 'have it' and also to reduce exposure to taxation, which would otherwise arise from transactions involving property; both of these were features of 'the Use', developed by equity in late medieval times. So why is it so significant that the trust was popularized during the nineteenth century, and what does any of this have to do with the increasing use made of trusts in commercial dealings?

The popularization of the trust and the emergence of the paradigm for modern trusts law

We know from Chapter 14 how and when the trust became popularized, and in that context how this provided the impetus for regulating the trust by making it clear what is expected of those who are entrusted with property that they have no entitlement to enjoy. As we learned then, modern trusts law also emerged to fulfil a facilitative agenda—that is, to ensure that those who wished to create trusts were able to do so, validly, and in the confidence that what they intended for their property would actually transpire.

Although we still see family settlements today, as early as Chapter 1 we learned that the trust can be found across economy and society, performing a range of functions. But it still has a number of applications for what might broadly be considered 'familial arrangements' concerning property. We can see this directly in family homes, where we saw trusts playing a vital function in determining ownership of what for most people will be the most important asset acquired in a lifetime. But, in some respects, this is not necessarily the most significant use of the trust in familial arrangements, any more than is the multimillion-pound settlement that we do still see in certain societal echelons.

In some ways, the most remarkable use of the trust can be seen in what we encountered much earlier in the text than home ownership. In Chapter 3, we could see the express trust as a wholly democratic institution that allows those who do not necessarily have very much in the way of property, and who do not necessarily come from socio-economic sectors in which specialist legal advice is available, very high levels of autonomy. Such an owner of property will, of course, be able to give his property away, or sell it, or (depending on its nature) use it as security, but such a person can also create a trust of it. This empowers such persons to make distinctions between property that is to be given absolutely and that which provides benefit subject to obligations as to how it is to be used, and is able to achieve this as readily as the societal groupings traditionally associated with family settlement trusts.

Property, ownership, and the trust as a democratic instrument

In the rules that have developed around certainty of intention, we can see that the obligations associated with the use of trust property can arise without an owner of property using the word 'trust'. And whilst Scarman LJ's references to the ordinary lives of 'simple folk' in *Paul v Constance* [1977] 1 All ER 197 might seem a little patronizing (and it was, of course, a borderline case), there seems to be a genuine attempt to make the trust accessible to those whose life circumstances mean that they cannot necessarily articulate their intentions regarding their property in technical language themselves, or afford the services of someone who can. So the law that has grown up around express trusts has developed to provide considerable flexibility around how owners of property can be found to have intended to create a trust. Here, equity's approach to requirements that must be met seeks to support this, whilst also reflecting that settling property on trust is a very significant arrangement, and one that will ultimately exclude an owner of property when it creates enforceable rights for the beneficiary and onerous duties for a trustee.

This can be seen as far as equity's own requirements have become shaped, such as the certainty rules, and also in the way in which equity has to coexist with law's requirements regarding dealings with property. In the latter regard, in the operation of the 'last act' doctrine for incompletely constituted trusts discussed in Chapter 5, we can see equity making genuine attempts to distinguish circumstances in which an owner-cum-settlor really has done everything that he can to ensure that his property will have a new owner and what remains outstanding are rigid legal requirements of 'form' of transfer from half-hearted (or less than so) attempts to vest the property in another.

It is from this model that we can understand how the law of implied trusts developed to facilitate a *formalized* approach to the creation of ownership in *informal* circumstances, under which there is no ownership of property at law and where there is no express trust.

Property ownership and the trust as a tool of social justice

As far as implied trusts are concerned, from Chapter 6 we can see the trust acting as an important tool to ensure that what owners of property appear to want can be effected in situations in which they do not make their intentions clear. This does, of course, empower owners of property, and does thereby empower ownership of property. With the resulting trust, equity will respond to what an owner can be presumed to have intended, given the circumstances, and once again this has the capacity to be democratic. Here, an 'incomplete disposal' resulting trust is equally capable of being applied to the fortune of one Tony Vandervell (considered in Chapter 4) and others who are considerably less wealthy. In this regard, we can see the implied trust as a tool of justice by ensuring that owners' wishes for their property are accommodated. But an even clearer case for seeing the trust as a mechanism for achieving a broader type of social justice can be seen in the use of implied trusts in determining shared home ownership. We do see the resulting trust (or at least something that appears to be very like it) here, but very significantly we see constructive trusteeship being imposed on those who own their homes at law, which will force them to use their property with regard to others who should have a proprietary interest in it on account of the circumstances.

What all of these situations have in common is that they are illustrations drawn from what might loosely be termed 'familial' dealings with property. It is the case that Vandervell's dealings arose from him seeking to benefit a charitable organization, but in common with a large number of trusts created, this was part of a conscious strategy to maintain wealth within his family. It is the case that constructive trusts are applied across economic spheres, and where constructive trusteeship arises in the context of 'lost property', as shown in Chapter 17, we do see a prominence of commercial, rather than familial, arrangements. This aside, the familial context for family home ownership is clear, but we can also find constructive trusts hard at work elsewhere to ensure justice in private arrangements, which are interpersonal and commonly familial. Indeed, in Chapter 9, and in materials looking at mutual wills, very briefly in Chapter 6 and more extensively on the Online Resource Centre, we have seen this in how constructive trusts arise in how property is dealt with after its owner's death, and a significant number of equity's interventions in incomplete property transfers encountered in Chapter 5 concern intended (or at least apparently intended) dealings with property to benefit family members. The strong familial context is equally evident in failed or incomplete disposal resulting trusts of the *Westdeutsche Landesbank Girozentrale* v *Islington LBC* [1996] AC 669 category B variety, and it is certainly very evident in those arising from a so-called 'voluntary conveyance' of title to property found within category A. Indeed, the development of the presumption of advancement alongside the presumption of the resulting trust is testament to the way in which equity perceives that the issues of ownership that arise here are highly likely to concern entitlements to property within close ties of kinship.

18.2 Introducing trusts in the commercial context

So it is the case that dealings with 'family' property—broadly configured—very much set the tone for the popularization of the trust, and in turn this would very much shape the development of modern 'trusts law' during the nineteenth century. Accordingly, it was such dealings that very much influenced how clear views on the entitlements of those intended to benefit emerged, and the concomitant ones of responsibility for those who hold property, whilst labouring under an imperative to use it for another. These arrangements also underpinned trust law's facilitative agenda, and taken together they have thus provided the structure and direction for much of this text.

The trust and celebration of its diversity

Alongside this, the text has given much emphasis to how the trust can be found across social and economic spheres in the twenty-first century. This, of course, includes anomalous arrangements governed by charity law (as discussed in Chapters 10, 11, and 12), but we have seen a large number of examples whereby private trusts—both express and implied—can be found across society and economy protecting the 'interests' of a number of parties through conferring upon them equitable ownership of property or the rights and entitlements which are those of persons who own property in equity. Most interestingly, we are seeing a significant use of trusts in contractual relationships arising from commercial dealings between parties. This is what we are focusing on in this Chapter, because increasingly 'trusts cases' are more about commercial dealings than familial ones. And in respect of this, trusts law is becoming more about commercial dealings than family ones, and is being developed through cases of this nature rather than traditional ones. This is one way in which we might regard commercial dealings as providing a new 'paradigm' for trusts law and its development. But the significance of commercial dealings for trusts law appears to be more significant still.

This is because, as commercial dealings started to incorporate trusts arrangements, they were facilitated by trusts law and traditional trusts principles. But we will now consider the proposition that the courts are actually developing different trusts principles for commercial trusts. Using illustrative examples drawn from express trusts and trusts that are implied, it will be suggested that this could have marked significance for the way in which trusts law is understood and studied. It might be that the law relating to private trusts will come to be defined by reference to 'commercial trusts', rather than private and broadly familial trusts, in the future. Another possible direction is that, from this, a distinctive body of 'trusts law for commercial trusts' could be developed in the same way as is currently recognized for 'implied trusts' or 'charitable trusts'.

18.3 Trusts arising in commercial dealings and the purpose of this chapter

As a matter of general observation, perception that the use *of* trusts *in* commercial dealings is increasing is clear from the Law Commission's 2006 report on *Trustee Exemption Clauses* (Law Com. No. 301, Cm. 6874). The Law Commission indicated that it was aware that this needed to be taken on board in forming its recommendations on the extent to which English trusts law should accommodate trustee exemption clauses (TECs). This has already been noted in Chapter 3, and Chapter 16 suggested that the Law Commission did take the view that those who create trusts in commercial dealings do not require the same protection (as far as establishing the existence of a TEC is concerned) as those who ordinarily create trusts, on account of market equality between the parties likely to be involved and widespread 'standard practice' already in commercial dealings. What can be added for the purposes of this chapter is how this is recognition that such arrangements raise different considerations from trusts as traditionally used, and might even actually require different principles of law as a result of this.

All of these themes are very significant for this chapter and also for the way in which it is being approached in this edition. Because the law relating to trusts continues to develop and evolve, and this chapter is completely new, it is not intended to be a definitive statement of anything in any way, shape, or form; instead it is seeking to set out how the state of trusts law currently appears and what its influencing forces might be. At this stage, it is not a comprehensive guide to trusts in commercial dealings, but instead focuses on a number of key areas in the law relating to private trusts in which the desire to use trusts appears to be particularly strong, and the desire to import trust principles into commercial dealings ordinarily governed by contract is reflective of this.

In this regard, much of the material can be found grouped around how financial distress in commercial dealings, and also property that becomes 'lost' in this context, are particular touchstones for appreciating the significance of trusts for commerce, and then the significance of commerce for trusts law.

18.3.1 The creation of trusts and 'signature events' in the context of commercial dealings

In Chapter 1, it was noted that the question of whether a trust exists in particular circumstances will often be precipitated by a signature event, which forces parties involved to consider who owns property. It was suggested at that time that a number of events will force questions of ownership into the parties' consciousness if they are not already there, and since then we have encountered death as a context for questions of proprietary entitlement (such as in *Jones* v *Lock* (1865) 1 Ch App 25 and *Richards* v *Delbridge* (1874) LR 18 Eq 11) and also relationship breakdown (in the materials relating to family homes), and even situations in which one party changes his mind about wishing another to have his property—in fact, and not simply in theory, in the case of *Mascall* v *Mascall* (1984) 50 P & CR 119. At the same time as we gave first substantive consideration to *Jones* v *Lock* and *Richards* v *Delbridge* in Chapter 3, we also came across what we will now analyse as a signature event: the imminence of financial failure. This event arises when one party is on the verge of becoming bankrupt or insolvent, which is a occurrence that will manifestly affect entitlements to property.

The imminence of bankruptcy or insolvency

This is because upon bankruptcy or insolvency, which is a legal term for a person being unable to fulfil his outstanding financial liabilities (that is, unable to pay his debts), a debtor loses ownership of his property, which becomes vested in those who are responsible for ensuring that as many of the debtor's outstanding financial liabilities as possible can be paid from this. Because this is triggered by inability to pay debts, it is almost always the case that there will be insufficient funds to satisfy all claims that could be made against the property by those who are owed by the debtor. Here, questions of how much is repaid to those who are owed and in what order are determined by insolvency law, which can currently be found in the Insolvency Act 1986, as amended. The policy of insolvency law is to ensure that as many creditors as possible can be repaid, but it also recognizes there will almost always be a shortfall. But once bankruptcy or insolvency occurs, this regime will automatically be triggered. This is why reference was made to imminent financial failure as a signature event for the role of trusts in determining ownership of property: once financial failure has occurred, it will be too late, and so any suggestion that a trust of property has arisen will have to relate to events that have occurred prior to this.

Before considering this any further, this observation does raise the question of why, in the face of imminent financial failure, the parties would wish to assert that a trust exists. The reason relates to two things, about one of which we know very little, and about the other we know rather more. The first matter is that, although we have not paid much attention to this up to now, commercial dealings between parties—whether these are both commercial parties, or as between a commercial party and its non-commercial client or customer—are governed by the law of contract. We have some idea that the law of contract and the law of trusts are different from looking at the way in which the trust has traditionally provided a way of giving third-party rights that could not arise using contract on the basis of the doctrine of privity, as explained in Chapter 1. When we looked at the loan as a way of providing benefits of property, we learned that although loans can be made on trusts principles, normally the loan of property from one person to another is governed by contract. This is the first step towards understanding why trusts might be attractive in imminent financial distress, because while contractual remedies are personal and arrangements arising under them will become subject to statutory insolvency law provisions upon financial failure, what we do know about a beneficiary's entitlement under a trust tells us that this will not happen where there is a trust. Under a contractual arrangement, a creditor can protect his position as such by requiring security from the borrower, but this assumes that a creditor is in a position to ask for it (given that creditor might be a local business, which supplies small-scale goods or services, or even a friend, as much as it can be a powerful creditor granting a large loan) and also that a borrower still has any property remaining to provide security.

Trusts protecting a creditor in a loan situation

In contrast, the existence of a trust will protect a creditor's position by virtue of the 'hard-nosed property rights' that beneficial ownership of property confers to a beneficiary. This is entitlement flowing from owning the property that arises as of right and does not depend on being 'fair, just and reasonable', and we also know that this entitlement is enforceable against anyone except a bona fide purchaser of that property. In the context of bankruptcy and insolvency, it means that, as a debtor loses legal title to his property, where this is owned by someone else in equity, it remains owned by him and entitles him to claim it. Assets subject to this type of arrangement will not—unlike loans made on contractual principles—become part of the pool of assets that are available to satisfy unpaid debts under insolvency law. But for this to happen, a trust will have to have arisen prior to an insolvency occurring, even it is only subsequently that this is argued by the parties and ultimately determined by the courts.

Beyond financial distress: the significance of lost property

We shall come to financial distress as a signature event, but prior to this we will also look at the loss of an owner's property as such. As anyone who owns property will understand, having property that belongs to him wrongfully taken is bound to concentrate an owner's mind on his ownership of property, because it is the first step towards being able to recover this from a person who wrongfully has this property because he is not entitled to it. This was the situation that we encountered in the previous chapter looking at actions that can assist an owner of property where this is taken from him. But, as it was stressed there, the actions at which we looked will only be able to assist someone who retains title to his property, even though it might now be in another's hands. This means that, to be able to use common law tracing rules, an owner who has lost his property must not have lost title to it, either through selling or pledging it, or through one of the exceptions to the *nemo dat* rule. Equally, equitable tracing rules will only ever come to the aid of a claimant whose equitable interest in property has not been lost to a bona fide purchaser of the legal title to that property. More will be said about this, including the way in which equity has made some adaptation of what is required for being entitled to use its tracing rules in recognition of growing demand for being able to do so largely from those in commercial relationships. And this starts with awareness that wrongful separation of property from its owner will force focus on who actually owns the property as a first step towards asserting ownership of it.

18.4 The influence of the commercial context on beneficiary actions for 'lost property'

It is very clear from the cases examined in Chapter 17 that commercial dealings have been enormously influential for the development of equity's beneficiary actions for 'lost property'. This can be seen for developments in who is entitled to use these actions and how the actions themselves are becoming developed as opportunities increase for those who own property to become wrongfully separated from it. This can be seen in relation to both the proprietary tracing action, and also equity's personal actions for knowing receipt and dishonest assistance.

We can see how the so-called commercial 'swap' agreements from the 1990s involving public authorities have been enormously influential in shaping the nature of the proprietary tracing claim for the twenty-first century. A number of cases—famously, *Westdeutsche*, but also *Guinness Mahon & Co.* v *Kensington and Chelsea RLBC* [1998] 2 All ER 272 and earlier *Hazell* v *Hammersmith* [1991] 2 WLR 372—became the battleground for competing views on proprietary entitlement and restitution. And in terms of how this was settled, the context in *Foskett* v *McKeown* [2000] 3 All ER 97 was a commercial building operation, albeit that this was building private dwellings. Today, virtually all of the cases that develop the proprietary tracing claim and the 'knowing' stranger personal actions are ones involving at least one party who is dealing as a commercial operator, and a relationship between him and the claimant that is a contractual one.

In this regard, the recent ruling of the Court of Appeal in *Starglade Properties Ltd* v *Nash* [2010] EWCA Civ 1314 is wholly typical of the way in which actions developed by equity are being used. These are, of course, actions designed to reflect both the strength of a beneficiary's ownership of trust property (as a right *in rem*), and also its key limitation that, ultimately, this right *in rem* could be lost to a purchaser of the legal interest in property for value and without notice. Today, these actions are not typically used by beneficiaries under a trust as traditionally understood, but by those whom equity is prepared to treat as if they were.

In addition to the way in which the right to trace can be lost even by a beneficiary in circumstances under which the property is destroyed and ceases to exist (and even in circumstances in which allowing tracing would be inequitable), traditionally the availability of equity's actions has been governed by the closely related criteria of the existence of a fiduciary relationship and that of an equitable proprietary interest in the property. This means that whilst equity might have developed the proprietary tracing claim, and the personal actions of knowing receipt and knowing (and now dishonest) assistance for a beneficiary under a trust, these are actions that have always been available in respect of corporate fiduciaries like the director in *Starglade*, and would be so in respect of a solicitor and client, executor and legatee, and agent and principal, all through the principle of availability to established categories of fiduciary relationship. In addition, as we discovered, there has been a great deal of emphasis on equity making these actions more widely available than this, with the impetus for this coming largely from parties in commercial dealings. This is on account of the limitations of common law actions that are available to those who own legal interests in property, and particularly the traditional restrictions of the common law tracing action.

The significance of commercial dealings for restating fiduciary obligations

As we know, this context has provided the opportunity for equity to reassert the core characteristic that a relationship must have if it is to be considered fiduciary: the obligation of loyalty, as set out in *Bristol and West BS* v *Mothew* [1998] Ch 1. However, it is significant that the context for this is strongly driven by commercial dealings, and it is this that provides the juxtaposition for the ordinary consequences of a contractual relationship between the parties and the special fiduciary relationship that is governed by equity's special expectations of fiduciaries. In the context of equity's beneficiary actions (as distinct from actions for undue influence, for example), virtually all of the litigation surrounding the ability of fiduciary relationships to arise from the circumstances has arisen where the parties are in a contractual relationship and at least one of the parties is a commercial actor, such as seen in *Halifax BS* v *Thomas* [1996] Ch 217.

In turn, the litigation reflects a strong desire to be able to establish a fiduciary relationship arising from the circumstances, because equity is both willing and also jurisdictionally able to extend beneficiary actions beyond established categories of financial relationships using its concurrent jurisdiction. In short, many parties wish to establish a fiduciary relationship precisely because they wish to use equity's actions for recovering property that is theirs, or for holding others responsible for its receipt or assisting in its loss. It is also the case that commercial dealings are commonly involved at some stage where equity extends the availability of its actions still further, to those who have been victims of fraud or theft, even outside the context of a contractual relationship.

The significance of commercial dealings for proposed future developments of tracing

With equity providing assistance to many commercial claimants who are not beneficiaries under a trust in this regard, it has come to pass that these cases have been extremely influential in how the law has developed. We can see this in the cases that characterized the key debate on the competing merits of proprietary entitlement and restitution as guiding principles for the proprietary tracing action. As that bigger question became settled in favour of proprietary entitlement, we can now see commercial cases at the heart of calls being made for a universal set of tracing rules. As this is envisaged by some of its key advocates, and centrally Lord Millett, this would seek to accommodate the proprietary entitlement of owners at law and in equity alike, and allow all of the benefits traditionally provided by equity's tracing rules and the simplicity of the common law's approach.

These are benefits that are also much fought over, as we can see with the fiduciary relationships litigation. Lord Millett's envisioned unified set of tracing rules would dispense with the fiduciary relationship requirement and, as we know from the previous chapter, it has a dubious pedigree. However, what has brought this very much into the open has been the huge volume of 'commercial fiduciary' litigation that has continued simultaneously to affirm and question the requirement. It looks likely that any further development of the law of tracing will be pursued through a case involving commercial actors, rather than an action arising from a beneficiary wishing to recover trust property missing as a result of a breach of trust committed by a trustee.

The significance of commercial dealings for the current state of 'stranger liability'

We can see a similar pattern in equity's actions of dishonest assistance and particularly knowing receipt. Indeed, in *Starglade Properties* v *Nash* [2010] EWHC 148 (Ch), as considered in the Court of Appeal in [2010] EWCA Civ 1314, we are reminded about how significant honesty or otherwise in commercial dealings is for mapping appropriate approaches to dishonesty generally in this regard, notwithstanding that this did involve a fiduciary in a conventional sense (albeit not a trustee). Similarly, although dishonesty was considered in relation to the conduct of a solicitor in *Twinsectra* v *Yardley* [2002] 2 WLR 802, the context was a commercial property deal. And in between these two key authorities, *Barlow Clowes* v *Eurotrust* [2006] 1 All ER 333 provides yet further reminder that breaches of trust that are occurring and being assisted are not paradigm arrangements involving trustees and beneficiaries in the trust arrangement that is of the familial arrangement type.

This is even more the case with liability for knowing receipt, where the significance of this action for commercial dealings has been crucial in the difficulties experienced in establishing the standard for liability to arise. Indeed as a number of cases prior to *BCCI (Overseas) Ltd* v *Akindele* [2000] 3 WLR 1423 demonstrate, it is the speed of commercial transactions that is seen as being responsible for difficulties in determining what degree of knowledge under *Baden Delvaux* [1983] BCLC 325 was required for liability to arise, and it is another commercial context case (albeit one involving an established category fiduciary) that ensures that *Starglade* provides the most current statement on the law relating to knowing receipt. We also know from the previous chapter that liability traditionally known as 'knowing receipt' is considered by many as a candidate for a '*Tan* moment' (after *Royal Brunei Airlines* v *Tan* [1995] 3 WLR 64), which would actually clarify the law by—if necessary—reconsidering its basis entirely. We can see this in Lord Millett's dictum in *Twinsectra* v *Yardley*, which calls for dispensing with the requirement of knowledge or notice, and replacing it with a restitutionary action. In this vein, it is interesting that this was considered as a possibility in *BCCI* v *Akindele* itself, in which Nourse LJ's view was that he was unconvinced that this would make a difference in the case of many commercial transactions.

Dissatisfaction in the law and sources for the impetus for change

At one level, this indicates why the law relating to knowing receipt remains so unsatisfactory. At another, more fundamental, level, it reveals what the courts understand to be the influences driving the law, and it is clear that this is not beneficiary trust arrangements that have evolved from family-type trust (broadly defined) and in respect of which equity developed these mechanisms for lost property.

What is happening in the area of missing or lost property is that the law is being developed by actions arising from commercial dealings rather than from traditional situations in which beneficiaries are equipped by equity to act where trust property in the conventional sense goes missing. It is not obvious from this analysis that rules are being developed for commercial dealings, which are different from traditional situations involving lost property. It is much clearer that the way in which the law approaches these traditional situations is being determined by developments concerning commercial dealings. It is important to make this point, because we have encountered developments in law that do suggest that different principles of law are being developed for applying trusts law beyond arrangements that have descended from family settlements. We can see this in relation to some of the requirements of a valid trust, and particularly legal rules governing satisfying certainty of intention and also constituting trusts through self-declarations of trusteeship.

18.5 Trusts arising from financial distress: determining loans that are trusts rather than contractual in nature

Having considered *why* trusts might arise in commercial dealings, we now need to consider *how* this happens. This is where we see that 'financial distress trusts' actually fall into two broad types, in terms of who is seeking to create them, which is key to understanding where we encounter them in trusts law and how they are significant for trusts law. So, in terms of who is seeking to create trusts in response to imminent financial distress, the person who most obviously might have an interest in doing this is a creditor who is seeking to protect his own position should bankruptcy or insolvency arise, but who cannot achieve this through taking security—either because his loan is not sufficiently sizeable, or because the borrower simply has no property left to levy. We shall see shortly how this can lead to the creation of express trusts and how this can give rise to a special type of resulting trust, and also what impact this might have on trust principles as traditionally understood. However, as we have seen in material relating to certainty of intention to create a trust, what we can now call 'financial distress trusts' can also arise from the insistence of the debtor himself that a trust should do so. This can be seen from the trust that was found to have been created prior to the insolvency of the mail order firm in *Re Kayford* [1975] 1 All ER 604, which also provides crucial insight into why a debtor would seek to do this. In a *Kayford* arrangement, a debtor is not seeking the creation of a trust to protect himself, but instead to protect his creditors against the consequences of him losing his property upon bankruptcy or insolvency. And, as we learned from *Kayford* itself, this is often to protect specific creditors against the general consequences that arise upon insolvency. We can see this also in the successful creation of a trust in *Re Chelsea Cloisters Ltd* [1980] 41 P & CR 98 and the failed attempt in *Re Multi Guarantee Co. Ltd* [1987] BCLC 257, and also *Re Farepak* [2007] 2 BCLC 1, which appeared to be a *Kayford* case even though *Kayford* reasoning was not applied.

18.5.1 The significance of creditor 'financial distress trusts' for understanding modern trusts law

In the course of not applying *Re Kayford* principles in *Re Farepak*, the court did suggest that the directors' execution of a deed of trust failed to establish the existence of a trust, and also rejected that a trust arose by way of an implied resulting trust. As we now discover, both of these mechanisms are ways in which a creditor can create a trust of a loan that he makes to someone whose insolvency is imminent. And by way of tying all of these factors together, although *Kayford* illustrates how debtors can seek to protect the (specific) positions of creditors, it is far more commonly the case that creditors will be instrumental in ensuring that their loans are more protected than would be the case on ordinary contractual principles.

More usually, trusts arise in the commercial context because those who lend money to others want to ensure that they *themselves* are protected from bankruptcy or insolvency, rather than are seeking (as in the *Kayford* situation) to protect *others*. In this more common situation, the best way in which to ensure the creation of a loan that is actually a trust *in favour of the creditor* is to require the debtor (who will acquire legal title to money lent) to declare himself trustee on behalf of the creditor. This express declaration can arise in circumstances under which a bank can protect itself against the bankruptcy of its customer by taking a trust receipt for money advanced or security released to the latter. Under this, the customer will typically declare himself trustee for the bank; the bank becomes both creditor and beneficiary under the trust. This means that the bank retains equitable title in the money advanced, or any goods that are subject to security, and the proceeds of sale where these goods are sold. In turn, this ensures that the bank is protected in the event of the debtor's bankruptcy or insolvency, provided that the property remains what is known as 'traceable', as considered in the previous chapter.

In addition to the loan that is an express trust deliberately created by financial institution creditors, there is also a special type of 'trust loan' that is found in business dealings. It is special because it involves using resulting trusts principles. Generally, a loan will be a 'trust' in circumstances under which it is intended that beneficial ownership of property will vest in someone other than the person holding legal title. In this special type of trust now examined, this arises where a loan is made on terms that ensure that if the money cannot be used for the purpose for which it is advanced, it will be returned to the creditor. This is known as a '*Quistclose* trust', from the leading case in the area, *Barclays Bank Ltd* v *Quistclose Investments Ltd* [1970] AC 567, embodying an early idea that where an identifiable sum of money is advanced by its owner to another for a particular purpose, the obligations of trusteeship will be imposed upon the latter.

Barclays Bank Ltd v Quistclose: *the facts*

At the heart of this case was Rolls Razor Ltd, a company in serious financial difficulties. Rolls Razor had an overdraft with Barclays Bank of £484,000, against a permitted limit of £250,000. If Rolls Razor were to stay in business, it would have to obtain a loan of £210,000, which was needed for paying dividends to shareholders that had been declared, but without the funds to pay for them. Rolls Razor was able to obtain a loan to do this, which it did from a company called Quistclose Investments Ltd. Quistclose agreed to make the loan on the condition that it was used only 'to pay the forthcoming dividend due on July 24, next'. The sum was paid into a special account with Barclays Bank, on this condition, which was agreed with the bank. Shortly afterwards, on 27 August, Rolls Razor went into voluntary liquidation. The dividend for which the loan had been secured had not, in fact, been paid and Barclays sought to count the money in the special account against Rolls Razor's overdraft, but the House of Lords held that the bank could not do this. The House of Lords' ruling was that Barclays held the money on trust for Quistclose, so that Quistclose was able to claim back the entire sum.

The essence of the decision is that, although the arrangement between Rolls Razor and Quistclose was essentially contractual (in ordinary contractual situations in which a debtor breaches a condition of the loan made, he is in breach of contract), alongside this there was also a primary and a secondary trust in existence: a primary trust arising in favour of shareholders for whose dividend the money was advanced solely; and a secondary trust arising for the original lender because this primary purpose could not be carried out. It was so held on the ground that, according to Lord Wilberforce at 582, there was no reason:

> ... why the flexible interplay of law and equity cannot let in these practical arrangements, and other variations if desired: it would be to the discredit of both systems if they could not. In the present case the intention to create a secondary trust for the benefit of the lender, to arise if the primary trust, to pay the dividend, could not be carried out, is clear and I can find no reason why the law should not give effect to it.

With its emphasis on practical commercial arrangements, it is clear from *Quistclose* that the rationale of giving effect to these arose from equity's longer-standing determination to ensure that those who hold legal title to property, but who are not intended to take its benefit, should be prevented from doing so; *Re Rogers* (1891) 8 Morr 243 achieving this by way of a resulting trust. These key ideas of the proper location of benefit within borrowing arrangements are captured in Lord Millett's capturing of the essence of a *Quistclose* trust in *Twinsectra* v *Yardley* [2002] 2 WLR 802, at [81]:

> ... the *Quistclose* trust is a simple, commercial arrangement akin ... to a retention of title clause (though with a different object) which enables the borrower to have recourse to the lender's money for a particular purpose without entrenching on the lender's property rights more than necessary to enable the purpose to be achieved. The money remains the property of the lender unless and until it is applied in accordance with his directions, and in so far as it is not so applied it must be returned to him.

A number of questions potentially arise from this, with two key ones now framing discussion of cases that have followed *Quistclose*.

(1) In what circumstances will an otherwise ordinary contractual loan be transformed into a 'primary trust' on *Quistclose* principles?

(2) In what circumstances can the original owner recover the money under the secondary trust arising from *Quistclose* principles?

Loans as Quistclose trusts: necessary conditions and key characteristics

In terms of what will transform a loan into a *Quistclose* trust, a central precondition seems to be that the money advanced is to be used for a specific purpose and that purpose alone, and that this (purpose) is known to the recipient; also, the money must be paid into a special account, which can be used for no other purpose. It is not clear whether the separate account is an absolute requirement, but at the very least the money must be earmarked for the particular purpose *and no other*. This was affirmed in *Re Farepak* [2006] EWHC 3272 (Ch) (albeit as rather a puzzling recourse to *Quistclose* reasoning, when quite clearly *Re Kayford* should have been considered), and its function is to negate any inference that it can be included in the debtor's general assets; in these circumstances, payment into a special dedicated account is the clearest way of evidencing this. This can also be seen illustrated in *Global Marine Drillships Ltd* v *Landmark Solicitors LLP* [2011] EWHC 2685, applied to money paid to a solicitor for a specific purpose.

Notwithstanding the core requirement of a specific purpose that is distinct from a debtor's general operations, it does seem that, where this inference is negated by some means, a special fund is not absolutely necessary. This can be seen in *Re EVTR* [1987] BCLC 646, in which an employee provided assistance to a company through depositing money with the company's solicitor and authorizing its release 'for the sole purpose of buying new equipment'. Although the money was not paid into a special fund, it was only ever paid out in pursuit of this purpose. Before the new equipment was delivered, EVTR went into receivership, and the Court of Appeal held that the employee lender was entitled to recover (an agreed proportion of) his money on *Quistclose* principles. This was explained by Dillon LJ at 392:

> [From] *Quistclose*, ... if the company had gone into liquidation, or the receivers had been appointed, and the scheme had become abortive before the £60,000 had been disbursed by the company, the appellant would have been entitled to recover his full £60,000, as between himself and the company, on the footing that it was impliedly held by the company on a resulting trust for him as the particular purpose of the loan had failed.

What this shows is that *Quistclose* principles do not strictly require a separate account in order to work, in circumstances under which the inference that it was intended to be included amongst 'general assets' could be negated by other factors. That having been said, the clearest way of raising the inference that money is to be used only for specific purposes is to locate it in a dedicated account, and this is what those considering making such a loan would be advised to insist on.

The advisedness of a separate account, even in absence of its essence, can be seen from the way in which *Quistclose* principles were not able to protect a lender in *Anglo Corporation* v *Peacock AG* [1997] EWCA Civ 992. However, it is difficult to see this as a definitive statement that a separate account is required, because there were other factors that suggested against the application of *Quistclose*. It was not clear that the recipient had taken the money on the understanding that it was to be separated from his general assets, and there was even some doubt that it was to be used only for a specific purpose.

But in terms of pointing to the usefulness of a separate bank account, even if it is not an absolute requirement, it is worth remembering that many of these cases will fall to be determined once the onset of insolvency has taken place. In these circumstances, there will be a number of claims against an insolvent's assets, which will become vested in either a liquidator or trustee in bankruptcy.

Here, a beneficiary's ability to assert his claim to the property rests on the property actually being traceable—that is, he must be able to point to a fund and say 'That property is property belonging to me'.

In this regard, the ruling in *Cooper* v *PRG Powerhouse Ltd* [2008] EWHC 498 that it is not necessary to segregate funds for a *Quistclose* trust to arise can be seen at work in *Mundy* v *Brown* [2011] EWHC 377 (Ch), in which the contents of an account held by an accountant alleged to contain the fruits of transactions at undervalue, and funds conferring preference and otherwise unauthorized (all contrary to insolvency law), were found to be held on a *Quistclose* trust even though they were not held in a separate trust account, and so could not have been payments of the company's money.

However, this text has always maintained that what matters is that the property remains traceable and, as we know from the previous chapter, equity has always permitted those entitled to use its tracing claim to trace property into mixed funds.

Quistclose *trusts: what must be intended and by whom*

Although we know from the previous chapter that a beneficiary can trace his property in a mixed fund, being able to point to an entirely separated body of money paid into a special account with no other funds moving in or out is going to provide the easiest way of establishing this. And, prior to this, as the agreement between the parties is being worked through, at the very least a lender's insistence on a separate bank account could well encourage fuller and clearer discussion about what is permitted use of the money and what is not, which is central to finding the existence of a trust on *Quistclose* principles.

This is very important given that, in *Peacock*, the Court of Appeal focused its determination on what the recipient had understood and accepted by the arrangement, and not on the lender laying down conditions: it is the latter that we might more readily associate with satisfying certainty-of-intention requirements.

Here, the lender was not protected by *Quistclose* principles, because the recipient 'did not believe it had reached any agreement about the basis on which it would accept the money'. Moreover, the judgment also stressed that 'unlike *Quistclose* and *Re Kayford* ... there was no identifiable trust property, such as money in a special account, on which the trust could be imposed'. This suggests that, at the very least, the value of a specific account is in inferring limited specific use of advanced moneys and thereby strong evidence in favour of a *Quistclose* arrangement. In a significant line of cases suggesting that a specific purpose can be identified without the physical segregation of money advanced from general assets, the key issue appears to be whether there is *intention* for the lender to retain an interest in the property that is advanced.

In linking issues on how specific purpose and 'earmarking' funds not for general use can be linked to establishing whether a *Quistclose* trust arises, intention is therefore central. On any reading, a lender's insistence on a separate bank account could well encourage fuller and clearer discussion about what is permitted use of the money and what is not, central to which is a lender's intentions in respect of it. This was elemental in the finding in *Peacock* that the lender was not protected by *Quistclose* principles because the recipient 'did not believe it had reached any agreement about the basis on which it would accept the money', as was the (absence of) communication of this to him.

The significance of this appears to be rather differently configured in *Twinsectra* v *Yardley*, which, whilst speaking of the intention of the settlor, also rather opaquely indicated that it was sufficient that he 'intends to enter into the arrangement, and not that he appreciates that they have the effect of creating a trust'. In terms of what must be intended and understood and by whom, *Du Preez Ltd* v *Kaupthing Singer & Friedlander (Isle of Man) Ltd* [2011] WTLR 559 summarizes this as a 'common understanding communicated to the recipient before or at the time of the transfer and accepted by the recipient', without which 'the monies vest absolutely in the recipient'. This latter observation reflects closely *Twinsectra*'s regard for the 'intention of the parties collected from the terms of the arrangement and the circumstances of the case'.

Does it matter where the money advanced actually comes from?

Although *Quistclose* principles will work only in relation to money advanced for specified purposes (which are most easily evidenced by the existence of a separate account even if this is not actually necessary), it does not appear to matter where the money comes from. In *Quistclose* itself, it was a loan made voluntarily by a third party; in *EVTR*, this was also by way of a voluntary disposition. There is also authority that moneys paid in furtherance of a contractual obligation to the debtor can be subject to a *Quistclose* trust—that is, *Carreras Rothmans Ltd v Freeman Mathews Treasure Ltd* [1985] Ch 207.

Carreras Rothman (CR) was a cigarette manufacturer, and it engaged FMT, which was an advertising agency that contracted as principal with a number of production agencies and advertising media. The arrangement was that CR paid a monthly fee to FMT, which was used as payment in arrears for FMT's services, and also to enable FMT to pay debts incurred to agency and media creditors. FMT got into financial difficulties, but needed funds to pay its production agencies and advertising media if it was to carry on acting for the claimant. CR also knew that if FMT were to go into liquidation still owing money to media creditors, the media creditors would have sufficient commercial power to compel CR to pay, and therefore (although it was not legally obliged to do so) it would in practice have to pay twice over. An agreement was therefore made between CR and FMT whereby CR would pay a monthly sum into a special account at FMT's bank, which was to be used only for the purposes of meeting the accounts of the media and production fees of third parties directly attributable to CR's involvement with the agency. So this was money owed by CR to FMT in any event and, on FMT's liquidation, a *Quistclose* trust was found notwithstanding this, as explained by Peter Gibson J at 222:

> if the common intention is that property is transferred for a specific purpose and not so as to become the property of the transferee, the transferee cannot keep the property if for any reason that purpose cannot be fulfilled ... True ... that if the defendant had not agreed to the terms of the contract letter, the plaintiff would not have broken its contract but would have paid its debt to the defendant, but the fact remains that the plaintiff made its payment on the terms of that letter and the defendant received the moneys only for the stipulated purpose. That purpose was expressed to relate only to the moneys in the account. In my judgment therefore the plaintiff can be equated with the lender in *Quistclose* as having an enforceable right to compel the carrying out of the primary trust.

Raymond Bieber v *Teathers Ltd (in liquidation)* [2012] EWHC 190 (Ch) illustrates how much what happens to money advanced subsequently *can* matter. Following a transfer of investors' moneys from a client account to a partnership account—made according to the terms of the subscription agreement—it was held that the firm's managing partner did not hold the money as trustee of a *Quistclose*-type arrangement, and that the investors' rights would instead be regulated by the partnership agreement in place.

The court held that, for a *Quistclose* trust to arise, it must be objectively verifiable whether funds transferred for an exclusive purpose have been applied for that purpose at the time of application, with this showing that actually issues of what happens to money after it is advanced speak directly to intention and the all-important 'specific purpose'.

Failure of the primary trust and the creditor's recovery under a secondary trust

The essence of the *Quistclose* trust is that where the 'stipulated purpose' for which money has been advanced cannot be carried out, the provider of the money can recover his property on the secondary trust that arises from the failure of this primary purpose. This requires us to think about when a primary purpose will be deemed to fail, and what must happen for a lender to be able to recover the property intended to be used for this under the so-called 'secondary' trust. This is essentially a question of enforcement, and embodies key questions of *who* can enforce a *Quistclose* trust and *when* can this be done. It also considers how resulting trust principles operate in these circumstances.

Lord Wilberforce's view in *Quistclose* itself was that there was a primary trust in favour of the shareholders and then, on the failure of the primary trust, a secondary trust in favour of the original provider. Since the provider of the money was able to claim it back, Lord Wilberforce had clearly come to the view that the primary trust had failed. Similarly, in *EVTR*, because the provider of the money was able to claim it back, the primary purpose of the trust must also be deemed to have failed. In both cases, the secondary trust was enforced, and because the original provider was both settlor and also beneficiary, this must have been by way of resulting trusts principles, as considered in Chapter 6.

In *Carreras Rothmans*, the primary trust (for paying the media advertisers) could still be carried out, and the order made was to that effect. But Peter Gibson J did express the view that the third-party creditors might themselves have had enforceable rights. However, in the trust scenario, enforceable rights are only ever given to beneficiaries, and so the clear implication is that whereas the beneficiary is the provider of the money once the primary trust has failed, the beneficiary under the primary trust is the person to whom payment is originally intended to be made (in *Quistclose* itself, Rolls Razor's shareholders).

However, there are problems with this view, as Lord Millett (then PJ Millett QC), who was counsel for Carreras Rothman, noted in his article based on the case at (1985) 101 LQR 269. It is not obvious why the primary trust had failed in *Quistclose* itself, because payment of the dividends *could* still have been carried out before the liquidation. It is not obvious that the payment became illegal even upon Rolls Razor's liquidation, and so we need to find another explanation of why the original lender could recover the money on a secondary trust because the primary one had failed. The facts in *Quistclose* and the decision do suggest an alternative, which asks instead whether the settlor's original motive has become frustrated, rather than whether it has become impossible to achieve, because it would make little 'commercial sense' in *Quistclose* to pay the dividend once Rolls Razor ceased business.

But there are still difficulties with this apparently simple explanation. There were no words of trust in *Quistclose*, and the only reason for inferring a trust was that the money had been lent for a specific purpose. So it does seem odd that, in deciding whether the trust has failed, the court ignored whether the specific (primary) purpose could still be carried out, and instead had regard to a different set of factors. Also, as Millett observed, nowhere else in trusts law does a *valid* trust fail because it no longer accords with the settlor's wishes; it fails only when performance becomes impossible or illegal, and that had not happened here.

The Millett article makes difficult reading, but there are numerous academic accounts. Several of these point to the difficulties in justifying the decision in *Quistclose* and subsequent authorities, whilst acknowledging 'policy considerations' that might guide the courts in the context that these situations almost always arise when money is lent to debtors who are not only experiencing financial difficulty, but who are also on the brink of insolvency or bankruptcy. From this, it is possible to find support for the view that the provider of the money can enforce the trust on *Quistclose* principles where:

the lender acquires an equitable right to see that [the money advanced] is applied for the primary designated purpose … if the primary purpose cannot be carried out, the question arises if a secondary purpose (i.e., repayment to the lender) has been agreed, expressly or by implication: if it has, the remedies of equity may be invoked to give effect to it.

(*Barclays Bank Ltd* v *Quistclose Investments Ltd* [1970]
AC 567, *per* Lord Wilberforce at 581)

In a number of respects, this passage is not the most convincing judicial statement and does not really say much beyond the view that, if the primary trust is not carried out, the lender acquires an equitable right to enforce the *secondary* trust. It certainly does not get to the heart of *why*, and indeed *when*, a primary trust will be deemed to have failed. However, on account of the 'policy' principles probably at work here, which do not necessarily reflect fully the strict operation of trusts law, Lord Wilberforce's analysis in *Quistclose* can probably be justified in spite of difficulties over why the primary trust had failed. And although it does contradict this in some respects, Millett's analysis is consistent with the *decisions* in all of the cases, including *Carreras Rothmans*, and ultimately it also avoids the problems of failure of primary purpose in *Quistclose*. Some of these policy considerations—as they may apply to current economic conditions and social constructions of financial liabilities, and the entitlements of those who respectively owe and are owed money under a loan arrangement—will be considered shortly.

Some thirty years on from the decision in *Quistclose* itself, *Twinsectra* reminds us that the crucial consequence of the loan found to be subject to a trust is that this property remains distinctive from other assets that might be applied to competing creditors' claims in a debtor's bankruptcy or insolvency. On *Quistclose* principles, this can be achieved on the basis of there being a resulting trust in favour of the provider of the property. However, it was argued in *Twinsectra* that there was no intention to create a trust and that there was no obvious 'specific purpose', and so there was no bar on the money being applied to unspecified purchases of property.

The House of Lords held that intention to create a trust (of the property held by Sims) could be found on the construction of the undertaking that the money was to be used for the acquisition of property and for no other purpose. In turn, this gave rise to a beneficial interest in the money to be held on resulting trust for the lender. This does appear to have been reiterated in *Re Farepak*, although it is not clear why *Quistclose* was considered at all, given that, as was suggested in Chapter 3, it appeared to have all of the hallmarks of an express trust that was valid on principles developed in *Re Kayford*. Furthermore, *Twinsectra's* views on when a trust will arise do not appear to be contradicted by thoughts in *Cooper* v *PRG Powerhouse Ltd* [2008] EWHC 498 or *Mundy* v *Brown* [2011] EWHC 377 (Ch) on segregation of a creditor's assets, and can now be seen in *Raymond Bieber* v *Teathers*, along with the consequences of finding that no trust has arisen.

18.5.2 What might *Quistclose* trusts reveal about the nature of modern trusts law and its current influences?

Quistclose trusts are very interesting because they reveal how the *constants* involved in a trust arrangement have given rise to new uses for trusts, and also how adaptable the traditional law of trusts has been in accommodating these new uses. For example, in explaining how a creditor under a *Quistclose* arrangement establishes certainty of intention, the separation of assets—actual or symbolic, or even merely 'still traceable'—is not a huge leap from the approach taken in *Re Kayford* [1978] 1 WLR 279, or even *Paul* v

Constance [1975] 1 WLR 527, concerning the establishment of irrevocable obligations to use the property in a particular way and for no other purpose.

It is true that, in the *Quistclose* arrangement, this purpose is not to provide benefit for a particular person, but it is property that is subject to obligations to use it in particular ways. However, the more interesting 'certainty of intention' issues are held over for discussion following an examination of *Re Kayford*. What is more interesting here is what *Quistclose* can tell us about how trusts actually work and whether, in seeing trusts being put to new uses, we are actually seeing some adjustments being made to traditional trusts principles.

The foregoing discussion has already started to encourage us to reflect on that fact that, whilst the function served by the *Quistclose* 'requirements' is clear, this alone does not explain satisfactorily *how* this arrangement works to enable a creditor to recover property that he advances subject to specific conditions on its use. The reasoning advanced in *Quistclose* itself is that the secondary trust arises from failure of the primary trust for which the money was advanced, but it is not clear that the primary purpose in *Quistclose did* fail. As the material has already asked, if it is not clear that *Quistclose* trusts arise only where a primary trust has failed, then *what is* happening?

We can see these questions being asked as long ago as 1985, extrajudicially, by Peter Millett, who called for a proper explanation of what is at work in the operation of *Quistclose* principles, and particularly conclusions that are reached in determining that a creditor can claim under the secondary trust because the primary one has failed. Millett suggested that this clarification was necessary for a number of reasons, and this chapter is particularly interested in those that he identified as relating to accepted understandings of the operation of trusts. In this vein, Millett suggested that, ordinarily, a trust that is actually valid (rather than not so *ab initio*) will fail only where it becomes illegal or impossible to carry out, which we saw at work in Chapter 6 on resulting trusts.

However, the rationale in *Quistclose* appeared to be not that it was actually impossible for the payment of dividends to be made, but rather that it was no longer commercially expedient for this to happen. If, in the case of a *Quistclose* trust, the court will be influenced by factors of 'commercial reality' rather than trusts law, this suggests that in commercial dealings the courts appear to be looking at different considerations from those that have traditionally governed trusts law. We know from studying certainty that a trust is a mandatory arrangement, which, once created, must be carried out, and yet this does not seem to be happening here.

On traditional trusts law principles, it should not be possible for the creditor to recover the property on the secondary resulting trust mechanism if it is still possible to carry out the trust. But the outcome in *Quistclose* suggests that things are working differently in such arrangements, which in turn suggests that we do need to try to ascertain exactly what is happening and why, by asking whether it is appropriate to adopt a different approach in these arrangements, and if so, whether this can be justified and even explained. To address these questions, we need to think back to the introduction to implied trusts for a reminder of what they are meant to do.

In Chapter 6, we learned that implied trusts have been developed as a mechanism to provide justice for those who might be disadvantaged by recognizing only legal ownership of property—and particularly in 'informal' arrangements. At that point, we learned that, in the case of the resulting trust, this deliverance of justice is generally anchored to ensuring that an original owner of property is not disadvantaged when he ceases to have legal title to property. It was also noted then that the modern *Westdeutsche* categorization of resulting trusts recognized *Quistclose* trusts within category B—that is, resulting trusts arising from failed express trusts (or incomplete disposal of equitable interest once a trust had been carried out).

In turn, this classification can be linked with the general idea that with the resulting trust equity provides a mechanism for a one-time owner of property to recover what was his at law once this is no longer the case, because the circumstances suggest that he should be able to recover it. In the case of a failed trust or partial exhaustion of equitable interests after a trust has been carried out, this is reasoned on the settlor's presumed intention that if the property cannot be applied as he originally intended, then it should be returned to him.

What *Quistclose* seems to add to this is that a settlor intends for the property to be returned to him if carrying out the primary trust is not expedient, even where it is technically possible. What might justify this special treatment of *Quistclose* trusts as resulting trusts that allow an owner to have his property returned even when the primary trust has not failed is as a matter of policy to look favourably on those who are prepared to lend property in these circumstances. As we can see from the cases, *Quistclose* trusts often arise as 'last ditch' attempts to defy financial failure by businesses for which the options for more conventional types of credit have long dried up, and perhaps the courts are mindful of this when ruling on when a creditor can recover under the secondary trust and are prepared to make some accommodation in these circumstances.

In these circumstances, it may well be *legally* expedient to encourage those with property to lend it, given that, even outside times of *economic* austerity, it is commonly short-term capital flows that will make the difference between whether a business on the brink of failure will go under or whether it can recover. The knock-on effects of this difference between survival and failure can be considerable for a business's employees and the local economy into which it is integrated. So there may well be justification on policy grounds for treating *Quistclose* arrangements differently from those that can more comfortably fit into *Westdeutsche*'s 'failed trusts' categorization.

Indeed, it is even arguable that Lord Browne-Wilkinson might have been acknowledging a different approach being applied to *Quistclose* arrangements by his specific reference to them in his explanation of category B. Following this line of thought, arguably *Quistclose* trusts can be accommodated within Simon Gardner's analysis of resulting trusts, in [1992] Conv 41, as mechanisms ensuring that 'property should be retained by its owner except to the extent that she voluntarily and effectively alienates it'. However, in doing so, we must also accept that *Quistclose* principles are quite different principles of trusts law from those found elsewhere in trusts law. In this case, we might have to regard *Quistclose* principles as not being part of the general law of trusts, and an example of (private) trusts law that is anomalous with this. This is considered at length in the Online Resource Centre materials, but following this logic here, we could suggest that *Quistclose* principles are an example of the development of principles of trusts law that operate differently from those that have evolved around private or familial arrangements, and that this development has been necessary because of the desire to use trusts in business dealings.

18.6 Financial debtor trusts and summarizing the significance of 'financial distress trusts' for understanding modern trusts law

There was an extended consideration of *Re Kayford* in Chapter 3, and attention paid to it here will be much briefer. For the sake of completeness, reference to *Re Kayford* at this point ties together our illustrative examples of trusts arising in the context of financial distress, but it has much more significance than for this alone.

The extended consideration of *Re Kayford* that was found in Chapter 3 regarded it as an authority for application to the business context of conduct-based certainty of intention, which allows an owner of property to establish through his actions rather than by using words that he intends to create a trust, and thereby manifest his understanding that this will create a permanent arrangement and one that will irrevocably deprive him of all beneficial interest in the property.

This is regarded as qualifying as Lord Langdale's imperative requirement, because it makes clear that property cannot be dealt with freely by its (apparent) owner, who is instead obliged to use it for another's benefit. Indeed, it was the presence of this intention and concomitant irrevocable commitment of particular 'earmarked' funds that made the difference between *Kayford* being applied to establish certainty of intention in *Re Chelsea Cloisters Ltd* [1980] 41 P & CR 98. It was the absence of this obligation to use property in a particular way that meant that *Kayford* was distinguished in *Re Multi Guarantee Co. Ltd* [1987] BCLC 257, in which no decision had been conclusively made about what to do with money that was separated from other assets.

Discussion in Chapter 3 of these 'commercial case' authorities on certainty of intention suggested that certainty of intention established on *Kayford* principles ought to have been able to establish the existence of a trust in *Re Farepak* [2006] EWHC 3272 (Ch). This discussion also noted that no trust was established and also surprise that *Kayford* reasoning was not actually applied. Indeed, the only reference to the possibility of an express trust was to the directors' execution of a trust deed that was incorrect, but which could be rectified. There was also reference to the possibility, which was dismissed, that a declaration might be implied from the circumstances, which seems to have been treated separately from the *Quistlclose* reasoning in this rather unclear judgment. The possibility of a constructive trust was also raised, on the basis that it would be unconscionable to retain the benefit of the customer contributors once the decision was made to cease trading. *Kayford* is, in any case, regarded as authority for an express declaration of trust, but this was not even mentioned.

So if a trust could have arisen on *Kayford* principles and yet *Kayford* was not even referred to in the decision, we do need to try to understand what was happening in the decision in *Farepak*. This might help us to determine whether *Kayford* is rightly regarded as classic authority for an express declaration of trust in the general law of trusts, or whether it suggests that the courts are treating certainty-of-intention requirements differently in commercial arrangements from those that are traditionally private familial ones.

Although it is not entirely clear why *Kayford* was not even mentioned, let alone followed, in *Farepak*, this is a decision that is regarded as being heavily influenced by considerations of policy. This was, of course, the case in relation to *Quistclose*, in which, in that type of arrangement, the policy was to encourage what were realistically last economic 'lifelines' for businesses on the brink of failure. In the course of explaining what these policy reasons might have been in *Farepak*, it will also be suggested that, just like in the case of *Quistclose* arrangements, these policy reasonings might actually be shaping the law and giving us trusts principles for commercial dealings that are different from trusts principles as generally understood. In this case, *Farepak* considerations are concentrated on certainty-of-intention requirements, and will be used to ask whether, in understanding how a debtor establishes certainty of intention, this is similar to or different from a settlor in private familial arrangements.

The policy considerations evidently at work in *Farepak*, even if they were not conclusively the reason for the failure to consider *Kayford*, were ones relating to insolvency law. We have encountered some references to insolvency law at various points in this text; we have even been acquainted with its key aim to provide a comprehensive regime for creditors to recover money that is owed to them once the borrower is unable to pay his debts and, in doing this, to treat creditors fairly through the operation of a 'workable system of clear priorities and ranking amongst creditors', as stated in the 1982 *Report of the Review Committee on Insolvency Law and Practice* (Cmnd 8558; the 'Cork Report'). In this regard, it is significant that, in *Farepak*, Mann J ruled that, even by rectifying the errors in the trust deed executed by the directors three days before cession of trading, the customer contributors would not be able to recover the earmarked money, because this was an intention on the part of the directors to confer a preference to one group of creditors over another.

This contravenes insolvency law's aim to treat creditors fairly by having a clear scheme of priorities, and Mann J felt that the directors were seeking to thwart the proper operation of insolvency law in executing the trust deed. As Chapter 3 suggested, *Pearson v Lehman Bros Finance SA* [2010] EWHC 2914 (Ch) establishes beyond doubt that these decisions are strongly influenced by the policy of seeking to ensure the proper operation of insolvency law, even if they are not actually decisions of *policy* rather than decisions of trusts law.

A decision made on policy, not on principles of trusts law

Farepak is not a sound judgment of trusts law, because, as we have suggested at numerous points up to now, property that is owned by a beneficiary under a trust never becomes part of the asset pool from which (other) creditors are paid, and so equally the ruling that such rights are held should not be regarded as thwarting the operation of insolvency law. However, this does reflect a more general concern that, precisely because this is the nature of a beneficiary's entitlement to (what is) trust property, the courts *should be* very conservative in allowing trusts to arise in commercial dealings at all.

This reflects a concern that, in a context in which most relations will be governed by contractual principles and their inherent limitations, it is inappropriate for anyone to be able to transform himself into a creditor with a protected interest. Creditor protection in the context of commercial dealings is normally achieved by the creditor taking security for his loan, while other creditors are able to achieve this by establishing that they are beneficiaries under a trust. Those who hold this view would argue that equity did not develop beneficiary protection to come to the aid of those involved in commercial dealings and that, because of this, importing trusts principles into commercial dealings should be conservative at any rate, and particularly so where there will be too many claims against available assets for all those who are owed money by the debtor to be repaid.

If, by reading what happened in *Farepak* and what has been said in *Lehman Bros* alongside what seemed possible from *Re Kayford*, it becomes clear that the courts might be seeking a more conservative approach in determining whether a trust has arisen, it might also be relevant that we are, at the time of writing, in the grips of recession and an era of austerity, which is likely to continue. However, this suggests that the courts will draw distinctions between what is required for commercial arrangements and what is accepted for familial ones. The decision in *Paul v Constance* shows us that the courts look for evidence of irrevocable commitment and recognition of an obligation to use property for the benefit of others.

The decision in *Paul v Constance* also shows us the scope of what is permitted in establishing this, and that having regard for the circumstances of the case will, on occasions, mean that the existence of a trust is upheld in borderline situations in which it is not actually possible to pinpoint a moment before property became subject to obligations that deprive its original owner of all beneficial interest and after which it was so.

The essence of commercial dealings and the operation of trusts principles

One can see why the courts would not wish to permit borderline decisions in commercial dealings, in which the parties are, in any case, dealing with each other at arm's length and without the moral obligations associated with family ties. Add to this the scope for commercial dealings to affect a multiplicity of other 'interests' and the justification for the 'borderline' case in commercial dealings vanishes still further.

However, it would seem, even in the clearest examples of irrevocability and recognition of obligation in commercial dealings, that the courts might not be willing to recognize certainty of intention to create a trust. In finding this, we can say for certain that the courts are not giving the same weight to the idea of an imperative and an irrevocable commitment in commercial dealings as would be the case in familial arrangements, and we can perhaps even conclude prima facie that the courts are looking for different things.

It may well be that *Farepak* is more a commentary on the courts' appreciation that, in what is likely to be prolonged economic austerity, the occurrence of insolvency is likely to continue to rise and that accompanying this the implications of business failure are likely to continue to hit the economy hard, and that this might be especially so for local economies. In this context, it is perhaps not surprising that the courts are mindful that insolvency law exists for a purpose, and it is perhaps especially important for the letter, as well as the spirit, of the statutory priorities to be complied with. Indeed, the distaste for conferring priority on particular creditors is plain for all to see within the judgment in *Farepak*.

But this does not alter the fact that, by doing this, the courts may be approaching questions of certainty of intention differently in the context of commercial dealings. What is interesting in this light is that although *Re Kayford* is regarded as classic authority for certainty of intention in the general law of trusts and is also a commercial context decision that is very pro-trust, its messages about finding certainty of intention in commercial dealings are more mixed than commentaries of it have suggested.

The essence of commercial dealings and the operation of policy

A number of things have been said up to now drawing on the commonalities between *Quistclose* and *Kayford* arrangements, and further 'shared observations' will be made about the law governing their creation shortly. And whilst it is the case that both *Kayford* and *Quistclose* arrangements attract criticism for interfering with the proper operation of insolvency law, it might also be possible, as a matter of policy, to distinguish them on grounds of meriting judicial and wider 'legal culture' support.

Whilst a *Quistclose* trust can transform the legal status and (quite literally) the fortunes of a creditor, 'creditor responsibility' is consistent with the spirit of insolvency law and is a core element of the law relating to companies, which it closely complements, albeit that reforms introduced by the Enterprise Act 2002 also acknowledge that some creditors are better placed to protect themselves than others.

It is also so that proactive asset management in the face of insolvency by a debtor might more readily attract association with transactions that confer preference, which expressly contravene insolvency law by virtue of s. 239 of the Insolvency Act 1986. And certainly where *Kayford* declarations arise once imminent insolvency becomes apparent, judicial tolerance of them could be legally problematic (where there is an apparent preference, unless a commercial argument can be made for showing this), which could inform a policy disposition against such findings.

However, it is also the case that the subsequent litigation against *Farepak* executives initially pursued and then dropped by the Insolvency Service produced an interesting reaction from the judge. This expressed tremendous sympathy for the savings scheme contributors and castigation of Farepak's bank, HBOS, as being 'aggressive' and 'proud' of the 'hard-ball approach applied' in maintaining Farepak's solvency in the face of likely failure, and continuing to collect deposits, knowing that these would likely be lost if failure were to transpire.

Peter Smith J maintained that Farepak directors were 'strong-armed' into attempting a solvent solution that could have saved all deposits, which reduced HBOS's own exposure by £4 million during that period. HBOS knew that deposits collected then would be lost if failure were to transpire, making it 'the only beneficiary of those deposits'.

In acknowledging that his judicial statement was a very unusual step, the judge urged HBOS to reconsider the 'pence in the pound' outcome of the collections made during its very aggressive pursuit of a solvent solution. More widely, this suggests that judicial attitudes towards *Kayford*-type arrangements are complex and that there is continuing recognition that such things will disproportionally affect those least able to bear losses.

Are there different certainty-of-intention considerations for commercial trusts?
This is because, long before *Farepak*, *Kayford* itself suggested that whether a trust is found might well depend on policy considerations and not simply whether the contemporary spirit of Lord Langdale's 'imperative' from *Knight* v *Knight* (1840) 3 Beav 148 could be found. In this regard, Sir Robert Megarry did regard the separation of funds for Kayford customers with unfulfilled orders as manifesting the necessary imperative, as evident from his submission that 'The whole purpose of what was done was to ensure that the moneys remained in the beneficial ownership of those who sent them, and a trust is the obvious means of achieving this'.

However, this was not the only significant factor for his conclusion that there had been a declaration of trust in respect of this property by the mail order company, and his judgment suggests particular significance being attached to those who stood to benefit from finding a trust in their favour. They were 'members of the public, some of whom can ill afford [the ordinary consequences of the insolvent liquidation] and all of whom are likely to be anxious to avoid this', and Megarry J continued in this vein by suggesting that 'Different considerations may perhaps arise in relation to trade creditors'.

It is, of course, the case that, in attaching particular significance to the mail order company's desire to protect customers with unfulfilled orders, Megarry J did not say definitively that he would have come to a different conclusion had the claimants been unpaid trade creditors. But that he suggested that this might have been the case is very interesting. It is the case that there is better protection today for members of the public, who can ill afford to lose out in the event of a liquidation, on account of the extensive statutory consumer protection regime, but it is also the case that even in the 1970s—before the modern regime for insolvency law was enacted—Sir Robert Megarry would have been aware that, in the event of an insolvent liquidation, there will be a number of ordinary trade creditors who supply businesses with goods and services who will be as unlikely to be paid as unpaid customers, and who will not be able to bear the consequences much better, if any better at all, than the customer contributors.

This is likely to be magnified in times of severe economic distress, which provided the background to *Re Farepak*. This may well embody judicial feeling that there is little to distinguish customers from a raft of other ostensibly business creditors for whom not being paid could make the difference between financial survival and financial failure, and who can also ill afford to be exposed to the ordinary consequences of an insolvent liquidation.

It is nevertheless very interesting that *Kayford* itself might have had a different outcome on entirely the same facts bar the persons who would be affected by the decision.

Given that *Re Kayford* is regarded as classic authority for certainty-of-intention rules within the general law of trusts, this raises very interesting possibilities. This is particularly so because, in his judgment, Sir Robert Megarry was satisfied that the assets were put to one side and could no longer be dealt with freely by the legal owner, which is classic establishing of imperative as required under *Knight* v *Knight* and, for familial-type arrangements, this appears to be all that is required (with *Paul* v *Constance* suggesting how much latitude can be given here).

If, in *Kayford*, the conduct itself was sufficient to establish that this was property that the legal owner understood no longer belonged to him (and there is every suggestion that it was), then perhaps the courts are looking at additional criteria where the existence of a trust is being asserted in the context of business dealings. Sir Robert Megarry indicated this in *Kayford*, by suggesting that the outcome could have been different if different parties had stood to lose from a trust not being found in their favour.

This does seem to be different from the ordinary familial arrangement under which certainty-of-intention requirements have grown up to ensure that all concerned know that there is a trust in existence from what the owner-cum-settlor actually says and does, rather than from looking at whether one should arise because a beneficiary is or is not a meritorious claimant. We can see in cases such as *Paul* v *Constance* [1977] 1 WLR 527 that the courts are keen to empower owners of property by enabling them to create trusts even when they cannot necessarily articulate this technically, and such an accommodating approach would not be appropriate in business dealings. Indeed, as the Law Commission suggests, commercial arrangements in which trusts arise are occupied by parties of equal strength and used to dealing in the course of business. But even as far as arrangements that are broadly familial are concerned, there is a consensus that, in *Paul* v *Constance*, the law had at least extended to the limits of its flexibility here, if not gone too far in what was a borderline case.

By contrast in *Kayford*, there *was* a clear point before which the mail order company could deal with the property as its owner and another after which it could not. And yet, by the admission of the presiding judge, a trust may well not have arisen if those affected had been from a different group of economic actors. One reading of this suggests that satisfying certainty-of-intention requirements where the trust is arising in commercial dealings is governed by different rules from those developed from the rules descending from family settlement arrangements during the nineteenth century. Traditionally, the courts have not considered who might be affected by a failure to manifest certainty of intention, as seen from the 'hard case' outcome of *Jones* v *Lock* (1965) LR 1 Ch App 25, and indeed being influenced by subjective considerations would traditionally be seen as undermining the core function of certainty of intention. This suggests that different considerations *do* attach to demonstrating this in the commercial context.

However, it may also be that we need to look at *all* certainty-of-intention cases *differently* as part of assessing what might be different about ones arising from commercial dealings. In this regard, perhaps *Paul* v *Constance* [1977] 1 WLR 527 and *Re Kayford* [1975] 1 WLR 279, and also *Jones* v *Lock* (1865) 1 Ch App 25 and *Richards* v *Delbridge* (1874) LR 18 Eq 11, require us to consider the significance of the rise of the ideology of consumer welfarism and its impact on the influence of market individualism in English *trusts law* in ways well established in the study of English *contract law* on account of the endeavours of Atiyah (1985) and Adams and Brownsword (2007). On doing so, it is at least possible that both *Paul* v *Constance* and *Re Kayford* are 'consumer welfarist' decisions, and that *Jones* and *Richards* might have different outcomes today. From this, it might be that the courts *are* looking at the implications of not finding a trust across family-type arrangements, as well as ones arising in commercial dealings. In this context, it is also interesting that *Lehman Bros* appears to suggest that the law should be flexible about giving effect to intentions by finding the existence of a trust and not too easily defeated by 'certainty' across the board. Indeed, in using as an example shared ownership of family homes, in this *Lehman Bros* judgment it was suggested that 'the law commonly recognises the creation of a trust' as a necessary consequence of parties' intentions regarding property in circumstances under which the parties themselves 'have given no thought at all to the terms of the consequential trust, if indeed they even recognised its existence'. In making this point about certainty of intention, this decision points to similarities in the role of trusts in new and traditional contexts. In doing so, it is also novel in attempting to join up analysis of trusts law responses to family situations and those arising in commercial dealings.

Shared observations from Quistclose *trusts and* Kayford *trusts*

This conclusion becomes harder to escape when these observations on *Re Kayford* and the other such cases are joined with the distinctive principles that appear to govern *Quistclose* trusts. In addition to the primary trust failure issues raised by these principles, there are issues surrounding establishing certainty of intention, which suggest that *Quistclose* trusts work differently from other trusts. This can be seen from *Anglo Corporation* v *Peacock AG*, *Twinsectra* v *Yardley*, and *Du Preez Ltd* v *Kaupthing Singer & Friedlander*, with all these decisions suggesting that the intentions and understandings of the debtor, as well as the creditor, are pertinent for establishing intention that a *Quistclose* trust should arise. This idea is closely bound up with establishing certainty of intention, in terms of what the parties understood from the arrangement, but mapping this approach onto traditional certainty-of-intention requirements is not entirely straightforward.

This is because, in terms of making the existence of a trust clear and certain, emphasis has traditionally been on the *settlor*'s words or conduct, rather than how these might be interpreted by others. We do know from *Richards* v *Delbridge* (1874) LR 11 Eq 11 that a settlor's words or actions have always been interpreted objectively in determining whether it is clear or certain from what he said or did that he intended to create a trust.

It is, of course, so that a prospective trustee's conscience must be affected for a trust ever to arise, with *Westdeutsche* providing authority for this position. But if these cases are suggesting that *someone other than a settlor* must intend a trust for a trust to arise, then this does signal some awareness that trust creation in this context might challenge traditional parameters. Indeed, *Twinsectra* deeming sufficient that there is intention to enter into an arrangement, and not necessarily requiring appreciation that this would have the effect of creating a trust, would seem to distinguish this situation from a conventional trustee awareness embodied in *Westdeutsche*, with *Du Preez*'s reference to 'common intention' perhaps also intimating a disposition to regard commercial parties as equal parties.

18.7 Trusts, trusts law, and commercial dealings: some tentative conclusions

We have seen that commercial dealings have been enormously influential across equity's beneficiary actions for lost property in every regard, from who can use them, to what they can achieve, and even determinations of their very basis. And, following on from this, the material on financial distress has suggested that commercial dealings appear to be providing a new paradigm for trusts law in the twenty-first century as they become applied across different social and economic spheres, and that they might even become more significant still.

Somewhere between these indices of significance of commercial dealings and current trends in trusts law is the discussion on the Online Resource Centre of why and how express trust arrangements may provide some creditors with better security for loans in the light of changing insolvency law—certainly as a matter of principle, given that criticisms of *Quistclose* arrangements, and now *Re Farepak* and *Pearson* v *Lehman Bros Finance SA* [2010] EWHC 2914 (Ch) (and subsequent *Lehman* litigation) suggest that the influence of insolvency law might provide a policy 'gloss' on the effective operation of traditional trust principles in commercial dealings in practice.

Given the rapidity of development in this sphere, and also that this type of analysis is an entirely new foray for this text, its conclusions now are brief and tentative, and are anticipated to become part of an ongoing narrative of how trusts principles developed around familial arrangements are being applied to commercial dealings ordinarily governed by contract law. What has been suggested so far is that, as far as requirements of a valid trust are concerned, these appear to be undergoing some modification to allow for this new reality to be accommodated and that this has some very interesting implications.

Indeed, the decision in *Lehman Bros* seems to acknowledge that the growth of trusts arising in commercial dealings will have very significant bearing on the future development of trusts law. This is apparent notwithstanding that Briggs J insisted that 'special care' is needed in importing trusts principles into business or commercial contexts, and that 'the law should not unthinkingly impose a trust where purely personal rights between [the parties] sufficiently achieve their commercial objective'. Briggs J also stressed that 'the law should not confine the recognition and operation of a trust to circumstances which resemble a traditional family trust', where finding a trust is an appropriate reflection of the parties' commercial objective. Moreover, in facilitating this, the courts are not to be hidebound by traditional rules about trusts derived from their origin in family settlements.

This particular case arising from the *Lehman Bros* insolvency does not claim to be the first case to be making these points, and in parts it also provides a number of restatements on 'fundamentals' of a trust. Most importantly, it is a very significant acknowledgement that the courts might be looking differently at trusts arising from commercial dealings, whilst it also appears to be the clearest judicial attempt to try to map these traditional and new contexts onto one another in terms of understanding the nature of trusts law.

This is very significant for the likely future direction for this chapter, but it is also the case that, from even a cursory glance at the high-profile *Lehman* litigation, we can see that this particular case is no ordinary one. Indeed, elsewhere, this extensive sprawl of litigation—including *Re Lehman Bros International (Europe) (No. 2)* [2009] EWHC 3228 (Ch), and in the Court of Appeal and Supreme Court, respectively, in *Re Lehman Brothers International (Europe) (in administration)* v *CRC Credit Fund Ltd* [2010] EWCA Civ 917 and *Lehman Brothers International (Europe) (in administration)* v *CRC Credit Fund Ltd* [2012] UKSC 6—makes much more extensive reference to the so-called Client Assets Sourcebook (CASS) rules within the Financial Service Authority (FSA) regime for regulated business relating to the segregation of a regulated firm's client assets.

The only reference to these rules and the statutory trust imposed thereby in *Pearson* is Briggs J's observation that the operation of CASS 7 'did not automatically mean that the statutory trust imposed by that regime was incapable of applying to client money until it had been segregated'. So it could be possible to downplay the significance of this litigation for ordinary trusts law. But Briggs J's judgment in particular does make some very interesting observations on the general law of trusts.

18.7.1 The role of trusts and equity more broadly in commercial dealings: is trusts law part of 'commercial' law?

This litigation might well also be deemed exceptional, or at least very unusual, in terms of its magnitude and its capacity for unsettling financial systems worldwide, but in any case it *is* part of a corpus of judicial commentary that now also includes *Crossco No 4 Unlimited* v *Jolan Limited* [2011] EWCA Civ 1619. Here, the Court of Appeal considered the central Supreme Court ruling in the cohabitation case *Jones* v *Kernott* [2011] UKSC 53 and the differences that, according to Etherton LJ, 'highlight a distinction between domestic and commercial cases'.

This remark was made in the context of applying proprietary estoppel and 'common interest constructive trusts', but this and the difficulties presented for the court by dealings between parties that are not 'a totally arm's length commercial transaction' allowed for observations to be made on the different behaviours of those who are in commercial relations from those whose relationship is what the Law Commission's Cohabitation Project 2006–07 termed 'intimate and exclusive'. This is part of a longer-standing judicial acknowledgement that 'the domestic context is very different from the commercial world' (*Stack* v *Dowden* [2007] UKHL 17, *per* Lady Hale), and could be a very exciting development for observing whether the courts are developing distinctive trusts law for parties in commercial relationships.

Certainly, *Pearson* itself is indicative of how trusts are increasingly being found at the heart of a number of complex financial transactions, and are popular as a structural basis for a range of investments and securitizations precisely because of the trust's attractions, as set out in the context of pensions. These are centrally the ability to pool assets and spread risks in an investment environment that is governed by fiduciary duties, where the standard of care is enhanced and the remedial regime is more extensive.

The more that we can understand about how trusts and associated fiduciary obligations operate in the commercial context, the better, given the increasing 'trust creation' that is being found here and given also that equity has a long tradition in operating alongside law in commercial dealings. Both observations may surprise, given that, whilst being focused on trusts specifically, this text has given considerable attention to equity's underpinning rationale of achieving fairness and justice, and conduct that is conscionable. We also know that trust and confidence are protected through equity's special governance of fiduciary conduct by means of the imposition of binding obligations that are 'enhanced' in comparison with those arising at common law.

Commercial dealings are not an obvious operating context for these core ideas, given that these are characteristically dealings 'at arm's length' governed by contract, involving an exchange between parties for profit, and in which considerable freedom is given to the parties by 'commercial law' to determine relations between them. But there are also *similarities* subsisting between equity and commerce.

There is some interrelatedness between these quite different ways of conducting interpersonal dealings. Trust and confidence are essential elements for contracting, because, notwithstanding all that has been said about commerce and its *raison d'être*, commercial parties will deal with only those whom they trust, even if this is at a 'threshold' level, and equally will want to be perceived as trustworthy, even if this is directed at profit maximization. This suggests that even very naked self-interest requires some fairness in exchange.

The key difference between them is the binding character of fiduciary relationships, which are quite different from those arising from the ordinary governance of commercial relations by commercial law. And we know from various points in this text—particularly from analysis in Chapter 17 of fiduciary relationships arising from 'the circumstances' (as summarized earlier in this chapter)—that commercial parties often go to some lengths to be accommodated by equity's governance in this regard.

In terms of comparing and contrasting fiduciary governance with commercial law, it is clear that commercial law is very effective in facilitating profit-making, through the mechanisms of contract and also the choices of form available for firms to organize their enterprises. We can see that the classification of contractual terms and law focused on 'governance' provides the framework for regulating the parties' interests in their dealings with one another, with also some restrictions on the scope of bargaining. However, there is one factor that is almost as fundamental to commerce as profit focus, which exposes the limitations of law as a mechanism for governing these arrangements.

Commercial dealings are highly dynamic. From the outset, contrasts have been drawn between the common law and equity in order to highlight equity's strengths. Centrally, this was a rationale rooted in justice and good conscience, but in Chapter 1 we learned that equity's strengths include flexibility. The common law is clear and certain, which has many advantages for contracting parties, with this being identifiable with its reluctance to change. But we also know that those who do have rights that law will recognize can be left frustrated by law's rigidity and limited responsiveness.

In a number of transactional arrangements that are intrinsically new, or operating in a new context by drawing in new market participants, we see an increasing recourse to equity, and its doctrines and mechanisms. In many respects, the favour for the trust mechanism and its associated equitable obligations that we have already encountered in our study of pensions can be seen as recognition of law's limitations. Certainly, the increasing number of investment funds and securitization 'products' that are structured around trusts are indicative of law struggling to keep abreast of dynamism and innovation, and also complexity and sophistication.

In this regard, contractual principles at the heart of commercial law may not be sufficient to deal with (new) issues arising, and, as briefly suggested in Chapter 1, the common law is reluctant to create new relationships to accommodate new ways of dealing. In contrast, equity has a long tradition of promoting flexibility alongside its other attractions. What we can see at work in the *Mothew*-type fiduciary relationships litigation is recognition that fiduciary relationships are much more flexible then contractual relations, and much more remedially generous in the event of a breach occurring. This helps to promote what might be termed 'threshold transactional stability', which is maintaining the elemental trust on which even the most profit-driven parties do rely. Central to this is the basis of fiduciary relationships in the duty of loyalty. And in fast-changing environments that are also highly sophisticated and complex, this provides for many an extremely useful mechanism for achieving 'fair play'—and this does fit with commercial rhetoric and intent: playing fair in the face of the unexpected.

The result of this is that equity can produce a workable framework of duties more easily than can law. The common law *is* good at managing the parties' intentions and also at allocating risk in transactions, whilst equity is more flexible for ensuring fair play in the face of rapid change. We see this in the increasing number of express trusts used in commercial transactions, in recognition of a theme recurrent throughout this text: 'express is best'.

This type of arrangement facilitates the creation of simultaneous interests in the same property (such as 'trust accounts' in secured finance), which we also know provide important protection in the event of insolvency. At the same time, the governance framework provided by fiduciary duties is also a useful regulatory tool for conflicts of interest and protecting confidentiality. Moreover, in sharp contrast with law, all of this 'works' without any need to imply terms or to detail express terms. And we have also just encountered *Quistclose* arrangements as a useful illustration of how this effect can be achieved less formally by virtue of equity being prepared to imply a trust where none is expressly created.

Given the popularization of trusts and fiduciary obligations, on the one hand, and the inherent nature of commercial dealings, on the other, it is also not surprising that some commercial actors seek to use the law of contract to exclude fiduciary duties. Using contract to limit the implications of fiduciary activity is something that we encountered in the discussion of trustee exemption clauses (TECs), and contracting parties being subject to, and being able to subjugate others to, elevated standards of care with significant remedial consequences will be a mixed blessing. Given that, ultimately, parties transact in the pursuit of profit, it is inevitable that a cost–benefit calculus will see some wishing to forgo the facility of this for themselves and be relieved of the burden of being on the receiving end.

This is why there is so much litigation around fiduciary relationships outside established ones, for every party that is keen to establish the existence of a fiduciary relationship another is fighting to avoid the imposition of one. Closely related to this, from our studies of the nature of trusteeship and also breach of trust, it should be clear that certain elements of fiduciary duties can never be excluded, such as liability attaching to the purchase or misappropriation of trust property, and more generally breach of the core obligation of loyalty.

In this way, we can see that the importation of fiduciary principles into commercial dealings could be a very significant factor in encouraging higher standards of dealing generally. But it is also the case that the English courts are rather cautious in doing so. We can see this in *Mothew*-type litigation on finding fiduciary relationships from 'the facts'; we can also observe it in the approach taken to 'finding' express trusts in *Kayford* arrangements and implied trusts in *Quistclose* ones, with a current policy regarding these (and perhaps particularly *Kayford*) arrangements as insolvency law avoidance devices also much in evidence. And for whatever else Briggs J's judgment in *Pearson* is authority, it is a message cautioning against law 'unthinkingly' imposing 'a trust where purely personal rights between [the parties] sufficiently achieve their commercial objective'.

Equity and commerce: innovation and tradition

So what can we tentatively observe from all of this? We can see how equity's key innovation—the trust and the obligations associated with it—can be extremely useful in commercial situations. We can find trusts structuring contractual obligations to be more adequate both *ab initio* and also *ex post*, making those that are inadequate *adequate*. But we also need to understand that the role of equity here is not unlimited. And indeed, in applying equity to commercial arrangements, we see respect for the primacy of commercial law generally, and contract specifically, and thereby equity being used as a supplement of law and not a replacement for it, and ultimately any role that equity has in commerce must make allowances for inherent risk in commercial transactions. Indeed, as Lord Browne-Wilkinson observed in *Westdeutsche*, some years prior to *Pearson*, 'wise judges have often warned against the wholesale importation into commercial law of equitable principles inconsistent with the certainty and speed which are central requirements for the orderly conduct of business affairs'.

But very interestingly, none of this is actually new. And in returning to what was said about the long tradition of equity's involvement in commerce, it is now appropriate to reference suggestion from law and society scholars W. R. Cornish and G. de N. Clark (1989: 95) that, during the nineteenth century, while the common law focused on sanctity of bargain and freedom of contract:

> equity ... would build up a protective jurisdiction of conscience as a refuge for those unfitted to a world of hard bargaining, or misled during their experience of it.
>
> (Cornish and Clark, 1989: 257)

Historians and contemporary commentary on the nineteenth century alike reflect on this as a time of rapid change and the emergence of significant 'market sophistication'. These were times when relative fitness for 'hard bargaining' could change very quickly indeed, leaving those hitherto well-equipped in this way in need of refuge. This sentiment is particularly resonant in the United Kingdom in the aftermath of the 2007–08 financial crisis. And in acknowledging the conversations about the applicability of general trusts principles generated by commercial dealings and bringing our discussions about the possible emergence of 'different trusts law' for such arrangements full circle, not only is it interesting to observe nineteenth-century recognition that equity was active in commercial dealings, but we can also observe the perception that any accommodation of this by law would have to reflect the key differences between commerce and 'conventional' trust arrangements. This can be seen in Hansard commentary dating from 1857:

> All mercantile transactions between men, generally speaking, were simple, short in duration, and easy of solution compared with, the relation subsisting between a trustee and his cestuique trust, spreading, as the latter often did, over a whole life, and generating in some cases feelings of respect and in others of animosity. Then, again, in mercantile life men entered into transactions for the sake of their own profit.
>
> (HC Deb, 9 July 1857, Third series, vol. 146, col. 1202, *per* Mr Rolt)

18.8 The changing context of 'conventional' trusteeship: a postscript for this text

Moving away from how commerce has adopted elements of trusts law both past and present, it is also the case that current trends in what nineteenth-century discourses on law termed 'conventional trusteeship' or 'trusteeship properly so-called' are likely to influence the content of this chapter, and in fact the nature of this text.

This is because it is also anticipated that future editions of the text will emphasize the way in which the law relating to express trusteeship (as considered in Chapters 13, 14, and 16) might even be becoming less about the trusts law developed in the context of (regulating and facilitating) family settlements, and more influenced by agreements between trusts services providers who operate by way of a business and in order to generate profit, and in which arrangements the scope of carrying out trusteeship is governed by tort and especially contract, rather than trusts law.

But this does also raise a further very significant point: while the desire to import trusts into commercial dealings might be increasing, the use of trusts in private and predominantly familial arrangements will not die out. This means that the principles developed by these arrangements for them will continue to remain relevant. This is because not all trustees will be paid professionals operating commercially, and, as we saw in *Bristol and West BS* v *Mothew* [1998] Ch 1 and even *Armitage* v *Nurse* [1998] Ch 421, ultimately even these operators are subject to limitations imposed by trusts law.

At this point, we can observe that different considerations are being applied to trusts arising in commercial dealings, and thus we can also ask whether this suggests that, over time, distinctive bodies of the 'general law of trusts' relating to express private trusts will emerge. This is a very exciting prospect, with far-reaching implications for trusts law—and it is hard to imagine what future editions of this text might look like if this were to prove the case.

 Revision Box

1. In relation to *Quistclose* trusts, ensure that you can explain:
   - what the essence of a *Quistclose* arrangement appears to be; and
   - what the key requirements of a *Quistclose* trust appear to be, drawing on *Barclays Bank Ltd* v *Quistclose Investments Ltd* [1970] AC 567 itself and subsequent cases.
2. In relation to the decision in *Twinsectra* v *Yardley* [2002] 2 WLR 802, ensure that you understand:
   - the spectrum of possible views advanced and the extensive analysis of why ultimately a resulting trust in favour of the lender was the one ultimately to be preferred;
   - how the resulting trust in favour of the lender operated subject to the mandate of the borrower to apply the sums advanced to the specified purposes and how this ultimately ensured that Sims did hold the money on (resulting) trust for Twinsectra; and
   - why, at that point, it did not matter that the money was advanced to be applied to a purpose rather than to benefit an identifiable individual.
3. In the light of questions 1 and 2, answer the following questions.
   (a) By way of a summary, what is the likely significance of key cases post *Twinsectra*?
   (b) What issues of *law* appear to arise from judicial recognition of *Quistclose* arrangements?
   (c) What issues of *policy* are associated with judicial recognition of *Quistclose* arrangements?
4. Ensure that you are able to explain where trusts and equitable obligations are to be found in 'commercial dealings', and that you are able to identify the apparent attractions of these mechanisms for contracting parties.

FURTHER READING

Adams and Brownsword (2007) *Understanding Contract Law* (London: Sweet & Maxwell).

Atiyah (1985) *The Rise and Fall of Freedom of Contract* (Oxford: Oxford University Press).

Bridge (1992) 'The *Quistclose* trust in a world of secured transactions' 12 Oxford Journal of Legal Studies 333.

Case Comment (2011) 'Final distribution ordered in *Farepak* case' Company Law Newsletter Co. 287, 7.

Collins (2006) '*Quistclose* examined' 12(7) Trusts and Trustees 15.

Cornish and Clark (1989) *Law and Society in England 1750–1950* (London: Sweet & Maxwell).

Gardner [1992] 'New angles on unincorporated associations' Conveyancer 41.

Glister (2004) 'The nature of *Quistclose* trusts: classification and reconciliation' 63 Cambridge Law Journal 632.

Kempster (2006) 'Quistclose trusts: offending the beneficiary principle?' 80 Trusts and Estates Law & Tax Journal 21.

Lee (2009) 'Rethinking the content of the fiduciary obligation' 73 Conveyancer 236.

Millett (1985) 'The *Quistclose* trust: who can enforce it?' 101 Law Quarterly Review 269.

Smolyansky (2010) 16 'Reining in the *Quistclose* trust: a response to *Twinsectra* v *Yardley*' Trusts & Trustees 558.

online resource centre

For summaries of a selection of these articles, please visit <http://www.oxfordtextbooks.co.uk/orc/wilson_trusts11e/>

INDEX

Introductory Note

References such as '178–9' indicate (not necessarily continuous) discussion of a topic across a range of pages. Wherever possible in the case of topics with many references, these have either been divided into sub-topics or only the most significant discussions of the topic are listed. Because the entire work is about 'trusts', the use of this term (and certain others which occur constantly throughout the book) as an entry point has been minimized. Information will be found under the corresponding detailed topics.